American
Medical
Women's
Association, Inc.

REPRESENTING WOMEN PHYSICIANS · SINCE 1915 ·

The Women's Complete Healthbook

THE WOMEN'S COMPLETE HEALTHBOOK

MEDICAL CO-EDITORS

Roselyn Payne Epps
M.D., M.P.H., M.A., F.A.A.P.
Expert, National Institutes of Health, Bethesda, MD
Professor, Howard University College of Medicine,
Washington, D.C.
Past President, American Medical Women's Association.

Susan Cobb Stewart
M.D., F.A.C.P.
Associate Medical Director, J.P. Morgan, New York City
Clinical Assistant Professor of Medicine, State
University of New York, Brooklyn
Past President, American Medical Women's Association.

Produced by
The Philip Lief Group, Inc.

Delacorte Press

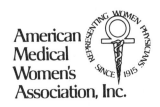

American
Medical
Women's
Association, Inc.

Published by
Delacorte Press
Bantam Doubleday Dell Publishing Group, Inc.
1540 Broadway
New York, New York 10036

Produced by
The Philip Lief Group, Inc.
6 West 20th Street
New York, New York 10011

Library of Congress Cataloging-in-Publication Data
The Women's Complete Healthbook/The American Women's
Association; medical editors, Roselyn P. Epps, Susan
C. Stewart

    p.cm.
    includes index.
    ISBN 0-385-31382-9
    1. Women—Health and hygiene. I. Epps, Roselyn Payne.
    II. Stewart, Susan C.
    III. American Medical Women's Association.
    RA778.W7481995
    613.04244—dc20   94-36851
                          CIP

Printed in the United States of America

Published simultaneously in Canada
June 1995

10 9 8 7 6 5 4 3 2 1

Contents

IV The Healthy Body: Symptoms, Diagnoses, and Treatments

Appendixes

Acknowledgments

Special thanks to our husbands, Duncan J. Stewart and Charles H. Epps, Jr., M.D., for their help and support, to AnnMarie Englese and Charlene Booker at J.P. Morgan, and to all the patients, who have taught us so much. The major participation of Eileen McGrath, J.D., C.A.E., Executive Director of the American Medical Women's Association is gratefully acknowledged. We thank the AMWA leadership, members and staff for their encouragement and assistance. We also thank reviewers Charles H. Epps, Jr., M.D., Charles H. Epps, III, M.D., Roselyn E. Epps, M.D., Howard R. Epps, M.D., and AMWA staff Marcia Saumweber, Lois Schoenbrun, Lisa McLendon, Sonia Ramamoorthy, Gillian Thomas, Regina Sanborn, Elizabeth Woods, Jacqueline DeSarno, and Marie Glanz, as well as Laurie Rockett, Esq.

Preface

When the American Medical Women's Association (AMWA) was founded in 1915, women did not have the right to vote, many medical schools did not admit women, and a physician could be arrested for discussing birth control with a patient.

Since that time, technology and social change have dramatically altered medicine in this country. AMWA has remained in the forefront of that social and technical change.

In the 1970s, American women began a grassroots movement in women's health. AMWA members were often among the leaders, empowering women to understand and take control of the health care decisions that affected their lives.

In the 1990s, this may be even more crucial. As parents live longer and child rearing becomes more complex, women are often at the center of their extended families. In this role, they not only make most of the health care decisions for themselves and their family, they are often primary caregivers.

The Women's Complete Healthbook is a resource to empower women who make health care decisions. The authors are women physicians who face the same challenges that you face. Like you, they make the health care decisions for their families and provide care when they are sick. Like you, they struggle for balance between their careers and personal lives. Like you, they sometimes need a place to find information.

On behalf of the 13,000 women physicians and medical students in the American Medical Women's Association, I encourage you to use this valuable resource.

Diana L. Dell, M.D., F.A.C.O.G.,
1995 AMWA President

Introduction

Health—the physical, mental, and social well-being of an individual—is a subject of interest to everyone. This is especially true of women. Most of the decisions about health care are made by women. They monitor their own care as well as that of their immediate and extended families. A woman's interest and involvement in health issues cover a broad spectrum: promoting family health, making decisions about care for aging family members, and being a wise consumer in using the health care system effectively. Now, in one valuable resource, a woman has the key information she needs when faced with important decisions about health care. *The Women's Complete Healthbook* was written by women physicians, for women, about women.

The Women's Complete Healthbook has been compiled by the American Medical Women's Association (AMWA) as another manifestation of its ongoing commitment to women's health. As the nation's oldest and largest medical organization of women physicians and medical students, AMWA represents women in every medical specialty and every type of medical practice. It is devoted to educating professionals, patients, and the public about important health care issues, specifically those that relate uniquely to women, as well as promoting women's health in general.

The authors represent the diversity in specialties and practice types of AMWA members. They are also women who understand the special concerns of women. These authors appreciate the need to treat the total woman, not just the disorder, and that sensitivity is reflected in the content of this book. It is designed to help women be educated, active participants in their health care and that of their loved ones.

The Women's Complete Healthbook is an authoritative, comprehensive reference to all aspects of women's health. It focuses on the special concerns of women. It eliminates the fragmented, inadequate information about women's health that often results when issues are addressed in isolation or the population is considered as a whole. This comprehensive women's health book has been written entirely by women physicians and other medical professionals. The authors represent leaders in their medical specialties, in medical education, and in public policy. Most of the authors are in practice and interact daily with patients. The result is a book that is scientifically based, contains the latest medical information, and yet is practical for the individual seeking personal information.

The emphasis of *The Women's Complete Healthbook* is on health and how to maintain it through prevention of disease and promotion of healthy behaviors. Diseases are a part of life, however, so it is important that women understand how disease affects the body systems and know when and how to obtain medical care. The book is organized in a manner intended to meet these goals and to enhance its use and value.

The content of *The Women's Complete Healthbook* is organized into four major sections. Part I, "Being a Savvy Consumer," focuses on the new national perspectives on women's health and the evolving health care system in today's environment of managed care. Part II, "Keeping Healthy," presents information on health maintenance of special significance to women, such as diet, exercise, mental health, and sexuality. Part III is devoted to a number of aspects of reproductive health. Part IV covers each of the body systems—structure and function, preventive measures, symptoms, conditions, and treatment—as well as special topics such as AIDS, cancer, pain control, and managing medications. An appendix describes diagnostic procedures.

The discussions of disorders and symptoms are geared to help readers analyze their problems logically and seek appropriate medical attention. Common medical conditions, especially those that occur more often in women, are highlighted. Because many conditions affect more than one system, there is some overlap in the content from one chapter to another. This overlap is intentional and designed to make the book easier to use. A book of this scope cannot cover every manifestation of every disease, however, and it should not be considered a substitute for the medical advice of the reader's doctor. The reader should consult the appropriate medical professional in all matters relating to her health. This book contains information about the training and expertise of various medical specialists to help in choosing the right physician. A safe rule to follow is to see a physician if symptoms persist. If the initial medical evaluation is unsatisfactory, seek further medical attention.

The Women's Healthbook is the collective effort of many individuals who contributed their time and their expertise to ensuring the quality of the content; their names appear at the front of the book and in the Editors and Contributors section at the end.

The Editors

PART I

BEING A SAVVY CONSUMER OF HEALTH CARE

CHAPTER 1

A New National Focus on Women's Health

Susan J. Blumenthal, M.D., M.P.A., F.A.P.A.

Over the last several decades, our society has witnessed tremendous changes in the lives of women. Today, women enjoy educational and professional opportunities never imagined a generation ago. For the first time in our nation's history, there are more women than men enrolled in colleges and universities, and more women than men now pursue graduate study. Women over the age of 18 make up 38 percent of the total populace and 45 percent of our nation's work force.

Thanks to general improvements in public health, women's average life expectancy has increased by almost 30 years since the beginning of the century. As of 1990, women made up 59 percent of Americans over the age of 65 and 72 percent of the group aged 85 and older. By contrast, in 1900, women constituted 49.5 percent of the population over the age of 65 and 55 percent of the group over the age of 85.

There's a darker side to this generally rosy picture, however. Although women are living longer, they are not necessarily living better. Women now face health problems that accompany old age—such as osteoporosis, depression, and Alzheimer's disease—in greater numbers than do men. Moreover, throughout their lives, women tend to suffer far more illnesses and chronic, debilitating conditions than do men. In fact, women's activities are limited by poor health approximately 25 percent more days each year than are men's activities, and women are bedridden 35 percent more days than men because of infectious diseases, respiratory problems, digestive diseases, injuries, and other chronic conditions.

Furthermore, work outside the home has become a necessity, not alway a choice, for many women with families. Since 1951, the number of women in the paid work force has increased by nearly 1 million workers per year, with the largest increase among married women who have children. Between 1977 and 1991, for example, the number of married women employed outside the home increased from 43 to 56 percent, and in 1990, 66.3 percent of women in the work force had children under the age of 18. More than ever before in U.S. history, women are essential to the economic survival of their families.

Despite the high influx of women into the American workplace and the increasing importance of women's contributions to the economic life of our country, women remain clustered in lower-wage and part-time jobs that do not provide health insurance or other benefits. Today, a woman still earns only 72 cents for every dollar earned by a man, an increase of only 3 cents since 1980. Of female-headed households in the United States, 45 percent have incomes below the poverty line compared with 8 percent of households headed by males.

The economics of many women's lives can have serious consequences on their health. Women who live in poverty—many of whom are women of color—suffer from more illnesses, have less access to health care, and have shorter life spans than other women. For example, the life expectancy for white women (79.4 years) is nearly 6 years longer than that of African-American women (73.6 years). According to the Centers for Disease Control and Prevention, between 1986 and 1988, the statistics for years of potential life lost before age 65 were highest for African-American women, followed by Native American women, white women, Hispanic-American women, Asian-American women, and Pacific Islander women.

Poor health care is often the reason for a lowered life expectancy. For example, while the incidence of breast cancer is actually lower among African-American women than among white women, African-American women have a higher mortality rate from breast cancer because of their more limited access to screening mammography, clinical breast examinations, and treatment. Simlarily, poor women in rural areas have less access to prenatal care than other American women, and homeless women have no regular source of health care at all.

WOMEN'S HEALTH AND THE MEDICAL COMMUNITY

With women now living longer and playing a more visible role in the public and economic life of our nation, the government, the medical establishment, and employers are beginning to pay more attention to the economic and social consequences of women's health.

Indeed, in recent years, the United States has experienced a virtual awakening about the importance of women's health and the deplorable dearth of verifiable scientific knowledge about the diseases and conditions that uniquely or disproportionately affect women. For example, we still do not know whether hormone-replacement therapy should be routinely provided to perimenopausal and postmenopausal women. We know that cardiovascular disease is the leading killer of women, yet we do not know definitively if estrogen—or aspirin, for that matter—can reduce the risk of heart disease for older women.

Part of the problem is that physicians and medical researchers have taken the Renaissance idea of "man as the measure of all things" in the most literal sense. It is true that women were sometimes excluded from medical research because of the fear of possibly harming a fetus; but in many cases, the exclusion clearly has reflected a social bias. For example, the Multiple Risk Factor Intervention Trial, a major study of heart disease (appropriately called "Mr. Fit"), looked at the influence of lifestyle factors on cholesterol levels and the development of heart disease among 15,000 men—and not a single woman. In short, women have not been seen as the measure of health, even for other women. Consequently, the medical community lacks hard data about the causes, risk factors, prevention strategies, and optimum treatments for such common diseases as cardiovascular disorders (the number one killer of women

in the United States) and osteoporosis. Not surprisingly, women have become increasingly disturbed and angry about the lack of attention given to *their* health problems.

It is particularly astonishing that women, who constitute a majority of the elderly in the United States, have even been excluded from studies of aging. For instance, the Baltimore Longitudinal Study on Aging, which was funded by the National Institutes of Health (NIH) and launched in 1958, did not include women until 1978, and the study's 1984 report, titled *Normal Human Aging*, contains no data specific to women.

The lack of scientifically sound information on women's health has negative repercussions for men, because research on women could provide comparative data for and insights into men's health. For instance, recent research on cardiovascular disease in women links high levels of estrogen with a lower incidence of disease among premenopausal women. These findings suggest that cardiovascular disease among men may be linked to their lower levels of estrogen. In fact, when it comes to studies of the human heart, perhaps women, who tend to develop such diseases later in life than men, should have been the model all along! (See Fig. 1.1)

RAISING AWARENESS ABOUT WOMEN'S HEALTH ISSUES

The women's health research movement emerged from a unique coalescence of factors. In the 1970s and 1980s, women began entering the work force, including the medical and health professions, in record numbers. Women also participated more in politics. At the same time, a nascent awareness among medical researchers of the gaps in knowledge of women's health led to the formation, in 1983, of the U.S. Public Health Service's (PHS) Task Force on Women's Health Issues.

Over the course of 2 years, this task force assessed the PHS's involvement in the area of women's health, including research. In 1985, the task force concluded that serious omissions existed regarding women's health and issued a series of recommendations to redress the inequities. These recommendations called for expanded biomedical research, with an emphasis on conditions and diseases unique to or more prevalent in women of all ages. The report also identified a need to increase women's representation in study populations of federally sponsored research. Responding to the later concern, the NIH developed a policy to encourage the inclusion of women in clinical research studies. How-

ever, this policy was not rigorously implemented until 1990.

Many groups are responsible for putting women's health on our nation's research agenda. In addition to advocacy groups like the Society for the Advancement of Women's Health Research and the National Breast Cancer Coalition, several members of Congress played and continue to play an important part in focusing attention on women's health. In 1977, the bipartisan Congresswomen's Caucus was established by 15 of the 18 women members of Congress. Four years later, with the admission of men, it became the Congressional Caucus for Women's Issues. Since its inception, the caucus has championed women's health research, increased health care delivery for women, and acted as an important catalyst in the establishment of two offices: the PHS Office on Women's Health (OWH) in the Department of Health and Human Services (DHHS) and the Office of Research on Women's Health (ORWH) at the NIH. With the establishment of these two offices, the days of focusing solely on men like "Mr. Fit" have become a thing of the past.

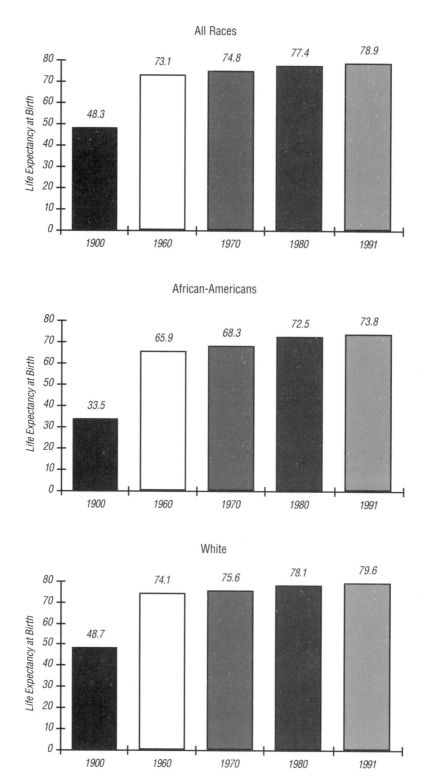

Figure 1.1. Women's Life Expectancy at Birth, 1900-1991.
Source: National Center for Health Statistics 1994.

The Federal Effort on Women's Health

PHS Office on Women's Health

The OWH was launched in 1991 to oversee and co-ordinate all women's health efforts on research, service delivery, education, and public policy undertaken both nationally and regionally by the agencies and offices of the U.S. Public Health Service. These agencies include the National Institutes of Health, the U.S. Food and Drug Administration, the Centers for Disease Control and Prevention, the Health Resources and Services Administration, the Agency for Health Care Policy and Research, the Indian Health Service, and the Substance Abuse and Mental Health Services Administration. That same year, the OWH issued *The PHS Action Plan for Women's Health*, which identifies goals and the necessary steps to achieve them for several top priority health issues, including women's access to general health care, participation in research, mental health, reproductive health, acute and chronic illnesses, and health-influencing behaviors. The OWH monitors progress in these areas and publishes a biennial progress review that includes a summary of achievements in meeting health needs of women nationally and regionally.

In 1993, the OWH was elevated within the U.S. Public Health Service with the appointment of the first deputy assistant secretary for women's health. The new prominence given to the PHS Office on Women's Health allows for greater coordination and collaboration of federal programs and enhances the opportunities for federal agencies to work together, with consumer health care professional and scientific groups, and with the private sector.

With its expanded mission and mandate, the OWH is undertaking a number of new efforts. These include coordination and implementation of the National Breast Cancer Action Plan (a major public-private partnership that should make significant progress in our fight against this disease), revitalization of women's health programs in the PHS regional offices, establishment of linkages between research institutions and service organizations in communities nationwide, initiatives to promote healthy behavior in young women, new efforts to improve the health of minority women by stimulating new progress to prevent domestic violence and to assist women who are the victims of such abuse, providing greater access to health care services, or fostering research and education and by innovative methods to disseminate information about women's health to women across the country, and strategies to recruit and promote women in science and the health professions.

In the coming years, the OWH will also initiate new efforts and activities to determine how environmental factors affect women's health and has established a coordinating group across the government to focus on these issues. Through collaboration with the NIH, the Health Resources and Services Administration, the Association of American Medical Colleges, and the American Medical Women's Association, the OWH will expand medical training in women's health issues and design a model curriculum to help medical schools incorporate a new approach to women's health into the training of future physicians and other health care professionals. In addition, the office will sponsor a series of continuing education seminars to inform health care professionals about new advances in women's health research.

Office of Research on Women's Health, NIH

In September 1990, the NIH established the Office of Research on Women's Health (ORWH) within the office of the NIH director. In 1991, Bernadine P. Healy became the first woman director of the NIH. During her tenure at the NIH, she became an important advocate for improving women's health. Around the same time, the NIH issued a new policy requiring the inclusion of women and minorities in clinical research. The policy stipulates that all grant proposals for clinical studies must include women in adequate numbers or have scientifically sound reasons for excluding women as research subjects.

ORWH is charged with monitoring and increasing the attention given to women's health research in projects supported by the NIH at institutions across the country and in the NIH's own laboratories in Bethesda, Maryland. The office supports new research initiatives that are important to the study of women's health, such as initiatives for endometriosis and uterine fibroids. The office also provides supplemental funding to the 24 institutes, centers, and divisions of the NIH to expand research into areas important to women's health and to promote the inclusion of women in clinical trials.

In fostering the involvement of more women in clinical trials, ORWH investigators must address factors such as child care and transportation to and from the trial site that may prevent many women from participating. In fact, the office, along with the Institute of Medicine, has been considering all the issues—including ethical and legal ones—to establish guidelines for the inclusion of women in clinical research.

Other PHS Agency Offices

Over the past two years, women's health offices have been established within other PHS agencies, including the Centers for Disease Control and Prevention (CDC), the Substance Abuse and Mental Health Services Administration (SAMHSA), and the Food and Drug Administration (FDA). Other agencies have designated women's health coordinators to weave a prominent focus on women's health into the fabrics of their organizations.

The Women's Health Initiative

The influence of social, cultural, and economic factors on the health of postmenopausal women will figure prominently in another major NIH effort, the Women's Health Initiative, which was launched in 1992. The initiative is a 15-year, $625 million study of major diseases and conditions—including heart disease, stroke, breast and colorectal cancer, depression, and osteoporosis—that affect women in the last third of their lives. Involving some 160,000 postmenopausal women at 45 centers across the country, this is the largest clinical study ever undertaken in the United States.

The Women's Health Initiative has three major components: (1) a surveillance study, which will involve approximately 100,000 women, to identify specific risk factors of disease; (2) a clinical trial, involving 45,000 participants aged 50 to 70, to study the role of diet modification, hormone-replacement therapy, and dietary supplements such as vitamins in the prevention of cardiovascular diseases, cancers, and osteoporosis; and (3) a prevention study, carried out in 60 communities nationwide, to determine the most effective methods for encouraging women to modify their diets and lifestyles and incorporate health-promoting behaviors, such as eating well-balanced meals, getting regular physical exercise, and stopping smoking. Particular attention will be given to reaching minority women and those who have not been adequately represented in research studies in the past.

The Women's Health Initiative, with its emphasis on studying the health of postmenopausal women, represents an important new approach to women's health care; an approach based on the recognition that women today have as many nonreproductive years of life as potentially childbearing ones. The initiative recognizes the fact that heart disease is the leading cause of death for women in the United States (as it is for men) and that women develop heart disease later in life than men, at a time when other health problems may complicate treatment. It recognizes the fact that women in the past have not received as aggressive an approach to the treatment of cardiovascular disease, which is reflected in the fact that almost 50 percent of women, but only 31 percent of men die within one year of suffering a heart attack. In seeking to answer questions about the possible benefits of hormone-replacement therapy for menopausal women, the Women's Health Initiative may help reduce the incidence of cardiovascular disease among postmenopausal women. The study will help identify risk factors for breast and colon cancer, and osteoporosis. This important study will also provide treatment recommendations to guide the care of older women for years to come.

CRITICAL ISSUES IN WOMEN'S HEALTH

The Younger Years

Adolescence and young adulthood (ages 12–24) are periods when individuals make important choices about lifestyle behaviors, including diet; physical activity; use of tobacco, alcohol, and other drugs; and sexual behavior, all of which influence a person's long-term health status. During this stage of life, lifestyle choices can also put an individual at greater risk for physical injury, and may even result in death.

- Violence has become a critical health issue for women during adolescence and early adulthood, costing thousands of lives, millions of dollars, and untold physical and mental suffering. In 1991, homicide was the second leading cause of death for young African-American women. Homicide is the number one killer of women in the workplace. Suicide became the third leading cause of death for young white women (aged 15 to 24) in that same year.

■ Infection with the human immunodeficiency virus (HIV), which causes AIDS, is a growing problem among women in the United States and around the world. In 1991 and 1992, women were the fastest-growing group afflicted with the AIDS virus, and there was a larger proportionate increase in reported AIDS cases among women (9.8 percent) than among men (5.2 percent). In some major U.S. cities, AIDS is now the number-one killer of women of reproductive age. In 1992, for the first time, the number of women who contracted AIDS through heterosexual contact exceeded those infected through intravenous drug use. Approximately 75 percent of women with AIDS are African-American or Hispanic-American.

■ The incidence of other sexually transmitted diseases (STDs) is rising partly because both women and men are becoming sexually active at younger ages and have more sexual partners. According to a study by the Guttmacher Institute, 39 percent of sexually active teenagers living in urban areas in 1988 had only one sexual partner, compared with 62 percent in 1972, and 17 percent had four or more partners, compared with 8.5 percent in 1972. The study estimated that over the course of a year 6.4 million women between the ages of sixteen and forty-four have direct contact with more than one sexual partner and an additional 5.5 to 11 million have indirect contact with multiple partners through nonmonogamous males. Thus between 11.9 and 17.4 million women are at risk of increased exposure to sexually transmitted diseases each year. Because STDs are frequently symptomless or hard to diagnose in women, such infections may go untreated until serious problems develop. Complications include pelvic inflammatory disease, which can result in infertility or ectopic pregnancies, the leading cause of maternal mortality among African-American women today.

BEHAVIOR AND HEALTH

A walk through a 19th-century cemetery or a review of mortality data from this time period reveals that 100 years ago women's lives were cut short by infectious diseases and the medical complications of childbearing. Medical progress during this century has resulted in a dramatic reduction in mortality caused by complications of childbirth. Additionally, overall improvements in public sanitation, antibiotics and other medical advances have played a large part in increasing women's life expectancy by almost 30 years since the turn of the century. Today, the medical community faces the challenge of keeping women healthy over the course of their longer life span.

As we look into the future, it is clear that environmental and behavioral factors figure prominently in the efforts to study and improve both men's and women's health. In setting a research agenda for the future, it is crucial that policymakers and the medical community take into account behavioral and lifestyle factors, including diet, lack of exercise, smoking, and substance abuse, that substantially contribute to the development of chronic illnesses and to all 10 of the leading causes of death in America (which include cancer, heart disease, diabetes, injury, violence, and suicide). Needless to say, behavioral factors also play a critical role in other major public health problems that are tearing at the fabric of our society, such as infant mortality, teen pregnancy, homelessness, substance abuse, and the reemergence of tuberculosis.

Any serious attempt to modify behavior must take into account the fact that most people need more than information to change their lifestyles. Information alone has not slimmed the obese, stamped out cigarette smoking, or substantially influenced what we transport on that short, yet important, journey from dinner plate to mouth. Nor has information alone encouraged enough sexually active young women to abstain, to practice birth control, or to protect themselves from the threat of sexually transmitted diseases.

The simple fact is that health-enhancing behavior by every American woman would have a far greater impact on preventing disease, improving the quality of life, and reducing the cost of health care than any other type of intervention. Therefore, the medical community must seek to understand better the behavioral, social, and environmental factors that contribute to a variety of behaviors and pose health risks to women. (See Fig. 1.2. A–C.)

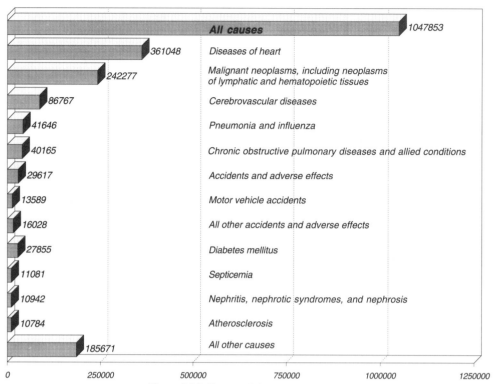

Cause	Deaths
All causes	1047853
Diseases of heart	361048
Malignant neoplasms, including neoplasms of lymphatic and hematopoietic tissues	242277
Cerebrovascular diseases	86767
Pneumonia and influenza	41646
Chronic obstructive pulmonary diseases and allied conditions	40165
Accidents and adverse effects	29617
Motor vehicle accidents	13589
All other accidents and adverse effects	16028
Diabetes mellitus	27855
Septicemia	11081
Nephritis, nephrotic syndromes, and nephrosis	10942
Atherosclerosis	10784
All other causes	185671

Figure 1.2A Causes of death - all women

Birth defects can also result from untreated STDs, with 100,000 infants dying or suffering birth defects as a result of STDs transmitted during pregnancy or at birth.

■ Between 1980 and 1990, the percentage of live births to unmarried women increased from 18 to 28 percent. The majority of these births was to unmarried adolescents. In 1991, some form of contraception was used by 81 percent of sexually active women between the ages of 15 and 19. Yet, of the 1.1 million women in that age group who become pregnant each year, 85 percent did not intend to get pregnant. The medical community not only must provide more effective methods of contraception but also must find more effective ways to encourage young women to practice abstinence or to use contraceptives correctly and consistently.

■ Behavior also plays a major role in a disease that now threatens the life of women during their adult years. Since the late 1980s, lung cancer has been the leading cause of cancer death among women in the United States. This is related to the increased rates of smoking among women. In the past 30 years, the death rate from lung cancer among American women has increased nearly 400 percent, almost exclusively because of cigarette smoking. In 1991, 51,000 American women died of lung cancer. It is estimated that by 1995 nearly 50 percent of the women in the world who die from problems caused by cigarette smoking will be Americans. And the majority of adult smokers began smoking during their teenage years.

The Later Years

Women's longevity puts them at risk for many diseases that are less prevalent among young women. Indeed, it is fair to say that women are pioneers of aging, and any study of the process of aging should focus on women. At present, women make up two-thirds of nursing home residents. Through advances from basic research into the causes and prevention of such diseases and conditions as Alzheimer's disease, coronary disease, osteoporosis, and cancer, the medical community could help make women's bonus years of life healthy ones.

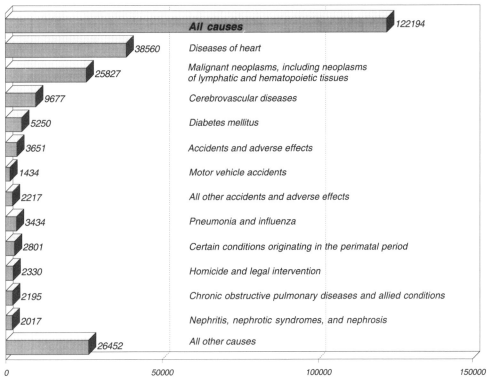

Figure 1.2B Causes of death - African-American women

■ Lung cancer is not the only form of cancer that takes the lives of American women. In fact, cancer is the second leading cause of death among American women of all ages, accounting for 250,000 deaths each year, and it is the leading cause of premature death. Today, approximately 27 percent of cancer deaths among American women are accounted for by cancers of the breast (44,000) and of the reproductive system, including ovarian (12,500), cervical (5,400), and uterine (5,500) cancers. Between 1979 and 1986, the death rate from breast cancer increased by 24 percent, and 1 in 8 American women will develop breast cancer during her lifetime, an increase from 1 in 20 women during the 1960s. It is estimated that only 5–10 percent of cases of breast cancer can be attributed to genetic predisposition and the recently discovered BRAC-1 gene; environmental and behavioral factors account for the rest. Recent evidence suggests that diet, pollutants, and other environmental toxins that may stimulate estrogen production may also play important roles in the development of breast cancer. Other factors, including lack of access to mammography screening, Pap tests,

and treatment services may also account for the fact that women of color have higher mortality rates for both breast cancer and cervical cancer.

■ Although women live an average of seven years longer than men, they are more susceptible to chronic health problems in their adult years. In fact, chronic and disabling conditions, especially such autoimmune diseases as rheumatoid arthritis and lupus erythematosus, are far more common among women than among men. According to a 1993 study by the Commonwealth Fund, 26 percent of women nationwide have been diagnosed with arthritis; 16 percent of women have a disability, handicap, or chronic disease that prevents them from fully participating in school or work-related activities; and 9 percent require assistance with such routine activities as shopping or household chores.

■ Osteoporosis affects an estimated 20 to 25 million American women, including 50 percent of women over the age of 45 and 90 percent of women older than 75. Osteoporosis causes more than 1.3 million fractures of the hip,

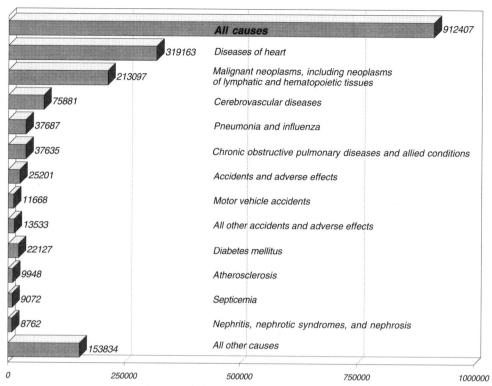

Figure 1.2C Causes of death - white women

wrists, and vertebrae and is responsible for 50,000 deaths each year.

- Urinary incontinence, which affects an estimated 10 million American adults, is two to five more times prevalent among women than among men.

- Women are also at greater risk than men for Alzheimer's disease. Researchers have identified a specific protein that appears to be responsible for the changes seen in the brains of those who suffer from Alzheimer's disease. This discovery could eventually lead to new drugs or therapies to prevent or delay the onset of the disease. The economic implications of being able to delay the onset of Alzheimer's make such research an especially important item on our nation's health agenda: Delaying the onset of the disease, which today affects four million Americans, by just five years could reduce the number of cases substantially and save our nation about $40 billion annually. Such research will not only help improve the lives of the women who suffer from the illness but will also help ease the burden of those

who care for the Alzheimer patient, the majority of whom are daughters, granddaughters, sisters, and other female family members. Although women remain the principal caregivers in our society, today's women have fewer traditional family and social supports available to them than their mothers had. Thus it is clear that we must respond as a society to the increasing demands placed on such women who are responsible all at once for their children and their elderly relatives.

What's Needed for the Future

Members of the medical community must focus new research efforts on discovering why gender affects the incidence, prevalence, level of disability, and death rates of disease. Biological sex differences may account for the predisposition to certain conditions and may explain why diseases affect men and women at particular phases of the life cycle. But psychological, social, and environmental factors, such as work patterns, lifestyles, and gender roles and beliefs, may override biology and change the inherent protection from and predisposition to particular physical and mental disorders for both men and women. When environmental and behavioral factors are modified, there may be a shift in the incidence of various diseases. Thus identifying and developing strategies to change health-damaging behavior and to eliminate environmental hazards should be critical components of future research and prevention efforts.

In coming years, basic research in human genetics will enable scientists to identify individual genes and to understand their roles in the onset and progression of disease. Genetic studies and development of strategies to repair genes hold the promise of transforming medicine in the 21st century and could result in a dramatic decline in the rates of a host of chronic diseases and conditions. Such research also holds tremendous promise for extending the boundaries of reproductive life. As more women marry later in life and give birth for the first time in their 30s and 40s, we must begin to address the ethical and legal issues raised by new reproductive technologies. At the same time, we must remember that new research findings and new medical treatments and technologies are only useful if they are widely available to all Americans.

As our society has become more ethnically, racially, and culturally diverse, the health of minority groups has become an important issue for our nation. Because of a lack of access to adequate health care and because of problems of cross-cultural communication, members of minority populations frequently experience more serious complications and higher mortality rates from some illnesses. When studying and treating members of a particular minority group, health care

professionals must have knowledge and understanding of the culture, its language, and attitudes about illness and the health profession. Physicians, nurses, and other health care providers must consider any culturally based differences that could affect the treatment of diverse groups of women.

To address these issues in a coherent fashion, it is imperative that a comprehensive research agenda is formulated. In addition to creating a list of diseases and conditions in dire need of further study, our society must reexamine the research processes and the institutions that conduct medical studies. In other words, it is not enough to focus solely on what should be researched. We must also examine how research is conducted in this country and how this affects our understanding of women's health issues. Some tough questions must be answered: By what criteria are priorities determined and who controls this process? Are women and minorities included in research studies and do they serve as the investigators on these projects? How are research advances disseminated to improve the medical care of women in communities across the nation?

Above all, we must relinquish a disease-oriented approach to the study of women's health and focus instead on discovering what constitutes optimal health for a woman throughout her entire life span. Such an approach requires that women's bodies be used as the medical model for women's health research. New policies mandating the inclusion of women in clinical research supported by the federal government are essential to establishing woman as the new medical paradigm. Additionally, clinical services must be available to all women and be provided in a way that is sensitive to the unique issues and needs of women patients.

STEPS TO GOOD HEALTH

Every woman needs to take responsibility for her own health. The first important step is education. The more you know about your body and how it functions, the better equipped you will be to safeguard your good health through prevention strategies, like eating a low-fat diet and exercising regularly. Knowledge will also enable you to detect the early signs of many illnesses and to ask your doctor better questions. Indeed, arming yourself with a deeper understanding of your mind and body can improve the quality of health care you receive.

The second step on the road to good health is taking action, based on knowledge and commitment. This may involve identifying the factors in your environment that could contribute to the development of disease and working to change them. Other actions are joining a self-help or support group, joining a smoking-cessation or weight-loss program, starting an exercise program, practicing relaxation training, wearing seat belts, getting regular mammography and pap smears, and simply getting enough rest.

Ultimately, taking action to promote good health

means making a commitment to yourself. That commitment means taking a proactive approach in dealing with your physician. Don't be afraid to ask questions. If you don't get satisfactory answers from your current doctor, find another one. Commitment sometimes includes taking action in your local community to improve health awareness and women's access to medical care and finding ways to increase funding for women's health research and service delivery programs. Remember that women's newfound economic and political power have put women's health on our nation's agenda, and this same power will keep it a vital issue.

Good health is as much process as end point. A healthy lifestyle is its own reward. An ancient proverb states, "He"—let's make that *she*—"who has health has hope. And she who has hope has everything." That is what the reward of adopting a healthy lifestyle is all about. While the medical community can conduct research and provide recommendations and guidelines on health-promoting behaviors, the ultimate responsibility for embarking on the road to a healthier and more hopeful life rests with you.

CHAPTER 2

How to Cope with the Health Care System

Jeanne F. Arnold, M.D., F.A.A.F.P

Today, women face challenges from all sides, from the demands of home and family to the pressures of work and the need for self-fulfillment. More than ever before, women have to make strong, informed decisions about their lives. No decisions are more important, however, than the choices we make about our personal health and well-being.

Of course, the most vital way you can protect and care for your own body is by observing the rules of good health. Eating a balanced diet, exercising regularly, and getting enough sleep are the building blocks of a strong, healthy body. Optimum health and energy also depend on a prudent lifestyle, which means not smoking, avoiding the excessive use of alcohol, and abstaining from illegal drugs. Finally, you must have reliable medical resources that you can turn to not only in times of crisis but also for regular preventive care. You must, in other words, become a savvy health care consumer.

WHAT'S HAPPENING IN HEALTH CARE TODAY

Our current health care system bears little resemblance to the system in place a few decades ago. Today, many more programs provide assistance with health care costs. Some employers offer health insurance to their employees and subsidize, to some extent, the cost of the premium that must be paid for the insurance. Government programs have been developed to provide health care for older persons and the poor. The quality of health care in the United States, despite publicized malpractice cases and product recalls, is high.

All of this has come at a cost. Ever-rising medical costs have affected the consumer's ability to choose health care that is right for her. For many people, the old doctor-patient relationship—a long-term, personal association with a family physician—is no longer possible. Now, we often must choose our doctors on the basis of their membership in a particular health care plan.

Health care plans vary tremendously in coverage, the options a patient has for treatment, and cost. The more procedures and types of care that are available, the higher the cost. The more freedom the consumer has to choose doctors, hospitals, and treatments, the more expensive the plan. The consumer may not pay all of the cost directly; government and employers often subsidize a portion. In the long run, the consumer ends up paying for health care, one way or another. Employees may find other benefits cut because of the high cost of health care. Taxpayers can see the rising health care costs in their rising taxes.

To cut their medical costs, many employers (and some consumers who pay for their own health care) have chosen to follow the *managed care* system of health care. Examples of the managed care system are health maintenance organizations (HMOs) and preferred provider organizations (PPOs). In return for lower costs, these programs limit the health care received:

- Doctors that can be seen
- Types of services performed
- Where services are performed
- Length of hospital stay

Of the different health care plans listed in the following sections, not all types are available to all people. Employers often offer several options to employees, who can pick the plan that best suits their needs (and pay accordingly).

Fee-for-Service Plans

In a fee-for-service plan, the patient or insurance company pays the doctor a fee for every service performed. Overall, the more services doctors perform, the more money they earn. This system is blamed by some for increasing health care costs. Because patients can see any doctor they choose, doctors have incentives to provide good service and develop relationships with their patients.

In fee-for-service plans, a premium is paid for the plan. Usually the patient must pay a certain amount of her own money for health care (a deductible) before the insurance company begins reimbursing the patient for care. After the deductible has been met, the company usually reimburses the patient for part of the total costs (often around 70 to 80 percent). Some expenses are covered in full, while others—perhaps medications—are not covered at all and must be paid for out of pocket.

Although fee-for-service insurance plans still exist, they are becoming more rare since they are the most expensive type of health care plan. Consumers are finding it more and more difficult to pay hundreds of dollars for out-of-pocket costs or to pay a large deductible before they are reimbursed. Employers find these plans less attractive because they lack built-in mechanisms to control costs. As employees' health care costs rise, the cost of insurance increases.

Health Maintenance Organizations

An HMO assesses a fixed monthly or annual fee for the medical coverage it offers. Covered services usually include medical, surgical, and hospital care as well as emergency, prenatal, prescription, and preventive services. Dental and vision services may also be provided, sometimes at an additional charge. There is usually no deductible, but you may pay a small fee, or copayment, for each visit to a doctor depending on the care provided.

Although they offer the advantages of lower costs, HMOs limit access to certain doctors. In an HMO, you choose a primary physician who acts as a gatekeeper and coordinates your total medical care. The gatekeeper's responsibility also involves reviewing and overseeing your need to see a specialist or to receive some types of therapy. HMOs try to lower costs by providing for more preventive and ambulatory care, recommending less surgery, and reducing the medical tests performed.

Some HMOs provide all their medical services at centralized locations. If your primary physician recommends a mammogram, it can be convenient to just go down three floors in the same building rather than driving across town. However, an HMO's few locations may be inconvenient for some people.

Other HMOs use a network of private physicians, urgent care centers, and hospitals. Only these facilities can be used, unless your primary physician authorizes use of another facility. This means you must learn which hospitals and other sources of care are affiliated with your HMO so that you go to the right one when you need care. If you become ill away from home, you must notify the HMO that you need care and get authorization to use another hospital. Even in an emergency, you may need to receive authorization to receive care; often this authorization can be requested after you've been admitted.

Preferred Provider Organization

Large insurance companies, hospitals, and some physician groups offer a type of medical coverage called a PPO. In many ways, PPOs are much like HMOs. The difference is that although certain doctors have joined a network sponsored by the PPO, you are not obligated to use them. When you see a physician in the PPO network, the fee for your care is lower. If you wish, you may choose your own nonmember physician; however, the fee for your care will be higher. All doctors who are part of a PPO have their own offices.

The advantage of a PPO over an HMO is the increased freedom to select physicians. In a PPO the fees are much higher if you seek care from a nonmember doctor or nonaffiliated hospital.

Federal Health Care Programs

Americans who are at least 65 years of age are covered by Medicare, a health insurance program run by the federal government. Basic Medicare insurance covers hospitalization; this coverage is free to anyone 65 or older. Persons eligible for Medicare also can purchase supplemental medical insurance from the Medicare program. For a small monthly premium, this supplemental insurance covers visits to a doctor's office. Because of restrictions on services and the costs reimbursed, however, many Medicare recipients buy additional private insurance, so-called Medigap because it fills the gaps Medicare leaves.

People in low income levels are eligible for another federal program, Medicaid. For both Medicare and Medicaid, efforts to save money have led to low fees being paid to doctors to reimburse them for their services. Because of this, many doctors do not participate in the program and don't accept patients covered by either plan.

WORKING WITH YOUR DOCTOR

Choosing a Personal Physician

Don't wait until you are sick to look for a personal or primary physician. Choose your doctor when you are in good health, feel in control of the situation, and are able to make judgments about your medical options. Doctors are not all alike. You might try several before you find a doctor you not only trust, are comfortable with, and respect but also treats you with respect and consideration.

To find the right doctor for your needs, get referrals from friends and relatives whose judgment you value. Make sure that the person who recommends a doctor has gone to that doctor several times.

With the growth of managed care, you may have less choice in selecting a physician. If you belong to an HMO and are limited to a particular roster of doctors, check around for referrals among colleagues at work or friends with the same plan. Has anyone else seen this physician? How did they feel about her manner, methods, and attitude? In any case, don't continue to see a doctor you are not satisfied or comfortable with; there are other doctors in the plan whom you can choose. If you are in a PPO or a fee-for-service plan, you may have more options in choosing your physician.

Once you have the name of a likely candidate, call the office and ask the doctor's assistant a few questions. Don't hesitate to ask questions; remember, you are paying the physician who is working for you. Some questions you might ask include

- Which hospital is the doctor affiliated with? What are the doctor's medical credentials, and how long has she been in practice?
- What are the doctor's fees? Does the doctor require payment immediately or will her office send you a bill? Verify that the doctor will accept your type of health insurance or is a member of your HMO or other managed care plan.
- If the doctor has an individual practice, who covers when the doctor is not available? If the doctor is a member of a group practice, can you ask for an appointment with the individual doctor of your choice or do you have to take whichever doctor is available?

- Is there a specific time of the day when patients can call the doctor and ask questions? Is the doctor there every day, or only a few days during the week?
- How does the doctor handle emergencies? Can you call anytime during the day or night to find out if you have a real emergency?

The attitude of the staff and their readiness to answer your questions promptly and courteously tells you a lot about the doctor before you even make an appointment. If you are satisfied with the information you receive, visit the doctor for a general checkup. At that time, bring up your health concerns with the doctor, ask questions, and make your evaluation.

Outside resources also can give you information on a physician's medical qualifications. All physicians should be licensed to practice by the state in which they practice. All states require doctors to show proof of graduation from an approved medical school and proof of certification in any special training. Physicians must update their state registration every 1–3 years, depending on the state.

Most physicians have 3 or more years of additional training, called residency, after graduation from medical school. Internists and family physicians have 3 years, while obstetrician-gynecologists have 4 years or more if they specialize in certain areas. These years of residency training make them eligible to take specialty board exams. A physician who passes these tests is board certified in the specialty. There are 24 specialty boards that are officially recognized as members of the American Board of Medical Specialties (ABMS). Of these, 20 boards require specialists to be recertified every 6 to 10 years to ensure that their knowledge is up to date.

The best way to learn whether your doctor has special expertise is to ask. To find a doctor with a particular certification, use *The Official ABMS Directory of Board Certified Medical Specialists* published by the American Board of Medical Specialties (708-491-9091) and Marquis Who's Who (908-464-6800). It should be available in your local library. Your state's medical society also may have a directory that lists credentials.

The First Visit: Establishing the Doctor-Patient Relationship

Ideally, you'll meet your new doctor for a general checkup or when you have a minor complaint that allows you time to ask questions and evaluate answers. Use this opportunity to get acquainted with the physician and to make sure this is the person you want to handle your health needs.

The doctor-patient relationship should be a mutually honest and open one, allowing for some differences of opinion. Be prepared to answer all the doctor's questions about your health and any symptoms you have. Orderly recordkeeping will help you to do this (see "Keep Track of Your Own Medical History").

Don't be afraid to offer your point of view, even if you worry that the doctor will think your objections are silly; the only stupid question in such a situation is the one that goes unasked. If you are not clear about something, ask for more information and further explanation. Be courteous, but be persistent.

The doctor should respond willingly to all of your questions. Make sure that you understand the diagnosis, the treatment, and any medication prescribed. If surgery is called for, the doctor always should be willing to have you seek a second opinion. If the doctor is not communicative, seems reluctant to discuss certain aspects of your treatment, or takes offense if you want a second opinion, find someone else to manage your health care.

Some problems may be resolved with a little straightforward communication. The doctor may not be aware, for example, that the front office puts patients on hold without asking whether it is an emergency or that sometimes your messages don't seem to get through. Also let the doctor know if you think the waiting time in the office is too long. You should not have to put up with long delays to see the doctor, unanswered telephone calls, or rude treatment from the office staff. If these problems persist, simply tell the staff and the doctor you are going elsewhere and ask them to forward your records to your new physician.

KEEP TRACK OF YOUR OWN MEDICAL HISTORY

Every doctor that you see, whether a primary physician or a specialist, will ask you questions about your past medical experiences and about your health in general. This information is important; a quick look at your medical history can give a practitioner a fairly accurate idea of your health risks and clues to help diagnose a current problem.

Because it's hard to remember all the dates of specific treatments, or the names of drugs you may have taken in the past, try keeping your own medical journal (see the sample form in Figure 2.1). Add any other facts about your health, no matter how minor, that you think may be of use to the doctor. Put copies of prescriptions, test results, notes, and your immunization records in the same file. If you are a computer buff, you may find it easier to store this history (and the medical histories of family members) in a computer for easy updating.

Take a copy of your health record with you every time you visit a new doctor. Keep this record in a readily accessible place, and update it regularly.

Medical Tests: The Routine Checkup

Even if you have no health problems, it's a good idea to see your doctor regularly for a periodic evaluation of your health. The exam should include measuring your height, weight, and blood pressure. Your breasts, abdomen, and neck (for thyroid gland) should be checked as a part of this exam. Each year, women who are sexually active or are older than 18 years of age should have pelvic exams, in which their genitals are examined. They should also have a Pap test to detect early signs of cancer of the cervix.

Certain tests should be done on a regular basis as a part of preventive health care. The recommended tests vary according to a woman's age. Likewise, different immunizations are recommended throughout your life to protect you from disease. These tests and immunizations are shown in Table 2.1. Other tests or immunizations are needed only for persons at risk of having an infection or other health problem. These are listed, along with who may need them, in Table 2.2.

FIGURE 2.1. YOUR HEALTH HISTORY

Birth and Childhood

Birth date: _____

Serious illnesses and treatments

Illness_____ Date_____ Treatment_____

Illness_____ Date_____ Treatment_____

Illness_____ Date_____ Treatment_____

Childhood immunizations (date):_____

_____

_____

Allergies

To_____ Symptoms_____

To_____ Symptoms_____

Medications

Medication taken_____ For_____

Medication taken_____ For_____

Medication taken_____ For_____

Chronic Illnesses

_____

_____

Tests and Immunizations

Most recent Pap test

Date_____ Result_____

Most recent mammogram

Date_____ Result_____

Other tests and immunizations

Date_____ Result_____

Date_____ Result_____

Date_____ Result_____

Date_____ Result_____

Date_____ Result_____

Date_____ Result_____

Operations and Hospitalizations

Date_____ Reason_____ Doctor (name, address, and phone number)_____

Date_____ Reason_____ Doctor (name, address, and phone number)_____

Reproductive History

Age at first menstruation_____

Length of menstrual cycle_____ days

Type of contraception used_____

Pregnancy history_____

_____

_____

Family History

Children

Name_____ Birth date_____ Illnesses_____

_____

Name_____ Birth date_____ Illnesses_____

_____

Parents (list cause of death if deceased)

Name_____ Birth date_____ Illnesses_____

_____

Name_____ Birth date_____ Illnesses_____

_____

Grandparents (list cause of death if deceased)

Name_____ Birth date_____ Illnesses_____

_____

Name_____ Birth date_____ Illnesses_____

_____

Name_____ Birth date_____ Illnesses_____

_____

Name_____ Birth date_____ Illnesses_____

_____

Brothers and sisters (list cause of death if deceased)

Name_____ Birth date_____ Illnesses_____

_____

Name_____ Birth date_____ Illnesses_____

TABLE 2.1   RECOMMENDED ROUTINE TESTS AND IMMUNIZATIONS FOR WOMEN BY AGE

Test/Immuniza-tion	13–18	19–39	40–49	50–64	65 or Older
Test					
Pap test	Yearly when sexually active or by age 18	Physician and patient discretion after 3 consecutive normal tests	Physician and patient discretion after 3 consecutive normal tests	Physician and patient discretion after 3 consecutive normal tests	Physician and patient discretion after 3 consecutive normal tests
Cholesterol	Not recommended	Every 5 years	Every 5 years	Every 5 years	Every 3–5 years
Mammography	Not recommended	Not recommended	Every 1–2 years	Yearly	Yearly
Fecal occult blood test	Not recommended	Not recommended	Not recommended	Yearly	Yearly
Sigmoidoscopy	Not recommended	Not recommended	Not recommended	Every 3–5 years	Every 3–5 years
Thyroid-stimulating hormone test	Not recommended	Not recommended	Not recommended	Not recommended	Every 3–5 years
Urinalysis	Not recommended	Not recommended	Not recommended	Not recommended	Yearly
Immunization					
Tetanus-diphtheria booster	Once between ages 14–16	Booster every 10 years	Booster every 10 years	Booster at age 50 if no immunization in last 10 years	Every 10 years
Influenza vaccine	Not recommended	Depends on chronic diseases, occupational exposure; see Table 2.2			Recommended
Pneumococcal	Depends on chronic diseases, special conditions; see Table 2.2				Recommended

Source: American College of Obstetricians and Gynecologists. *The Obstetrician-Gynecologist and Primary-Preventive Health Care.* Washington, D.C.: ACOG, 1993; *Annals of Internal Medicine,* October 1, 1994.

HOSPITAL CARE

Just as there are many kinds of health plans today, there are many types of hospitals that meet the needs of different patients. Despite the various kinds of hospitals, your choice may be limited. Many insurance plans contract not only with specific doctors but also with specific hospitals and other facilities that provide health care (see "Alternatives to Hospitals"). If you receive care from a facility that is not approved by your health care plan, you may have to pay much or all of the bill yourself. To avoid this, find out which hospitals and other facilities are approved by your insurance. If you have a choice of several health care plans, think about the choice of hospitals and physicians they offer.

Choose a plan affiliated with a hospital that you want to use.

Managed care insurance plans often require precertification before any hospital stay except for emergencies. Usually, your primary doctor has to authorize your stay. In addition, your doctor may have to get advance approval from the insurer for some types of care. Again, if you do not precertify your stay, you may find yourself holding the bill.

When you need more than a doctor's visit or can't wait for an appointment, you may be able to use one of the new alternatives to hospitals, ambulatory care (walk-in) centers or urgent care centers (see "Alterna-

TABLE 2.2 TESTS AND IMMUNIZATIONS FOR WOMEN WITH RISK FACTORS

Test or Immunization	Risk Factors
Test	
Skin exam	Increased exposure to sun due to recreation or work; family or personal history of skin cancer; precancerous skin changes
Blood test for hemoglobin	Caribbean, Latin American, Asian, Mediterranean, or African descent; heavy menstrual periods
Urine test for infection	Diabetes
Sexually transmitted disease (STD) testing	Having multiple sexual partners or a partner with multiple partners; sexual contacts with persons who have an STD; history of STDs
Human immunodeficiency virus (HIV) testing	Seeking treatment for STDs; past or present drug use by injection; prostitution; having a past or present sexual partner who is HIV positive or bisexual or who injects drugs; birth or long-term residence in an area where HIV is common; blood transfusion during 1978–85
Genetic testing/counseling	Women of reproductive age exposed to substances that could harm the fetus; women 35 years old or more planning pregnancy; personal, family, or partner history of birth defect or genetic disorder; African-American, Eastern European Jewish, Mediterranean, or Southeast Asian ancestry
Tuberculosis (TB) skin test	Infection with HIV; living or working with someone known or suspected of having TB; having a medical condition that increases the risk of disease if infection has occurred; birth in country where TB is common; having low income and poor access to health care; alcoholics and intravenous drug users; living in long-term care facilities (such as nursing homes or mental institutions) or prison; working in high-risk health care facilities
Blood test for type of lipids (cholesterol)	Having a high cholesterol level; having a parent or brother or sister with a high cholesterol level; having a brother, sister, parent, or grandparent younger than age 55 with heart disease; diabetes; smoking
Mammography	Being 35 or older and having a mother or sister who had breast cancer before menopause
Fasting glucose (sugar) test	Family history of diabetes; being very overweight; having had diabetes in pregnancy
Thyroid-stimulating hormone test (for thyroid function)	Family history of thyroid disease; having an autoimmune disease
Colonoscopy	Personal history of inflammatory bowel disease or polyps in the colon; family history of colon cancer
Immunization	
Rubella vaccine	Women of childbearing age without proof of immunity to rubella
Hepatitis B vaccine	Use of intravenous drugs; receiving blood products; working in health care or with blood; living or having sex with someone who has hepatitis B virus; prostitution; having sex with multiple partners in the past 6 months
Fluoride supplement	Living in area with poor water fluoridation
Influenza vaccine	Living in chronic care home; having chronic heart or lung disease; having metabolic disease (such as diabetes, sickle cell anemia, suppressed immune system, or kidney disease); older people
Pneumococcal vaccine	Risk factors for influenza vaccine plus Hodgkin disease, asplenia, alcoholism, cirrhosis, multiple myeloma

Source: American College of Obstetricians and Gynecologists. *The Obstetrician-Gynecologist and Primary-Preventive Health Care.* Washington, D.C.: ACOG, 1993.

ALTERNATIVES TO HOSPITALS

Hospitals are expensive. Costs are high because they offer a lot: extensive staff, a wide variety of costly equipment, and a large building with many beds. Often, a woman who doesn't need all the services that a hospital provides can receive appropriate care elsewhere at a lower cost.

For example, some relatively simple operations can be done in a doctor's office or clinic. At some walk-in clinics, patients can seek treatment for a medical condition without an appointment. When a procedure requires recovery of a short stay (up to 24 hours), a short-term surgery center may be suitable. These centers can handle simple surgeries in patients at low risk for complications.

When a medical condition is more serious, an urgent care center may be a good alternative to a hospital emergency room. Urgent care centers are less expensive than emergency rooms and can provide appropriate care for many patients with non-life-threatening conditions.

Patients needing special care also may find an alternative to a hospital. For example, pregnant women may be able to give birth in a birthing center run by either doctors or nurse midwives. Persons who are terminally ill may prefer hospice care to a hospital. The goal of a hospice is to allow a terminally ill person to spend her final days in a supportive setting, free from pain. Hospices provide basic medical services, especially those aimed at relieving pain, but they usually avoid taking extraordinary measures. In other cases, consumers may be able to receive some home care that would normally require hospitalization.

community hospital—a type of voluntary, not-for-profit hospital—may be in a rural setting and have few beds with a volunteer, part-time physician staff. Compare this with a large, bustling city hospital that has many beds with an extensive, full-time staff of doctors.

Hospitals also vary in the type of care they provide. Community hospitals serve as general hospitals. Even though they provide basic medical care, community hospitals may not have the staff or equipment to treat some high-risk or complicated conditions. *Specialized hospitals* treat a particular family of diseases, such as diseases of the eye, pulmonary diseases, or cancer. Other specialized institutions limit their patients to a certain group or members of a particular organization.

Teaching hospitals train medical students and residents who are receiving additional training in a specialty. Residents spend long hours at the hospital caring for patients under the supervision of an attending physician who is experienced in the specialty. A teaching hospital can operate under any type of funding mechanism—not-for-profit, for-profit, or government—and it can be a specialized or general hospital.

A teaching hospital is usually affiliated with a medical school, and most of the physicians on staff at the hospital also hold teaching or research positions at the medical school. Some staff physicians in teaching hospitals are experts in their fields, with years of experience. Patients at teaching hospitals are frequently cared for by a number of physicians, some of whom are residents, even if they have primary physicians responsible for their care.

Many teaching hospitals are well known for their excellence in certain specialties and for their advanced medical technology and equipment. Teaching hospitals are often located in large urban centers, so they also provide primary care in the hospital's clinics.

tives to Hospitals"). Although they are usually less expensive than hospitals, they, too, must be accepted by your insurance plan before you can be reimbursed. As with hospitals, it is best to know in advance which centers and procedures are covered by your plan.

Types of Hospitals

finances—how they are funded and what types of payment they accept (see Table 2.3). Size and staffing are other factors that set hospitals apart from each other. A

If Hospitalization Is Necessary

surgery, you have the time and opportunity to gather information about the procedure and the services available at the hospital. Your doctor and the office staff should give you the details about your upcoming stay. The hospital admitting office also should instruct you about directions, visiting hours, parking facilities, types of rooms, and so on. Ask about special programs related to your situation. For example, many hospitals now offer classes to prepare a pregnant woman for labor and childbirth and other educational programs.

TABLE 2.3   A HOSPITAL PRIMER

Type	Administration	Funding Source	Types of Patients	Payment Accepted
Voluntary, not-for-profit	Nonprofit groups, religious groups	Payments for care and government funding; aim is to balance costs	All patients, including those who cannot pay	Cash, insurance, government programs, uncompensated (charity) care
Private, for-profit	Private corporation	Payments for care; aim is to make profit	Patients with money or private insurance	Cash, private insurance
Public	City, state, county, and so on	Payments for care; subsidized by government	All patients, including those who cannot pay	Cash, insurance, government programs, uncompensated (charity) care
Federal (military, Veterans Administration)	Federal government	Subsidized by federal government	Veterans or persons with current military service; their dependents	Federal government

You and your family may benefit from knowing whether the hospital has a *patient advocate*, a person who acts as a liaison between you and the hospital staff. By law, you have certain rights as a patient. Among others, you have the right to:

- Know the name and function of any health care professional who is treating you. Never allow yourself to be treated or examined by anonymous people. Always ask the name and specialty of any residents who say they are taking part in your care. Don't be afraid to ask them questions.

- Give informed consent. Informed consent means that before you agree to a procedure, your physician provides you with complete current information concerning diagnosis, treatment, and prognosis in terms you can be reasonably expected to understand. You should be told about the specific procedure or treatment or both, the risks involved, and any alternatives to treatment.

- Refuse treatment to the extent permitted by law and to be informed of the medical consequences of your action.

The Complete Patient's Bill of Rights, as established by the American Hospital Association, should be made available to you on admission to the hospital. Copies also should be posted in conspicuous places within the hospital.

THE ROLE OF THE EMERGENCY ROOM

The emergency room of a hospital or medical center is designed to provide rapid assessment and initial treatment of seriously ill and injured people. In many communities, however, emergency rooms have become overcrowded with patients who have no health insurance and no regular doctors they can consult about health problems.

Making the emergency room your family doctor strains the staff and equipment of the emergency room. Plus, it has the following drawbacks for you:

- Little continuity of care, that is, treatment by one doctor who is familiar with your health problems and needs

- Long waits for nonemergencies, which are treated after emergencies

- High fees

Some people think that all sudden illnesses and injuries, no matter how minor, should be handled in the emergency room. The reality is that most of these

FIGURE 2.2.   LIVING WILL

This Living Will has been prepared to conform to the law in _____ *as set forth in* _____ .
In that case the Court established the need for "clear and convincing" evidence of a patient's wishes and stated that the "ideal situation is one in which the patient's wishes were expressed in some form of writing, perhaps a 'living will.' "

I, _____ , being of sound mind, make this statement as a directive to be followed if I become permanently unable to participate in decisions regarding my medical care. These instructions reflect my firm and settled commitment to decline medical treatment under the circumstances indicated below:

I direct my attending physician to withhold or withdraw treatment that merely prolongs my dying, if I should be in an **incurable or irreversible mental or physical condition with no reasonable expectation of recovery.**

These instructions apply if I am (a) **in a terminal condition;** (b) **permanently unconscious;** or (c) **if I am minimally conscious but have irreversible brain damage and will never regain the ability to make decisions and express my wishes.**

I direct that my treatment be limited to measures to keep me comfortable and to relieve pain, including any pain that might occur by withholding or withdrawing treatment.

While I understand that I am not legally required to be specific about future treatments **if I am in the condition(s) described above I feel especially strongly about the following forms of treatment:**
  I do not want cardiac resuscitation.
  I do not want mechanical respiration.
  I do not want artificial nutrition and hydration.
  I do not want antibiotics.

However, I **do want** maximum pain relief, even if it may hasten my death.

Other directions:

These directions express my legal right to refuse treatment, under the law of the state of _____. I intend my instructions to be carried out, unless I have rescinded them in a new writing or by clearly indicating that I have changed my mind.

Signed _____   Date _____

Address _____

I declare that the person who signed this document is personally known to me and appears to be of sound mind and acting of his or her own free will. He or she signed (or asked another to sign for him or her) this document in my presence.

Witness 1 _____

Address _____

Witness 2 _____

Address _____

FIGURE 2.3.   HEALTH CARE PROXY

(1) I,_____

hereby appoint _____
(name, address, and telephone number)

_____

as my health care agent to make any and all health care decisions for me, except to the extent that I state otherwise. This proxy shall take effect when and if I become unable to make my own health care decisions.

(2) Optional instructions: I direct my proxy to make health care decisions in accord with my wishes and limitations as stated below, or as he or she otherwise knows. (Attach additional pages, if necessary.)

_____

_____

_____

(3) Name of substitute or fill-in proxy if the person I appoint above is unable, unwilling, or unavailable to act as my health care agent.

_____
(name, address, and telephone number)

_____

(4) Unless I revoke it, this proxy shall remain in effect indefinitely, or until the date or conditions stated below. This proxy shall expire (specific date or conditions, if desired):

_____

(5) Signature _____

Address _____

Date _____

Statement by Witnesses (must be 18 or older)

I declare that the person who signed this document is personally known to me and appears to be of sound mind and acting of his or her own free will. He or she signed (or asked another to sign for him or her) this document in my presence.

Witness 1 _____

Address _____

Witness 2 _____

Address _____

---

problems could be managed more efficiently and certainly a lot faster in doctors' offices and clinics. In fact, most insurers have specific lists of conditions that they consider to be emergencies worthy of treatment in an emergency room. If you receive care at an emergency room for a condition that your insurance company does not consider to be a true emergency, the company may not pay the bill.

So, when should you go to an emergency room? In general, go to the emergency room if your condition can't be safely and quickly treated elsewhere. For more specific information, ask your doctor and your insurance company what they consider to be an emergency. Throughout this book, you can read about symptoms and conditions that require urgent care. The emergency room is always appropriate for these life-threatening conditions:

- Heart attack
- Poisoning
- Loss of consciousness
- Severe breathing problems
- Seizures
- Severe injury, such as from a car crash

To make your own use of emergency rooms more efficient, take the following steps:

- Establish a regular relationship with a health care provider that you can contact 24 hours a day. If you have severe symptoms, your doctor

or the doctor on call can tell you whether you need to go to the emergency room.

- See your doctor for regular recommended preventive care.
- If you have a medical condition, follow the treatment your doctor prescribes. Tell your doctor about any changes in your condition or reactions to medication you are taking for it. Your doctor can tell you which symptoms are signs of a true emergency.
- Have a plan. In an emergency, know whom to call and where to go. Have the ambulance service number nearby.

Instead of making random visits to the emergency room because there is nowhere else to turn, you'll receive more comprehensive and thorough treatment from a physician who knows your medical history and health status.

THE RIGHT TO DIE: LIVING WILLS AND HEALTH CARE PROXIES

If life is more complicated these days, so is death. Even though medical technology saves more lives than ever before, it also prolongs the lives of terminally ill or injured people who cannot speak for themselves.

You may have strong feelings about how much technical intervention you want to keep your body functioning when there is no hope of survival or no hope for an acceptable quality of life. To make sure your wishes in this important matter are followed—and to make the process easier for your family and friends—we strongly recommend that you prepare what is called an advance directive, or a *living will*.

A living will is a document that tells your family and your doctor that you do not want your life to be prolonged by invasive procedures or artificial life-support systems when you are terminally ill and your chances of regaining a meaningful life are nonexistent. By law, hospital admissions offices in most states must ask incoming patients whether they have such a will (this doesn't mean you have to have one). Most hos-

pital admissions offices and hospice programs (a program offering care and support for the terminally ill) can provide a blank form that you can fill out at any time. (See Fig. 2.2 for an example). Free forms are also available from Concern for Dying (250 West 57th Street, New York, NY 10107; 212-246-6962.

In conjunction with the living will, you might want to prepare a Durable Power of Attorney for Health Care Decisions, or a *health care proxy*. This is usually a part of the living will form. When you complete this part of the living will, you give a designated person authority to make medical decisions for you when you are unable to do so. (See Fig. 2.3).

Two adults who are not related to you must witness the living will, and a health care proxy or power of attorney must be notarized. When you have completed the living will, make copies for your close relatives and ask your physician to place it in your medical file for future reference. Keep the original signed document with your private papers in an accessible place.

PART II

KEEPING YOURSELF HEALTHY

CHAPTER 3

Diet, Nutrition, and Healthy Weight

Elaine B. Feldman, M.D., F.A.C.P

"You are what you eat." Like many most popular phrases, this one has some merit. Everything that the body needs to function—from building materials for bones, muscles, and organs to the energy to run complex systems and processes—comes from and reflects the food and drink that make up our daily diet. Unhealthy diets lead to unhealthy bodies.

What is a healthy diet? New studies about the benefits and risks of eating certain foods are in the news nearly every day. It's difficult, though, to read between the lines and get the whole story. For example, huge quantities of a particular food may have had to be consumed for the reported results to take place. Or perhaps only a few people were studied, or the evidence was sketchy or preliminary. Some dietary habits are definitely linked to disease, however. We know that high levels of fat and cholesterol in the diet increase the risk of heart disease and stroke. Lack of fresh fruits and vegetables can promote disease, including cancer. On the other hand, a healthy diet can prevent disease and even ameliorate it.

GUIDELINES FOR A HEALTHY DIET

What makes a healthy diet? One of the best sets of recommendations is the U.S. government's *Dietary Guidelines for Americans.* Updated in 1990, these seven easy rules provide for a varied and well-balanced diet.

1. Eat a variety of foods.
2. Maintain healthy weight.
3. Choose a diet low in fat, saturated fat, and cholesterol.
4. Choose a diet with plenty of vegetables, fruits, and grain.
5. Use sugars only in moderation.
6. Use salt and sodium only in moderation.
7. If you drink alcoholic beverages, do so in moderation.

Women who make habits out of these seven guidelines will reduce their risk of disease, feel better, and live longer. It's never too soon—or too late—to start.

Guideline 1: Eat a Variety of Foods

Different foods are good sources of different nutrients. By eating a varied diet, you increase your chances of getting all the nutrients your body needs. Plus, eating many different foods makes dinnertime a lot more interesting. The problem is choosing which foods to eat for basic health maintenance.

Choosing from Food Groups

You may remember learning about the "Four Food Groups" in school. There were four categories: milk and dairy products, meat and protein foods, fruits and vegetables, and grains and cereals. Unfortunately, this grouping seems to put too much emphasis on the first two categories. Most Americans get more protein in their diets than they may need, and dairy products and meats are high in fat.

In 1992, the U.S. Department of Agriculture introduced the "Food Guide Pyramid" as a way to give Americans a better guide to food selection (Figure 3.1). More servings per day are recommended of the foods at the bottom of the pyramid, and fewer servings per day are needed of those at the top. The pyramid is divided into the following basic food categories:

1. Bread, cereal, rice, and pasta (6 to 11 servings per day)
2. Vegetables (3 to 5 servings per day)
3. Fruit (2 to 4 servings per day)
4. Meat, poultry, fish, dry beans, eggs, and nuts (2 to 3 servings per day)
5. Milk, yogurt, and cheese (2 to 3 servings per day)

The fats, oils, and sweets, which are found at the top of the pyramid, should make up only a small part of the healthy diet. Fats and sugars are found in the other groups of the pyramid, too. Some occur naturally, such as the sugars in fruit or the fats in meat or milk. Others are added, such as the fats and sugars in baked goods.

You should eat foods from each group on a daily basis. How many calories you need each day depends on your age, your size, how active you are, and whether you are pregnant or breast-feeding. Here is a general guide:

- Women who get little exercise and small older women: 1,600 calories per day

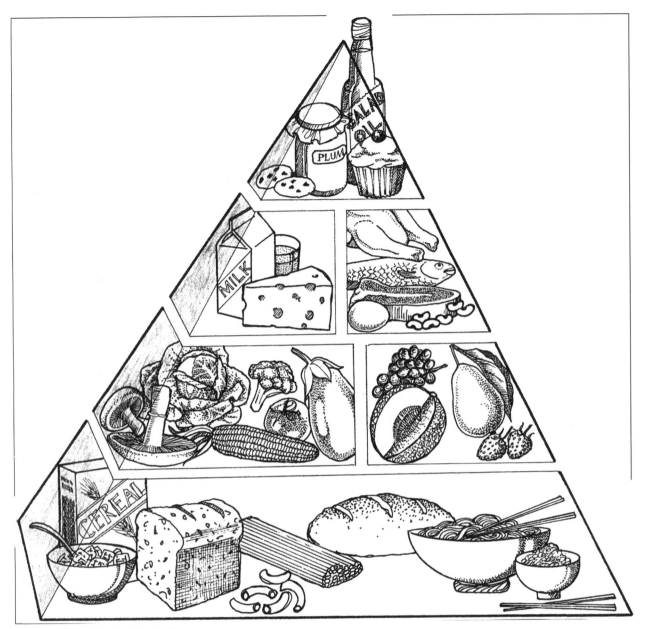

Figure 3.1. The Food Guide Pyramid.

- Most children, teenage girls, and active women (women who are pregnant or breast-feeding may need more): 2,000 or more calories per day
- Very active women: 2,400 or more calories per day

Once you know about how many calories you need, you can choose the right number of servings from each food group (Table 3.1).

Serving sizes are important, too. If serving sizes are too big, even of nutritious food, the extra calories may lead to weight gain. If too small, the foods may not provide all of the needed nutrients. Table 3.2 gives examples of serving sizes for each food group.

Nutrients

Nutrients are the basic components of food. Nutrients fall into six categories: proteins, carbohydrates, fats, vitamins, minerals, and water. All of these are a part of a healthy diet, but the body needs more of some nutrients and less of others.

TABLE 3.1 CHOOSING THE RIGHT NUMBER OF SERVINGS

Food Group	1,600 Calories	2,200 Calories	2,800 Calories
Breads (servings)	6	9	11
Vegetables (servings)	3	4	5
Fruits (servings)	2	3	4
Dairy products* (servings)	2	2	2
Meats (ounces)	5	6	7

Source: Modified from the U.S. Department of Agriculture, *The Food Guide Pyramid* (Home and Garden Bulletin No. 252), Washington, D.C.: USDA, 1992.

* Women who are pregnant or breast-feeding, teenagers, and young adults (up to age 24) need 3 servings of dairy products per day.

Proteins

Proteins are the building blocks of the body. They form muscles and organs and are responsible for the repair and maintenance of tissues. Some hormones, especially the polypeptide type like insulin, are made from amino acids. Important as they are, only about 15 percent of the calories in the average woman's diet must come from proteins.

TABLE 3.2 WHAT COUNTS AS A SERVING?

Food Group	Serving Size
Breads	• 1 slice of bread • 1 ounce of ready-to-eat cereal • ½ cup of cooked cereal, rice, or pasta
Vegetables	• 1 cup of raw leafy vegetables • ½ cup of other vegetables, cooked or chopped raw • ¾ cup of vegetable juice
Fruits	• 1 medium apple, banana, or orange • ½ cup of chopped, cooked, or canned fruit • ¾ cup of fruit juice
Dairy products	• 1 cup of milk or yogurt • 1½ ounces of natural cheese • 2 ounces of process cheese
Meats	• 2 to 3 ounces of cooked lean meat, poultry, or fish • ½ cup of cooked dry beans • 1 egg • 2 tablespoons of peanut butter

Source: U.S. Department of Agriculture, *The Food Guide Pyramid* (Home and Garden Bulletin No. 252), Washington, D.C.: USDA, 1992.

Animal foods, such as meats and milk, are good sources of complete protein. A complete protein contains all of the *essential amino acids* our bodies need. Amino acids are the building blocks of proteins, and essential amino acids are the ones that we must obtain from our diets because our bodies cannot manufacture them. Proteins are found in plants as well. Legumes are a particularly good source of plant protein. Legumes are beans and peas such as kidney beans, lentils, soybeans, garbanzo beans (chick-peas), and black-eyed peas. Grains, such as corn and wheat, are also good sources of plant protein. Different types of plants have different amino acids. Thus vegetarians can get enough of the essential amino acids if they eat the appropriate variety of plant proteins.

Carbohydrates

Carbohydrates come in two kinds: simple and complex. Simple carbohydrates, or sugars, are easily digested by the body and provide a source of quick energy. Complex carbohydrates, or starches, are made up of long chains of molecules, and provide a long-lasting energy and dietary fiber. Breads, pasta, grains, cereals, and some vegetables are complex carbohydrates. Carbohydrates should make up at least 55 percent of the calories in the average woman's diet.

Fats

Fats are the four-letter words of the nutrition world, but they do serve a purpose—in small quantities. A certain amount of fat is vital to maintaining good health, and fats are packed with energy (and calories). While proteins and carbohydrates contain 4 calories per gram (31 grams equal 1 ounce), fats have more than twice as many calories per gram—9 in all. Fats help the body absorb the so-called fat-soluble vitamins. Because of their tendency to raise blood cholesterol levels, fats should make up no more than 30 percent of the calories in the average woman's diet, and saturated fats—those that solidify at room temperature—should make up no more than 10 percent. Saturated fats include butter, hard cheese, the fats from beef and other meats and the vegetable fats of coconut, palm kernel, and palm oils.

Vitamins and Minerals

Vitamins are organic substances that are essential to a wide variety of body functions, including the biochemical conversion of protein, carbohydryates, and fats into energy. Minerals are inorganic substances that help control many metabolic processes. The body needs both vitamins and minerals to realize its full po-

READING LABELS

Recent federal regulations require that all labels on packaged foods provide information on the number of calories and amount of fat, saturated fat, cholesterol, sodium, carbohydrates, dietary fiber, sugar, and protein that food contains. The information is related to a normal daily diet that contains 2,000 calories, 65 grams of fat (30 percent of calories), 20 grams of saturated fat, 300 milligrams of cholesterol, 2,400 milligrams of sodium, 300 grams of total carbohydrates, and 25 grams of fiber. The percentage of the daily values that one serving of the food provides is given, along with a percentage of the daily value for vitamin A, vitamin C, calcium, and iron.

Use the information on food labels to limit the amount of your fat consumption. Here's how to find the percentage of calories from fat in one serving of a food:

1. Multiply the number of grams of fat in a serving, as shown on the label, by 9 (there are 9 calories in each gram of fat) to find the number of calories from fat.
2. Divide the number of calories from fat by the total number of calories, on the label, shown for one serving.
3. Multiply this amount by 100 to get the percentage of calories from fat.

If you look at any package label, you will see that one serving of pretzels has 1.5 grams of total fat and 180 calories. (1) The total number of calories from fat is 1.5 × 9, or about 14 calories from fat. (Total calories from fat is often shown on food labels.) (2) Divide 14 by 180 (the number of calories in one serving), which comes to 0.077. (3) Finally, multiply by 100. About 8 percent of the calories in these pretzels come from fat.

Be alert to serving sizes, which are also listed on the label. If the label specifies two cookies as one serving, and you eat four cookies, you'll need to multiply all of the nutritional information by two to get the nutrient content of the food you consumed.

Fresh meat, fish, poultry, and produce are not required to carry labels with this information. Sometimes this information is available at the produce or meat counter of grocery stores.

tential. The Recommended Dietary Allowances (RDAs) issued by the U.S. government show how much of each nutrient the average healthy woman needs (Table 3.3). Women who are pregnant or breast-feeding have special needs and require more of some nutrients in their diet.

Different foods contain different amounts of vitamins and minerals, so consuming a variety of foods is the best way to get all these nutrients (Table 3.4). Some commercial foods are enriched to provide more nutrients, including white flour, cereals, and pasta. Fruit juices may have added calcium, and vitamin D is usually added to milk. To preserve vitamin value, do not overcook foods, especially vegetables.

Vitamin and mineral supplements may benefit some women. If you are pregnant or breast-feeding or if you are a vegetarian, you may have special needs or dietary inadequacies that can only be met by supplements. Note that consuming large amounts of some vitamins and minerals may be dangerous, however; and there are few proven health benefits to "megadosing." Therefore, do not take much more than is suggested by the RDAs. This is especially true of vitamins A and D, which are fat soluble and stored in the body. Consuming too much of vitamins A and D can poison the body. Therapeutic or high-potency vitamins may have two to three times the RDAs for the B vitamins and vitamin C. They may be helpful if you have had recent illness, weight loss, or surgery. However, in most cases, you should get the bulk of your vitamins and minerals from the food you eat.

Guideline 2: Maintain a Healthy Weight

Today women are bombarded by advertisements and the media to cultivate a slim waist, slender legs, and shapely breasts. The attainment of this "ideal" figure is generally unrealistic, and often downright unhealthy. But it is important that you maintain a healthy weight—one that is right for your age, size, and body structure. Not only will you look and feel better but you will reduce your risk of disease, particularly diabetes, heart disease, and hypertension.

Remember, being a few pounds overweight is not the same thing as being obese. Obesity means being more than 20 percent over your optimum weight. Where you carry the weight matters, too. Muscles weigh more than fat. If you are large and muscular, you may not have much body fat and may weigh more than recommended for your height and age, but this is not unhealthy. If you do have excess fat, note where it is stored in your body. Fat carried around the hips and thighs—the so-called pear shape—is considered to be

TABLE 3.3   RECOMMENDED DIETARY ALLOWANCES FOR WOMEN

Nutrient	Nonpregnant (years old)				Pregnant	Breast-Feeding
	15 to 18	19 to 24	25 to 50	51+		
Protein (grams)	44	46	50	50	60	65
Vitamins						
Vitamin A (micrograms)	800	800	800	800	800	1,300
Vitamin B$_1$* (milligrams)	1.1	1.1	1.1	1.0	1.5	1.6
Vitamin B$_2$† (milligrams)	1.3	1.3	1.3	1.2	1.6	1.8
Vitamin B$_3$‡ (milligrams)	15	15	15	13	17	20
Vitamin B$_6$§ (milligrams)	1.5	1.6	1.6	1.6	2.2	2.1
Vitamin B$_{12}$‖ (micrograms)	2	2	2	2	2.2	2.6
Vitamin C (milligrams)	60	60	60	60	70	95
Vitamin D (micrograms)	10	10	5	5	10	10
Vitamin E (milligrams)	8	8	8	8	10	12
Vitamin K (micrograms)	55	60	65	65	65	65
Folic acid (micrograms)	180	180	180	180	400	280
Minerals						
Calcium (milligrams)	1,200	1,200	800	800#	1,200	1,200
Iodine (micrograms)	150	150	150	150	175	200
Iron (milligrams)	15	15	15	10	30	15
Magnesium (milligrams)	300	280	280	280	320	355
Phosphorus (milligrams)	1,200	1,200	800	800	1,200	1,200
Selenium (micrograms)	50	55	55	55	65	75
Zinc (milligrams)	12	12	12	12	15	19

Source: Adapted from National Academy of Sciences, *Recommended Dietary Allowances,* Washington, D.C.: National Academy Press, 1989.

* Thiamin.
† Riboflavin.
‡ Niacin.
§ Pyridoxine.
‖ Cobalamin.
Some medical authorities recommend 1,500 milligrams.

less of a health risk than the apple shape—the big belly look seen in men and some women. The apple shape has been linked to heart disease, high blood pressure, and diabetes.

How Obesity Affects the Body

Too much poundage increases your risk of heart disease and hypertension. In fact, heart disease occurs two to three times more often in obese women than in women of normal weight. One reason for this is that many obese women have high levels of cholesterol in their blood. Cholesterol, a fatty substance, clogs the blood vessels, eventually causing a heart attack. Strokes are also more likely to occur if you have high cholesterol levels. Women who are obese are more likely to have a sedentary lifestyle and high blood presssure, both of which raise the risk for cardiovascular disease.

The obese are more likely to have the most common type of diabetes, which is the inability of the body to metabolize sugar properly. Other risks of obesity include varicose veins; bloodclots in the legs; arthritis in the knees; gallbladder disease; hernias; breathing problems; and cancers of the uterus, breast, colon, and rectum.

What Is a Healthy Weight?

A healthy weight depends on several factors: your height, your body frame size, and your age. Taller women, women with larger bone structures, and older

TABLE 3.4   SOME VITAMINS AND MINERALS

Nutrient	Function in Body	Diet Source
Vitamins		
Vitamin A	Needed for normal vision in dim light; prevents eye diseases; needed for growth of bones and teeth	Liver, fish liver oils, butter, carrots, spinach, cantaloupe, sweet potatoes
Vitamin B_1 (thiamin)	Helps body digest carbohydrates; needed for normal functioning of nervous system	Enriched or whole-grain cereals, pastas, peas, nuts, beans, meats
Vitamin B_2 (riboflavin)	Helps body release energy to cells; promotes healthy skin and eyes	Liver, milk, yogurt, cottage cheese, eggs, leafy vegetables
Vitamin B_3 (niacin)	Promotes healthy skin, nerves, and digestion; helps the body use carbohydrates	Liver, peanuts, chicken, salmon, tuna
Vitamin B_6 (pyridoxine)	Helps form red blood cells; helps body use protein, fat, and carbohydrate	Liver, meat, fish, poultry, peanuts
Vitamin B_{12} (cobalamin)	Maintains nervous system; needed to form red blood cells	Liver, meat, eggs, shellfish
Vitamin C	Speeds healing of wounds and bones; increases resistance to infection; needed to form collagen	Citrus fruits, melons, strawberries, green pepper, broccoli, brussels sprouts, turnip greens
Vitamin D*	Helps body use calcium and phosphorus; needed for strong bones and teeth	Fortified milk, fish liver oils, fish, egg yolks
Vitamin E	Needed for use of vitamin A; helps body form and use red blood cells and muscles	Vegetable oils, margarine, meat, peas, nuts
Vitamin K	Aids in making blood-clotting factors	Green tea, turnip greens, broccoli, leafy vegetables
Folic acid	Needed to produce blood cells and protein; helps some enzymes function	Liver, leafy vegetables, oranges, peanuts
Minerals		
Calcium	Needed for strong bones and teeth; helps in blood clotting; needed for normal muscle and nerve function	Milk, cheese, sardines (with bones), tortillas, almonds, broccoli and other green vegetables
Iodine	Needed to produce thyroid hormones that regulate body's energy use	Seafood (haddock, cod, lobster), iodized salt, dairy products, bread
Iron	Needed to make hemoglobin; prevents anemia; increases resistance to infection	Meat, calves' liver, poultry, fish, beans, raisins
Magnesium	Needed for nerve and muscle function; helps body use carbohydrates	Milk, meats, seafood, cereal, peanuts, bananas, dark green leafy vegetables
Phosphorus	Needed for strong bones and teeth	Milk, bologna, liver, hamburger, cheese
Selenium	Prevents breakdown of body chemicals	Seafood, organ meats, muscle meats, whole grains
Zinc	Needed to produce some enzymes and insulin	Red meat, shellfish (oysters), eggs

Source: Data in columns 1 and 3 from E. B. Feldman, *Essentials of Clinical Nutrition,* Philadelphia: F. A. Davis, 1988. Data in column 2 from American College of Obstetricians and Gynecologists, *Planning for Pregnancy, Birth, and Beyond,* Washington, D.C.: ACOG, 1990.

* Also manufactured in the body when the skin is exposed to ultraviolet radiation (sunlight).

CHOOSING AND PREPARING FOODS SAFELY

Natural foods and organic foods generally do not have special nutritional value. They also are more expensive than foods grown by commercial methods. Fertilizers used on commercially grown foods contain chemicals similar to those that appear in manure (used in organic farming) and the soil and plants themselves.

Pesticides are found on many foods, but the amounts present are usually very small. The U.S. government sets allowable limits for pesticide residues in food, and in 1987, only 1 percent of the food products sampled had residues higher than the limits. To limit your exposure to pesticides, make sure you wash vegetables and fruits thoroughly before eating them.

To prevent foodborne infections, handle certain foods and kitchen tools with care. Store raw meat, poultry, and fish separately from cooked foods or foods that will be eaten raw. Wash your hands well after handling raw meats, poultry, and fish and before working with other foods. Thoroughly wash cutting boards and surfaces used to prepare raw meats. For added protection, wipe cutting boards and countertops with a watered-down bleach.

Cook meats thoroughly, especially ground meat. Cook poultry until the juices run clear. Fish should be cooked until it is translucent; overcooking will cause a loss of flavor. It is not recommended that you eat raw fish, because it may harbor parasites. Use products by their expiration date or freeze them for later use.

The proper storage of food is also important. Do not leave cooked foods at room temperature for long periods of time. Bacteria can multiply and toxins can form that will be present in the food, even if reheated. Refrigerate leftovers promptly.

women have higher weight allowances. Table 3.5 lists recommended body weights based on height and age. Another way to calculate the suggested weight for a given height is the body mass index (BMI) (see "Calculating Your BMI").

Controlling Your Weight

The United States is fortunate in that it has an abundance of available food and its population is one of the best fed in the world. Malnutrition certainly exists in

HEALTH RISKS OF OBESITY

If you are 20 percent or more over the recommended weight for your age, height, and body frame, you run the risk of developing

High blood pressure
Cardiovascular disease
Stroke
Diabetes
Arthritis (hips, knees, and ankles)
Gallstones
Cancer (uterine, breast, colon, and ovarian)

TABLE 3.5	USDA SUGGESTED WEIGHTS FOR WOMEN*	
	Age	
Height	**19 to 34 years**	**> 35 years**
60"	97–128	108–138
61"	101–132	111–143
62"	104–137	115–148
63"	107–141	119–152
64"	111–146	122–157
65"	114–150	126–162
66"	118–155	130–167
67"	121–160	134–172
68"	125–164	138–178
69"	129–169	142–183
70"	132–174	146–188
71"	136–179	151–194
72"	140–184	155–199

Source: American College of Obstetricians and Gynecologists, *Weight Control: Eating Right and Keeping Fit* (ACOG Patient Education Pamphlet AP064), Washington, D.C.: ACOG, 1993.

* Height, in inches, is without shoes. Weight, in pounds, is without clothes. The lower weights more often apply to women, who have less muscle and bone.

our society, but the greater problem is obesity. Unfortunately, there is much confusion in the public perception of body image—women who are only minimally overweight struggle to lose weight, while many obese women, tired of dieting, give up and decide to live with their problem, however severe.

Women who are greatly overweight or obese can improve their health and lower their risk of disease by rejecting calorie-counting diets and by sticking to a sensible plan of weight control. Weight control means not only losing pounds but keeping the pounds off. Permanent weight loss, then, requires a change in life-

CALCULATING YOUR BMI

You can calculate your body mass index (BMI) by using the following formula:

$$\frac{\text{Weight (in kilograms)}}{\text{Height (in meters) squared}}$$

To convert your weight and height to metrics, note that 1 pound is equal to 0.45 kilogram and 1 inch is equal to 0.0254 meter. For example, a woman who weighs 120 pounds and is 64 inches tall also weighs 54 kilograms (120×0.45) and is 1.63 meters tall (64×0.0254). Her BMI would be $54 \div (1.63 \times 1.63)$, or about 20.3, which puts her in the normal range. Normal, overweight, and obese ranges for BMIs vary, but in general, a BMI of 20 to 25 is considered normal, 25 to 30 is considered overweight, and over 30 is considered obese. Using these ranges, up to 33 percent of the U.S. population should be considered obese. Obesity is more common in women than in men.

---

style and a new attitude toward food and eating. It means not thinking in terms of "dieting" at all. Dieting is merely a temporary restriction of all your favorite foods, which comes to an end as soon as a particular weight goal is met. Making permanent changes certainly is more difficult, but the benefits pay off for a lifetime. These changes include focusing on the right foods, engaging in regular exercise, and perhaps finding the right support system.

Dietary Changes

A sensible plan for weight loss means losing about 0.5 to 1 pound a week. More rapid weight loss may be achieved by starvation-type diets, but these regimens don't work in the long run. Furthermore, there are physiological reasons for the failure of most of these kinds of diets. When the body suddenly stops taking in the accustomed amount of calories, it acts as though it were starving. The rate of metabolism, or how fast your body burns the calories needed to maintain daily functions, slows down. If the diet is still restricted, weight loss occurs slowly if at all (the so-called plateau of dieting). The dieter becomes discouraged and may begin to sneak in some extra calories. After the weight is gained back, she begins dieting again. This on-again, off-again *yo-yo* dieting is counterproductive—the weight is gained back rapidly, and each time a new diet starts, the body's metabolism slows down still more. The pounds are harder to lose each time you try.

Generally, reputable plans for weight loss do not restrict calories to less than 1,200 a day. On a sensible lifetime plan, foods can be chosen from all the food groups. There is even room for most of your favorite snacks—including chocolate—if portions are kept small and the fat content is minimal (Table 3.6). The best plans emphasize a gradual weight loss that, ideally, is combined with a real desire to make changes that will eventually become part and parcel of a new, healthier lifestyle.

Exercise

Regular exercise not only burns fat but also helps raise the body's metabolic rate, and it increases the size and tone of the muscles. In addition, regular exercise increases your overall fitness and improves your sense of well-being and self-esteem.

Because regular exercise is so essential, it is important to choose a workout that you enjoy and will pursue often. Choose some activity that is convenient and readily accessible. Although downhill skiing can be fun and is great for burning calories, it's difficult for most women to build a regular exercise program around skiing. Instead, choose jogging, brisk walking, swimming, biking, or aerobic dancing as the core of your exercise program, with other sports added for fun.

Aerobic exercise works the heart and lungs, and it is the best exercise for weight control and overall fitness. Your workout should up your heart rate into your target heart rate zone (Table 3.7). The target heart rate is 60 to 80 percent of your maximum heart rate. (You can determine your maximum heart rate by subtracting your age from 220.) After checking with your doctor, start slowly, aiming for the low end of your target heart rate zone. Exercise three times a week for 20 to 30 minutes at a time. As you become more fit, you can work out every day for 45 to 60 minutes at a time.

Weight Loss Support

Although most women who lose weight successfully do so on their own, some of us need guidance and support. There are many professionals and organizations who can help you in your weight loss venture. Doctors and nutritionists can plan a weight loss program or refer you to a reputable organization. Many commercial weight loss programs may be a good source of education and support. Weight Watchers and Overeaters Anonymous are two well-known programs. University-based health or wellness programs also exist. If you are interested in joining a weight loss program, do some reseach. Find out how each program

TABLE 3.6   EATING SENSIBLY

Food Group	Choose More Often	Choose Less Often
Breads	Whole-grain breads; whole-grain and bran cereals; rice; pasta	Refined-flour breads and cakes; biscuits; croissants; crackers; chips; cookies; pastries; granola
Vegetables	Dark green, leafy vegetables (spinach, collard, endive); yellow-orange vegetables (carrots, sweet potatoes, squash); cabbage; broccoli; cauliflower; brussels spourts	Avocados; vegetables prepared in butter, oil, and cream sauces
Fruits	Citrus fruits (oranges, grapefruit); apples; berries; pears	Coconut; fruit pies; pastries
Dairy products	Low-fat or skim milk; low-fat or nonfat yogurt and cheeses (ricotta, farmer, cottage, mozzarella); sherbet; frozen low-fat yogurt; ice milk	Whole milk; butter; yogurt made from whole milk; sweet cream, sour cream, whipped cream, and other creamy toppings (including imitation); ice cream; coffee creamers (including nondairy); cream cheese; cheese spreads; Brie; Camembert; hard cheeses (Swiss, Cheddar)
Meats	Low-fat chicken or turkey (white meat without skin); fresh or frozen fish; water-packed canned tuna; lean meat trimmed of all fat; cooked dry beans and peas; egg whites and egg substitutes	Beef, veal, lamb, and pork cuts with marbling, untrimmed of fat; duck; goose; organ meats; luncheon meats; sausage; hot dogs; peanut butter; nuts; seeds; trail mix; tuna packed in oil; egg yolks; whole eggs

Source: Adapted from American College of Obstetricians and Gynecologists, *Cholesterol and Your Health* (ACOG Patient Education Pamphlet 101), Washington, D.C.: ACOG, 1993.

operates, what type of weight loss it recommends, and how much it costs. Some programs require that participants purchase some or all of their food from the program. This may seem convenient, but these foods are usually more expensive than similar foods purchased in the grocery store or cooked at home. Relying on a preplanned diet of special foods can also make it difficult for you to maintain your weight loss after you reach your ideal weight. Learning to choose foods wisely is a vital part of remaking one's lifstyle, and this important skill may not be learned as readily in programs that rely on special foods.

Women who are severely obese need more than supportive programs to lose weight. They need medical help. Weight loss programs for severely obese women should be developed and monitored by a doctor or nurse.

Eating Disorders

It's dangerous to be overweight, but it's also risky to eat and weigh too little. Some women, especially teenage girls, have a distorted image of their bodies. Even if their weight is normal, they may see themselves as grossly overweight and may embark on strict diets and rigorous exercise programs. These women may be suffering from

an eating disorder that can have grave effects on their health, both physically and psychologically.

Particularly devastating is *anorexia nervosa,* a chronic eating disorder. Women with anorexia, no matter what their weight, believe they are overweight and severely cut down on the amount of food they eat. Sometimes these women starve themselves to the point of emaciation. They also may exercise to extremes, led on by their pathological fear of gaining weight. Teenagers as well as models, gymnasts, dancers, and long-distance runners are at risk for this serious condition, which can lead to severe malnutrition, even death.

Binge eating, or *bulimia,* is closely associated with anorexia. Women with bulimia eat huge amounts of high-calorie foods—usually sweets—at one sitting, and then undergo self-induced vomiting so they won't gain weight. Many of these women use laxatives or diuretics to force fluids quickly out of their systems. This overuse of medications can seriously disrupt the body's chemical balance and increase the chances of heart problems, including fatal arrythmias. Like anorexia, bulimia can lead to death. Unlike women with anorexia, however, women suffering from bulimia recognize that their eating habits are abnormal. They often become severely depressed after a bulimic episode and may seek help more quickly than do women with anorexia.

DIETARY MYTHS

The most common dietary myths relate to food and its effects. Books, magazines, and TV talk shows are prime sources of the latest food fads, usually for losing weight. Some fad diets promise quick results, which don't last. Other fad diets are so unbalanced that they could actually harm your health if prolonged. The cruelest food hoaxes are those aimed at persons who have cancer or other serious diseases. Women who believe that concoctions of peach pits can cure their cancer will *not* benefit from such treatment, and they may delay seeking medical care early, when their conditions are most treatable.

Remember, if something sounds too good to be true, it probably is. Watch out for these dietary myths:

- Starchy foods are especially fattening.
- Cottage cheese and grapefruit are slimming.
- Special wraps, lotions, and pills can promote weight loss.
- Some diets, like the extremes of the Zen macrobiotic diet, carry no serious health risks.
- Tests for nutritional status based on hair analysis (or other unorthodox strategies) are sound and accurate.
- Taking tryptophan is a safe way to relieve insomnia.
- Vitamin C prevents colds.
- Special foods promote sexuality or act as a "fountain of youth."
- Some special foods or vitamins can cure cancer or mental illness.

There is a strong psychological compulsion connected with these illnesses, and both medical and psychological help is necessary to treat them successfully (see Chapter 8). Treatment may be long term, as it can take some time to relearn healthy patterns of eating.

Guideline 3: Choose a Diet Low in Fat, Saturated Fat, and Cholesterol

A healthy diet includes reducing your fat intake to 30 percent or less of your total daily calories. Keep in mind that saturated fat—the kind of fat that is solid at

TABLE 3.7   TARGET HEART RATE

Age (years)	Beats per Minute
20	120–160
25	117–156
30	114–152
35	111–148
40	108–144
45	105–140
50	102–136
55	99–132
60	96–128
65	93–124
70	90–120

Source: Adapted from National Heart, Lung, and Blood Institute, *Exercise and Your Heart* (NIH Publication No. 81-1677), Washington, D.C.: U.S. Government Printing Office, 1981.

room temperature—has the worst effect on the blood cholesterol. However, it is important to note that cholesterol levels in the blood are not 100 percent diet related: There is also a genetic component at work. Some women have low cholesterol no matter what they eat, while others have high levels of cholesterol despite a low-fat diet.

The Health Risks of a High Fat Diet

There is a strong association between diet and the development of heart disease and cancer. The consumption of too much fat may increase the risk of developing these diseases, but other foods may actually reduce your risk.

Heart Disease

Cardiac problems are the leading causes of death for American women. Heart disease tends to occur later in women than it does in men, presumably because premenopausal women produce estrogen, a hormone that seems to provide some protection against heart disease. The level of estrogen, however, drops drastically at menopause, when menstrual periods stop. Without the protection of estrogen, a woman's risk of heart disease begins to climb.

If you consume high levels of saturated fat and cholesterol, sticky lumps may build up in your arteries, leading to a condition called *atherosclerosis*. Eventually, the arteries may clot off or become completely blocked, causing a stroke or heart attack.

Not all blood cholesterol is bad, however. When you consume fat, it is digested and bound into fatty packages called lipoproteins. Lipoproteins carry the fat through the blood vessels for use or storage in other parts of the body. There are three main types of lipoproteins:

- Very low-density lipoproteins (VLDLs)
- Low-density lipoproteins (LDLs)
- High-density lipoproteins (HDLs)

The VLDLs carry fat and cholesterol through the bloodstream to fat tissue. After they drop off some of the fat, they become LDLs. LDLs are sometimes called carriers of "bad cholesterol" because this type of cholesterol builds up in the blood vessels. HDLs are called "good cholesterol" particles because they pick up the cholesterol that has been deposited in the blood vessels and carry it back to the liver where the body can get rid of the cholesterol. Trouble arises when there is not enough good HDL to carry the LDL cholesterol deposits away. To keep down the level of your LDLs, choose a low-fat low-cholesterol diet. Exercise increases the amount of HDLs in your body, another reason why it's important to exercise regularly.

Cancer

A diet high in fats seems to increase the risk of some cancers, although the exact reasons for this are unknown. In particular, a high-fat, high-calorie diet is believed to increase the risk of cancer of the breast, uterus, colon, and ovaries. One theory postulates that fats may increase a woman's production of some estrogen products that promote cancer. While estrogen does help prevent heart disease, too much estrogen is believed to be a prime cause of reproductive cancer in older women. Some authorities recommend a diet of less than 20 percent of calories from fat to reduce the risk of breast cancer.

Finding and Preparing the Right Foods

Today, it is easier than ever to make low-fat foods part of a delicious, healthy diet. From nonfat ice cream to crackers and cookies, low-fat foods are a major growth industry in this country. Restaurants, too, have gotten on the low-fat bandwagon (see "Eating Out").

When shopping, read food labels carefully, especially noting when a product is called "low-fat" or "90 percent fat-free." These claims may not reflect the true calories from fat in the food. The problem with figuring the percentage of fat in a product is that the percentage is based on weight, including water. For example, ground meat is about 70 percent water. So, even if the meat is labeled "10 percent fat by weight," it still derives over 50 percent of its calories from fat.

As with other types of dietary changes, the key word in reducing fat intake is *moderation*. Drastic changes in the diet are much more difficult to accept and maintain. Instead, adopt the concept of choosing low-fat foods more often and high-fat foods less often. Limit the use of saturated fats in general, and use vegetable oils such as olive and canola oils. Watch the portion size of protein-rich foods. You only need about 6 ounces for the entire day. Vegetables and grains (starches) are filling and low in fat, so make them the center of a meal, and use protein-rich foods for accent.

EATING OUT

When newspaper articles report on the high amount of fat in Chinese, Italian, and Mexican foods, you may think it's impossible to find a low-fat restaurant meal. Just as at home, though, healthy meals can be had by selecting low-fat options and avoiding the high-fat items.

- At Chinese restaurants, eat more rice and vegetables and less meat and sauce. Skip the fried appetizers and choose steamed dumplings or soup instead.

- At Italian restaurants, select pastas with tomato-based sauces instead of pastas topped with heavy cream and cheese sauces. Pick a salad (with dressing on the side) instead of garlic bread.

- At Mexican restaurants, rice and beans, if not refried in fat, are a healthy part of your meal. Chicken soft tacos and fajitas are acceptable too. Skip the fried taco shells and taco salads, and limit your intake of sour cream, cheese, and guacamole.

- At fast-food restaurants, choose a plain burger over one with the works, and hold the cheese. Grilled chicken sandwiches are a good choice if not breaded. Try a salad bar instead of fries, but keep the portion reasonable and choose raw vegetables instead of prepared pasta or bean salads.

Instead of red meat, choose chicken (without skin), fish (fish oil may help protect against heart disease), and plant proteins (such as peas and beans).

Many of your favorite foods can be easily adapted to provide the same flavors with lower calories. Try making salad dressings with a tomato or yogurt base instead of oil or mayonnaise. Nonfat yogurt can substitute for high-fat sour cream. Milk shakes can be made with fruit and nonfat frozen yogurt or ice milk. Try an angel food cake instead of a layer cake.

Be alert to methods of food preparation, too. Avoid frying, or pan fry in a skillet sprayed with a nonstick vegetable oil. Grilling, broiling, and microwaving are good low-fat methods for cooking meats, poultry, and fish.

Guideline 4: Choose a Diet with Plenty of Vegetables, Fruits, and Grains

As shown in the Food Guide Pyramid (see Fig. 3.1), vegetables, fruits, and grains are the foundation of a healthy diet. Fortunately, these foods are inexpensive and an excellent source of vitamins, minerals, and fiber. Fiber helps the body feel full, improves bowel function, and also seems to protect against cancers of the colon and rectum. Vegetables, fruits, and grains are naturally low in fat and sodium and contain no cholesterol.

Try to build meals around these healthy foods and go easier on dairy and meat products. Vegetable soup, whole-grain bread, and a salad for instance, make a great low-fat meal that is loaded with fiber, vitamins, and minerals.

Guideline 5: Use Sugar Only in Moderation

Foods high in sugar tend to have *empty calories*—calories without other nutrients. Besides adding calories, sugar may also take the place of healthy foods in the diet and prevent you from getting all the nutrients you need. Digested rapidly by the body, sugar provides a quick energy source that may be used up just as quickly. Consuming complex starches instead provides a more even,

longer-lasting energy source. Finally, foods high in sugar, especially sticky sweets, promote tooth decay.

Try making healthy substitutions when the sweet tooth strikes. Fruit or fruit juice is a healthy option, for example. If you do indulge in an occasional dessert, keep the portion small. Cereals, processed foods, and baked goods are often high in hidden sugars, so check the label before buying. Another tip: Put fruit on your breakfast cereal instead of sugar.

Guideline 6: Use Salt Only in Moderation

The average American diet is too high in salt—over 9 grams a day. Your daily salt intake should be no more than 6 grams (1½ teaspoons). Sodium can increase blood pressure in susceptible people. A few studies have indicated that sensitivity to salt increases with age, so get in the habit now of moderating your salt intake. Try to avoid using salt when cooking or at the table. Instead, use herbs and other spices to perk up a dish. Many processed foods are high in sodium, so check labels before buying. Some manufacturers now offer products containing low or no sodium.

Guideline 7: If You Drink Alcoholic Beverages, Do So in Moderation

Women who use alcohol should limit their daily intake to no more than 2 drinks and to no more than 10 drinks spaced throughout a week. Pregnant women should not drink at all, because of possible damage to the fetus.

The evidence linking alcohol use with disease is strong. Excess alcohol increases the risk of liver damage, high blood pressure, and some forms of cancer. Like sugar, alcohol contains empty calories. Alcohol can kill the appetite for healthy food and affect how the body absorbs and uses nutrients in foods. Malnutrition is common in alcoholics. Protein and vitamin deficiencies can occur, resulting in anemia, neurological damage, and skin problems.

Even in moderate quantities, alcohol can affect balance, coordination, and judgment. Never drink before driving or operating machinery.

SPECIAL NUTRITIONAL ISSUES FOR WOMEN

Women have different nutritional needs at different ages and stages of their lives. Younger women need to replace iron loss from menstruation, while menopausal women must increase their calcium intake to compensate for the loss of the mineral that occurs during and after menopause. Pregnant and breastfeeding women need increased nutrients to nourish a growing baby. Understanding your nutritional needs allows you to avoid disease and be at your best throughout your life.

Menstruation

Women who are having monthly menstrual periods may need more iron in their diet, because they lose iron with the blood they shed each month. After women go through menopause, their RDAs for iron are the same as those for men. Meat, eggs, vegetables, and fortified cereals are good sources of iron. Some women may benefit from taking a daily multivitamin supplement that contains iron.

Before, During, and After Pregnancy

Pregnant women need to make certain changes in their diet to support both their own nutritional needs and that of the growing fetus. Making the correct nutritional changes before as well as after pregnancy can improve the health of mother and baby.

The Prepregnant Diet

A healthy diet in the period before conception is important. Carefully planned pregnancies allow women to make any necessary modifications to their diets before they become pregnant, ensuring that their babies will get the best possible start in life.

Many times a woman is pregnant for several weeks before she even suspects it. The first few weeks of fetal growth and development are critical; during this time, all the major organ systems are forming. Evidence is growing that birth defects affecting the spine and brain (neural tube defects) may be caused by a lack of folic acid in the earliest weeks of pregnancy. Some doctors recommend that women planning a pregnancy be sure to get enough folic acid from foods in their diet, or take a daily supplement of 0.4 milligrams. Folic acid is found in liver, leafy vegetables, oranges, peanuts, peas, beans, and lentils.

Pregnancy can strain your body's reserves of nutrients, especially iron and calcium. Build them up before pregnancy, if possible.

The Pregnancy Diet

Women who eat a well-balanced, healthy diet need to make only a few changes in their food intake during pregnancy. In particular, a moderate increase is needed in the number of calories and amount of iron, protein, folic acid, calcium, and phosphorus consumed.

It's not necessary to "eat for two," as the old adage says. Most pregnant women need about 300 calories per day extra to meet the needs of the growing baby. The exact amount depends on a recommended weight gain, which varies from woman to woman. If your weight was normal before you became pregnant, you should plan to gain 25 to 35 pounds. Underweight women can gain more—28 to 40 pounds—as can women carrying twins (35 to 45 pounds). Overweight women should gain less—about 15 to 25 pounds. Pregnancy is not the time to try to lose weight, either. Most of the extra nutrients needed can come from your regular diet (see Tables 3.1 and 3.4 for sources of these nutrients). To get the extra calories and nutrients, choose a moderately high number of servings from each of the food groups in the Food Guide Pyramid (See Fig. 3.1):

- Breads: 9 servings
- Vegetables: 4 servings
- Fruits: 3 servings
- Dairy products: 3 servings
- Meats: 3 servings

You may find it more comfortable to eat several small meals or snacks rather than eating three large meals.

For some nutrients, especially iron, it may be difficult to get all the needed amount from the diet alone. Your doctor may prescribe multivitamin supplements with iron. If you are a vegetarian, work with your doctor to plan a beneficial diet. If you eat milk and eggs, you may still be able to provide for all the baby's needs.

Complete vegetarians, however, may need to take supplements.

Some women, especially African-Americans, have a condition called *lactose intolerance,* which means their bodies are unable to digest the sugar in milk products. Women who are lactose intolerant may need to limit their intake of dairy products to avoid possible gas and cramping. Instead, they should take a calcium supplement that provides about 1 gram of calcium per day.

In general, though, do not exceed the RDA for any nutrient, because some vitamins can be harmful if taken in excess. Too much vitamin A, for example, can cause birth defects.

As stated previously, avoid alcohol if you are pregnant. If you drink, you increase the risk that your child will be born with *fetal alcohol syndrome,* a condition that includes facial defects and varying degrees of mental retardation. The more you drink, the higher the risk. Because no one knows what constitutes a "safe" level of drinking during pregnancy, it's best not to drink alcohol at all.

Some women feel strong urges to eat nonfood items such as laundry starch or clay. This type of craving is called *pica.* If you experience this compulsion, discuss it with your doctor. Pica can be a sign of a nutritional deficiency, or it may cause deficiencies.

The Postpregnancy Diet

Once the baby is born, many women wonder how soon they can drop to their prepregnancy weight. Although women lose about 18 to 20 pounds within 10 days after birth, many women do end up weighing more than they did before. Weight gain is not absolute, however, if you begin a sensible weight loss plan right after birth. If you are not breast-feeding, choose low-fat options and keep to the low end of the recommended number of servings indicated by the Food Guide Pyramid. Include regular exercise in your fitness program.

If you are breast-feeding, you may need the same or even more nutrients than you did during pregnancy. Do not plan to lose much weight while you are breast-feeding. You can, however, lose a little weight slowly, perhaps 2 pounds a month, and still produce enough milk for your infant. (A nursing mother needs 500 to 600 more calories per day than she needed before she became pregnant.) Additional amounts of some nutrients are needed for breast-feeding (see Table 3.3), but these can usually be obtained from a well-balanced diet. Women who are lactose intolerant, vegetarians, or who cannot get the vitamins they need from their diet may need supplementation.

Generally, whatever you eat and drink is passed into your breast milk. Nutrients in the milk provide for the baby's growth and development. Harmful substances can end up in the milk as well, however. Alcohol can affect the baby if you have three or more drinks per day. Too much caffeine may also be harmful to your child. If you consume more than three cups of coffee (or the equivalent) per day, your breast-fed baby may be irritable and have trouble sleeping. Just about any medications you take can be found in your breast milk, too. If you are taking medication, check with your doctor before you begin breast-feeding your baby.

Menopause

By the time a woman reaches her early 50s, her periods become erratic and gradually end. For women in the United States, the average age at the last menstrual period is about 51 years. Women who have had their ovaries removed by surgery go through an immediate menopause, called a surgical menopause.

After menopause, a woman no longer produces as much of the female hormone estrogen. Estrogen provides some protection against heart disease. Once estrogen production slows down, it is especially important to eat a diet low in fat, saturated fat and cholesterol.

The loss of estrogen also affects the bones. Around and after menopause, the rate of bone loss increases, and may cause a condition called *osteoporosis.* If too much calcium and protein are lost, bones can become spongy and brittle. Risk factors for osteoporosis include being thin and being white or Asian. Smoking and a sedentary lifestyle or excessive exercise also increase your risk for bone loss. Many doctors recommend that postmenopausal women get 1,500 milligrams of calcium each day. The main sources of calcium in the diet are dairy products, but calcium is also found in green leafy vegetables, tofu (bean curd), and fish with bones. Women who are lactose intolerant or who are vegetarians may be able to get enough calcium from nondairy sources. For some, supplements are a good idea. Avoid eating too much protein, which can even be harmful because it causes the body to flush out needed calcium. Also minimize drinking carbonated soft drinks that are high in phosphorus (which flushes calcium from the system) and limit caffeine. You need enough vitamins to keep the minerals in the bones.

Exercise during the postmenopausal years is still vital. It helps burn fat and strengthens the heart. It also strengthens bones, which protects against osteoporosis, and strengthens muscles, which improves balance and prevents falls.

THE LATER YEARS

Women who are 65 years or older have special dietary needs of their own. For one, older women need fewer daily calories than younger women, because the body's metabolism tends to slow down as people age. Older women also tend to be less active than younger women. The foods that provide the calories needed to maintain a healthy weight may not be enough to provide enough nutrients, so a multivitamin supplement is a good idea.

Osteoporosis continues to be a major health risk for older women. Approximately 33 percent of women over age 65 will suffer a fracture of the spine, and by age 90, 33 percent of all women will have experienced a hip fracture. Older women should be sure to get enough calcium in their diets, keep up with moderate exercise, and be careful to avoid falls.

Although good nutrition is key for an older woman's health, changes in the body present special dietary challenges. The senses of taste and smell may decline so that foods seem less appetizing, for example. Different seasonings may need to be used, but it is a good idea to try herbs and spices rather than just adding more salt. If older women have lost some teeth or have poor-fitting dentures, they may find it difficult to eat. Careful attention should be paid to dental care and proper denture fit.

Loss of appetite may be a problem in the very elderly, causing malnutrition. In severe cases, food supplements or feeding through a tube may be necessary. Older women may not be outside enough to produce adequate amounts of vitamin D, so they may need supplements of this vitamin, too.

VEGETARIANS

Women may adopt a vegetarian diet for reasons of religion, moral beliefs, or health. Those who eat dairy products and eggs in addition to plant foods are called *lacto-ovo vegetarians.* Those who eat foods only of plant origin are called *vegans,* or *complete vegetarians.*

If you are a vegetarian, choose your foods carefully to be sure that you get all the essential amino acids (the protein building blocks that your body does not manufacture) from your diet. If you eat a variety of foods daily all the needed amino acids will likely be provided. For example, beans or peas can be combined with rice; grains plus legumes and nuts plus seeds are other good combinations. Because soy protein has the best amino acid makeup of the vegetable protein sources, use products made from soy, such as tofu.

Vegetarians should be especially alert to the presence of iron, calcium, and vitamin B_{12} in their diets. Beans, seeds, nuts, green leafy vegetables, dried fruits, and grains are good sources of iron, as are fortified cereals. Calcium can be found in green leafy vegetables and tofu in addition to dairy products. Because vitamin B_{12} is found naturally only in foods from animals, you may wish to eat more fortified breads and cereals or, better, take a daily supplement.

CHAPTER 4

Exercise and Physical Fitness

Janet Emily Freedman, M.D.

t's official: Regular exercise can help women live longer, healthier lives. In the fall of 1992, the American Heart Association formally designated inactivity as one of the top four risk factors for the development of heart attack and stroke—the nation's number-one killer of women every year. Along with high blood pressure, cigarette smoking, and high cholesterol, the lack of exercise is a contributing factor in cardiovascular disease.

Women and exercise did not always go together. Historically, women were not encouraged to go "all out" physically. Certainly it was viewed as unfeminine for women to actually sweat. Fortunately, we have come a long way in just about every sport and physical activity you can name.

Due in part to Title IX of the Educational Assistance Act (which requires all educational institutions receiving federal monies to offer equal opportunities to women and girls to train and compete in sports) more and more women have entered professional sports in the past few decades. In l970, two years before Title IX, no woman had ever finished in the New York City Marathon. In 1994, the top woman finisher ran the course in 2 hours, 27 minutes—just 16 minutes behind the male finisher. In recent Olympic games, American women have brought home more medals than their male colleagues.

Most women have neither the time, the training, nor the desire to compete in sports on the level of the highly trained "elite" athlete, but we can all enjoy the proven benefits of an exercise program.

WHAT EXERCISE CAN DO FOR YOU

The Health Connection

The news is easy medicine to swallow: Exercise prevents disease. By exercising regularly, you can significantly lower your risk of a myriad of diseases that are influenced by obesity and inactivity.

Exercise appears to help prevent cardiovascular disease, including heart attacks, stroke, and high blood pressure, by lowering low-density lipoproteins (the so-called "bad" cholesterol), increasing high-density lipoproteins (the "good" cholesterol), and lowering resting blood pressure and heart rate. There is some evidence that consistent exercise may be related to decreased rates of certain cancers, specifically breast and ovarian cancer, but strong scientific evidence is not yet available.

One of the most widespread diseases in the United States, diabetes mellitus, is also affected by physical inactivity. Recent studies show that regular exercise cuts in half the risk of developing adult-onset diabetes; burning just 500 extra calories a week decreases the risk of developing the disease by as much as 6 percent. (For more information about diabetes, see Chapter 30.)

The Emotional Connection

Exercise has been called nature's tranquilizer because it has been shown to break up stress patterns in the body. Exercise affects the brain and the emotions in many complex ways. Many exercisers report feeling good after a workout. This is due to the release during vigorous exercise of body chemicals called endorphins, which are known to dull pain and produce a mild euphoria.

Exercise and Weight Control

Exercise and weight control are often linked together, and it's easy to see why. Your body weight is the result of a complex interaction between the food you consume, your physical activity, and your body's metabolism. Exercise alone, or exercise in combination with a sensible diet, can help you lose weight and keep it off. Exercise can also help you maintain your ideal weight even as your metabolism slows down as you age. (After the age of 35, it takes fewer calories and more exercise to avoid putting on weight.) Women who are only 10 percent above their ideal weight may be able to achieve weight loss with exercise alone. Twenty minutes of vigorous exercise can burn up as much as 300 calories per session.

Exercise promotes weight loss in several ways.

- *Exercise increases your metabolic rate.* Between the ages of 20 and 50, about 70 percent of your body's energy expenditure is to main-

BENEFITS OF REGULAR EXERCISE

- promotes weight loss and decreased body fat
- decreases risk of cardiovascular disease
- lowers blood pressure
- decreases insulin use in diabetics
- prevents osteoporosis
- lowers serum cholesterol
- raises serum HDL
- slows aging of heart and lungs
- slows age-related muscle loss
- reduces back pain
- improves self-image

Possible Benefits of Exercise

- lowers rates of breast cancer
- lowers rates of ovarian cancer
- lessens labor pain
- lessens menstrual cramps/PMS
- strengthens immune system

tain the resting metabolic rate—the sum of all processes or chemical reactions in the body, such as digesting food and maintaining body temperature. Thirty percent is used for physical exertion. Exercise not only increases energy use for physical exertion, but also causes an increase in the resting metabolic rate, which may last as long as 48 hours after exercise. A regular exercise program burns calories, therefore, even on your "off" days.

In addition, the single biggest factor in producing a higher resting metabolic rate is the amount of your lean body, or muscle, tissue. Muscle tissue is highly active, even when at rest, eating up a great deal of energy to sustain itself. On average, it accounts for five times as

WHY DIETS DON'T WORK

Most weight-loss plans are poorly designed and don't result in permanent weight loss. In fact, diets based on limiting your caloric intake for a certain period of time—especially fad diets and crash diets—are doomed to failure. You may lose a few pounds by starving yourself, but as soon as you stop the dieting, your body will return to its previous weight. Even worse, repeated weight loss and weight gain from dieting—called the "yo-yo syndrome"—makes it harder to lose weight the next time around and may be dangerous to your general health.

The only recommended way to lose weight and to keep it off is to change your eating habits permanently (behavior modification) and increase your physical activity on a regular basis (exercise).

much of our total daily energy expenditure as fat. So the more total muscle you have, the higher your metabolism and the less fat you accumulate.

- *Exercise preserves muscle.* Dieting alone causes loss of body fat and muscle mass equally. Exercising *plus* eating a nutritious low-fat diet shifts the balance toward reducing fat and keeping muscle—the desired effect. This important shift occurs because active muscle tissue burns more fat for its energy needs and because the fibers are using the available food supply more efficiently.
- *Exercise may be an appetite suppressant.* Many women who exercise believe they eat less and feel less hungry. It has been suggested that if you exercise about two hours before a meal, you may actually eat less. It has not been proven that exercising actually diminishes your appetite—perhaps you eat less because you are "revved up" and feeling good. Research also suggests that mild exercise *after* meals may also help in controlling weight gain. A light exercise, such as walking, allows digestion to continue and can aid in the movement of food through the digestive tract.

TYPES OF EXERCISE

There are two basic types of exercise: aerobic and anaerobic.

Aerobic exercise improves cardiovascular health by forcing the body to deliver larger amounts of oxygen to working muscles. (The word *aerobic* is derived from a Greek word meaning "air.") With regular aerobic exercise, your heart increases its ability to pump blood and deliver oxygen to your body's tissues efficiently. In addition, your muscles will develop a greater capacity to use this oxygen and your heart will become stronger. It also allows your heart to rest longer between beats even when exercising.

Anaerobic exercise, or exercise "without air," strengthens individual muscles that draw on their own sources of energy and do not require the body to increase its supply of oxygen. Anaerobic exercise, which includes muscle conditioning or weight training, builds muscle mass while keeping the body strong and flexible.

Since a major health concern among women is the threat of osteoporosis (loss of bone mass), it is important to add another term to the physical fitness lexicon: *weight-bearing exercise.* These exercises provide the stress of muscles contracting or pulling on bones, in effect adding to the force of gravity. Exercises such as walking, running, aerobic dancing, and weight training all help to maintain or build bone mass.

THE EXERCISE PRESCRIPTION: TRAINING

The benefits of exercise come as the result of training, which means adapting the body to exercise over time. It is important to note that when it comes to exercise, men and women are not created equally. We must train longer and harder to achieve equal capacity for prolonged exercise.

Women should train to improve in several areas:

- *Strength.* Strength is the ability of a muscle to apply or resist a force. It determines how much weight a weightlifter can lift at any one time, or how steep a hill a bicyclist can pedal. Because women produce little of the male hormone testosterone, we have less strength than men with the same body weight. We also have a higher percentage of body fat, so we have proportionally less muscle. Our muscles do respond well to strength training, however, so strength training should be a part of your exercise program. You can develop strength and muscle tone by practicing repeated muscle contractions against resistance.

- *Endurance.* Endurance is the ability to repeat an activity over an extended period of time—to bike or run longer distances or lift a weight repeatedly. Surprisingly, women have a greater ability to train for endurance than do men. This phenomenon is not clearly understood, but many exercise experts believe that once all barriers to equality in training disappear, women will surpass men in some endurance activities.

- *Flexibility.* Flexibility is the ability of the muscles, tendons, and ligaments to move easily at the joints. Women are more flexible in this area than men, whose larger muscles can inhibit movement of joints. This ability may be hormonally related—we know, for example, that flexibility increases during pregnancy. Also, flexibility is not tied to strength—witness some weight lifters who have difficulty touching their toes.

- *Aerobic capacity.* This refers to the ability of the heart and lungs to deliver oxygen to the muscles, and the ability of the muscles to use that oxygen efficiently. Women have smaller hearts and lungs and generally begin training with less aerobic capacity than do men of similar size. Your aerobic capacity can be improved by increasing the heart rate through steady, sustained exercise for at least 20 minutes three times per week. It is not necessary to do exercises faster but rather to do them over a longer period. The heart becomes stronger and more efficient; it beats more slowly, but each beat pumps more blood. The lungs become larger and stronger, moving more oxygen in and more carbon dioxide out.

HOW TO PLAN A GOOD EXERCISE PROGRAM

To achieve a healthy balance, it is important to maintain a balance between too much and too little exercise. Not exercising frequently enough will greatly lengthen the time needed to achieve the beneficial effects of exercise. On the other hand, workouts need not be complicated or exhausting to be effective. The truth is that more is not always better when it comes to exercise (see box below). Beginners in particular may err on the side of overdoing it, perhaps trying to make up for lost time. And exercising too frequently will not improve aerobic capacity, strength, or endurance any faster and may, in fact, lead to more frequent injuries. Working too hard can also cause fatigue and muscle cramping.

If you wish to exercise daily, alternate types of activity between an aerobic day and a stretching or weight training day. Or alternate swimming, which is almost injury-proof, with some other aerobic activity. (If you use weights, it is recommended that you lift no more than two or three times a week, because muscle fibers need 48 hours to recover.) You need one day every week without vigorous exercise so that your body can rest and recover. You can walk on an "off" day, but don't run.

Conventional wisdom used to be to check with a physician before starting any exercise program, but it is now believed that the benefits of pre-exercise exami-

TOO MUCH OF A GOOD THING: THE EXERCISE ADDICT

As healthy as exercise can be, for some women it becomes an unhealthy addiction. A portrait of an exercise addict includes exercising to the point of hating the activity, ignoring injuries ("My knee doesn't hurt that much"), preoccupation with attaining an unrealistic appearance ("I could never be too thin"), and the inability to take a day off from the activity without emotional distress or depression. You are an addict if exercise literally runs your life; you talk, think, and dream about exercise all the time; you lie about how often you exercise; you crave the addiction and deny it ("I really don't exercise that much"). This particular addiction is more likely to strike women who, as a group, are more likely to be dissatisfied with their appearance. The recommended treatment is counseling with a professional who is experienced in dealing with addictions.

nations have been overstated. Generally it is not necessary to get a doctor's approval if you are in good health, unless you are over 35 and sedentary or in a risk category because you are a heavy smoker, overweight, or have diabetes, hypertension, or high cholesterol. Your doctor may then recommend an exercise cardiogram, which measures heart electrical function, but even that test is sometimes misleading as it rarely detects abnormalities in women who have no obvious symptoms of heart disease.

Sample Workout

1. *Warm-up.* Warming up is an essential part of any exercise program, regardless of the level of difficulty. It is as important to warm up before a brisk walk as before a marathon. At rest, the large muscles of the body have very little blood flow, and a sudden increase in the demand on these muscles requires an increase in blood and oxygen. Similarly, muscles, tendons, and ligaments are at their shortest length while at rest, and exercise can suddenly stretch them, causing injuries.

Warming up consists of gentle stretching of the body parts that will be exercised, followed by a *gradual* increase in activity. Runners, for example, should warm up with stretches for the legs (Figure 4.1), then do some walking or slow running; bicyclists may warm up with walking or pedaling slowly on a level surface. Most exercisers develop their own warm-up routine, which should be longer on cold days. (It is also a healthy idea to dress in layers that can be taken off during warm-up.)

Pay particular attention to certain areas of the body that may be abused over the normal course of a day. For example, wearing high heels may cause shortened Achilles tendons, and sedentary desk jobs can also result in shortened hamstring muscles. If you do keyboard work, you may experience shortness and tension in the muscles of the neck. You need to lengthen these muscles during warm-up and stretching. Some simple rules:

- Stretch until tension is felt. The feeling should be tightness or mild burning, but never pain. Hold for 10 to 20 seconds. (Figure 4.2.)

- Do not bounce; stretch out like a cat. Bouncing can cause tears in muscles and can lead to

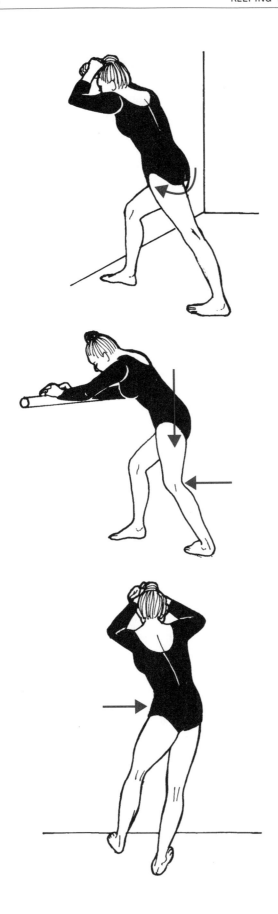

Figure 4.1. Stretching out before any type of exercise can help prevent injuries. Here are some general guidelines:

• *Never stretch a cold muscle.* Do some brisk walking or jogging slowly in place to warm up your muscles before stretching them.

• *Don't bounce.* Hold the stretch to a count of 30, release, and then repeat. Bouncing during the stretch can cause muscle injury.

• *Don't forget to breathe!* Breathe in deeply and then exhale slowly as you go into the stretch. Don't tense up—relax into the stretch, breathing deeply, slowly, and regularly.

Top: Calf stretch. To stretch the gastrocnemius (calf) muscle, stand facing a wall with your right knee bent and your left leg stretched out straight behind you. Push in toward the wall, keeping your back straight, your left leg straight, and your heel flat on the floor. You should feel the stretching sensation in the back of your calf and knee. To prevent injury during this stretch, do not let your right knee extend forward past your toes. Repeat with the other leg.

Middle: Soleus stretch. The soleus muscle lies underneath the gastrocnemius. To stretch it, bring your left leg in toward the wall, bending your left knee and keeping your heel flat on the floor, and press your left leg down into the floor. This stretch is a little harder to get right than the calf stretch; practice adjusting your position until you feel the stretch deep in your calf muscle. Like the calf stretch, the soleus stretch should not cause your right knee to extend forward past your toes. Repeat with the other leg.

Bottom: Hip stretch. To stretch the muscles that surround the hip, lean your upper body against a wall with your weight on your right leg. Place your left leg slightly forward with the knee bent, and push toward the right with your hips. Repeat on the other side.

scars, calcium deposits, and ultimately decreased flexibility.

■ Stretch every day, at least to start. After several months, flexibility can be maintained with stretching every other day. (Some women choose to incorporate yoga into their routines. Yoga strengthens, stretches, and relaxes the body.)

2. *Aerobic Exercise.* The bulk of your exercise program should be devoted to an aerobic workout. The eventual goal is 20 to 30 minutes of aerobic exercise that increases the heart rate. Beginners should exercise aerobically only 5 to 10 minutes, building up their endurance over six or more weeks. Running, stair climbing, cross-country skiing, bicycling, rowing, aerobic dance, and brisk walking all are good workout choices.

In order for aerobic exercise to have a healthy effect, it must be of sufficient intensity. Exercise at your target heart rate (see box).

YOUR TARGET HEART RATE

Your maximum heart rate is calculated by subtracting your age from 220. As you exercise, try to achieve your *target heart rate,* which is 60 to 80 percent of your maximum heart rate. (Figure 4.3.)

TRAINING HEART RATES BY AGE

Age	60%	80%
30	114	152
35	111	148
40	108	144
45	105	140
50	102	136
55	99	132
60	96	128

For example, if you are an average 50-year-old, your maximum heart rate is 220 minus 50, or 170. Your target heart rate is from 102 to 136 beats per minute, 60 to 80 percent of your maximum heart rate.

3. *Muscle Conditioning.* Although a level of physical fitness can be maintained with aerobic conditioning alone, many women find the benefits of weight training to be well worth the extra time and effort. A weight-training and muscle-conditioning routine involves about 30 minutes of slow but constant stress on different muscles of the body. An adequate weight-lifting routine can be formulated with an exercise specialist in a gym, but generally speaking it should consist of about a dozen exercises: six for the upper body and six for the lower.

4. *Cool-down.* When you finish exercising, it is crucial to have at least 5 to 10 minutes of slowly decreasing activity followed by stretching so that your heart rate, breathing, and body temperature can return to rest levels. In a proper cool-down, more blood is delivered to the skin, which helps eliminate heat and literally cools you off. Cooling down also helps the body rid the muscles of waste products—chemicals produced by the muscles during exercise—that are in part responsible for the achy "charley horse" feeling the day after strenuous exercise.

HOW TO PREVENT INJURY

Two decades ago, women athletes suffered injuries at rates far higher than those of male athletes. This dismal record led to the incorrect conclusion that women were more prone to injury and unable to participate in sports at the same level as men. The truth is that women were (and sometimes still are) denied the thorough training afforded male athletes and that successful training techniques used by men are not always directly applicable to women. With proper training, women athletes' injury rates are dropping to a level roughly equivalent to that of men.

But, no matter what exercise you choose, no exercise is injury-proof. Name a body part and there is probably a sports-related concern, from swimmer's ear to tennis elbow. Blisters, bumps, and strains are common to most sports. Different types of activities also stress different parts of the body. For example, running stresses the lower leg, bicycling taxes the upper leg, and tennis and squash involve sudden stops that can hurt the knee, ankle, and lower back.

Some exercises are safer than others. For example, swimming (despite some ear problems) is generally considered a safe exercise for just about everyone—even the disabled. Similarly, brisk walking can be undertaken by almost any able-bodied woman. Jogging, on the other hand, puts pressure on weight-bearing body parts and can be particularly unsafe if you run regularly on hard surfaces such as concrete or asphalt.

Exercise-related injuries are of two kinds: *acute* injury, which occurs suddenly as the result of a single accident or misuse (such as a twist or fall), and *overuse* injury, which occurs as the result of an activity that is constantly repeated and strains the body over a long period of time. A proper exercise program should include injury prevention activities. Several elements are involved.

For one, exercise and physical activity should *never* be painful. Don't accept the oft-repeated saw "No pain, no gain." Any pain experienced during or after exercise deserves investigation and should be eliminated. Such pain is usually due to improper mechanics or, more commonly, to overuse of muscles not yet strong enough for internal activity. The solution is to slow down the rate of progression of the exercise program. Also spot-strengthen specific muscles to help them catch up with the demands of the exercise.

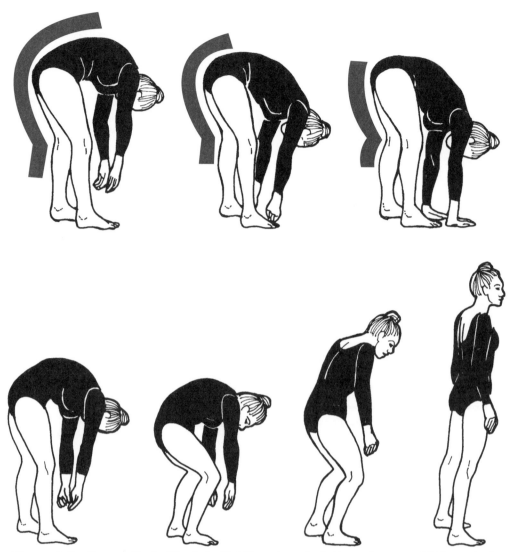

Figure 4.2. Lower-Body Stretch. Stretching out your back, hips, groin area, and thigh muscles is a good idea before any type of exercise.

Top: This stretch will loosen your hamstrings, the group of muscles in the backs of your thighs. From a standing position, slowly bend forward and over as far as comfortably possible. Don't lock your knees—allow them to bend naturally. If you can, continue the stretch until you touch your toes, and then place your hands flat on the floor. Do not force this stretch, or you may pull a muscle in the back of your leg. Hold for 30 seconds and release; as with all stretches, do not bounce.

Bottom: After holding the stretch, slowly rise to a standing position with your head down and arms hanging forward. Think of your spine as "uncurling," and feel the stretch work up your back.

Consider consulting an athletic trainer for advice on injury prevention and for help in designing a healthy fitness program. The trainer should have a degree in physical education and experience in prescribing exercise workouts for all types of students.

As previously discussed, warm-up and cool-down are absolutely essential to injury-free workouts. They may seem to be boring and unproductive parts of exercise, but if you are cool, stiff, or out of shape you can tear a ligament or tendon if you skip warm-up. If you

eliminate cool-down, the abrupt shift after strenuous exercise can cause fainting or worse. When first beginning an exercise program, the warm-up and cool-down periods should nearly equal the actual vigorous exercise in duration. As you get in shape and become better trained, these segments can drop in duration but should never be less than 10 to 15 minutes.

Be careful not to push yourself too fast and too far when first beginning an exercise program. Do half of what you think you can for at least three exercise ses-

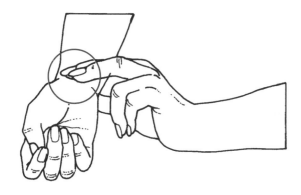

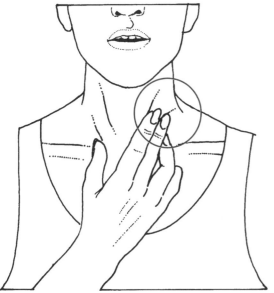

Figure 4.3. Taking your pulse can be done most easily by feeling it on the inside of your wrist (top) or in the carotid artery in the side of your neck (bottom). Press lightly with two fingers on one of these two pulse points; you may need to move your fingers around a little to find your pulse. Once you do, count the beats you feel for six seconds, then multiply by 10 to get the number of beats per minute; this is your heart rate.

sions. This gives you the opportunity to test for areas of weakness and pain before overuse sets in. View increasing the level of exercise as a process that will take months, not weeks.

It is also important that you do not exercise if you have a fever or a viral infection. A mild workout will not make a cold worse, but exercising tends to raise body temperature and you don't want to exercise if you are already feeling hot. It is a myth that exercise "flushes" out illness, and overdoing it may be harmful to your muscles and heart.

Dehydration is a common cause of fatigue during workouts. As a rule, drink water before each workout and then drink several gulps of water every 10 to 15 minutes during the workout. The rule of thumb is: If you feel thirsty, it's too late—you're dehydrated.

Although exercise has an accumulated positive effect, unfortunately it can't be stored up to be used later. If you miss more than three consecutive exercise sessions, you will need to decrease the amount of exercise you have been doing and build up again. Your body loses improvement from exercise at a rate of between 5 and 10 percent per week of rest, and completely stopping exercise for one month results in a 50 percent decline. If you know in advance you have to reduce your exercise program, try to decrease the time spent during each session rather than decreasing the frequency—this will better preserve your gains.

To treat injuries, the general advice is RICE: *r*est (stop the activity); *i*ce (apply cold, which constricts blood vessels and limits swelling); *c*ompress (wrap a towel or cloth around the injury part); and *e*levate (raise the injury above the level of your heart). Do not immediately put heat on a wound. It increases blood flow, which causes swelling—but after 24 hours you can apply moist heat on a tear or sprain.

Several parts of a woman's body are highly susceptible to injury due to overuse, improper training, inadequate warm-up, poor flexibility, or inadequate equipment.

Knee Injuries

Knee injuries are especially common. The knee is a complex joint that undergoes tremendous stress during activities requiring repetitive bending (flexing) and straightening (extending) or a constantly flexed knee (such as volleyball, racquet sports, and downhill hiking). The major stabilizers are the quadriceps and hamstrings, the large muscles of the thigh. If very strong, these muscles can protect the knee joint from injury. Unfortunately, in many women these muscles are not strong enough, and knee pain and injury result.

When you seek a physician's opinion about knee pain, the knee should be thoroughly examined and a complete history of the pain taken, including the type and location of pain, aggravating activities, swelling, locking, and heat sensations. X-rays may or may not be indicated. You should be examined sitting and standing, with legs and feet completely undressed.

The *patella,* or kneecap, is a common site of knee pain. The patella is a small oval bone embedded in the tendons of the quadriceps muscle, and it rides over the knee joint as the knee bends and straightens. The line of movement of the patella is unique in each woman and is determined by the angle formed between the *tibia* bone of the lower leg, the *femur* in the thigh, and the strength of the quadriceps muscle. This line of movement is called the *Q angle.* The Q angle is larger in women than in men and if very large may result in abnormal patellar movement and pain.

The degeneration of the cartilage and the pain of chondromalacia is not a disease in itself but a response to abnormal or excessive forces on the knee. In virtually all but the most severe cases, the most important treatment is strengthening of the quadriceps and hamstring muscles. Surgery is generally not recommended until a complete trial of exercises has been completed.

Chondromalacia

Chondromalacia is a condition in which the cartilage on the undersurface of the patella is degenerating. In the early stages of the condition, the cartilage swells and softens, and cracks form on the surface. Pain increases when the knee flexes beyond 90 degrees, and the sufferer will find going downstairs more painful than going up. Extending the knee generally decreases the pain. On physical examination, there may be pain on the underside of the edge of the patella. Abnormal movement of the patella may or may not be seen.

Achilles Tendinitis

Achilles tendinitis is injury to or inflammation of the Achilles tendon, also called the heel cord, located in the back of the ankle. Achilles tendinitis is common in running and jumping activities. Women who have been wearing high-heeled shoes for many years may have shortened Achilles tendons and may be prone to developing tendinitis. The pain is located at the top of the back of the heel and increases with ankle movement. It may be worse in the morning.

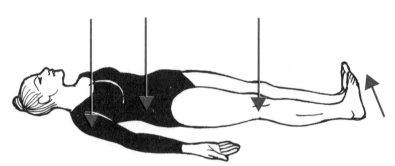

Figure 4.4. Foot Stretches. Gently stretching an injured Achilles tendon—after swelling and pain have been reduced—can help return it to normal length. Lie flat on your back with your shoulders, hips, and knees touching the floor and your legs straight. Slowly bring your toes up toward you as far as you can without pain.

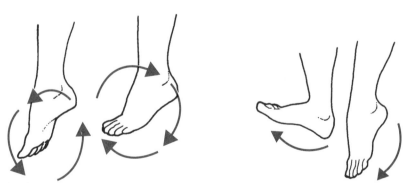

Figure 4.5. Treatment for shin splints includes stretching the tibialis anterior (shin) muscle in the front of the lower leg. These stretches can be done while sitting or lying down.
Top: Raise your toes as far up toward your upper body as possible; hold, then stretch them downward as far as they will go.
Bottom: Rotate your ankle in either direction, making a circle as large as possible. Repeat in the other direction.

Treatment includes rest and, if severe, crutches and a cast or ankle splint. Local heat or ice and anti-inflammatory medication are helpful. In the acute phase, a heel lift will shorten the tendon and relieve pain. Once pain is reduced, gentle stretching is started to return the tendon to normal length (Figure 4.4). Prevention of Achilles tendinitis includes avoiding high heels and thorough stretching of the Achilles tendon prior to exercise.

Shin Splints

Shin splints are the occurrence of pain along the front and middle of the lower leg, felt during or after running, walking, or hiking. Shin splints are caused by many tiny tears in the muscles attaching to the tibia, the large bone of the lower leg. The problem is caused by the impact of the foot on the ground and is worsened by running on a hard surface, wearing worn or insufficiently padded shoes, weak leg muscles, and insufficient warm-up stretching. Treatment includes rest, local heat and/or ice, well-padded shoes, and proper stretching (Figure 4.5). Persistent shin splint pain that does not go away quickly should be evaluated by a doctor.

Stress Fractures

Stress fractures are far more common in women than in men. The most common sites for stress fractures are the bones of the foot and leg. In older women who have experienced menopause, stress fractures may be due to the bone weakness that results from osteoporosis (see Chapter 11). Except in highly trained athletes, stress fractures in young exercising women are the result of incomplete training or a too rapid increase in the amount of activity before the muscles are properly strengthened. As improper training occurs more frequently with women than with men, women have greater rates of stress fracture. Stress fractures can be prevented by gradual training to allow bone strength to increase at the same rate as the activity stressing the bones.

The pain of a stress fracture is generally limited to the area of the broken bone and increases with continued activity. There may not be swelling, and X-rays may not show the fracture until 2–3 weeks after injury. Treatment involves rest. A cast is generally not required, although crutches or a cane may be. Recovery and return to activity should involve a muscle strengthening program. (For more information about injuries, see Chapters 21 and 34.)

STICKING WITH YOUR EXERCISE PLAN

Beginning an exercise program is easy; maintaining it is the difficult part. Women who smoke, are overweight, have little free time, or begin an overambitious program are at highest risk of dropping out. To improve your chances of maintaining your exercise program, keep these tips in mind:

- Any exercise is better than none. Although aerobic training requires at least 15–20 minutes three times per week, any vigorous exercise burns calories and increases circulation, flexibility, and endurance.

- To avoid boredom, select an activity that is suited to your personality. Exercise can be social (aerobic class, running with a partner, hiking trips) or solitary (jogging, swimming, stair climbing). Increasingly women are exercising their competitive side by joining teams. There are now women's leagues in just about every

sport, including basketball, softball, bowling, and karate.

- Set reasonable goals. A program that is too strenuous is at best discouraging and painful; at worst, it may cause injury. Start slowly and build gradually; expect the first stages to be awkward, boring, and even frustrating.

- Do not expect noticeable gains for at least 4 to 6 weeks. The good news is that unfit people enjoy fast initial improvement: unused muscles and tissues react swiftly to regular workouts. But increasing muscle strength and endurance requires actual changes in the muscle tissue, which takes time.

- Do not begin exercising with a male partner. Even an out-of-shape man has greater strength and endurance than an out-of-shape woman of the same age, size, and general health. A man will be able to do more and advance faster

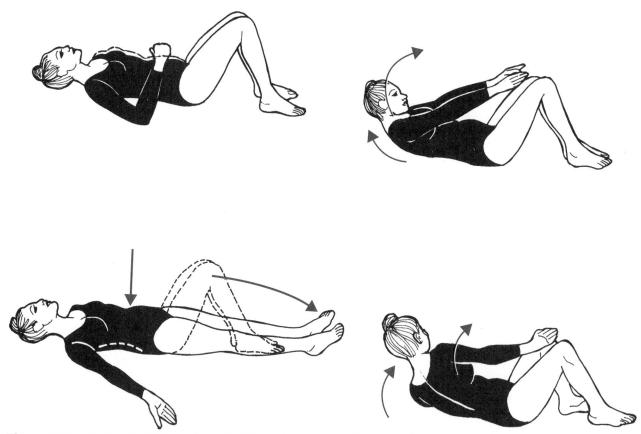

Figure 4.6. Abdominal Stretches. Stretching and strengthening the abdominal muscles is safe during the early part of pregnancy. All of these stretches are begun lying down with your hips, shoulders, and feet flat on the floor and your knees bent.
Top left: Back presses: Press your lower back into the floor without raising your hips or shoulders; hold and release, then repeat.
Bottom left: Leg lifts: Lift your feet off the floor and slowly straighten your legs all the way out and down. Then lift up your feet and bring your knees up again into the original position. To prevent lower back strain, be sure to use your abdomen, not your lower back, to raise and lower your legs during this exercise.
Top right: Straight curl-ups: Tuck in your chin and reach your hands up to your knees, allowing only your shoulders to lift off the floor. Keep your lower back in contact with the floor during this exercise.
Bottom right: Reach with your right hand up and over to your left knee, keeping your left shoulder on the floor. Repeat on the other side.

than you will, which may frustrate you. If you want to exercise with someone, choose a partner of the same sex, age, and ability.

■ If you are significantly overweight, try not to set yourself up for almost certain failure. It makes sense, for example, not to join a gym that caters to primarily fit, thin women. Begin instead by walking or working out with another overweight buddy.

■ Put your best foot forward, literally, by buying well-fitting athletic shoes. Highly specialized shoes—for tennis, walking, or basketball—are popular but are often unnecessary and costly.

Make sure whatever shoe you choose is cushioned, gives you enough toe room, and has a padded insole and good arch support. If you exercise regularly, have a pair of shoes devoted only to exercise and allow them to dry completely before each use.

■ Do not spend a fortune on unnecessary or inappropriate clothing. Wear clothing that is comfortable and loose, such as sweats. Fabrics should be stretchy, absorbent, and made of natural fibers or fiber blends. One-hundred-percent artificial fibers can, in fact, increase your risk of dehydration.

- Similarly, do not spend a great deal of money on exercise machines and specialized equipment. Most home exercise equipment sits collecting dust or winds up in your next tag sale. If possible, try out any equipment you are considering buying at your local gym. (You can test an exercise tape by renting it first from your local video store.) Be particularly wary of equipment advertised on television that claims to help firm specific parts of your body. This equipment is often no better than a general exercise program, and some of the items may actually increase your risk of injury. Watch out for any exaggerated claims ("Lose eight inches overnight without breaking a sweat!"); there is no substitute for physical activity.

EXERCISE AND MENSTRUATION

Menstruation itself does not affect athletic performance. World records and Olympic medals have been won by women in all phases of their menstrual cycle. In fact, exercise tends to ease cramps, and many women athletes experience less pain at that time. Unless you suffer from excessive bleeding, you can exercise as hard as you like during menstruation.

Severe changes in the menstrual cycle occur rarely, and only among women who are training at collegiate or Olympic levels. Certain sports have been more closely associated with disruption of the menstrual cycle—running, gymnastics, and figure skating. Although the cause of menstrual cycle changes in athletes is not well understood, it is believed to be due to a combination of an extreme amount of exercise, increased lean body mass, inadequate nutrition, and competition-related stress.

Menstrual changes include amenorrhea (no periods); oligomenorrhea (light periods); cycles without ovulation; and delayed menarche (late age of onset). Exercise-induced menstrual dysfunction generally resolves once training decreases. There are, however, long-term consequences to prolonged exercise-related menstrual cycle disruption. Amenorrheic athletes suffer bone loss at a rate similar to that of women in menopause, and they may have a greater risk of fractures later in life.

It must be stressed that these potentially serious consequences are experienced by a very small number of highly trained athletes. The average exercising woman experiences no menstrual changes and, as noted, usually benefits greatly from exercise. Do not assume that menstrual irregularities are caused by exercise. If you are exercising and experience menstrual changes, consult your physician. In addition, any vaginal bleeding that occurs between menstrual periods, no matter how strenuous the workout, is abnormal and should also be discussed with your physician.

EXERCISE AND YOUR BREASTS

Some women are concerned—in part due to some misconceptions—about the effect strenuous exercise can have on their breasts.

There is no evidence that contact sports result in any serious breast trauma. If anything, the fatty parts of the breast protect the other parts from becoming injured. When trauma to the breast does occur, it does not cause anything more than a bruise, which rarely requires any treatment. It does not lead to the development of breast cancer, cause difficulty in breast feeding, or promote any other breast disease or condition. Women with breast implants, however, should avoid contact sports, as trauma may cause rupture of the implant or bleeding of breast tissue.

The nipples are more vulnerable, however. "Runner's nipples" is a condition of abrasion and irritation of the nipples caused by the rubbing off of the outer layer of the skin as the exerciser runs or bounces during exercise. You can prevent this condition by wearing a supportive bra without seams, putting Band-Aids or nursing pads over the nipples during exercise, and wearing warm outer clothing in cold weather. You can also give the nipples a chance to heal by switching exercise activities, using a different type of movement on alternative days.

There is no evidence that exercise either enlarges or reduces the actual size of your breasts. Because the breast consists of predominantly fatty tissue, loss of overall body fat leads to some fat loss from the breasts as well.

The myth persists that exercise involving bouncing will cause the breast to sag. This is not true. This misconception may be based on the fact that the connective tissue that attaches the breast to the body does not seem to offer structural support. Sagging, when it does occur, is a result of breast size, weight, and age. It *is* a fact, though, that large-breasted women may find physical activity uncomfortable unless their breasts are supported by a well-fitting sports bra. Sports bras should be snug and strong enough to hold you and keep you from bouncing but light enough to breathe. Avoid bras that ride up or have bones or wires.

EXERCISE AND PREGNANCY

In the past, the ideal activity during pregnancy was rest or "confinement." The general consensus today is that most activities can be safely continued during and after pregnancy. Even women who have never exercised before can begin a limited exercise program when they are pregnant.

The health benefits of mild to moderate exercise are generally positive for the mother. Active women gain less weight and have less subjective distress during labor, although the length of labor is unchanged.

You need to make some concessions to your burgeoning size, however. For example, there are changes in the cardiopulmonary system: the heart rate is faster, the volume of blood larger, and the stroke volume (the amount of blood pumped per beat) increased. The growing fetus puts an additional demand on your energy. It is as if the body is already performing mild exercise, so there is less reserve left for additional exertion. You will also be more easily fatigued and find you have a decreased exercise tolerance.

In the beginning of your pregnancy, you can continue your pre-pregnancy exercise program with only a few modifications. All exercise should include warm-up and cool-down periods to prevent injury to lax joints: muscles stretch, ligaments soften, and joints loosen to make room for the baby. Stretching and strengthening (particularly of the abdominal muscles) and weight training are acceptable for uncomplicated pregnancies (Figure 4.6). Exercise performed in the supine position (lying on the back) should be limited by the second trimester. This position not only causes back pain, but also results in the uterus compressing the large blood vessels and decreases blood flow to the

WHO SHOULD NOT EXERCISE DURING PREGNANCY

The American College of Obstetricians and Gynecologists suggests the following as contraindications to vigorous exercise during pregnancy:

- any heart or lung disease;
- history or risk of premature labor;
- history of three or more miscarriages;
- incompetent cervix;
- multiple gestation (twins, etc.);
- ruptured membrane.

In addition, consult a doctor before starting an exercise program if you are hypertensive, overweight, or extremely sedentary.

uterus. Similarly, the Valsalva maneuver (increasing abdominal pressure while holding the breath) decreases blood flow to the uterus and should be avoided. Activities which may result in Valsalva include weightlifting and rowing.

Walking and swimming can continue throughout pregnancy and are excellent choices if you are just beginning to exercise: They build endurance, strengthen muscles, and improve circulation and res-

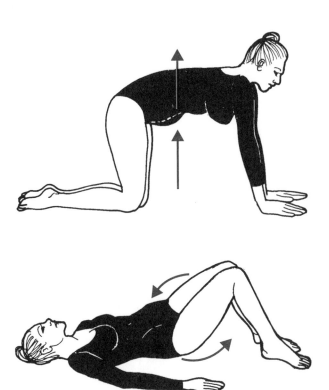

Figure 4.7. Abdominal muscles can be firmed up and returned to their normal shape after delivery by exercises that strengthen the muscles in the pelvis.
Top: Tummy tucks: On all fours with your hands directly beneath your shoulders and your knees under your hips, tighten your abdominal muscles by rounding your back and curling inward.
Bottom: Pelvic tilts: Lie on your back with your knees bent and your feet on the floor. Press down your lower back by contracting abdominal muscles; tilt your hips upward.

piration. Avoid activities such as fencing. Jogging, volleyball, and tennis—activities that involve impact and balance—need to be reduced and stopped altogether by the third trimester. Bicycle riding and cross-country skiing should also be tapered off by the third trimester.

Some guidelines for exercising during pregnancy are based on the knowledge that hyperthermia (high body temperature) can be dangerous to both mother and fetus. We know that exercise, in general, raises body temperature; sustained strenuous aerobic activity can increase maternal body temperature, often to as high as 102° F. To be safe, then, it is advised you check your temperature at the end of each exercise session. If it exceeds 101° F, take immediate steps to stay cool. To further prevent hyperthermia and reduce the risk of injury due to fatigue, a limit of 15 minutes of exercise at maximum level of exertion (see box on "Your Target Heart Rate") is recommended for all but the highly trained athlete. (Since body temperature can also rise in hot tubs, saunas, and whirlpools, avoid them or limit your bathing time to no more than 5 minutes.)

You can resume exercising after a normal vaginal delivery as soon as you have been given consent by your doctor. It is generally easier to recover from childbirth if you establish a regular exercise regime. Exercise can help restore those abdominal muscles that don't just pop back into shape without effort (Figure 4.7). Choose any physical activity as long as it doesn't cause pain. The only exception is swimming, which can cause bacterial infection, because the cervix needs time to close.

EXERCISE AND AGING

For a woman entering or past the age of menopause, exercising may be the single best thing she can do for her emotional and physical health. Whether or not she takes estrogen replacement (see Chapter 11), the active postmenopausal woman has a much better chance of keeping her heart healthy, her bones strong, and her body fit than her more sedentary sisters (Figure 4.8). The woman over 60 who exercises at least 30 minutes three times per week has the heart, lungs, and muscles of the woman ten years younger.

It can actually be dangerous to your health *not* to exercise. A serious concern for the older woman is the threat of osteoporosis, a degenerative bone disorder.

Women reach a peak bone mass at age 35, after which bone gradually decreases until menopause, when a rapid decrease occurs if replacement hormones are not administered. Along with nutritional factors (not eating adequate dietary calcium), lack of exercise may be an important promoter of accelerated bone loss.

In addition, women well past the age of menopause may be able to increase their bone mass by performing weight-bearing exercises. Remember, even if you are returning to exercise after a period of inactivity, you are not starting from zero. Muscles may in fact have "memory." Being active in any way will do a lot to improve overall health in the later years.

Since older joints become stiff and inflexible there may be a need to do a longer warm-up and modify your exercise—perhaps by doing fewer repetitions. Work toward your own target heart rate (see box on heart rate). And always be alert to any danger signs: lightheadedness, chest pain, or shortness of breath. In terms of specific exercises, calisthenics promote flexibility, weightlifting promotes muscle strength, brisk walking is beneficial and convenient, and stationary bicycling and swimming strengthen the heart muscles and bones. Jogging may not be a good choice: the jogger's foot lands with a force equal to several times body weight, which can injure older bones, tendons, ligaments, and joints.

Again, it's never too late to start exercising. A 1987 survey on exercise, diet, and bone loss in the *Journal of the American Geriatrics Society* found that sedentary nursing home residents in their eighties experienced more than a 4 percent increase in density of the forearm bone when they performed mild exercises three times a week for three years. A group of nonexercisers underwent a 2.5 percent decline in bone density over the same time period.

Exercise will also help you maintain your weight or lose weight, even as your metabolism slows as you age. Not only will staying fit directly help you avoid developing serious diseases, such as diabetes and heart disease, but by exercising you will look and feel younger and more energetic. You may find that exercising alleviates some menopausal symptoms such as annoying hot flashes, and that your complexion looks and feels younger as more blood is pumped into the tiny capillaries that feed the skin. Improved circulation will also help your digestive sys-

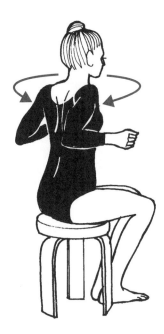

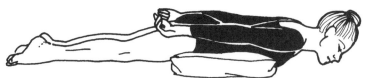

Figure 4.8. Back-Strengthening Exercises. Strengthening your back muscles can help avoid the back pain that often accompanies aging.
Top: To strengthen the trapezius muscles in the upper back and shoulders, sit with your back straight and your feet on the floor. With your arms relaxed and bent, pull back your shoulders as far as they will go.
Bottom: Lie face down with a cushion under your hips and torso, your arms at your sides, and your legs straight. Lift your head and feet off the floor at the same time and hold, then relax and repeat.

tem stay healthy and keep your immune system strong.

It's no wonder that the National Institutes of Health refer to exercise as "the most effective anti-aging pill ever discovered."

No one has found the fountain of youth—but you can certainly increase your odds and live longer and better by exercising. Staying physically fit should be a lifetime commitment.

CHAPTER 5

Living in a Healthy Environment

Diane L. Adams, M.D., M.P.H.

Our home environment has numerous health risks, many with the potential to cause health problems. There are potential biological hazards inside, such as mold or fungi, and outside, such as ticks that carry Lyme disease; there are physical hazards in and around the home, such as broken steps that could eventually collapse, or even a violent thunderstorm, with damaging winds and hail. Many of these hazards are easy to do something about; others are difficult for the individual to counteract. Being aware of the ones that can be dealt with is the first step toward improving health in and around the home.

Not all health hazards around the home lead to a health problem. In fact, most physical, biological, or chemical hazards can easily be coped with through proper use, cleanliness, and, in the case of chemicals, careful use and following of manufacturer's instructions. Ultimately, the majority of health problems caused by the effects of our surrounding environment—from inside the home to the backyard—can be controlled by our own choices.

BIOLOGICAL RISKS AROUND THE HOME

Microorganisms, such as viruses and bacteria, can be biological risks in and around the home. Most are harmless, while others can cause allergies, colds, and other respiratory ailments. Tiny organisms that cause respiratory ailments can be spread from person to person by air, water, bodily fluids; in most cases, allergens are carried by dust through the air. Molds and fungi can form from excess humidity and cause upper respiratory problems as they lodge in the lungs. Even setting out meats and certain foods on the counter for long periods of time invites microorganisms: *Campylobacter jejuni* (a bacteria that infects poultry, beef, and lamb) and *Staphylococcus aureus* (a common bacterium) are two disease-causing bacteria that proliferate under such conditions and can cause food poisoning.

There are other biological concerns outdoors, including plants and bugs. The best way to cope with the potential health risks from them is to be aware of the hazards.

Outdoor Biological Hazards

■ *Poisonous Common Wild Plants:* Many plants are poisonous—do not eat any plant unless you are sure it is not poisonous. In particular, keep chldren from eating such plants as nightshade, wild mushrooms (to be safe, never eat any wild mushrooms), oak tree leaves and acorns, pokeweed, May apples (especially the fruit), and horse chestnuts. (See Fig. 5.1 A-D)

■ *Poison Ivy, Poison Oak, Poison Sumac:* Up to 80% of the population is allergic to the oils in the leaves, roots, and stems of these plants. The oils cause itchy rashes and blisters if they are touched (the oils can also be on clothes if you brush past the leaves). For outbreaks of poison ivy, oak, or sumac (sumacs are only found in the eastern United States), consult your doctor, who will probably prescribe a special lotion and medication if necessary. (See Fig. 5.2). In addition, do not scratch the rash or blisters. You risk infecting the damaged skin.

■ *Poisonous Common Garden Plants:* While most garden plants are harmless, there are some (plants, fruits, or leaves) that are poisonous to eat (unless noted, all the plant and its parts are poisonous): geranium, English Ivy, hyacinths (bulbs), daffodils, Lily-of-the-Valley, yew (seeds within the berry), rhododendron (even the honey from the flowers can make you ill), morning glory (seeds), holly (berries), mistletoe, tomatoes (vine and leaves), potatoes (green spots and sprouts—even cooking does not destroy the poison in the green spots), and seeds (also called pits) of most fruits (cherries, apples, peaches, plums, and apricots). (See Fig. 5.3 A-C).

■ *Common Insects and Outdoor Creatures to Watch:* Most backyards have no real harmful insects or creatures (unless you are allergic to certain bites or stings); most of the insects just cause irritating bites. With thousands of species of insects and outdoor creatures, it is impossible to list all those that can be obnoxious or dangerous. A very general list follows, and many of the insects and creatures overlap from one part of the country to the other (you can find out about other types of harmful insects in your area by contacting your local home cooperative extension agency):

Around the Country

- *mosquitos:* A mosquito bite causes an irritating, itchy welt (use over-the-counter anti-sting medication to stop the itching); in the tropics, mosquitos can carry malaria and yellow fever. (See Fig. 5.4).

- *bee, wasp, and hornet stings:* Bee, wasp, and hornet stings can cause a large irritating, itchy welt. The stinger may also be left in the skin (remove with tweezers). Those who are allergic to bee stings should see a doctor immediately after being stung (some people allergic to such stings carry medication with them when they are outdoors). To stop the itching, use over-the-counter anti-sting medication. (See Fig. 5.5).

- *flies (greenbottle, bluebottle, and houseflies are most common):* These flies do not sting (blackhorse, deer, and black flies do—see below), but can spread filth and disease if they land on exposed food. They lay their eggs anywhere—on manure, garbage, or carcasses. Try to keep flies away from food at picnics or inside the house. (See Fig. 5.6).

- *snakes:* Although most species of snakes are harmless, there are several in various parts of the country that are poisonous. For instance, in the south, water moccasins (cottonmouths) and coral snakes are poisonous. To avoid snakes, be careful around open spaces in rock or wood piles and along garden paths. See a doctor immediately if you are bitten by a snake. (See Fig. 5.7).

Northeast

- *deer, black, and blackhorse flies:* The bites cause large, irritating, itchy welts; some people will have allergic reactions to such bites (consult a doctor if excessive swelling occurs).

- *deer ticks:* Deer ticks suck blood from their hosts. They are found in the woods (usually

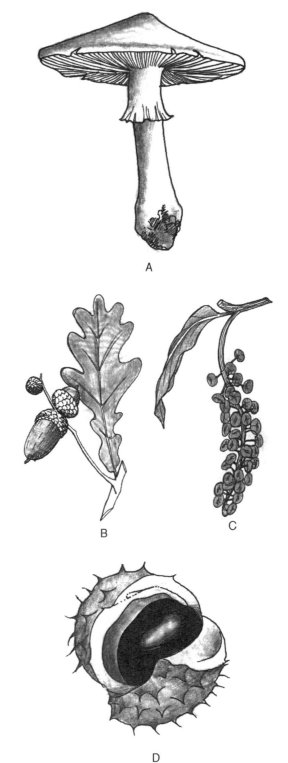

Figure 5.1.   Some common wild plants are poisonous if eaten. Wild mushrooms (A) should never be eaten under any circumstances, even if you believe you know what species they are. Accidental poisonings and deaths can occur in experts who are knowledgeable about mushroom species. Oak tree leaves and acorns (B), pokeweed (C), especially the berries, and horse chestnuts (D) are also poisonous if eaten.

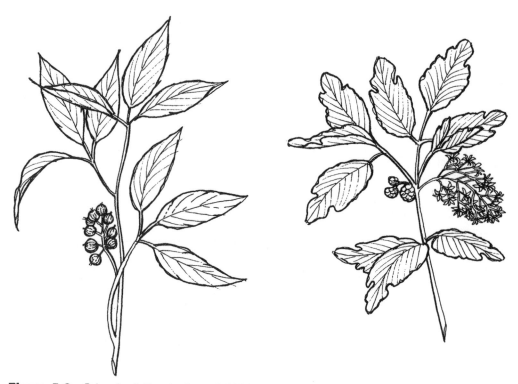

Figure 5.2. Poison ivy (left) and poison oak (right) are abundant species that exude an oil (urushiol) from the stems and leaves that causes painful rashes upon contact. The oil can be carried on clothes, shoes, or pets that touch these plants.

in deer territory, thus the name) from the spring to fall, peaking in the summer months. Some deer ticks carry Lyme disease, a bacterial infection that often begins as a simple rash (another symptom may or may not be a bullseye rash, flu-like symptoms, and muscle pain). If you find a tick (they are usually about ⅛ inch or smaller in diameter), use tweezers and pull the tick straight out (do not twist). Put the tick in a bottle, and contact your doctor. (See Fig. 5.8).

Southeast

■ *ticks:* Many ticks in the Southeast (and some to the west) carry Rocky Mountain spotted fever. If you find a tick (they are usually brown with spots on the back, and about ¼ inch in diameter—an engorged tick may be up to ½ inch in diameter), use tweezers and pull the tick straight out (do not twist). Put the tick in a bottle, and contact your doctor. (See Fig. 5.9).

■ *fire ants:* Fire ants give painful stings, causing an irritating, itchy welt (use over-the-counter anti-sting medication to stop the itching). In particular, watch children playing in the backyard—they can be badly stung by a nest of fire ants.

Southwest

■ *scorpion:* Scorpions, about an inch long with a curled tail, have a very painful sting. Watch for them under stones and around wood and rock piles. The stinger, on the end of the tail, can cause severe swelling; contact your doctor if you have been stung by a scorpion. (See Fig. 5.10).

Indoor Biological Hazards

■ *Common Poisonous Plants:* Although most indoor plants are harmless, there are several plants that are poisonous to eat, including

TERMS IN ENVIRONMENTAL HEALTH

In order to understand the potential dangers around us, it is necessary to understand the terms that are used in describing environmental conditions and health:

Allergens: Substances that cause physical reactions in persons sensitive to them through touch, inhalation, or ingestion. The most common forms of allergens are from dust, pollen, animal dander, and insect parts.

Carcinogens: Carcinogens are cancer-causing chemical compounds. Exposure to a carcinogen does not mean that a person will develop cancer, but that the risk for cancer increases. For example, tobacco has a mixture of carcinogens, and people who smoke have a higher risk of developing a number of different cancers.

Contaminants: In reference to pollution, contaminants are chemical substances that change the composition of the air, water, and soils by their presence and may or may not affect humans in an adverse way. It is often used interchangeably with *pollutant;* although a pollutant is usually a harmful substance, whereas a contaminant may not be harmful.

Epidemiological studies: Epidemiological studies look at groups of people in the same (or similar) localities to determine existing reasons for a health problem within the group. For example, looking at clusters of cancers within a community may help determine why certain cancers are prevalent and identify the cause.

Exposure: Exposure is defined as coming into contact with a health hazard, which may or may not affect the human body. Exposures to potential health risks can be one-time occurrences or a number of occurrences over an extended duration. The human body's reaction can be immediate, or a period of time may elapse between the exposure and onset of the health problem. A continual high- or low-level exposure to a hazard can also lead to a health problem after a long period of time, such as long exposure to excessive amounts of natural radon gas, which has been linked to lung cancer in some people.

Hazard: An event, structure, or substance that has potential to harm the human body in some way. Major hazards can be physical, biological, or chemical. For example, chemical hazards include carcinogens (chemicals that cause cancers), teratogens (chemicals that cause birth defects), and toxins (chemicals that are harmful or fatal to humans in low doses).

Pesticides: Pesticides are chemicals used to eliminate pests from commercial or residental crops or from homes. There are thousands of pesticides known to exist, many of which are not banned or registered with the Environmental Protection Agency. Pesticides are divided into several groups: insecticides (which kill insects), herbicides (which kill plants), fungicides (which kill fungi), and rodenticides (which kill rodents).

Particulate matter: Very small pieces or particles of substances in the air we breathe, including smoke, soot, ash, dust (includes human dander and microscopic insect parts), and aerosol sprays. Particulate matter comes from many sources, including industrial processes, burning of fuels, volcanoes, dust storms, aerosol cans, burning of vegetation and wood; it occurs as residue from grinding, quarrying, demolition, and milling operations; and it is associated with some homebased hobbies, such as woodworking.

Radiation: Radiation is the emission of energy in the form of certain electromagnetic rays, including microwaves, ultraviolet light, and X-rays. The sun is the greatest source of naturally occurring radiation, but radiation is also produced by man-made sources such as microwave ovens and power lines.

Risk: A risk is the perceived harm an event, substance, or entity can have on a human. Risk usually has to do with statistics and the population; that is, what percentage of the population would be affected by the exposure to a potential hazard and the resulting health problems from such an exposure. It is difficult to interpret risk based on a hazard's effects on people because everyone responds differently to an exposure. Although there are some hazards known to affect all humans in relatively the same way, everyone is chemically different: Some people may be more genetically inclined toward being affected by a substance, and some can tolerate a greater exposure than others.

Toxin: Toxins are any substances that are harmful or fatal to humans at a high enough dosage. There are thousands of potential toxins, for many of which it has been difficult to evaluate the health hazards. The level of a toxic dose of each toxic substance is difficult to pinpoint, as the toxic dose to a human is usually derived from animal studies or from the health records of individuals actually exposed to the substances.

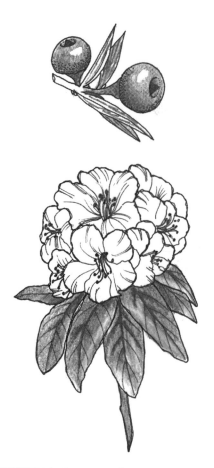

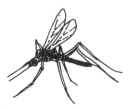

Figure 5.4.   The bite of the common mosquito can cause an irritating, itchy welt; in tropical areas, mosquitoes may carry malaria.

Figure 5.5.   Bee stings are painful and, in people who are severely allergic, can be dangerous or fatal. Shown here is a honeybee, one of the least aggressive bee species that can deliver a painful sting if disturbed.

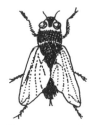

Figure 5.6.   Houseflies are extremely common. Although they don't sting or bite, they can spread disease.

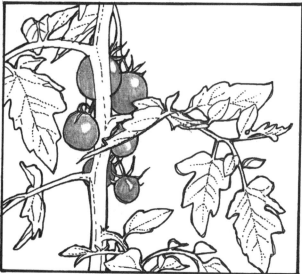

Figure 5.3.   Common garden plants that are poisonous if eaten include the berries of the yew (A), any part of a rhododendron (B), even the honey from the flowers, and the vine and leaves of the tomato (C).

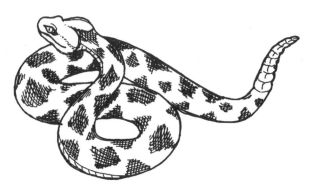

Figure 5.7.   Most snakes found in the wild are harmless, but among those that aren't are some species of rattlesnakes. Depending on the species, a rattlesnake bite can cause a range of serious reactions, from respiratory distress to death.

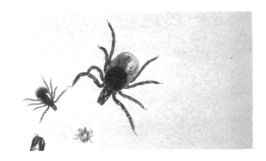

Figure 5.8. The deer tick has three stages of development: larva, nymph, and mature adult. Most cases of lyme disease are caused by the nymph. Because it is only the size of a pin head, the nymph is difficult to see or feel, and it is most active in the spring and summer, when people are outside.

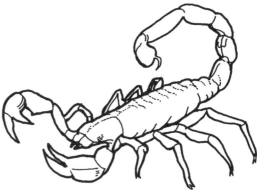

Figure 5.10. Nine species of scorpion inhabit the United States. Most are found in the Southwest, but they range as far north as Idaho and as far as east as Colorado. Few are dangerously poisonous, but the sting of at least one species can be fatal.

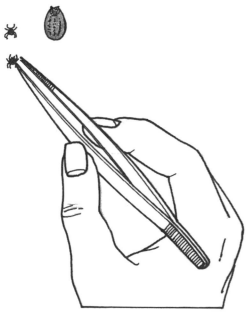

Figure 5.9. Ticks swell to many times their normal size (top right) when engorged with a host's blood. They should be removed by grasping them with tweezers (bottom) and pulling straight out, without twisting.

poinsettia, philodendren leaves, dieffen-bachia (or dumbcane) leaves, and Jerusalem cherry. (See Fig. 5.11).

■ *Common Insects to Watch:* Common in-door insects can come from outdoors, or from insects that are found on humans and animals.

■ *bed bugs:* Bed bugs are found in rugs or bedding. At night, they crawl (they never fly or jump) to feed on humans or animals. They are smaller than ¼ inch in diameter and are brownish, broad, and flat. Both males and females bite, leaving a painful rash of small welts. Bed bugs can be elimi-nated by washing linens; for more extensive cases, exterminators must be called in to eliminate the bugs.

■ *fleas:* Fleas are most often carried by indoor animals. There are 1,000 different kinds of fleas, depending on the hosts (dogs, cats, mice, etc.). They have no wings, but can hop from about 8 to 13 inches. A flea bite can leave a painful rash of small welts. Fleas can be eliminated by using special flea sprays or by bug exterminators (to lower the risk of further infestation, have dogs, cats, and other animals wear flea col-lars). (See Fig. 5.12).

■ *lice:* There are three types of lice found on humans: head, body, and crab. The lice are wingless, have brown to gray bodies, and cause an irritating itch. Head lice are found mostly in the scalp, or around any body-hair; washing with special shampoo helps to eliminate head lice. Body lice occur in any part of the body; a special soap helps to eliminate most body lice. Crab lice oc-cupy certain hairy parts of the body, espe-cially the groin area; they thrive in moist conditions. To eliminate crab lice, use a special soap.

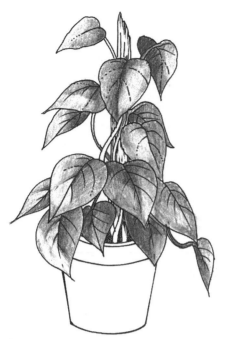

Figure 5.11. The philodendron, a common houseplant, is poisonous if eaten by people or pets.

■ *dust mites:* Dust mites are microscopic creatures that live in the dust of your home.

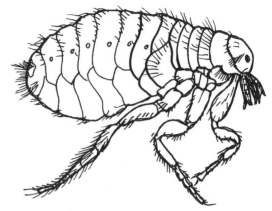

Figure 5.12. Fleas can be carried indoors by dogs or cats, and their bites can cause welts or a rash on human skin.

They live off particles in the home, most commonly human dead skin cells. They pose no real health threat unless you are allergic to the mites—allergic reactions include sneezing, runny nose, and cough. The best way to eliminate dust mites is to keep dust (including the notorious "dust bunnies") to a minimum by vacuuming and dusting.

PHYSICAL RISKS AROUND THE HOME

Many major risks around the home are physical, and are usually easily taken care of or repaired: broken stairs, loose electrical lines, or unsecured rugs. These hazards can lead to abrasions, fractures, lacerations, and burns. Protecting yourself from physical hazards in the home is mostly common sense: fix damaged stairs and broken floorboards to prevent tripping; use rugs with rubber backing to prevent slipping on smooth floors; hide loose wires and long cords to prevent tripping; and place rubber mats in the bathtub and rubber-backed rugs on the bathroom floor to stop slipping.

Other physical risks are found outside the home, including improper use of lawn machines (lawnmowers, electric hedge clippers), and tripping on uneven walkways or stairs. Sunburn—caused by the burning of the skin by the ultraviolet rays of the sun—is a major risk because of its link to skin cancer, especially in fair-skinned people. The average number of skin cancer deaths each year is 8,500 (and many researchers believe it is on the rise because of the destruction of atmospheric ozone). People can reduce their chances of skin cancer by wearing light protective clothing and sunscreens, preferably with a sun-protection factor (SPF) of 15 or higher.

CHEMICAL RISKS AROUND THE HOME

Chemicals in the environment are all around us and are virtually inescapable. Chemicals are found in and on the foods we buy at the store; in our clothing, cosmetics, and furniture; and in the air, water, and soil. Most of these chemicals create few problems for hu-

man health. Others cause health problems ranging from allergies and skin rashes to cancer and poisoning.

Chemicals can affect health immediately over the short-term or cumulatively as chemicals build up in the body. Some chemicals appear to have a particular effect on women, especially those who are pregnant or in their childbearing years; other chemicals affect women, men, and children alike. The following list describes the chemicals that are of most concern to us in and around our homes, and possible symptoms of exposure (an asterisk [*] marks those chemicals that are common in many homes):

Arsenic: Arsenic is a highly poisonous metallic element when digested, although long ago people ate small quantities daily for medicinal reasons with no ill effect. Arsenic is found in weed killers, insecticides, and in combinations of metals. It is of most concern to families living around mines and in rural areas where use of insecticides is widespread. Symptoms of arsenic exposure include nausea, vomiting, restlessness, darkening of the skin, headaches, memory loss, and convulsions. Arsenic has also been linked to cancer of the lungs and liver. *If you suspect that you have been exposed to arsenic, see your doctor immediately.*

Asbestos Fibers: Asbestos is a fire retardant and was once (and still is, in some cases) used in brake linings, hair dryers, fireproof fabrics, asphalt, shingles, pipe insulation, and home insulation. In 1980, after asbestos was reported to cause lung cancer in asbestos workers and mesotheliomas in people living near asbestos plants, the Environmental Protection Agency promoted the removal of asbestos from buildings. Recent studies have shown that such removal may not have been necessary: more problems occurred when the asbestos material broke up on removal. In addition, the wastes from the removal process were difficult to get rid of, as landfills were closing or refusing to allow asbestos on site.

Carbon Monoxide: Carbon monoxide is the odorless, colorless gas that is released in car exhaust; from a kerosene heater or stove; in vapors released when stripping paint or varnish with methylene chloride; or in cigarette, pipe, and cigar smoke. It is also one of the leading causes of death by poisoning in the United States. Carbon monoxide can enter the bloodstream by inhaling or skin absorption, the gas attaching itself to the hemoglobin in red blood cells and preventing oxygen from reaching vital parts of the body. Symptoms of low dosage include headache, lethargy, nausea, and fainting; higher amounts can lead to bizarre behavior, and for prolonged periods, it may be fatal, as the body is "starved" of oxygen. If you suspect carbon monoxide poisoning, get to fresh air as soon as possible (open a window, or go outdoors). Keep kerosene heaters or stoves in proper working condition; use paint strippers or varnishes in a well-ventilated area; and use air filters to filter out cigarette, pipe, and cigar smoke (or stop smoking).

Carbon Tetrachloride: Carbon tetrachloride is a solvent and cleaner found in many households and has been widely used for many years. It is a known liver toxin as well as a hepatocarcinogen (cause of liver cancer); it is also considered a central nervous system depressant.

Dust and Particulate Matter: Dust is all around us, and it carries particulate matter in the form of molds, bacteria, mites, soil, gases, lead, soot, and ash. Small amounts of particulate matter are common in most households, usually entering the house through open windows or air conditioning units. Larger amounts of particles are more of a concern for those living near quarries, mines, dusty fields, or demolition sites. Some hobbies are also associated with larger particles, including home machine shops and woodworking. Smaller particulate matter inside or outside of the home is of particular concern to those who have allergies to mites, molds, or pollen. Dust may also hold lead particles, often from lead paint from older buildings, which in excess can lead to health problems. Long-term exposure to certain types of dust may cause scarring (fibrosis) of the lungs, resulting in shortness of breath (called pneumoconiosis), although this condition is usually found in association with those who work in certain fields, such as sandblasting, mining, or welding. If you are concerned that you have a health problem associated with dust or particulate materials, try purchasing an air filter for your home; air conditioners often eliminate dust from the outside but should be properly maintained. For hobbies that create larger particles, wear protective face masks and have proper ventilation. If your condition worsens (especially upper respiratory problems), see your doctor.

Fluorocarbons: Fluorocarbons are chemical compounds of carbon and fluorine. They are most often found in solvents and as propellants in spray cans, lubricants, and insulators. Inhalation of fluorocarbons, especially in spray cans, can cause nausea or even unconsciousness. To eliminate possible contamination by fluorocarbons, use all chemicals in a well-ventilated area, and follow manufacturers' suggestions for use.

Food Chemicals: Many of our foods contain certain chemicals that can be harmful, especially in excess. Cured meat, smoked fish, and some beers contain sodium nitrite to prevent bacterial growth associated with botulism; but when sodium nitrite combines with nitrosamine, found in other foods, it becomes carcinogenic. Other chemicals are in foods as additives, preservatives, and flavorings. Most that have been proven to be harmful to humans have been banned from use; others have a negative health affect on people who are sensitive to the chemicals. In most cases, it is up to the consumer to decide what chemicals they want to avoid. If you realize you have an adverse reaction to a chemical, read labels and avoid products that would cause you to react.

Formaldehyde: Formaldehyde is found in fabrics (clothing, drapes, rugs, and upholstery); both the home and car contain the chemical. It is also used in particle board, plywood, and some foam insulation (it was banned from use in insulation in 1982, but older homes may still have such insulation). Formaldehyde is a suspected carcinogen; in excess, it is an irritant to smell and can hurt the nasal membranes, eyes, throat, and lungs. To lower the risk of exposure to formaldehyde (especially fumes), wash new fabrics; choose other types of paneling, not particle board or plywood (when purchasing such products, ask how the wood was processed); open the window after installing new rugs; and vacuum new cloth-covered furniture. If you still suspect that formaldehyde is a problem, seek medical attention.

Lead: Lead is a known poisonous element. It is used to line storage tanks and pipes; it is also used in batteries. Certain types of industry release lead in particulate form from smokestacks, although there are strict government laws that regulate the amounts released.

Exposure to lead in the home is usually from the air from nearby industry. Hobbyists who make ceramics (glazes), solder stained glass, or target shoot are all exposed to higher levels of lead. Although it was banned from paints in the last decade, there are still homes with old lead paint on the walls. Such paint poses the most serious threat to children and animals, who tend to eat the pieces of the paint that flake from the walls.

Lead can hurt a fetus, whose nervous system is vulnerable to the toxic effects of lead; exposure to the metal can cause permanent learning disabilities, hyperactivity, and mental disorders in children. The metal is particularly harmful to young children, who often exhibit learning disabilities after long-term exposure; in adults, lead exposure can cause irritability and mental confusion. Highest doses can cause severe brain damage and death. *If you suspect lead poisoning, see your doctor immediately (there are blood tests that can be administered to determine lead levels in the blood).*

Mercury: Mercury is a poisonous heavy metal similar to lead. It is used in chemical pesticides, barometers and thermometers, mercury lamps, antiseptics, and germicides. Photographers are exposed to mercury in the development process; painters who use certain pigments in paints also are exposed to small amounts of mercury; metalworkers are susceptible to mercury poisoning, either by direct contact or by breathing particles of mercury. Seafood lovers should also be concerned about mercury: in 1976, dumping of mercury into waterways was banned because fish had particu-

larly high levels of the chemical in their bodies. The concern was not the fish (they are not affected by the metal), but to humans who ate the fish.

Mercury poisoning has many symptoms. Organic mercurials cause dizziness, slurred speech, diarrhea, and convulsions; inhaling mercury oxide fumes cause flu-like symptoms. Mercury is readily absorbed into the skin when touched; never try to pick up the mercury from a broken thermometer with your bare hands. A major debate is whether mercury amalgam used in dental fillings is a health problem. The choice of using mercury amalgam for fillings is the consumer's choice; if you suspect exposure to mercury, seek medical attention.

Perchloroethylene: Perchloroethylene is the chemical you smell when you enter a dry cleaning establishment. It is a central nervous system depressant and can cause dizziness and nausea in some people. It has also been found to cause cancer in animals, but such a connection to humans has not been proven.

Polychlorinated Biphenyls (*PCBs*): Almost all living things have PCBs in their tissues. These chemical compounds have been used in generators, transformers, and large electrical equipment for years; in 1979, because they were suspected of being carcinogenic, PCBs were banned from use in equipment. Even so, other countries still use PCBs in the manufacture of lubricants, adhesives, and solvents. The problem with PCBs is their long lives: they take years to break down into a harmless substance. PCBs are soluble in the fatty tissue of humans and animals and remain for years in the body, but little is known about their effects on the body. It is unlikely that PCBs will be a problem within the home, but there are still some areas that have not eliminated transformers or other electrical equipment with PCBs. In most states, PCB-containing equipment must have warning signs that the substance is in use.

Polyvinyl Chloride (PVC): PVC is found in the plastics that surround us: credit cards, furniture, shower curtains, computers, cars, garden hoses, and some plumbing pipes. It is a known carcinogen, and the particles can be harmful if you file, cut, or sandpaper plastics containing PVC; such work should be conducted in a well-ventilated area, and a face mask should be worn.

Radon: Radon is a colorless, odorless gas that occurs naturally from the decay of radioactive elements (especially uranium). It is found everywhere in the soil, including material made from soils, such as brick, stone, adobe, tile, concrete, and cinder blocks. The distribution of the gas varies throughout the country, being more abundant where uranium exists underground. In very large amounts, radon can cause lung cancer over time. Smaller amounts appear to do no appreciable harm.

Tobacco Smoke: More than 4,000 chemical compounds—mostly irritants and carcinogens (about 43 of them are carcinogens)—have been identified in cigarette smoke, including carbon monoxide, benzene, nitrosamines, nicotine, and nitrogen dioxide. Smoking has been linked to lung cancer and emphysema in smokers and a range of ailments in those exposed to secondhand smoke, especially children. Children of smokers suffer from a higher incidence of respiratory infections than children of nonsmoking parents; 6- to 11-year-olds who live around a parent who smoked had lower heights and weights than children from households with nonsmoking parents. If you are concerned that you have any health problem associated with cigarettes, stop smoking. If your condition worsens, see your doctor.

Trichloroethane and Trichloroethylene: Trichloroethane is used as a chemical intermediary for hundreds of products and in aerosol waterproofing sprays. Trichloroethylene was widely used as a degreaser. Both chemicals are known to be central nervous system depressants.

HOW TO HELP YOUR HOME ENVIRONMENT

Healthy Air

Although most air in and around the home falls within safety standards, it can contain carbon monoxide, particulates, sulfur oxides, nitrous oxides, and photochemical oxidants from nearby industry or cities. Inside, pollutants can come from cigarette smoke, furniture, carpeting, certain interior structural materials (such as pressboard), household chemical products, and radon. Outside, air pollutants come from auto exhaust, emissions from fossil fuel power plants, industrial processes, and forest fires.

Smog is probably the major outdoor air pollutant. Smog is the result of a chemical reaction caused by sunlight acting on hydrocarbons (methane, benzene, and other products of combustion), nitrogen oxides, and other pollutants. The results include ground-level ozone, aldehydes, ketones, peroxyacetyl nitrates, organic acids, and sulfuric acids (a source of acid rain), carbon oxides, sulfur oxides, and particulate matter are also prevalent as air pollutants.

Inside the Home

1. Tobacco: Tobacco is one of the largest single sources of indoor air pollution. Recent studies have shown that passive smoking, or breathing someone else's smoke from cigarettes, cigars, and pipes, can also increase a bystander's chance of contracting lung cancer or developing respiratory ailments. Quitting smoking immediately can avoid future health problems and allow your body to recover from previous intake of tobacco and the bystanders smoke.

2. Furnishings: The best way to lower the problem with formaldehyde is to have adequate ventilation and wash fabrics to eliminate much of the formaldehyde fumes.

3. Radon: There are simple radon kits on the market that will measure the amount of radon in your home. In many states, the health department can tell you more about your choices. The interest in energy conservation in the 1970s, which included making homes airtight and energy efficient, may have exacerbated the levels of radon in homes. Since it is impossible to prevent radon from occurring, the best way to cope with elevated levels is to improve circulation within the home, repair cracks in the basement floor or walls, and vent the gas to the outside.

4. Household Products: Substitute water-based or "environmentally safe" household products for the home; others may contain hydrocarbon gases that could cause upper respiratory ailments. Do not combine cleaning products (or any other household products) unless suggested by the manufacturer. Especially dangerous is the combination of bleach and ammonia. These chemicals react with each other and can cause upper respiratory ailments, fainting, or even damage to the lungs.

5. Filtering the Air: Air filters may be the answer to cleaning the air sufficiently to eliminate possible particulates from your home. Air cleaners often help people who have asthma attacks and allergies from pollen or dust. Air conditioners may also help people with allergies; but caution must be taken to keep the air conditioner clean to prevent disease-causing bacteria and mold.

Outside the Home

1. Smog: Smog is the biggest concern outside the home. Smog alerts—when air quality degrades to dangerous levels—often occur when hot, humid high pressure systems stagnate over a region. The weather system acts like a cap, holding the smog over the area; the smog increases as cars, industry, and other processes continue to pump chemicals into the air. During smog alerts reduce your activity (to decrease the amount of smog entering the lungs); remain indoors when possible and keep windows closed or partially closed; keep an eye on children, the elderly, and people with respiratory ailments, and advise them to stay inside.

2. Electromagnetic Fields: Electromagnetic fields (EMFs) are of major concern to those who live near high-power electrical wires. The effects of the EMFs are questionable, but in 1990 the Environmental Protection Agency announced that EMFs were "possible" human carcinogens because of several reports that linked electromagnetic fields with leukemia, lymphoma, and brain cancer in children; adult health problems were only in association with working in the electrical fields. The information on EMFs is contradictory: one recent study suggested that women who work in the electrical trades run a 38 percent greater risk of dying from breast cancer than other working women, yet other studies show no such connection between human health risk and EMFs.

Healthy Water

About 90 percent of the U.S. population relies on city water supplies, which are monitored for safety and contaminants. City water is usually not subject to contamination. There are many sources of water pollution, including leaking gasoline tanks and landfills, pesticides, chemical dumping (often illegally in rivers, lakes, and oceans and along highways), and vehicle and industrial emissions. Every source of water on the planet—groundwater, lakes, oceans, rivers, and streams—contains some type of pollution, which may or may not cause health problems. The threat of water pollution is mainly to rural private wells, which get their water from groundwater sources; and many of the sources are close to agricultural centers, landfills, or dumps.

TOO MUCH NOISE

One of the most ignored, yet troublesome, environmental health problems is noise pollution. It does not involve particulates or dangerous chemicals; noise pollution is caused by sound that can cause damage to the ears, increase stress, and may lead to behavioral problems.

Excessive noise—mainly associated with large cities (vehicles are the major source), airports, and recreational noise—can cause damage to the ears: tinnitus (ringing in the ears, which can occur for years even after exposure to one loud noise); loss of high-, middle-, or low-pitch hearing; and physical damage to the eardrum. Case study upon case study has shown that noise does cause certain levels of stress, anxiety, and insomnia in some individuals, depending on the person and loudness and pitch of the noise. Loud noise can lead to physiological changes, such as hypertension (high blood pressure); some sounds can be addictive (sounds from "boom boxes" could elevate levels of adrenaline in the body); and certain behavior has been reported to be caused by noise.

The simplest way to reduce your exposure to noise in the home is to turn down the volume to radios, televisions, and stereos. Bothersome noise coming from outside the home can often be subdued by "white noise," a soft, constant noise to block out the outdoor sounds, for example, radio static. Protect your ears from loud noises, especially in hobbies such as boating, snowmobiling, and hunting. Protective earmuffs or earplugs can protect you from ear damage.

Inside the Home

1. Test Water: It is important to be aware of possible contamination; people with wells near landfills, agricultural fields, and old chemical plants or dumps should be particularly watchful. Contact the local health department for possible contamination reports around your home. If you have any suspicion of contamination, hire independent state-certified laboratories for testing (not laboratories that sell water treatment equipment, as their results may not be objective). Test the water at least once a year in any case. Test for contaminants such as organic and inorganic chemicals, radon, and bacteria. To interpret the test results, consult the office of the Environmental Protection Agency near you.

2. Keep Water: If your city or town reports water contamination, be sure to follow the health department's directions (including boiling water); if harsher contaminants are found, do not drink the water or use it for bathing, as per the direction of the health department. Those who live near flood-prone areas should keep extra jugs of water in storage in case of emergency; change the water frequently to keep it fresh.

3. Lead from Pipes: There are several ways to lower the presence of lead in the water: do not use hot tap water for cooking or drinking (hot water dissolves lead in the plumbing more readily); let water run from the tap for about 30 seconds before taking a drink, for about 3 minutes in the morning, and for about 5 to 7 minutes after more than a week-long vacation, as lead levels are higher in standing water in pipes.

Outside the Home

1. Dumping Pollutants: One of the ways to prevent contamination of water supplies (especially in rural areas where most homes use wells for drinking, bathing, and cooking water) is not to dump pollutants in gutters, in the backyard, or in rivers, lakes, or streams. Contaminants such as motor oil or concentrated lawn chemicals should be disposed of at specified recycling centers.

2. Pesticides and Lawn Care: Another way in which groundwater is contaminated is by the excessive use of pesticides and lawn care chemicals, especially in rural areas that depend on groundwater for their water supplies. A solution is to use organic alternatives to pesticides; older pesticides and chemicals should be brought to specified recycling centers.

3. Septic Systems: Septic systems in rural areas should be installed by certified septic system companies. The systems should be located so as not to contaminate nearby water wells and must be sealed from corrosion, watched for leakage, and not allowed to overflow.

Healthy Land and Outdoors

Soils are of concern to many homeowners, as grounds can carry and hold toxins or chemicals for long periods of time. If soils are contaminated, there is a chance that young children playing in the yard, or even the avid gardener tending her flowers and vegetables, could be exposed to toxins.

Contamination of the soil may have many sources: chemicals from landfills leach into the soils; chemicals sprayed on gardens and lawns seep into the soil; old or used oil or chemicals are often wrongly thrown into the backyard or gutters; and emissions from industry, automobiles, and chemical plants deposit chemicals, heavy metals, and particulates into the soil.

Inside the Home

1. Recycling and Precycling: One way to cut back on what is sent to the landfills is to reuse or recycle newspapers, plastics, glass, cans, and other recyclable materials. Most of these materials do not decompose in the landfill for years, if at all, and may produce harmful chemicals that can leak into the soil and groundwater. Precycling is choosing products that use the least amount of disposable packaging.

2. Used Oils and Chemicals: Dispose of used oil at a recycling center or gas station—never dump it into the sewer system or in the backyard. Get rid of old, unusable chemicals (such as household cleaners, solvents, or pesticides) at special recycling centers or at chemical recycling drives held by local governments or environmental groups.

Outside the Home

1. Lead in Soils: A major concern is soil contaminated with lead. Chips or particles of old lead-based house paint is the most common source of the metal contaminant. Soils near busy roads may also contain lead from the days of leaded gas. Children playing in the soil near homes or around buildings can be exposed to toxic levels of lead. One of the best ways to avoid exposure to lead in the soil is not to let children play around flaking paint or close to the road of a busy street. Getting rid of lead in the soil is more difficult, requiring the expensive removal of the soils.

2. Testing the Soils: If you suspect your soil to be contaminated (for example, if you live near an old chemical plant or a major industry), have the grounds tested by a certified laboratory (look under "soil testing" in the telephone directory). The laboratory will also provide options if your soil is found to be contaminated.

3. Rural and Urban Pesticides and Chemical Sprays: Rural locations have an even more insidious problem with chemicals: agricultural fertilizer and pesticides that enter the soils. Urban lawns also commonly have pesticides. Because these chemicals can remain in the soil for a long time, modify their use and research more natural alternatives to the pesticides you use on your garden, bushes, trees, and lawn. Use alternatives to chemical fertilizers, especially natural composting.

Healthy Food

The most common concerns about the safety of food are residue pesticides, chemicals and additives, poor preparation, and raw foods.

Inside the Home

1. *Clean Foods:* To rid fruit and vegetables of pesticides and other contaminants, clean them with mild soap and water, then rinse. Purchase fruits and vegetables that were grown organically to lower your exposure to chemical pesticides.

2. *What Is Added:* Not all foods with additives or chemicals cause problems; the consumer must make her own decisions about the ingestion of additives and chemicals. In most cases, food additives have no adverse effects on people. The best way to protect yourself from possible health problems from additives and chemicals is to know how your body reacts to certain products.

3. *Proper Handling:* Be sure to refrigerate meats until they are ready to be prepared. The cold stops the growth of microbes, and proper cooking of food kills biological contaminants. Always clean your hands before handling any food. When handling meats, be sure to cut with a clean knife on a clean cutting board and cook with uncontaminated equipment. Common contaminants are the bacteria *Salmonella* and *Campylobacter,* both of which produce gastroenteritis, evidenced by vomiting and/or nausea. To control these bacteria, food should be not be kept out of the refrigerator for more than 2 hours. Meats, eggs, and dairy products should be put in the refrigerator as soon as possible after use.

4. *Raw Food:* Eating raw food is not recommended, especially raw eggs, milk, fish, raw cheese, and meats. These foods are more susceptible to microbial contamination. For example, eggs may contain the *Salmonella* bacterium, which can cause food poisoning; cooking the eggs until they are solid (such as hard-boiling) kills the bacteria.

Outside the Home

1. *Labels:* When grocery shopping, read labels (now a law for most foods) to determine the additives, chemicals, and preservatives added to processed foods. Make your own decision as to the amounts of such chemicals you want you or your family to ingest.

SPECIAL CONCERNS FOR WOMEN

Beside avoiding hazards in the air, water, soil, and foods, women—especially those in their childbearing years—must watch for other hazardous exposures that could lead to health problems, mainly in the reproductive system. Of particular concern is the developing fetus, who is more susceptible to environmental hazards during the various stages of its life before birth.

Prenatal Conditions

There are several stages of fetal development when the fetus is most susceptible to agents that cause birth defects. During the first two weeks, certain hazards,

mostly chemical, can cause the fertilized egg not to implant itself on the uterine wall. At this point, some chromosomal problems may occur from the exposure to the hazard, which may result in a spontaneous miscarriage.

At 3 to 8 weeks, the developing embryo forms most of the major organs. At this point, the fetus is very vulnerable to environmental teratogens (drugs that cause abnormal fetal development and are responsible for birth defects), which can interfere with, or even stop the functioning of, the formation of organ structures and could cause a miscarriage. In general, after the eighth week, environmental hazards have less of a physical effect on the fetus. But because the nervous system is still growing, certain environmental hazards can damage the fetus's mental development and lead to retardation. Of course, a major hazardous exposure, such as a massive dosage of radiation, would be harmful to both the mother and child.

The Fetus and Children at Risk

Most children are born healthy, even when born to mothers exposed to certain hazards in and around the home. As with adults, fetuses and children are affected by exposure to environmental hazards based on characteristics such as genetic susceptibility, the nature of the hazard, the dosage received, and the exposure time. It is estimated that 95 to 97 percent of children born in the United States each year have no sign of birth defects; of the 3 to 5 percent who do, about 2 to 10 percent of the birth defects are caused by chemical exposure, drugs, or environmental hazards.

There are certain "controllable" chemicals that a woman should be aware of during her pregnancy that have the potential to harm the fetus:

- *Alcohol:* It is known that alcohol contains ethanol and acetaldehyde, two toxins that easily pass through the placenta to circulate in the fetus. Alcohol consumed during the first trimester, when fetal organs are forming, is the most damaging; and acetaldehyde is thought to contribute to the disruption of cell growth and metabolism. Researchers still do not know if moderate drinking (one to two drinks per day) has an negative effect on the fetus, but women are cautioned to avoid all alcohol consumption during pregnancy. Heavy or frequent drinkers face twice the risk of miscarriage; the child may have fetal alcohol syndrome, including delay in growth, abnormal features of the face and head, and nervous system abnormalities. A lesser effect from excessive alcoholic consumption during pregnancy is called fetal alcohol effect, which includes some eye and heart defects, impairment of certain organs, slowed growth, and behavioral problems such as hyperactivity and excessive irritability.

- *Tobacco:* Women who smoke run the risk of adversely affecting not only their own health but also the growing fetus. Cigarettes increase the amount of carbon dioxide entering the fetal system, reducing oxygen to the growing baby. Some of the effects on the fetus appear to be smaller lung development (which may make the child more susceptible to respiratory ailments); smaller size; and premature birth. As to be expected, the more the cigarettes smoked per day, the greater the problems resulting in the fetus. There are also studies that connect passive, secondhand smoke to low birth weight, although these studies are not conclusive.

- *Drugs:* Almost all recreational drugs (cocaine, marijuana, and heroin and other opiates) are connected with possible developmental effects in unborn children. Cocaine can remain in the fetus much longer than in an adult (sometimes a single dose lasting for five days); the affected baby is jittery, has low birth weight, and is usually born prematurely. Marijuana, like cigarettes, can reduce oxygen flow to the fetus; other studies, although not conclusive, show that affected babies have lower birth weights. The effects of heroin and other opiates are more difficult to determine—because in many of these cases other substances are also in use—but one of the major threats to babies born to heroin-using mothers is withdrawal: some 60 to 90 percent suffer from withdrawal, including tremors, fever, seizures, and irregular breathing. Most babies born to heroin addicts have serious medical problems, such as respiratory ailments and brain hemorrhages, and are at risk of having HIV (the virus that causes AIDS).

- *Over-the-counter and Prescription Medications:* Medication can have an adverse effect on the growing fetus. Every pregnant woman should consult her doctor before taking any medication, even if it is an over-the-counter drug. In addition, if she believes she is pregnant, she should tell her doctor, dentist, or specialist— especially if her doctor is going to prescribe a medication. One of the best ways to determine if a drug may harm a fetus is to read the warnings on the medication bottle. If you are pregnant, it is best to consult your doctor before taking any medication, even for such medications as aspirin, cold and allergy medicines, and laxatives.

HEALTH WATCH

Federal, state, and local governments help in the regulation of hazards within our environment. If you are concerned about a possible health problem in or around your home and want to become involved in mitigating an environmental health problem, you may want to contact certain health services for information concerning the environmental health problem:

- *Public Health Service:* Public health departments inspect the meat, poultry, and fish industry for any violations of health regulations; keep restaurants, markets, and hospitals within health safety guidelines; and enforce regulations that are designed to prevent the contamination of food, drugs, beverages, and cosmetics. They include six major divisions: the National Institutes of Health (NIH), which provide funding for medical research studies; the Food and Drug Administration (FDA), which oversees the wholesomeness of the products (except meat, poultry, and eggs) consumed in the United States and are responsible for the control and prohibition of harmful chemicals (natural or synthetic) in food, drugs, and substances; the Centers for Disease Control and Prevention (CDC), a collection of centers that provide information on communicable diseases around the country and collect epidemiology studies of certain diseases; the Substance Abuse and Mental Health Services Administration (SAMHSA), which provides research and services aimed at reducing or controlling substance abuse and mental health problems; the Agency for Toxic Substances and Disease Registry (ASTDR), which prevents exposure to and adverse effects from hazardous substances; the Health Resources and Services Administration (HRSA), which oversees projects aimed at improving health services for mothers, infants, and children.

- *United States Department of Agriculture:* This federal government agency is responsible for the safety of meat, poultry, and eggs. It is responsible for the "USDA inspection" stickers often found on meats. The USDA Meat and Poultry hotline is 1-800-535-4555.

- *Environmental Protection Agency (EPA):* This federal government agency is in charge of protecting public health by controlling air and water. It is also in charge of regulating the production, use, and disposal of toxic chemicals in the environment.

- *State and Local Health Departments:* The state and local health departments have a variety of duties. Many state health departments disseminate information to the public concerning major environmental health concerns, such as radon gas. Cities or towns are in charge of sanitary engineering departments (including garbage collection and landfill maintenance) and sewage treatment (including sewage treatment plants and sewer lines).

CHAPTER 6

Working in a Healthy Environment

Rosemary K. Sokas, M.D., M.O.H., F.A.C.P.

What does work mean for a woman? Research has shown that women work longer hours for less money than men and devote a greater proportion of time, energy, and income to child rearing. At the same time, women in industrialized countries live longer than men; women working outside the home in these countries are also healthier and happier than those not in the paid work force. Work that is valued enables the individual to participate as a contributing member of society, achieve self-respect and financial security, and develop a network of supporting relationships.

The key word here is *value,* which is not synonymous with *money;* unpaid work in the home may be highly valued and provide all the personal benefits already mentioned. In our society, however, secure support systems and income security (including retirement benefits, health insurance, etc.) require conscious planning. Americans have traditionally assigned high worth to individualism and to material self-improvement, presenting additional hurdles for the woman who remains outside the paid work force. Finally, work outside the home is a financial necessity for growing numbers of women in both single-parent and two-parent households.

The benefits of work are many, but certain occupations co-exist with serious hazards, stemming from our shameful history of considering the worker as a "thing"—literally true during the age of slavery and virtually true during the Industrial Revolution. Industrial accidents and epidemics of lead poisoning and silicosis scarred the first part of this century; pockets of similar troubles exist to this day. Women died horrific deaths as garment workers in the Triangle Shirtwaist fire of 1911, in which 140 New York City sweatshop workers were killed in the space of a few minutes. Eighty years later, 25 poultry processors were killed in the Imperial Foods fire in Hamlet, North Carolina. Both tragedies involved poor, mostly female workers; blocked safety exits; and in the former, abysmal or no regulations, and, in the latter, disregard for regulations. Both were entirely preventable. Women in "pink collar" activities experience hazards from neglect and abuse, while those entering traditionally male fields have faced hostility and inflexible workplace designs.

Occupational hazards are, by definition, the result of human activity. The creative solutions to overcoming them will also be the result of careful, energetic human activity. What, then, are the health and safety hazards women face as workers, and what are the social, economic, and biological issues contributing to these problems? What health and safety resources are available, and what resources need to be developed?

WORKPLACE HAZARDS

Workplace problems are not exclusively gender identified; similarly, solutions will benefit both sexes. Smaller-size safety equipment designed for women will benefit smaller men; on-site day-care facilities will benefit fathers as well as mothers. Nevertheless, there are areas that disproportionately affect women and problems that are recognized only when women enter the labor force in substantial numbers. The three major issues are those based on size and shape differences, those concerning reproduction and pregnancy (some of which fall into the "size and shape" category), and those stemming from social factors. Women encounter these problems whether they work in traditional women's jobs or in jobs previously reserved for men.

The general differences in physical design and strength between men and women are the easiest to address. Traditionally, activities requiring occasional bursts of extreme physical strength have been separated from those requiring repetition or dexterity (hunt- ing versus gathering, if you will). If you walk through an average manufacturing plant, you'll probably see areas of assembling or packaging where women are using small amounts of force with great frequency. Nearby there may be several men lifting boxes, hauling equipment, or resting during the slack time between the need for less frequent but more force-requiring activity. Needless to say, the chances are good that the men are paid nearly twice what the women are paid.

What about the old argument that each gender is doing what suits it best? The average man does have greater lifting capacity than the average woman, but there is considerable overlap across the male and female population. Furthermore, since lower back injuries are directly proportional to the lifting requirements of the job—and since they represent the single greatest work-related injury expense—better engineering to minimize these requirements makes obvious sense. When the need for sporadic strength is less predictable (during fire fighting or policework, for example), then specific strength requirements must be defined and applied equally to women and men. The Americans with Disabilities Act of 1992 strictly limits the use of physical requirements in job placement. The requirements must legitimately reflect the needs of the job, and there has to be no reasonable way to alleviate the job's strength requirements.

The reverse argument, that women were somehow better suited for repetitive handwork, has resulted in a massive wave of upper-extremity repetitive strain injury, including carpal tunnel syndrome (pain or numbness from pressure on the nerve passing through the wrist) and a variety of types of tendonitis (inflammation of the tissue that connects muscle to bone). This type of injury now threatens to exceed back injury as the most expensive work-related injury, because it is no longer confined to factories but is seen among clerical workers who spend entire workdays glued to their computer keyboards. The abuse of physical capabilities is unacceptable for either men or women and cannot substitute for proper work process design.

What design changes are needed? Machine controls; operating heights; reach distances; and safety equipment such as masks, goggles, and gloves must be made to accommodate the range of body types in the population. Women who work in traditionally male industries often have to deal with ill-fitting gear that may actually increase rather than decrease hazards. Women who work in traditionally female fields, on the other hand, are assumed to have no safety problems and thus are generally ignored. This is foolish, since ergonomics (including the science of adapting the workplace to the worker) has shown us how to increase not only safety but also efficiency. As in any engineering field, new designs for the workplace require careful planning, and there must be prototype trials to ensure that the designs are safe and effective. What's more, subsequent monitoring under actual use is required to make sure the designs remain helpful. American industry's failure to attend to safe equipment design affects the entire work force, but its impact is greatest on women. (See Fig. 6.1).

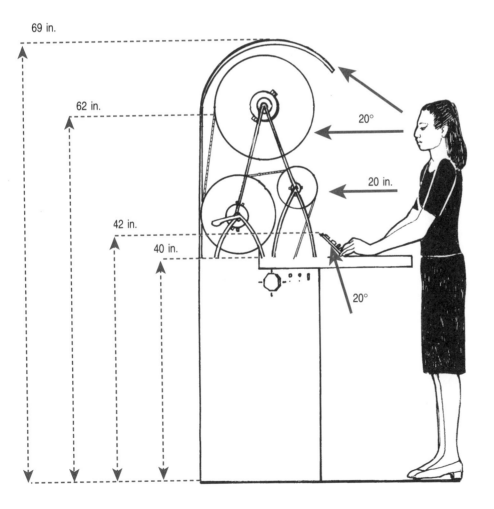

69 in.

62 in.

42 in.

40 in.

20°

20 in.

20°

Figure 6.1 A Well-Designed Work Station
Research in the field of ergonomics—the science of adapting the workplace environment to the physical attributes of the worker—has focused increasing attention on the safety and comfort of work stations. Critical angles and heights are taken into account in relation to the worker in the design of an ergonomic work station.

There are other differences between men and women that are assumed to affect where women work and at what. Women have a different body composition, with a higher proportion of fat to muscle, and hips and elbows that are angled slightly differently from men's. Women also have a keener sense of smell. Some studies have shown slight gender-based differences in heat tolerance and stamina as well as in absorption, metabolism, and storage of some chemicals. None of these differences is absolute, and men and women outside the "average" range will overlap.

Furthermore, by law in this country each worker is entitled to a safe and healthful workplace. There are mandated margins of safety for exposures to chemical, biological, and physical hazards, and trivial differences between men and women should not matter. In areas in which such differences might be important, such as space exploration, women would be favored more often as not.

Nowhere are the problems of workplace safety and health more emotionally charged than when childbearing is discussed. Historically, the social and public health and reform movements that ended child labor and other abuses saw women also as victims. Hence, women were covered under protective legislation. It was only after pressure from the women's movement, in fact, that some states removed restrictions on night work or double shifts for women.

Today, there is an increasing concern for the health of developing fetuses. Curiously, this concern is exhibited only when women attempt to enter traditionally male work areas and never seems to take into account the economic needs of the mother or child. No one has ever seriously argued that we bar women of reproductive age from working in child-care settings, where the risk of infections that may cause birth defects and miscarriage (such as measles and rubella) is quite real. Similarly, women have not been barred from work as nurses or hospital technicians, even though they may be exposed to gases, radiation, and medications that can adversely affect pregnancy.

The issues of pregnancy and fertility in the workplace have brought about court actions. In the late 1970s, the Oil, Chemical, and Atomic Workers Union sued the American Cyanimid Company on behalf of five women who underwent surgical sterilization in order to keep their jobs. They lost the case; the courts upheld the right of American Cyanimid to require women in lead-exposed work areas to document surgical sterility. And it wasn't until 1991 that the U.S. Supreme Court ruled that policies barring fertile women from a work area are discriminatory.

What are the issues here? Certainly no one wants knowingly to expose her child to poisons. But such poisons can affect men as well and have been shown to cause infertility and cancer in men and fetal deformity and cancer in their offspring. Policies that focus exclusively on women fail to protect children fully because they ignore critical paternal factors. Furthermore, these policies deny a woman control over her own reproduction and prevent her from making choices in her own or her family's best interests. The demise of women-focused policies will allow standards that minimize toxic exposures to everyone.

Of course, there are legitimate circumstances in which both women and men considering having a child may want to take greater precautions at work. For example, no one should have to tolerate the lead levels currently permitted in factories and construction by the Occupational Safety and Health Administration's (OSHA's) standards. But the risks to adults are considerably less than to children born of those adults, since exposure affects sperm, crosses the placenta, is excreted in breast milk, and targets the fetus's developing nervous tissue. The answer, however, is not to sterilize all workers in these industries but rather to encourage flexibility, such as allowing lateral transfers to nonexposed areas for workers starting a family. Many hospitals allow nurses and pharmacists to avoid mixing chemicals when pregnancy is planned, for example. It would be better to use special equipment to minimize everyone's exposure, because many chemicals that damage the developing fetus may also cause cancer in adults.

There are pregnancy workplace issues as well. At one time, women who worked outside the home were expected to resign when pregnant for social and cultural reasons. We know now that pregnant women can safely engage in moderate activity up to the time of delivery. On the other hand, some pregnant women entering the skilled trades have been subjected to an all-or-nothing approach to their work performance. Reasonable modifications can be made to accommodate the physical demands of pregnancy. As the center of gravity and balance changes later in pregnancy, climbing and lifting requirements need to be altered. Metabolic demands may require activity modification and may limit the use of respirators and other protective gear.

These accommodations are reasonable, yet they— and adequate maternity leave—are contested by some employers and co-workers, especially in the traditionally male professions and the blue-collar trades. We should see our children as a societal resource and responsibility. When the child arrives, parents have new concerns. Adequate leave for mother and/or father; good, safe, reliable child care; and ease and acceptability of breast-feeding are important issues for parents. To work full-time and to breast-feed with no supplemental formula feedings require enormous effort; a woman needs both privacy and time during the workday to express milk. This can be nearly impossible in many job settings, particularly industrial ones.

Another breast-feeding concern is toxic substances in the milk. A number of known hazards, such as lead and PCBs (a chemical now banned but once used in paints, in adhesives, as a machinery lubricant, and as an insulator), may enter the milk from storage sites in bone and fat or from ongoing exposure. If there are serious concerns, breast milk can be analyzed for toxic substances. The benefits of breast-feeding are overwhelmingly clear, and women should discontinue breast-feeding only when toxic contaminants are confirmed.

Economics may be another issue. Because some employers have been inflexible concerning the need for maternity leave, child care, flexible shifts, and so on, women have been forced to drop in and out of the work force in response to the needs of their families. Some "women's work" is thus characterized by low pay and few or no chances for promotion. When women leave and reenter the work force, they lose seniority and benefits. In the past, it was expected that men's work would be subsidized by women willing to assume all household duties.

As women enter the work force, the stress of home management and conducting family affairs often escalates. The need to perform as parent, tutor, laundress, chauffeur, cook, and housekeeper as well as breadwinner may be the result of single parenthood, a negotiated distribution of responsibilities, or a simple need to keep the peace. Women may be unable to negotiate equitable sharing of family responsibilities or to identify and enlist sources of help and support, and so they end up tired and resentful.

The options available for each one of us to cope with balancing home and work may differ markedly, but options do exist. Children can perform meaningful chores if rewarded by an appreciative parent (who is not inclined to step in to do the task herself). Simple meals and housekeeping just sufficient enough to prevent the spread of disease may in fact be the price of sanity. The point is, each woman must decide where her priorities lie and which battles are worth fighting. If dirty windows depress you, you may get more benefit from paid housekeeping help than from a family vacation.

Men have been excluded from this discussion, not because they're exempt from these responsibilities but because it is a matter of individual choice how much any woman wishes to negotiate with her mate. We must learn to respect each other's decisions.

Physical violence most often occurs in the home and must not be tolerated under any circumstances. However, it can also be an occupational hazard and is the leading cause of on-the-job death for women. Women in traditional jobs, such as working in a store, and in less traditional ones, such as driving a bus, have been killed and injured in the line of work. For most of these crimes, the gender of the victim is immaterial, although some may involve sexual harassment or rape. The threat of violence disproportionately affects women. We need to respond to it with specific preventive measures. Safety issues, which affect men and women alike, include adequate lighting, security personnel, acrylic partitions, emergency call buttons, and training in self-defense.

Much more specific to women is the issue of sexual harassment, a form of physical and psychological violence. It is encountered in female and male settings. Occasional cases of vicious, concerted, criminal activity have been reported. It requires courage and self-confidence to report and stop sexual harassment, and the good news is that courageous, self-confident women are reshaping the face of American institutions from the military to industry to academia.

Women in the workplace can face an array of obstacles to safety, serenity, and success. While emotional and psychological obstacles to an ideal workplace may not seem quite as great a challenge as exposure to toxic chemicals or dangerous equipment, the danger is still real. Archaic values and institutions as well as emotional and psychological assaults not only can create an environment that overlooks or even fosters danger but can also create terrible stress, a threat to health and well-being that must be considered (see Chapter 9).

ON-THE-JOB RISKS

Men and women, for the most part, face the same hazards in the workplace. On-the-job risks can be categorized as safety hazards (those that cause injury) or health hazards (those that cause disease). This distinction isn't absolute, and some conditions, such as lower back pain, might be considered either an injury or a disease.

(These categories were initially set up to address industrial accidents but now include other problems.)

Safety Hazards

Safety hazards cause injury and death in obvious, often dramatic ways. Less obvious is the fact that good safety engineering and careful administration and inspection can prevent most of these tragedies. The term *accident* implies that an occurrence is unforeseen. Actually, careful evaluation of the worksite not only can foresee such problems but can often eliminate them.

Accurate statistics of deaths due to trauma in the workplace are difficult to ascertain, because different sources of information give different results. But approximately 10,000 workers die on the job each year, while another 22 million lose work because of a work-related injury (ranging in severity from mild sprains to permanent total impairment). Men greatly outnumber women in occupational mortality statistics, since they predominate in the more dangerous industries of mining, construction, and heavy-equipment operation. However, women who have entered these fields over the last 20 years have died these same preventable deaths. Because young workers are injured and killed disproportionately, the impact of this loss is far greater than the numbers themselves indicate. If we consider years of life lost (using the standard life expectancy for those killed), trauma, including motor vehicle, falls, and workplace injuries, causes greater losses than either heart disease or cancer.

The leading cause of death on the job is motor vehicle accidents, involving workers who drive as a part of their job. A review of motor vehicle safety gives us an opportunity to look at the *hierarchy of controls* that safety experts bring into play whenever safety issues are addressed. The first, best-level of response to a known hazard is to eliminate it. With auto safety, this would mean finding another work process—for example, communicating by fax or teleconference instead of traveling. The second level in the hierarchy is to substitute specific material or equipment, such as using the train instead of the automobile.

Since these solutions are often not feasible, the third choice for prevention—engineering control—becomes a very important one. This includes environmental engineering, such as safe roads with adequate lighting, entry ramps, and dividers, as well as safety engineering for the vehicles. Vehicle safety starts with design and materials and concludes with specific parts such as dashboards, steering columns, and airbags. The engineered parts must be tested for safety and efficacy; what's more, it's critical that there be follow-up evaluation under actual road conditions.

The last level of the hierarchy of controls involves protective devices that rely on individual cooperation and participation, such as wearing a seatbelt.

All occupational safety can be considered under this hierarchy of controls. Overall issues need to be considered first, such as whether a particular plant is safe enough to build (e.g., a nuclear power plant), and how far from housing or schools certain facilities need to be. Next, safety must be built into the design and materials of a plant as well as into each item of equipment. Each procedure that needs to be performed should also be examined in terms of safety. Scrupulous attention to detail, including railings, machine guards, lock-out procedures, routine inspection and maintenance, safety and fire drills, and housekeeping is part of a safe working environment. As the old poster said, "Safety is no accident!" To ensure that a high safety standard is maintained, facilities need a joint labor-management committee to evaluate the working environment and to solve safety problems.

Mining, construction, and agriculture, for which environmental engineering is difficult, have extremely high death and disability rates. Yet, even in these industries, careful consideration of equipment design, administrative practices, job training, safe work practices, and appropriate personal protective equipment can improve work site safety. Personal equipment (safety shoes, goggles, etc.) must fit properly, should not interfere with the worker's ability to function and communicate, and should be comfortable. Anyone who has ever been required to wear such equipment can testify that there is enormous room for improvement.

Health Hazards

Health hazards are often less obvious than safety hazards; the diseases they cause may take years to develop and often resemble diseases of nonoccupational origin. Occupational exposures may cause disease, join with other factors in developing disease, or may simply exacerbate a preexisting disease. All of this makes it difficult to measure the exact number of deaths and disabling conditions brought about by health hazards in the workplace. Conservative estimates attribute approximately 5 percent of cancer deaths to workplace carcinogen exposure. Job-related deaths from respiratory failure, poisoning, and renal and liver failure bring the estimated annual death toll to around 200,000. The toll of nonfatal disease is much higher. Common complaints include repetitive musculoskeletal injury (carpal tunnel syndrome, tendonitis, and the like), noise-induced hearing loss, dermatitis (skin inflammations), asthma, headaches, and stress-related symptoms (see Chapter 9). These problems impede functioning at work and at home. They often require medical care and interfere with the joy of living.

Health hazards are organized into four broad categories: biologic, mechanical, physical, and chemical. Biologic hazards include workplace-acquired infections such as hepatitis B and allergies to materials found at the job site. Mechanical hazards include repetitive lifting, pushing, pulling, and carrying as well as movements that require the individual to use awkward postures with varying degrees of force and repetition. Physical hazards consist of heat, cold, noise, vibration, light, high and low ambient air pressures, and various forms of radiation. Chemical hazards are ubiquitous in our workplaces and include both natural and synthetic substances such as solvents, metals, caustics, pesticides, catalysts, and acids.

In general, we need to consider whether a worker is actually being exposed to harmful substances and if it is possible to isolate the worker from such substances. Biologic and chemical hazards usually enter the body through breathing, swallowing, and/or skin absorption. Clouds of fine particles from grinding and heating (as when welding or burning) are inhaled. Workers who have inadequate hand-washing facilities or who eat or smoke at their work stations may ingest toxic material. Some substances are absorbed readily through the skin. For all categories of hazards we speak of a *dose-response* relationship. Within a normal range of varia-

tion and depending on the substance, there seems to be a connection between the amount of a substance a worker is exposed to and the severity of the symptoms or disease that results.

Disease can be prevented in much the same way accidents can. Safer procedures and substances can be substituted, as in agricultural practices that eliminate the need for pesticides and the use of fiberglass or rock wool insulation instead of asbestos. It is important to determine that the new substance doesn't have problems of its own, as has been the worry with fiberglass.

Engineering controls are also extremely important for disease prevention. Industrial hygienists—the engineers who usually address health hazards in the workplace—measure noise, chemicals, and other potential problems and design and implement machine modifications to protect the worker. Examples include sound-proofing the booth a machine operator works in and installing exhaust ventilation close to a welding or grinding operation. Similarly, ergonomists evaluate mechanical hazards and develop and monitor means for preventing diseases such hazards can cause. The sources of safety problems that affect both men and women aren't limited to the factory floor.

No discussion of workplace hazards would be complete without mentioning child labor—still a fact of life throughout the world. In the United States child labor problems are evident in apparently innocuous jobs such as working in a fast-food restaurant. In many of these facilities, improper safety standards expose our teenage children to burns and worse. Children are killed working on farms, where machinery can be frighteningly complex and is underregulated. Certain marginal industries, particularly ones that rely heavily on illegal aliens, also hire children.

YOUR LEGAL RIGHTS AND RESOURCES

You have a legal right to work in a place and in a manner that is safe and healthy. Some threats to this, such as blocked exits, may be obvious, will affect everyone who works with you, and are regulated. Other problems, such as allergies to office indoor air pollution that is worse than established standards, may appear to be unique to you. You will have to rely on your own instincts and observations about what you can change yourself (making sure to choose the safest possible car if you're in sales, for example) and what will require outside intervention.

Depending on your circumstances, there are many avenues to pursue in search of relief of workplace dangers or of health problems you suspect are work-related (see "Where to Go for Help"). You can turn to both government and private agencies for help in correcting and preventing occupational hazards. Government programs for occupational safety and health include federal, state, and local governments, with most of the resources being federal. OSHA was created by the Occupational Safety and Health Act of 1970. It is part of the Department of Labor and is charged with developing and enforcing regulations to ensure that every U.S. employee works in a safe and healthy environment.

Although the law says that the right to a safe and healthful workplace is absolute, in practice this right is often compromised. Employers balance workers' right against financial considerations. Supreme Court rulings have instructed OSHA to demonstrate the cost/benefit ratio of new regulations; improvements in work environments are usually restricted to what is feasible and what will not cause industry undue hardship.

Complicating things still further, the process of setting standards is slow. Public hearings on proposed regulations are held, and some of the presented ideas are then incorporated into the final standard. And once regulations are established, they are frequently challenged in court. Moreover, groups of workers, such as those employed by small businesses (less than 10 employees), domestic workers, agricultural workers, construction workers, and government employees, are exempt from part or all of OSHA protection. Some OSHA regional offices, however, implement the "general duty" clause when a more specific regulation is lacking. This clause requires that employers have a general duty to provide a safe and healthful workplace. A number of states have developed their own plans that may be substituted for OSHA's as long as basic federal requirements are met.

OSHA has recently begun to focus on hospital safety and health, which is important because of concern about bloodborne diseases and multiply resistant tuberculosis. Standards exist for bloodborne disease transmission and use of ethylene oxide and formaldehyde (disinfectants and preservatives).

Repetitive strain injury has also been targeted by OSHA. The musculoskeletal complaints associated with computers are more difficult to address. Some obvious adjustments in seating, posture, arm, and screen heights can be made. The federal government says that the number of people with these injuries may be as high as 282,000. In response, OSHA is initiating proceedings to create regulations requiring all employers, including those in office settings, to do more to prevent these repetitive strain disorders.

The worst office environment is likely to have fewer measurable toxic exposures than most industries, even during office renovation. However, because of the nature of office work, even these levels of exposure may produce symptoms. Paint thinner can cause headaches, and nose and throat irritation, for example. Cigarette smoke is another irritant often found in the office building.

Hazard Communication gives workers the right to know about any potentially hazardous materials in the workplace. The standard requires employers to arrange training and to keep copies of a *Material Safety Data Sheet* (MSDS) for each potentially hazardous material at the job site. MSDSs list the specific chemical names for materials and emergency and toxicity information. They are provided by the manufacturers and distributors and may be kept in the purchasing department or in the company's safety office. If you are concerned about an exposure at work or have an illness that may be work related, ask for an MSDS for each substance you work with. Your doctor or your union health and safety specialist can independently check on the health effects of the chemicals. The manufacturer's contact number is also provided on ths MSDS, along with a 24-hour hot line number to call in case of emergency spills. In case of a spill, the emergency response team or physician will be able to call the manufacturer directly and speak with a chemist or toxicologist so that proper medical attention can be provided.

IMPROVING THE WORKPLACE

Your workplace is a significant part of your life; what goes on there can affect your health in equal measure. Occupational health and safety is your right and the right of every working woman. Know your rights and resources, but be aware that those resources may be limited. The workplace is already better because of our input. We need to work both individually and together to make sure that improvements continue to be made.

WHERE TO GO FOR HELP

Association of Occupational and Environmental Clinics (AOEC). AOEC can refer you to the nearest clinic so that your work-related health problem can be attended to. It can be reached at 202-347-4976, Monday through Friday, 9:00 A.M. to 5:00 P.M., Eastern Time.

CHEMTREC. CHEMTREC operates a hotline (800-262-8200) to assist the general public with nonemergency health, safety, and environmental questions about chemical products. It also distributes *Material Safety Data Sheets,* which include information about particular chemicals that workers may be exposed to. The hotline is open Monday through Friday, 9:00 A.M. to 6:00 P.M., Eastern Time.

Equal Employment Opportunity Commission (EEOC). EEOC will discuss, or help you file a report on, workplace challenges to your health and well-being from any kind of discrimination, including sexual harassment. It can be reached 24 hours a day at 800-669-4000.

National Institute for Occupational Safety and Health (NIOSH). Part of the Center for Disease Control, NIOSH was set up to research occupational health and safety. If you have an unusual problem or one that OSHA cannot address call the institute at 800-356-4674. NIOSH can inspect a work site and make recommendations but has no enforcement powers. It can provide information on a variety of subjects and has a continuing education program.

Occupational Health and Safety Administration (OSHA). OSHA can inspect and enforce workplace safety regulations. It also offers free consultations to small businesses. Look in the government section of your telephone book under "Department of Labor" or "Labor Department."

Office of Occupational Medicine. The Office of Occupational Medicine is an OSHA consulting service for physicians who want more detailed information about an occupational illness or injury. You may want to mention this service to your doctor. It can be reached at 202-219-5003, Monday through Friday, 8:00 A.M. to 5:00 P.M., Eastern Time.

Union. Find out if your union has a health and safety officer. That person may know of other local, national, and international resources.

Workers Compensation. Workers compensation provides income support and medical expenses for workers disabled by work-related injury or illness. It may offer help if your problem is not yet regulated or you have problems that fall under official guidelines. Look in the government section of your telephone book under "Department of Labor" or "Labor Department."

CHAPTER 7

Substance Abuse in Women

Roselyn Payne Epps, M.D., M.P.H., M.A., F.A.A.P., and
Anne Geller, M.D.

Over the centuries, drugs have been used for rituals, for pain relief, for social bonding, and to help people function day to day. When used properly, some drugs are not harmful. If abused, however, mind-altering drugs can pose serious health risks, cause dependency, and interfere with work and relationships. Women should be aware of the risks of drugs. They can then make informed choices about using them and know when to seek help at the first signs of trouble.

Statistically, women are less likely than men to abuse drugs, but substance use among women is increasing at an alarming rate. Cigarette smoking, for example, has decreased overall but has increased among women aged 16–22, who are more likely than their male counterparts to smoke. Estimates indicate that of the 15.1 million Americans who abuse alcohol or are alcohol-dependent, 4.6 million are women. This means that roughly one-third of alcoholics are women.

Women are prone to special problems linked with drug use. Although they may drink less than men, the health impact on women is greater. They are more subject to alcohol-related liver disease, experience menstrual disorders associated with alcohol use, and are more likely to become victims of aggressive acts when under the influence of alcohol. Over twice as many women as men are admitted to emergency rooms as a result of the overuse of tranquilizers. More than 80 percent of cases of acquired immune deficiency syndrome (AIDS) in women are associated with intravenous drug use. And the use of cigarettes, alcohol, and other drugs during pregnancy can cause serious harm to the fetus, especially in the first weeks of gestation, when a woman may not know she is pregnant.

HOW DRUGS AFFECT THE MIND AND BODY

Messages are sent from the body to the brain by means of electrical signals that are conveyed to the nerve cells in the brain through neurotransmitters. Any substance that interferes with these neurotransmitters, such as mood-altering drugs, can short-circuit these messages. Different drugs have different effects, but they all affect brain chemistry. Even small changes can greatly affect one's mood.

There are four types of mind-altering drugs: sedatives, narcotics, stimulants, and hallucinogens (see Table 7.1). All have the potential for psychological dependence and physical addiction. Because these drugs affect the part of the brain responsible for pleasure, euphoria, or pain relief, they can easily lead to abuse. The risk increases with the strength of the drug,

the amount, the speed with which it reaches the brain, and how often it is taken. In order of increasing risk, drugs can be taken by mouth, by sniffing or snorting, by smoking, and by injecting into a vein.

The effects of drugs vary with the individual. Men seem to process alcohol in their bodies faster than women, for example. The very young and the very old are more intolerant of drugs. Weight is also a factor; those who weigh less are affected more. Many drug takers use more than one substance at a time—either an illegal drug, alcohol, or tobacco. Older women especially are not only more susceptible to alcohol but also often take multiple medications that can interact with even small amounts of alcohol to produce a harmful reaction.

WHO IS AT RISK?

Women who are at higher risk for substance abuse include those with the following history:

- Biologic daughter of an alcohol- or drug-abusing parent
- Spouse of an alcoholic or drug abuser
- Women who have recently experienced traumatic life events, such as

  Divorce or separation
  Death of spouse or significant other
  Job loss
  Retirement
  Rape or sexual abuse
  Witnessed a traumatic event

- Women with a physical handicap or disability

TABLE 7.1.   TYPES OF MIND-ALTERING DRUGS

Sedatives	Narcotics	Stimulants	Hallucinogens
Drugs in Everyday Products		Alcohol Caffeine Nicotine	
Prescription Drugs			
SLEEPING PILLS Amytal Dalmane Doriden Halcion Nembutal Placidyl Quaalude Seconal	Codeine Darvon Demerol Dilaudid Lomotil Methadone Morphine Percodan Talwin	Benzedrine Control Dexedrine Dexatrim Methedrine Preludin Ritalin Tennate	
TRANQUILIZERS Ativan Librium Miltown Serax Tranxene Valium			
Street Drugs Blues Downs Goofballs Nembies Red devils Yellowjackets	Heroin (skag, horse, junk, stuff) Methadone (dollies) Darvon (pinks and greens)	Bennies Cocaine (crack, snow, flake, coke) Crystal Dexies Hearts Speed	Marijuana (grass, pot, weed) Hash LSD (acid, cube, D) PCP (angel dust, hog, peace pill)

- Health care professionals
- Women who have a psychiatric disorder (depression, psychosis, anxiety, hyperactivity)

There are both physical and psychological signs of drug abuse. Some physical signs include tremors, slurred speech, irregular heart beat, cough and runny nose, and nervous mannerisms. Psychological problems can include memory loss, panic, paranoia, unexplained mood swings, and personality changes. Vague complaints such as fatigue, insomnia, headaches, sexual problems, and loss of appetite can be early red flags that a person may have a drug problem.

TYPES OF DRUGS AND THEIR EFFECTS

Tobacco

Cigarette smoking is the single most preventable cause of disease and death in the United States. The statistics are grim:

- The average cigarette smoker shortens her life by 5–8 years.

- One of every six deaths in the United States is related to smoking.
- Cigarette smoking now contributes to 30 percent of all cancer deaths.
- Smoking is responsible for over half of the deaths from cardiovascular disease in women less than 65 years old.

■ Smoking is linked to various types of cancer, chronic lung disease, and reproductive problems.

Despite these serious health risks, 26 percent of reproductive age women (18–44 years old) smoke an average of 18 cigarettes per day. Smoking is also on the rise among young women; the number of smokers aged 12–18 years has doubled in the past 10 years. More teenage girls than boys now smoke. This trend toward early initiation of smoking behavior is ominous because many of the health risks associated with smoking increase both with earlier onset of smoking and duration of the smoking.

The number of women smokers is almost the same as the number of male smokers because more men than women have stopped smoking. But women are as susceptible as men to the harmful effects of tobacco. In addition, smoking during pregnancy poses special concerns to a woman and her fetus.

What Is in a Cigarette?

Cigarette smoking became popular among women after 1940 as more and more women entered the work force. During 1953–54, there was a decline in the num-

TABLE 7.2.   WOMEN SMOKERS

Characteristic	1992 %
Race/Ethnicity	
White	25.9
African American	24.1
Hispanic	18.0
American Indian/Alaskan Native	39.8
Asian/Pacific Islander	4.0
Education level (yrs)	
<12	27.5
12	28.2
13–15	23.1
16	14.6
Age group (yrs)	
18–24	24.9
25–44	28.8
45–64	26.1
≥65	12.4
Socioeconomic status	
All above poverty level	23.8
Below poverty level	31.7
Unknown	22.1
Total	24.6

ADDICTIVE PERSONALITY TRAITS

Certain personality types appear to be linked to drug abuse:

■ Impulsiveness
■ Difficulty in delaying gratification
■ Sensation-seeking
■ Rebelliousness
■ Weak commitment to social goals
■ Sense of alienation
■ Low tolerance for stress

Other characteristics (may appear in combination with above):

■ Low self-esteem
■ Vulnerability to anxiety and depression
■ History of conflicting parental expectations

ber of cigarettes smoked as reports began to emerge linking cigarette smoking and lung cancer. The Surgeon General has identified ways in which smoking cigarettes poses risks for lung cancer and other lung disorders. The Surgeon General's 1988 report warned that nicotine, a main ingredient in cigarettes, is as addictive as heroin and cocaine. Smoking, the report stated, must be viewed as a life-threatening addiction and not merely an unhealthy habit. In 1992, the Environmental Protection Agency (EPA) classified tobacco smoke as a class A carcinogen, placing it in the same category of cancer-causing agents as asbestos and benzene.

These early warnings led to the increased use of filter cigarettes and brands with less tar and nicotine. Lower tar and nicotine cigarettes are not the answer, however. The reported amounts of these harmful substances do not necessarily represent the smoker's actual intake. Also, evidence is mounting that individuals who switch to these brands inhale more deeply, smoke a greater proportion of cigarettes and, in some cases, smoke more. Many conventional filter cigarettes may, in fact, deliver more carbon monoxide than nonfilter cigarettes. Even the lowest yield cigarettes present health hazards that are very much higher than not smoking at all.

More than 4,000 chemicals have been identified in tobacco smoke, including carbon monoxide, oxides of nitrogen, ammonia, polycyclic aromatic hydrocarbons, hydrogen cyanide, vinyl chloride, and nicotine. Many of these substances are known carcinogens.

Nicotine is the addictive substance in cigarettes. Nicotine affects all major organs and systems in the body, including the nervous system, voluntary muscles, stomach, intestines, heart, brain, and oral cavity. Nicotine is distributed throughout the body and processed by several organs, including the liver. Eventually, it is cleared through the kidneys.

Nicotine is an addictive substance that reinforces and strengthens the desire to smoke. Nicotine stimulates the release of the brain's opiates, the endorphins, which have a number of effects on the brain. Smoking can alter brain chemicals to promote feelings of reward and well-being, reduce anxiety, and reduce hunger. For these reasons, nicotine creates a psychological as well as a physical dependence.

IMPACT OF SMOKING ON WOMEN

The lack of large-scale studies that focus specifically on female populations makes it difficult to fully assess the impact of smoking on women. However, women show the same responses to cigarette smoking as men. Depending on the number of cigarettes smoked per day, the age of beginning cigarette smoking, and the amount of inhalation, women have death rates similar to men.

In general, women who are smokers experience more illness and chronic conditions than women who have never smoked. According to the American Cancer Society, women who smoke heavily have nearly three times more bronchitis and emphysema, 75 percent more chronic sinusitis, and 50 percent more peptic ulcers than nonsmokers. The incidence of illness, such as influenza, for women smokers is 20 percent higher for women who smoke than for those who don't. Currently employed women smokers report more days lost from work due to illness and injury than working women who do not smoke. In addition, women under 65 years of age who smoke have more limited physical activity than those who have never smoked. More than that, women smokers show an increased rate of heart attacks, cancer, oral diseases, and lung conditions.

Cardiovascular Disease

Coronary heart disease, including heart attacks, is the major cause of death among women in the United States. In general, cigarette smoking doubles the risk: Carbon monoxide slows the transfer of oxygen from the blood to the body. Nicotine increases the heart rate by 15–25 beats per minute, and blood pressure goes up by 15–25 points. When combined with high blood pressure and high blood cholesterol, smoking multiplies the risk of having a heart attack.

Women smokers who also use oral contraceptives are 10 times more at risk for having a heart attack. Additionally, smoking increases the risk for hypertension and brain hemorrhage.

Cancer

There has been a rapid increase in the number of lung cancer deaths among women. Women who are heavy smokers are 24 times more likely to develop lung cancer than those who have never smoked, and lung cancer is now the leading cause of cancer deaths in women, exceeding even breast cancer.

The warning signals of lung cancer are:

- A cough that won't go away
- Sputum (secretion coughed up from the lungs streaked with blood)
- Chest pain
- Recurring attacks of pneumonia or bronchitis

Lung cancer is often discovered in advanced stages of the disease, when it is difficult to treat and when it is too late to be cured by surgery. Only 13 percent of lung cancer patients live 5 or more years after it is diagnosed (see box on "The Problem of Passive Smoking").

Cigarette smoking also is linked with cancer of the larynx, the mouth, the esophagus, and the pancreas. Heavy alcohol intake combined with cigarette smoking increases the risk of oral, laryngeal, and esophageal cancer. In women, smoking is associated with cancer of the cervix.

Oral Cavity Diseases

Tobacco use is a prime cause of oral diseases, including cancer and other serious conditions. Smoking also increases dental treatment management risks and problems. Those who use tobacco show slower healing of wounds, and periodontal disease treatment may be negatively affected by smoking.

THE PROBLEM OF PASSIVE SMOKING

Cigarette smokers are not the only ones to suffer from cigarette smoke. Tobacco smoke in the environment, also called passive, secondhand, or environmental smoke, is harmful to anyone around the smoker. In fact, studies have shown that environmental tobacco smoke is a cause of lung cancer in humans, responsible for about 3,000 lung cancer deaths annually in the United States. Women who live or work with smokers are especially at risk.

Exposure to tobacco smoke also causes tissue irritation. The main effects are in the eyes and mucous membranes of the nose, throat, and lower respiratory system. Children who are exposed to passive smoke are more likely to suffer from respiratory illness, severe asthma, and middle ear problems.

Lung Disease

There is a rising death rate due to chronic obstructive pulmonary disease (COPD) among women who smoke. The prevalence of chronic bronchitis varies directly with the number of cigarettes smoked per day. A close relationship also exists between cigarette smoking and chronic cough and sputum production, which increases with the number of cigarettes smoked.

Smoking also causes emphysema, a progressive disease that destroys the elasticity of the lungs and makes it difficult to breathe. Almost 80 percent of people with emphysema smoke or once smoked.

SMOKING AND REPRODUCTION

Studies in women and men suggest that cigarette smoking may impair fertility. In women, substantial data demonstrate that smoking lowers the age of menopause. The average age of menopause in nonsmokers is 50; among women smoking one-half pack a day, it is 49; in those smoking one or more packs a day, 48. Evidence suggests that the earlier menopause of smokers is not related to weight differences between smokers and nonsmokers but rather is a direct result of some component of cigarette smoke. Smoking also increases the risk of osteoporosis, a condition that causes the bones to become brittle and break, in menopausal women.

Smoking during Pregnancy

Smoking during pregnancy increases the risk of miscarriage, stillbirth, preterm delivery, and low birth weight. When a pregnant woman smokes she risks her own health and that of her baby, before, during, and after birth.

Babies born to women who smoke during pregnancy weigh, on the average, 7 ounces less than babies born to nonsmoking women. The relation between smoking by the mother and lower birth weight is separate from other factors that can influence birth weight, including race, number of previous births, maternal weight, socioeconomic status, sex of the child, and length of the pregnancy. If a woman gives up smoking early in her pregnancy, her risk of having a low-birth-weight baby approaches that of a nonsmoker.

The risk of spontaneous abortion, fetal death, and neonatal death increases directly with levels of maternal smoking during pregnancy. Increasing levels of smoking result in a significant increase in the risk of early separation of the placenta, which connects the mother and fetus, and rupture of the membranes, which surround the fetus and contain the amniotic fluid. There is also a higher risk of complications during pregnancy for women who smoke.

Babies of smokers seem to be more susceptible to diseases. Sudden infant death syndrome (SIDS) occurs 2½ times more often among babies of smoking mothers.

HOW TO QUIT SMOKING

The benefits of not smoking start within days of quitting. As the carbon monoxide level in your blood decreases, the oxygen level increases. The heart beat slows to normal, and the lungs begin to clear and heal.

After 1 or 2 years of not smoking, your risk of a heart attack drops sharply and gradually returns to normal after about 10 years. The risk of cancer is gradually reduced, coming close to that of nonsmokers after 10–15 years. In addition to health benefits, quitting smoking also creates a healthy environment for others in the household. Spouses of nonsmokers have half the lung cancer risk of spouses living with smokers, and infants are less apt to experience respiratory and ear problems.

Despite all the incentives, smoking is not easy to overcome. But every year more than 3 million Americans quit smoking. Nearly half of all adults who ever smoked have quit for life.

The Steps to Smoking Cessation

First, decide to quit. Try to avoid negative thoughts about how difficult it might be (see "Ways to Quit Smoking"). Some ideas that will help are:

- List all the reasons you want to quit and review the reasons every day.
- Begin to condition yourself physically: Exercise, drink more fluids, get plenty of rest, and avoid fatigue.
- Set a target date for quitting—perhaps your birthday, your anniversary, or some other day of personal significance.
- On the day you quit, throw away all your cigarettes and matches, and hide your ashtrays and lighter.
- Visit the dentist to get your teeth cleaned of the cigarette stains.
- Ask your family and friends to help you over the rough spots.

The first few days after quitting, spend as much free time as possible in places where smoking isn't allowed. Develop a clean, fresh, nonsmoking environment around yourself at work and at home.

Many people who are considering quitting, especially women, are concerned about gaining weight.

Quitting doesn't necessarily result in weight gain, however. About one-third of ex-smokers gain weight, but another one-third actually lose a few pounds. When ex-smokers gain weight, it is usually because they eat more. On average, expect to gain anywhere from 5 to 20 pounds. Your weight gain can be minimal if you eat low-fat foods and exercise.

Many smokers have withdrawal symptoms when they quit. Symptoms usually occur within 24 hours of stopping smoking: Some of the more common symptoms are lack of concentration, anxiety, irritability, insomnia, fatigue, constipation, and hunger. These are signs that the body is recovering from smoking and clearing itself of nicotine, a powerful addictive chemical. Be patient. Most of the nicotine is gone from the body in 2–3 days and withdrawal symptoms usually end within 2–4 weeks. The urge to smoke will last longer however.

Some people find it easier to quit by using a nicotine patch or nicotine gum. These forms of nicotine replacement deliver small doses of the drug to the body in an attempt to help smokers wean themselves off cigarettes. Although nicotine replacements may relieve the symptoms of withdrawal, they may not completely relieve the craving for cigarettes.

Both the gum and the patch are considered medications and must be prescribed by a physician or dentist. The dose varies with the individual's previous level of smoking. Do not continue smoking after starting the medication. Nicotine replacement should not be used by pregnant or breastfeeding women, or by people with certain heart conditions or health problems.

The unpleasant aftereffects of quitting are only temporary. They signal the beginning of a healthier life. The benefits of giving up cigarettes far outweigh the drawbacks.

The Relapse Factor

Most relapses occur in the first week after quitting, when withdrawal symptoms are strongest and your body is still dependent on nicotine. Gird yourself against the urge to resume smoking by calling on all your willpower, family, and friends to get you through this critical period. Other relapses occur during the first 3 months after quitting, when certain stressful situations may have you reaching automatically for a cigarette—your old pathway to relaxation. Keep alert to these relapse potentials, and avoid them.

If the urge to smoke is overwhelming, remind yourself that you've quit and you're now a nonsmoker. Then analyze your sudden urge to smoke. Ask yourself these questions:

- Where was I when I got the urge?
- What was I doing at the time?
- Whom was I with?
- What was I thinking?

Typical triggers to smoking include working under pressure, feeling blue, finishing a meal, watching tele-

WAYS TO QUIT SMOKING

Many people go cold turkey when they throw away their cigarettes—it's a tried and true method that might work for you. If you prefer a more gradual approach, try these steps:

- *Switch brands.* Try a brand that you find distasteful, or change to a brand that's low in tar and nicotine a few weeks before your target date for quitting. Don't smoke more cigarettes, however, or inhale more often or more deeply.

- *Cut down on the number of cigarettes you smoke.* Smoke only half of each cigarette, or decide that you'll smoke only during particular times of the day. Or decide beforehand how many cigarettes you'll smoke during the day. There's no substitute for quitting, however. If you're down to five or six cigarettes a day, quit.

- *Think before you light up.* Smoke only those cigarettes you really want. Don't smoke only out of habit. Make yourself aware of each cigarette you smoke—put the pack in an unfamiliar location or look in the mirror each time you light up. You may decide you don't need it.

- *Make smoking inconvenient.* Stop buying cigarettes by the carton. Wait until one pack is empty before buying another. Don't carry cigarettes with you at home or at work. Make it tough to get one.

vision, having a drink, and watching someone else smoke. Anticipate these triggers and prepare to avoid them. Find activities that make smoking difficult. Exercise. Avoid places where smoking is permitted. Reduce your consumption of alcohol, which often stimulates the desire to smoke. And reward yourself for not smoking—treat yourself to a concert, a movie, or a new dress.

ALCOHOL

Alcohol has long been an integral part of most societies, although it is a custom that has not always included women. As women left the home and increasingly entered the work force, they also faced decisions about what constitutes an acceptable level of drinking. The line between alcohol use, or social drinking, and abuse may be hard to draw. In general, alcohol use is light to moderate drinking—one or two drinks at different times. Abuse is drinking in large amounts or in binges.

The number of women in the United States who drink alcohol has increased significantly over the past 40 years. About 60 percent of adult women in the United States drink, and nearly half drink once a week or more.

According to one survey, 3.5 million American

women are using alcohol inappropriately and may be classified as suffering from alcoholism. Young women (age 21–34) report the highest rates of specific drinking-related problems. About 16 percent of young, employed women are heavy drinkers, consuming 3–5 drinks per day. Women age 35–49 have the highest rates of chronic alcohol problems. It is also estimated that 10–15 percent of the elderly women in this country abuse alcohol, many of whom developed the problem after age 60.

Drinking varies among women of different racial or ethnic backgrounds. African-American women are less likely to drink than white women. Hispanic women drink infrequently, less than African-American or white women, although this may change as they enter new social and work arenas. Marital status also influences

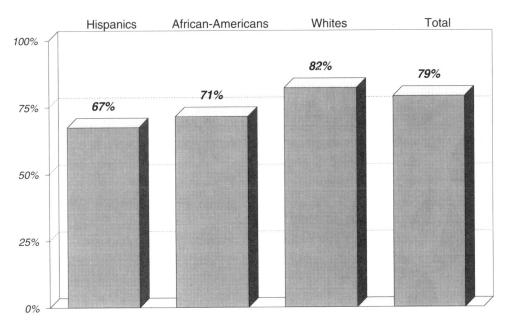

Figure 7.1. U.S. Women Who Have Used Alcohol (%, 1992).

drinking habits. Single, divorced, or separated women are more likely to drink heavily and experience alcohol-related problems than women who are married or widowed. Unmarried women who are living with partners are most likely to develop drinking problems. Alcoholism tends to run in families, and alcoholics often marry other alcoholics. (See Fig. 7.1)

A drinking problem can develop over time. For some women, alcohol problems take 10–20 years to develop; in others such problems occur in a matter of months. Abuse can also arise as the result of a life crisis, such as the loss of a loved one, or stress imposed by marriage and family problems or financial difficulties. Alcohol can cause problems when used as a means of combating low self-esteem or to overcome loneliness or shyness. Women may become addicted to alcohol to help them deal with a physical loss, such as a miscarriage, mastectomy, or hysterectomy.

There is no single profile of a problem drinker; it occurs at all ages, in all types of people. Likewise, there is no one single factor that causes problems with alcohol. Alcohol use is affected by a variety of factors, including the physical and psychological effects of dependency.

The Effects of Alcohol

Alcohol is a drug that depresses the central nervous system. The initial effect is to stimulate thought, action, and sociability, or to induce a pleasant emotional state.

If drinking continues, the depressant effects on the brain take control, disrupting thinking and coordination and resulting in mood swings, irritability, and depression.

The strength of alcohol's effect is directly related to the amount of alcohol in the blood. Alcohol is metabolized at a rate of 3/4 ounce of absolute alcohol per hour. This is equal to one drink that contains 1 1/2 ounces of 100 proof hard liquor, 4 ounces of wine, or 8 ounces of beer. If a person drinks faster than this rate, the blood and brain alcohol levels rise and mood and behavior changes occur.

Women generally weigh less than men and also have a higher proportion of body fat to water. Thus, a woman achieves a higher level of alcohol in her blood faster than a man of the same size who drinks the same amount. The effect of alcohol also can vary with the stage of the menstrual cycle due to changes in the amount of body fluid. Just before menstruation, a woman retains fluid. There is more water in the body for the alcohol to be distributed in, thus the alcohol has less effect. In the middle of the menstrual cycle, when a woman is losing fluid, the same amount of alcohol can have a much stronger effect.

Those who are alcohol dependent have no ability to control their alcohol intake. Drinking takes place in response to intense internal mental and physical demands of which the drinker is often not aware. When this occurs, alcohol can disrupt relationships and pose serious health risks.

In addition to the personal misery and social distress suffered by a woman who abuses alcohol, her life span is about 15 years shorter than that of the average woman because of accidents that occur while drinking and as a result of damage to organs in the body. Not only does alcohol increase the risk of injuries from falls and driving accidents, it also makes a women vulnerable to being the victim of robbery, physical abuse, and date rape. Alcohol abuse damages the heart, liver, ovaries, brain, nerves, muscles, and blood cells, and can lead to certain types of cancer. It causes damage directly by attacking the delicate membranes surrounding cells and indirectly because of the poor nutrition that usually goes along with heavy drinking. In addition to death from liver failure, hemorrhage, or severe brain damage, alcohol causes illnesses such as inflammation of the liver (hepatitis), inflammation of the pancreas, heart failure, damage to the bone marrow causing anemia, and severe memory loss. Alcohol also has effects unique to women that result in risks to her health as well as that of her future children.

ALCOHOL AND THE SPECIAL CONCERNS OF WOMEN

Most studies on alcohol and alcohol-related problems are based on men, and the results are different when these studies are repeated in women. Physically and mentally, women respond differently to alcohol than do men, and the impact of alcohol appears to be greater on women than men:

- *Depression.* People who abuse alcohol often feel depressed, and alcohol can increase depression. The incidence of suicide attempts is higher in alcoholic women than in the female population as a whole.

- *Liver damage.* Women are more susceptible to alcohol-related liver damage. They develop liver disease in a shorter time and at lower levels of consumption than do men. The number of alcoholic women who develop alcohol-related liver disease is higher than among alcoholic men.

- *Cancer.* Alcohol has been linked to cancer of the breast, although the relationship is unclear. There does seem to be an association between alcohol use and hormone levels, causing changes in a woman's menstrual function.

With excess drinking, menstruation may become irregular or stop, and fertility is decreased.

- *Fetal damage.* Drinking during pregnancy can pose serious risks to the fetus. The more a woman drinks, the greater the danger, especially in the early stages of pregnancy. When a woman drinks, the alcohol quickly reaches the fetus through the placenta and can damage its delicate systems while they are being developed. Alcohol also increases the risk of miscarriage.

The most serious risk of drinking during pregnancy is *fetal alcohol syndrome.* This is the most common cause of mental retardation in babies. Babies are shorter, weigh less, have heart and facial defects, and have poor control over body movements. Children with fetal alcohol syndrome often are hyperactive; they are nervous, jittery, and have poor attention spans. It is not known how much alcohol can cause fetal alcohol syndrome, so it is recommended that pregnant women do not drink any alcohol.

WHEN DRINKING BECOMES A PROBLEM

It is difficult to know how much alcohol is too much or when use becomes abuse. The effects vary with the individual and depend on a variety of factors such as what motivates her to drink, her patterns of drinking, and how long and how much she drinks. Certain tests can show signs of a drinking problem (see boxes on CAGE and T-ACE questionnaires). There are also some warning signs of a drinking problem:

- Having an auto accident after leaving a party in a state of intoxication

- Missing work or being late to work because of a hangover
- Not being able to perform housework or daily functions
- Having memory lapses or blackouts
- Having intercourse with someone to whom you would not ordinarily be attracted
- Fighting with friends or hitting one's children
- Being preoccupied with drinking and organizing activities and social functions around it
- Having marriage or family problems in which drinking could be a factor

CAGE QUESTIONNAIRE

A positive response to only one of the first three questions may be an early sign of a drinking problem. A positive response to the last question is considered a sign of a more serious problem that requires treatment.

C   Have you ever felt you ought to **C**ut down on your drinking?

A   Have people **A**nnoyed you by criticizing your drinking?

G   Have you ever felt bad or **G**uilty about your drinking?

E   Have you ever had a drink first thing in the morning to steady your nerves or get rid of a hangover (**E**ye opener)?

Source: J. A. Ewing, Detecting Alcoholism: The CAGE Questionnaire. *Journal of the American Medical Association* 252 (1984): 1907.

Some drinking patterns may be a sign of trouble with alcohol:

- Being intoxicated more than once or twice a year
- Drinking more than a glass of wine or an occasional beer when alone
- Drinking to relieve stress or to allay anxiety
- Drinking to relieve insomnia, tension, depression, or pain
- Drinking after a party is over or the next morning to relieve a hangover

A person who has a problem with alcohol use may be reluctant to think about it or to seek advice for fear of being labeled an alcoholic. The label is not as important, however, as the effect on that person's life. Alcoholism is a disease that needs treatment. A woman who is drinking more than she would like to, who is having difficulty controlling her alcohol intake, or who finds that alcohol is having a disruptive effect on her life should seek help.

Getting Help

More and more women are seeking professional help for alcoholism as they confront the incompatibility between the economic reality of gainful employment and

T-ACE QUESTIONNAIRE

For the TOLERANCE question, an answer of more than two drinks is considered a positive response. A score of 2 is assigned for a positive response to the TOLERANCE question, and a score of 1 is assigned to all others for positive responses. A T-ACE score of 2 or greater is considered a sign of a drinking problem.

T   How many drinks does it take to make you feel high (TOLERANCE)?

A   Have people ANNOYED you by criticizing your drinking?

C   Have you felt you ought to CUT DOWN on your drinking?

E   Have you ever had a drink first thing in the morning to steady your nerves or get rid of a hangover (EYE OPENER)?

Source: R. J. Sokol, S. S. Martier, J. W. Ager, "The T-ACE Questions: Practical Prenatal Detection of Risk-Drinking." *American Journal of Obstetrics and Gynecology* 160 (1989): 865.

the compelling need to drink. One in every three members of Alcoholics Anonymous (AA) is now a woman; many women attend employer-sponsored alcoholism treatment programs.

Alcoholics Anonymous has led the way in demonstrating the effectiveness of self-help. Meetings are held throughout the United States and Canada and the 2 million members are committed to the common goal of maintaining their sobriety one day at a time.

Alcoholism is a family problem and can arise in any member. The alcoholic should be confronted with the problem and directed to help. In addition to Alcoholics

Anonymous, other groups such as Al-Anon, Al-Ateen, and the National Association for Children of Alcoholics may be helpful.

Professional treatment is available through physicians and counselors such as psychiatrists, psychologists, and social workers. Their services may be available privately or through clinics, hospitals, or rehabilitation centers. Other sources of help include community mental health centers or programs available through employers. In major cities the National Council on Alcoholism has affiliates that maintain a list of treatment sources.

PRESCRIPTION DRUGS

It is estimated that up to 2 percent of Americans use psychotherapeutic drugs—tranquilizers, sleeping pills, stimulants, and pain killers. Because of the mind-altering capability of these drugs, they have a potential to be misused. Misuse becomes abuse when these drugs are used in greater amounts or for purposes other than those for which they were prescribed. Misuse can result in a psychological or physical dependency or both. Although these drugs can bring relief of symptoms such as anxiety, sleeplessness, and pain, they also have side effects and hazards that should be weighed against their benefits.

Tranquilizers

Properly used, tranquilizers can provide short-term treatment of anxiety and stress caused by emotional conflict or a sudden trauma. They should be considered a bridge to other, more long-term forms of therapy and should always be used under the direction of a doctor.

The effect of tranquilizers on the brain is similar to that of alcohol. Low doses bring a feeling of relaxation and cheerfulness, while higher doses cause intoxication. Long-term use can lead to dependency similar to alcohol. When the drug is stopped symptoms such as severe anxiety, jitteriness, and insomnia can appear. Some women experience severe withdrawal symptoms, including emotional distress, dizziness, restlessness, headaches, and gastrointestinal upsets.

Women who are at risk of abusing drugs should not use tranquilizers. Signs of abuse include using more of the drug than prescribed, increasing the dose, or using tranquilizers to get intoxicated.

Sleeping Pills

Drugs to relieve insomnia are barbiturates and hypnotics. Although these drugs may have a value in certain short-term circumstances, long-term use can cause more harm than good. Prolonged use of sleeping pills can lead to dependency and side effects that continue after the person stops taking the drug. Tolerance can develop quickly and it becomes necessary to increase the amount of the drug to achieve the same effect. With increasing use, the effects of these drugs persist the next day and can result in mental cloudiness, poor concentration, memory difficulties, mood swings, anxiety, depression, and irritability. Withdrawal effects are similar to tranquilizers but more severe.

Amphetamines

Stimulants such as benzedrine and dexedrine were once prescribed for weight loss. These drugs increase energy and depress appetite, which makes them appealing and, at the same time, subject to abuse. The body adapts quickly to these drugs, however, so after an initial weight loss, appetite returns and the weight is regained. For this reason, as well as because of their tendency to produce psychological and physical dependence, these drugs have been banned for weight-reduction purposes by the Food and Drug Administration. Often they are used illegally, however, to boost the effects of other drugs. Long-term use can result in agitation and insomnia, and they have a high potential for overdose.

Pain Killers

Addictive pain killers are related in some way to opium. Some are derivatives of morphine, whereas others share some of its properties. They include prescription pain relief drugs as well as heroin and methadone. Pain killers have long-lasting effects, mainly on the brain, nervous system, and muscles, producing a sense of well-being, relaxation, and decreased sensitivity to pain. Side effects include constipation, kidney disease, and overdose. Pain killers are highly addictive and, when withdrawn, cause physical and mental symptoms that can be serious.

ILLICIT DRUGS

Illegal drug use is widespread and affects people of all backgrounds. According to a recent survey, 7 percent of Americans use illegal drugs, such as marijuana, cocaine, and opiates. Of the nearly 60 million women of childbearing age (15–44 years), over 5 million (9 percent) use marijuana or cocaine monthly if not more frequently. (See Fig. 7.2 and 7.3)

In addition to the effects of the drugs themselves, drug use poses other risks that relate to an unhealthy lifestyle. Female drug abusers have a higher incidence of sexually transmitted diseases, believed to stem from the practice of trading sex for drugs. Drug abusers also have poor nutrition, making them susceptible to illness. Drug users who share needles are at risk of getting infections such as hepatitis B virus and human immunodeficiency virus, which causes acquired immune deficiency disease (AIDS).

Abuse of illicit drugs during pregnancy can pose serious problems for the fetus. Both cocaine and heroin can cause preterm birth and fetal death. When a woman uses drugs during pregnancy her baby can become addicted to them just as she can. Babies born with an addiction show signs of withdrawal from the drug soon after birth.

Cocaine

Derived from the coca plant, cocaine can be snorted, injected, or smoked. The availability of crack cocaine, a pure form of the drug that is smoked, has led to its widespread use. It is estimated that about 5 million men and women in the United States are regular users.

Shortly after it is ingested, cocaine produces an intense sense of euphoria and well-being that lasts about 30 minutes. Other effects include heightened self-confidence, a rush of energy, increased sensuality, and loss of appetite. The high is rapidly followed by a low, which increases the urge to repeat the drug and leads to addiction. Prolonged use results in nervousness, insomnia, inability to concentrate, fatigue, anxiety, and depression. The crack form of cocaine, because it is the quickest and most effective way to achieve the high, is the most popular form of the drug. It is also the most addictive, with addiction occurring within 6 months of use.

Regardless of how it is ingested cocaine affects all the major body systems. It causes an effect similar to a burst of adrenaline, increasing the heart rate, blood pressure, breathing rate, and temperature. This type of

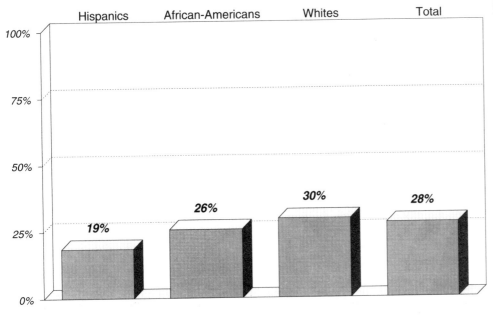

Figure 7.2. U.S. Women Who Have Used Marijuana (%, 1992).

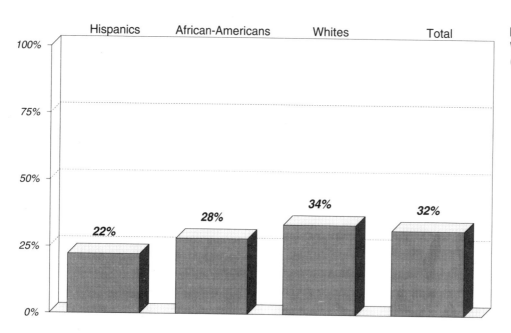

Figure 7.3. U.S. Women Who Have Used Illegal Drugs (%, 1992).

body stress places a great demand on the heart and blood vessels and can lead to chest pain, heart attack, or stroke. Cocaine also stimulates the brain and can cause seizures and convulsions. When used repeatedly, cocaine causes cells to die from lack of oxygen. When it is snorted, for instance, the dead cells in the nose become irritated and swell, causing congestion. Eventually, so many cells may die that a hole appears in the membrane separating the nostrils, which requires corrective surgery.

Narcotics

Opiates, also known as narcotics, are drugs distilled from opium that dull the senses, relieve pain, and produce sleep. They are used as pain relievers (see ''Prescription Drugs'') and abused as illegal drugs such as heroin. Heroin can be ingested by snorting or injection. The latter method produces prompt effects that last from 3 to 4 hours. Heroin addiction can develop quickly and serious health problems result with chronic use. An overdose can suppress the central nervous system to the point where the heart and lungs cease to function.

Withdrawal symptoms—sweating, tremors, cramps, anxiety, and an intense craving for the drug—occur soon after a person stops taking the drug. Methadone, a synthetic substitute for heroin, is sometimes given to heroin addicts to help them function without heroin. Information and referral for methadone programs and

other types of treatment as well as support groups can be obtained through hospitals and social service groups in the community.

Hallucinogens

Hallucinogens include substances derived from organic materials, such as marijuana and hashish, as well as synthetic agents such as LSD and PCP (angel dust). They all produce effects on the central nervous system that alter perception and body function. The effects are more long lasting with some forms of drugs than with others.

Marijuana and hashish produce a mood that is calm, reflective, and detached. Hallucinations are rare with these substances, but they can occur, as can panic attacks. Marijuana is retained in the fatty tissues for several days before it is processed by the body, although there is no evidence that prolonged use causes permanent damage. Chronic heavy use may cause loss of energy and drive and result in psychological dependence, which is indicated by a preoccupation with the drug and an inability to control its use.

The hallucinogens PCP and LSD share many similar properties. They produce vivid changes in sensation and perception, conveying euphoria, or alteration in the sense of passage of time. Both agents are thought to worsen latent schizophrenia. Their use may lead to chronic psychosis, flashbacks, and violent behavior.

INFORMED AVOIDANCE OF SUBSTANCE ABUSE

An increasing number of contemporary women are using psychoactive substances, ranging from nicotine and alcohol to tranquilizers, stimulants, and opiates. The reasons for this trend are varied and complicated but no doubt are connected to the pressures that today's society places on women to juggle the demands of job and family. Fortunately, women have access to information and resources to help them make informed decisions. Women can take control of their health and that of their families by being fully informed, active participants in decisions about drug use. This means awareness of certain key concepts:

■ Nicotine can end a life before its time.

■ Alcohol can cause a woman to lose control of her life and lead to major health problems

■ Drugs can cause physical and mental dependency.

By being alert to warning signs and doing something about it, women can avoid the problems associated with drug use. Counseling and treatment are available at local and national levels; these programs are effective in helping women help themselves to lead healthier lives free of the mental and physical effects of drugs.

ADDITIONAL RESOURCES

American Cancer Society
  800-ACS-2345

American Heart Association
  800-AHA-8721

American Lung Association
  800-Lung-USA

National Heart, Lung, and Blood Institute
  301-251-1222

National Cancer Institute
  800-4-CANCER

Office on Smoking and Health
  Centers for Disease Control
  800-CDC-1311

American Society for Addiction Medicine
  301-656-3920

Also see the list of Associations and Organizations on page 681.

CHAPTER 8

Mental Health

Leah J. Dickstein, M.D., F.A.P.A.

Throughout the life cycle, the psychological development of women differs substantially from that of men. The modern woman must contend with a changing image and conflicting societal demands that impose varying degrees of stress on her mental and emotional resources. As a young woman, for example, she may find that an abnormal concern for the perfect body as depicted in the popular media may lead to a lifelong dissatisfaction with her own body and perhaps even to an eating disorder. In her twenties and thirties, as the stresses of work outside the home and family life merge, she may experience acute anxiety and exhaustion as she attempts to do everything. In her forties and fifties, menopausal symptoms, the fear of growing older, and being part of the sandwich generation caring for elderly relatives as well as her young adults and possibly grandchildren, in addition to her home and outside work, may trigger depression or the onset of anxiety.

Fortunately, most of these symptoms of mental upheaval do not affect the majority of American women, who seem to manage their emotional ups and downs successfully themselves. And, certainly, it is not necessary to seek the help of mental health professionals at every sign of mild, short-term episodes of anxiety or the "blues." Occasional moodiness or a depressed feeling are not likely to be symptoms of mental disturbance, but merely a part of everyday functioning.

If you are trying to gain control over your emotions and your life, take advantage of the resources around you. It helps to sit down quietly and sort out the stresses in your life that are disturbing you. Don't blame others for your problems. Instead, take a good look at your responses to daily events and see how you can make adjustments that might make a substantial difference in your life. Cultivate some strategies that will help you get through your life with fewer complications and frustrations. Above all, after reviewing your issues, communicate clearly with the important people in your life.

STRATEGIES FOR IMPROVING YOUR EMOTIONAL HEALTH

We know that to succeed in the world we must have inner discipline and a sense of control over our lives. This doesn't mean that we always accomplish what we set out to do, or that we don't suffer disappointments and losses along the way. Here are some suggestions to prevent the stresses and strains of everyday life from adversely affecting your mental and emotional health:

- *Have a physical check-up.* Often what appears to be a mental disorder is actually the result of a physical problem. For example, if you are chronically tired and depressed, you may be suffering from a thyroid condition that is sapping your energy. If you are experiencing panic attacks—when your heart races and you break out in a sweat—you may have the symptoms of hypoglycemia. It's always best to rule out physical causes first.

- *Exercise regularly.* Your physical well-being is the basic foundation of your mental and emotional well-being. Daily vigorous exercise helps lower the level of triglycerides in the blood and stimulates the production of endorphins, a morphine-like chemical that helps to counteract feelings of anxiety and depression. Many women also find that exercise can help alleviate the symptoms of premenstrual syndrome (PMS), perhaps because PMS has been proven to create sudden drops in the levels of endorphins released in the brain. Regular exercise also will help you relax throughout the day and sleep better at night. Before beginning an exercise program you should have a complete physical examination.

- *Eat the right foods.* A nutritious diet—with lots of fruit, vegetables and whole grains and low-fat meats and fish—is essential to good health. But it's also important to avoid foods that have a strong effect on your moods and can disrupt the body's smooth functioning. Caffeine in coffee, tea, and soft drinks, for example, is a stimulant that produces anxiety and interferes with sleep and many medications in many people. Caffeine stimulates the locus coeruleus, which is located in the medulla oblongata, the site in the brain that is responsible for "fight or flight," a primitive human reaction to any sign of danger, real or imagined.

  Sugar is another culprit. You may crave sugar at certain times of the day because your blood sugar is low. But eating sugar on a daily basis just increases your blood sugar highs and lows. If you cut sugar out of your diet, you will find that you no longer have the urge for it; your energy level and your mood will also remain constant throughout the day. Women tend to crave sugar during PMS, but studies have shown that women who remove sugar from their diets experience fewer PMS symptoms, including less anxiety and depression. And, of course, avoid smoking, drugs, and the excessive use of alcohol.

- *Take control of your life.* It is our attitudes and response to the events and vicissitudes of life that determine our life story. Use your losses as a means of enriching your life experience and as a learning opportunity. Review your lifestyle choices and their effect on your well-being. Sometimes changing some aspect of your life, although difficult, may be the best path toward a positive mental outlook. If you hate your job, for example, seek out another one—remaining in a demeaning situation will only make your anxiety and depression worse. Be cautious, however. Although moving, changing jobs, and leaving destructive relationships all have the potential to change your state of mind for the better, it is not always a solution. If you do not clearly identify the source of your problems, you may find yourself in a new job or in a new relationship with all the same anxieties and frustrations. As the old adage says, "You can change your skies, but not yourself." It is absolutely essential that you try and understand the specific sources of your distress before you make radical changes in your life, especially if others will be adversely affected, such as children or other loved ones.

- *Keep busy, but not too busy.* Certainly one of the best ways to avoid depression is to keep active. Many women find that when they are engrossed in their work, they tend to be happier. It is important to work, plan for the future, and set goals, but it's vital to enjoy life's pleasures, too. Use your leisure time for a hobby or acquiring a new skill, and take the time to relax. Relaxation—whether through yoga, meditation, relaxation tapes, or biofeedback—is another tool you have to control your state of mind. After practicing a method for a few weeks, you will more than likely be able to lower your anxiety level.

- *Become socially involved.* A balanced life is one that incorporates personal and social activities equally. Friends, especially, can help in times of mental or physical distress. If you can relieve your tensions by talking to a friend who experienced a similar situation, you may find that you are not alone and that you are more normal than you think. Trying to figure out all of your problems alone may be a fruitless task because in isolation you can lose perspective.

If you experience increasing anxiety and depression, whether realistic or irrational, you may gain some insight and help from a good self-help book or from interaction with a self-help group. Sometimes, however, our problems are too overwhelming or severe for the more simple solutions. When that happens, you will need the advice and counsel of a competent mental health professional.

MENTAL HEALTH SPECIALISTS

Several kinds of professionals, with different types of training, can provide treatment for a wide range of mental and emotional needs. *Psychiatrists* are licensed physicians who specialize in the mental health field. They are the only mental health professionals who can take a complete medical history and understand the interactions of physical illness with emotions, and prescribe drugs. Their form of psychiatric treatment often combines drug therapy with psychotherapy. *Psychologists* have academic doctoral degrees in the field of psychology. They are not medical doctors, however, and cannot prescribe medication. Psychologists often use psychotherapy in treating their patients and refer patients to psychiatrists if and when they believe psychotherapy alone is not the correct treatment. *Psychiatric social workers* have academic degrees in the field of social work with advanced training in psychotherapy. Many of these practitioners are excellent counselors, but they do not have the depth of psychological training that psychologists do.

When you consult a professional, don't be afraid to ask as many questions as you wish. Remember, a consultation is not a commitment. The practitioner should help you understand your problem and should make a number of suggestions as to the alternative therapies available. A preliminary consultation will also give you a sense of what it would be like to work with that particular person.

TYPES OF THERAPIES

Psychotherapy—also called "one on one"—takes place between you and your therapist. Its goal is to make you feel better as you share your personal life experiences with the therapist and gain insight and understanding into your behavior and emotions. There are a number of different types of psychotherapy.

Psychoanalysis is an intensive form of psychotherapy that enables you to explore your conscious and unconscious thoughts, as well as your childhood conflicts and early relationships. Psychoanalysis is usually a long-term therapy that takes several years to complete. *Cognitive therapy* can help you to correct negative thinking patterns and explore how you view yourself in your environment. This type of therapy is short-term, usually requiring a minimum of 10 to 12 visits. *Behavioral therapy* is based on the principles of operant conditioning, the reinforcement of behavior by reward and punishment. Psychotherapists engaged in behavior modification use varied techniques to retrain your impulses and mode of thinking, including systematic desensitization and counterconditioning. *Marriage and family or dyadic therapy* attempts to resolve conflicts within the family setting. Members of the family come to the therapist either singly or together and talk openly about the problems experienced within the marriage and/or family or relationship structure. Usually short-term, this type of counseling attempts to find reasonable alternatives and solutions to destructive family and relationship dynamics. Group therapy is also a very useful form of therapy. All of these therapies, or variations of them, are used to treat anxiety, depression, phobias, and other mental and emotional disorders.

ANXIETY

Anxiety is a vague kind of fear or tension that occurs when you sense something unpleasant or threatening is about to happen. Some anxiety is a normal reaction in certain situations—a sense of anxiety may even improve performance—but persistent, irrational anxiety can cause physical symptoms such as rapid heartbeat, dry mouth, dizziness, intestinal problems, an inability to concentrate, irritability, insomnia, and even a fear of impending doom.

Anxiety can appear in several forms. Psychiatrists classify anxiety into the following types: generalized anxiety disorder, obsessive-compulsive disorder, panic disorder, simple phobias, and post-traumatic stress disorder.

Generalized Anxiety Disorder (GAD)

This type of anxiety can spread throughout many areas in a person's life, creating a constant state of tension and worry called "free-floating" anxiety. GAD makes one feel as if something terrible were going to happen at any moment. This state of dread often causes a secondary anxiety that makes the sufferer worry that the anxiety itself will cause her to lose her job or develop an illness or even "lose her mind." GAD most commonly occurs in young adults, often following a period of major depression. The physical symptoms can include palpitations, diarrhea, chronic muscle tension, nervous twitches, breathing problems, headaches, sweaty hands, insomnia, and the general "jitters." In half the patients who experience an anxiety disorder mild to moderate depression can also accompany the anxiety. A number of antidepressants have antianxiety features as well; thus one medication can alleviate depressive and anxiety symptoms.

Treatment: After a physical examination and a complete history is obtained to rule out any other medical disorder, a psychiatrist can prescribe the appropriate medication to relieve this anxiety and depression. You will also be encouraged to begin therapy. The treatment of anxiety disorders varies, but a combination of drugs and behavioral therapy seems to be most effective. Behavior therapy focuses on the specific patterns of behavior that are distressing to the patient or interfering with daily functioning; psychoanalysis has been found overall to be less effective in these cases.

Psychiatrists treat anxiety disorders with a group of drugs called anxiolytics. These medications must be used with caution because of their addictive qualities. Most of these drugs are from the family of benzodiazepines that includes alprazolam (Xanax) and diazepam (Valium). Usually taken in pill form, anxiolytics have potential side effects, including confusion, lethargy, and an inability to coordnate muscle movement. Clonazapan (Klonopin) and buspirone (Buspar) are newer antianxiety agents. If you are taking any of these medications, don't drink alcohol, or use caffeine, and watch your driving and other use of machines early in treatment. Never use over-the-counter medications without checking with your physician first. In some cases, the drug may cause you to develop new anxieties. If that happens, check with your physician; she or he will probably reduce or discontinue the drug treatment. It is also important to gradually decrease the dose of anxiolytics: if treatment is stopped abruptly, serious withdrawal effects can occur, including severe nightmares, insomnia, and seizures.

Obsessive-Compulsive Disorder (OCD)

The symptoms of obsessive-compulsive disorder usually appear first during adolescence or early adulthood. The obsessive part of the disorder is characterized by an idea or impulse that recurs involuntarily, despite the attempt of the afflicted person to stop or suppress these thoughts and impulses. The compulsive behavior is demonstrated by a compelling urge to repeat a behavior or ritual to eliminate or counteract the obsession, even though that behavior appears to be senseless. For example, an individual may be obsessive-compulsive about cleanliness and wash her hands dozens of times during the day. Or she may check countless times to make sure she has completed a specific task, such as turning off the stove or locking the door.

OCD affects about 1 to 2 percent of the population. Anxiety disorders, like many other medical illnesses, have a genetic predisposition; that is, they run in families. Those who suffer from the disorder tend to have rigid and orderly personalities. If they are not allowed to perform their daily rituals and obsessive actions, they usually become overwhelmed with anxiety and fear.

Treatment: As with generalized anxiety disorder, OCD usually responds to behavioral therapy. The idea is to gradually expose the OCD patient to the situation that provokes the undesirable behavior. In most cases, a combination of drug treatment and behavioral therapy can reduce or eliminate the obsessive-compulsive impulses and rituals. Specific antidepressants may be used to counteract the anxiety disorder as well as the accompanying depression.

Panic Disorder

Panic disorder starts with a sudden feeling of intense dread, apprehension, and a sense of impending doom. Physical symptoms include heart palpitations, shortness of breath, dizziness, weakness, sweating, choking, nausea, and a numbness or tingling sensation in the extremities. The symptoms can be so severe that a sufferer may rush to the hospital thinking she is having a heart attack. In fact, because of its physiological symptoms, panic disorder is often misdiagnosed as a respiratory or cardiac problem.

People who suffer from panic disorder often link their attacks to the specific place where they occurred. For example, if they have an attack in a crowded elevator or in an airplane, they will avoid elevators and planes as possible triggers of further attacks. As a result, many sufferers severely limit their activities; some eventually develop a fear of going out of their homes at all, developing a phobia known as agoraphobia. Women in particular are more likely to suffer from panic disorder with agoraphobia.

Researchers have found that panic disorder, like generalized anxiety disorder, has a genetic component. It is thought that panic attacks originate in the locus coeruleus, which produces norepinephrine, a chemical used for the "fight or flight" response. Too much of this substance produces anxiety and fear. As people age, the locus coeruleus produces lower levels of the chemical, so older people tend to have fewer, if any, panic attack episodes.

Treatment: The medications commonly used to relieve panic attacks are either the tricyclic antidepressants or the selective serotonin reuptake inhibitors. Antianxiety drugs may also be effective to relieve the initial fear of the attacks themselves. Behavior modification combined with relaxation therapy can be a valuable alternative or complement to medication.

Phobias

Among the most common anxiety disorders, simple phobias are characterized by a constant irrational fear of a particular object, activity, place, or situation. The phobic person may have a clear understanding of how senseless the phobia is but still have a persistent desire to avoid its cause. Many types of phobias exist, including:

- *Ailurophobia*—a fear of cats.
- *Belonephobia*—a fear of sharp objects.
- *Claustrophobia*—a fear of enclosed spaces.
- *Monophobia*—a fear of being alone.
- *Acrophobia*—a fear of heights.
- *Sitophobia*—a fear of food.
- *Pterygophobia*—a fear of flying.
- *Ocholophobia*—a fear of crowds.
- *Acaraphobia*—a fear of small insects.
- *Agoraphobia*—a fear of public or open spaces.

Although minor fears exist in everyone, a true phobia can alter a person's behavior and lifestyle. For example, if you live in the country and you are afraid of a city subway system, it's not a real problem because you can manage quite successfully without having to take a subway. But if you need to move to the city to take the job of your dreams, you may find that your fear of subways seriously restricts your life.

Treatment: Phobias can often be successfully treated with behavior modification therapy, using a technique called systematic desensitization. In desen-

sitization therapy, you are repeatedly exposed to the anxiety-provoking stimulus while in a deep state of relaxation. During repeated visits to the therapist, you are led through a process of increasing exposure until your fear and anxiety gradually diminish. Many people require medication as well.

Post-Traumatic Stress Disorder (PTSD)

If you have witnessed or experienced an intensely traumatic situation or event, you may later suffer from post-traumatic stress disorder (PTSD). This disorder is characterized by a chronic reexperiencing of the traumatic event in the form of nightmares, hallucinations, and recurring flashes of memory. You may suffer from insomnia, decreased sexual drive, heightened sensitivity to noise, depression, anxiety, and intense irritability. You may also feel isolated from other people and withdraw socially. Victims of PTSD can relive the stressful event for weeks, months or years at a time while showing a numbness to their present surroundings.

Not surprisingly, most of the knowledge of PTSD comes from research conducted on veterans of World War II and the Korean and Vietnam conflicts. Survivors of rape and other crimes may also suffer from this condition. Although PTSD is classified as an anxiety disorder, it is a response to an actual experience and is therefore considered to be more of a normal reaction to an overwhelming trauma and shock. The severity of PTSD is directly linked to the psychological strength of the person before the event took place. Symptoms usually appear shortly after the trauma, but in some cases the disorder is not apparent until after an incubation period of several months. The symptoms typically disappear after about six months, but in some cases they can recur for years afterward.

Treatment: A psychiatrist can prescribe the appropriate medications to relieve your depression and anxiety. You will also be encouraged to begin therapy to talk out the problem and to formulate ways to control your thoughts and inner reactions.

DEPRESSION AND OTHER MOOD DISORDERS

Depression is a common psychological condition that affects millions of Americans to varying degrees. It can occur without any apparent reason, although current research supports the belief that complex psychologi-

cal, environmental, and biochemical changes may trigger the initial mood swing. Depression also may be an inherited condition.

Sadness, grief, and a depressed feeling are all normal reactions to a serious loss or tragic event. And everyone suffers now and again from a mild case of the "blues." Major depression, however, persists to the point where it interferes with your daily tasks, impairing your ability to live a normal life. In many cases, the cause of major depression is unknown. A sad or traumatic event is often the trigger. Some medications can bring on a bout of depression. A severe lowering of mood can even occur as a reaction to a lack of sunlight during the fall and winter months.

Symptoms of Depression

Often it is difficult for physicians and patients to recognize a case of major depression. A true depression is characterized by the following signs and symptoms.

- *Negativity in all aspects of life.* You have a feeling of pessimism and the belief that nothing can make your life better.

- *Changes in sleep patterns.* Typically, there is initial insomnia or you wake up in the middle of the night and can't get back to sleep again. Or you have early morning awakening at 2:00, 3:00, or 4:00 A.M. Or you sleep more than is necessary.

- *Change in eating patterns.* You have a lack of or change in appetite and eat either too little and lose weight, or too much and gain weight.

- *Fatigue.* You experience a lack of energy that permeates everything you do, including a declining interest in your work, leisure activities, and sex. You have difficulty concentrating or making decisions.

- *Isolation.* You feel anxious or disinterested in social situations and gradually withdraw from people. You may neglect your appearance.

- *Persistent sadness and self-loathing.* You develop a lack of self-confidence and feel a sense of worthlessness. You have frequent bouts of crying for no reason. Your feelings of hopelessness may lead to thoughts of and plans for suicide.

Studies have shown that individuals are more prone to depression at certain times of life. Depression in women first may occur in adolescence when the pressures of becoming a young woman in our society to-

WINTER BLUES

Although many people find the dark, dreary days of January and February to be depressing, there are some who suffer much more deeply at this time of the year. They experience what is called seasonal affective disorder (SAD). More women than men have this condition, which typically occurs in the winter months when sunlight is at a minimum.

During the colder part of the year, the pineal gland, located at the bottom of the brain, secretes a hormone called melatonin. This hormone is associated with drowsiness and lethargy. Although most people are not affected by the surplus of melatonin in their brains, SAD sufferers cannot tolerate the excess hormone and become severely depressed and debilitated. Researchers have found that light therapy—the use of specially designed fluorescent lights that mimic the sun's rays—can enable most of these people to recover their normal energy and emotional stability.

gether with school and the issues of breaking away from the family and facing adulthood often cause teenagers to doubt themselves and turn inward. Divorce, sexual problems, a limited work horizon, personal disappointments, and past unresolved grief and abuse issues may bring on depression in the middle years. Depression among the elderly is also common and may be attributable to the death of friends and family, physical and mental limitations, and thoughts of impending death. Women especially are liable to experiencing depression associated with hormonal changes in the body. Women experience depression twice as frequently as men.

Hormonal Depression

Chemical depression, or hormonally induced depression is common among pregnant women and among those who suffer a spontaneous abortion or undergo a hysterectomy. Some women suffer from postpartum depression after childbirth (see Chapter 17). Women in their thirties and forties may experience premenstrual syndrome (PMS). Premenstrual Dysphoric Disorder (PMDD) is the feeling of tension, irritability, and depression that occurs every month for up to two weeks before menses. Although PMS is still poorly understood, it is thought to be the result of hormonal changes in the body and seriously affects approximately 5 percent of women.

SUICIDAL THOUGHTS

Severely depressed people often have thoughts of committing suicide. Although these thoughts may not be necessarily connected to actual plans to end one's life, they are a common symptom of major depression and center around a person's feeling that life is not worth living and they see no future for themselves. Because thoughts of suicide are the most serious symptom—and sometimes outcome—of clinical depression, people expressing these wishes must be taken seriously. Physicians often will not raise the issue of suicide for fear of introducing the idea to the patient, so it is important to inform the physician if suicide has been mentioned by the patient. In fact, asking a patient if she has thought about suicide and if she has a plan can relieve this preoccupation and lessen the chances of suicide. Furthermore, asking the patient what would keep her from committing suicide can be lifesaving.

The elderly suffer most from depression-induced suicide. Often an older person's low spirits are confused with senile dementia and polypharmacy (the prescription and self-medication of too many medications) and the underlying depression goes untreated. Suicide is also more common among those suffering from alcoholism and those who live alone. Suicide is one of the nation's primary causes of adolescent death, and its incidence is on the rise. The rate of suicide among the elderly is three times that of adolescents. Women make far more attempts to kill themselves, but men are more likely to die from the act because they choose more lethal methods, such as a gun. Unfortunately in recent years woman are also choosing more lethal methods. It is impossible to know for sure if a person who threatens suicide is actually serious about dying. If you know someone who has expressed a suicide wish, don't criticize or dismiss the behavior. Instead, make contact with a suicide hotline, a physician, or your local hospital. Wait until the depressed individual is under a physician's care before you leave her alone.

Treatment: At least one out of five Americans will suffer from severe depression in their lives and only one of every five depressed adults will seek treatment. It is therefore important to realize the available options for treating this serious mental disorder. A common treatment includes both the use of antidepressant medications and psychotherapy.

Within 4 to 6 weeks of the initial drug therapy, you should begin to feel the benefit of the prescribed antidepressant. (Many physicians are inclined to prescribe a moderate dosage, but some of these chemicals are more effective in greater quantities.) Drug treatment for depression usually lasts between 6 months and a year. Recent research has shown that many people benefit from continuing the use of antidepressants after recovery because it can help avoid another depressive episode. When the drug therapy is seen as no longer necessary, tapering off the dosage gradually is best or serious side effects may result. Typical medications used in the treatment of depression include the tricyclic antidepressants, monoamine oxidase inhibitors, SSRIs, and lithium. Tricyclic antidepressants, unlike amphetamines, do not raise your mood artificially, but simply relieve the depression. The type of tricyclic chosen depends upon which side effects you can handle most easily. Some of the drugs in the amitriptyline (Elavil) class will make you feel somewhat lethargic and thus may be a good choice if you are nervous or overanxious or have problems with insomnia. Common side effects of these antidepressants may include constipation, dry mouth, temporary blurred vision, minor urinary tract problems, and dizzy spells. Elderly people may suffer from short-term memory loss and temporary impotence. Antidepressants affect different people in varying ways, and each drug must be given an allotted amount of time before it is expected to take effect.

Other popular antidepressant treatments include the following:

- *Fluoxetine (Prozac).* One of the most useful of the new antidepressants on the market, Prozac (fluoxetine) takes effect in about three weeks and works with a standard dose level. Known side effects include anxiety, a decrease in appetite, headache, and nausea. Sertraline (Zoloft) and paroxetine (Paxil) are two other very effective SSRIs.

- *Monoamine oxidase (MAO) inhibitors.* MAO inhibitors are used when the tricyclic or SSRI antidepressants don't work, especially for what is called atypical depression. These drugs are very effective and work quickly, but their side effects can be more dangerous than the tricyclics. One disadvantage is that MAO inhibitors react dangerously with a number of different foods, including aged cheese, red wine, pickled herring, and beer.

- *Electroshock therapy (EST).* Formerly thought to be dangerous, electroshock therapy is now considered a very safe and effective treatment for major depression. It is one of the fastest ways to get results and is also painless. EST is usually administered to severely depressed or suicidal patients in a hospital setting, but it can be used on an outpatient basis as well. Short-term memory loss is the major side effect of EST, but most disruptions of memory are resolved within 6 to 9 months after treatment. EST is usually followed by psychotherapy and antidepressant medication under a psychiatrist's care.

Bipolar Disorder

Bipolar disorder is the scientific name for manic-depressive disorder, a mental condition characterized by bouts of depression followed or preceded by manic exuberance and enthusiasm. The change in mood is often accompanied by irrational thoughts and periods of anger or rage. The manic phase includes irritability, grandiosity, and a sense of elation. The person is sleepless, talks a great deal, displays impulsive behavior, and often is irresponsible with money and goes on spending sprees. In some people the manic episodes are more frequent, while others experience more depression.

Bipolar disorder differs from major depression in a number of ways. It is much less common. It occurs with equal frequency among men and women, and they do not generally display the low self-esteem or obsessive thinking that those suffering from major depression do. Also, while major depression can occur at any time during the life cycle, bipolar disorder usually occurs before the age of thirty. Finally, bipolar disorder is characterized by frequent short outbursts, while major depression lasts longer and occurs less often. For all these reasons, researchers believe that major depression and bipolar disorder spring from different roots although both have a genetic basis, that is, occur in other family members.

Dysthymia and Cyclothymia

People who pass through phases of depression throughout their lives but otherwise function normally may have dysthymia or cyclothymia. These mild disorders are characterized by patterns of repetitive depression, but the patient may fail to display enough symptoms to be classified as suffering from major depression or from bipolar disorder. *Dysthymia* is a chronic mild depression marked by introversion, a perpetually gloomy outlook, and an apparent inability to experience much joy or pleasure from life. Dysthymics often are sluggish and have low self-esteem. The disorder is twice as likely to occur in women as in men. *Cyclothymia* is also a chronic mental condition that often becomes a way of life. A cyclothymic will never go for more than a few months without a phase of moderate manic or depressed behavior. Often they come to depend upon the manic periods, which are full of intense bursts of energy and heightened creative and mental acuity.

Treatment. Lithium is the drug of choice for those who suffer from bipolar disorder, although it doesn't work for everyone. Lithium is not used to correct an existing state of mania but rather to prevent future occurrences. Most physicians prescribe it in conjunction with another antipsychotic drug that is used to control the current manic attack. Lithium has common side effects, however, including weight gain, lethargy, twitches, nausea, hand tremor, and vertigo. It can also affect the thyroid and the kidneys, so the patient must be monitored regularly.

Two new medications are now being used to treat bipolar disorders: valproate (Depakote) and carbamazepine (Tegretol). Used for more than a decade for treating epilepsy, these medications do not cause cognitive impairment (one of the possible side effects of lithium), but they may have other serious side effects. Nevertheless, these two drugs are viable alternatives for people who cannot tolerate lithium's side effects.

DISSOCIATIVE DISORDERS

The dissociative disorders all involve disconnections of the personality, which means that at times memory for certain events, identity, and ability to handle situations are missing from the conscious mind. The person has usually suffered severe abuse in the past and learned to run away in her mind when she couldn't in actuality. The most common dissociative disorders are dissociative identity and dissociative amnesia.

Dissociative Identity Disorder

Dissociative Identity Disorder, formerly called multiple personality disorder, is characterized by the existence of two or more personalities in the same individual, each with her own memories, experiences, behavioral patterns, and relationships. The number of different personalities existing in one body have been documented to range from two to one hundred, although more than half of these cases involve fewer than 10. Not as rare as once thought, dissociative identity disorder almost invariably develops in childhood. It is often the result of sexual abuse or severe trauma and is usually not diagnosed until years later. Women are more likely to have the disorder than men, and it is more common in those who are related to others with the disorder.

Dissociative Amnesia

Not to be confused with the amnesia due to a general medical condition, dissociative amnesia is a loss of memory caused by a sudden shock or traumatic event. There are four forms of this type of amnesia.

- *Localized amnesia*—All of the events during a particular time frame are erased.
- *Selective amnesia*—Only certain experiences during a period of time are blocked out.
- *Generalized amnesia*—An entire life's past is forgotten.
- *Continuous amnesia*—All events following a certain period of time are blocked out, along with experiences that occur after the amnesia has begun.

Another form of amnesia is called *dissociative fugue*. This fairly rare condition occurs when a person assumes a completely new identity, forgetting the old one completely. While most with generalized amnesia may wander around confused, not knowing who they are, the person with dissociative fugue pursues her or his new existence with complete confidence and certainty.

Treatment: Generally, treatment for persons suffering from dissociative disorders involves support and psychotherapy with experienced therapists. Patients are encouraged to remember as much of their past as possible and to make the necessary adjustments to their present condition.

PERSONALITY DISORDERS

Problems of the personality often are the result of unresolved emotional problems experienced during childhood. Many people exhibiting the symptoms of a personality disorder fail to seek treatment, preferring instead to blame others for their persistent difficulties in marriage, work, and relationships. Psychotherapy is the treatment of choice for these problems, although occasionally medications are also used. Generally the following disorders reflect a person's inability to exist within the limitations and demands of the outside world.

Avoidant Personality Disorder

Individuals with avoidant personality disorder withdraw socially. They may want to experience close relationships but fear rejection. People with avoidant personalities usually suffer from low self-esteem and tend to blame themselves for their social failures.

Borderline Personality Disorder

People with borderline personality disorder have a poor self-image. They have unstable personal relationships, tending to focus on erratic or intense friendships. Extremely fearful of abandonment, these individuals suffer from frequent mood changes, a lack of inner control, anger, and an inclination to fight. Their self-damaging, impulsive behavior, sometimes accompanied by drug abuse, casual sex, and binge eating, usually estranges these people from peers and family. Recent research has shown that for many diagnosed with borderline personality disorder, their behavior is a consequence of underlying post-traumatic stress disorder consequent to abuse.

Dependent Personality Disorder

As the name indicates, people with dependent personality disorder tend to depend on others to make the major decisions in their lives. Most common in domestically abused women, the disorder is closely linked with a fear of abandonment. A woman suffering from this syndrome can easily fall into a no-win cycle of asking her partner for advice on every aspect of her life, then finding she suffers from low self-esteem and depression because of her lack of independence.

Histrionic Personality Disorder

More common in women than men, histrionic personality disorder is manifested by an exaggerated display of emotion. These people often display an overwrought and inappropriate demeanor in order to get the attention they crave. They may appear to be lively and warm at first meeting, but their relationships with others deteriorate swiftly as they become increasingly demanding and needy. Constantly seeking attention and praise these individuals have a low frustration tolerance.

Narcissistic Personality Disorder

The narcissist combines a sense of grandiose self-importance with bouts of inferiority. These people tend to brag about themselves while constantly checking what others think of them. People with this disorder demand full attention but are indifferent to the emotions and needs of others. If they are rejected, they tend to display excessive anger and envy.

Obsessive-Compulsive Personality Disorder

People with obsessive-compulsive personality disorder spend most of their energy cultivating a sense of efficiency. They make lists and follow self-imposed rules, but they usually end up accomplishing very little. Preoccupied with the details of a trip, for example, an obsessive-compulsive will spend so much time worrying about the itinerary that she fails to enjoy the trip itself. Because of their excessive preoccupation with details these people often spoil the experiences of people close to them.

SOMATOFORM DISORDERS

The term *somatoform* refers to physical ailments that are either caused or strongly influenced by your emotions and current mental state. The label *psychosomatic* often has a negative connotation, implying that the illness is a product of your imagination rather than an actual ailment. To you, however, the pain and discomfort of a migraine, a skin rash, or an intestinal problem are real enough for you to seek relief and medical help.

Although the nature of somatoform illness is still not clearly understood, it is currently accepted in all of medicine that psychological factors can influence genetically predisposed people to succumb to a particular ailment or disease. For example, migraine attacks and eczema outbreaks—both diseases with genetic roots—are often triggered by fatigue and stress. If you have an illness that does not respond to standard medical therapy, your physician may ask you questions about your lifestyle and current frame of mind and possible life experiences. It is possible that counseling, relaxation techniques, and medications may help to lessen your symptoms and reduce the frequency of your attacks.

Paranoid Personality Disorder

People with paranoid personality disorder are overly suspicious and sensitive to perceived injuries and slights from others. They frequently blame others for their difficulties and have an exaggerated sense of their own importance. They appear cold and humorless, may show a limited range of emotional expression, and turn hostile if their defects are pointed out to them.

Passive-Aggressive Personality Disorder

Passive-aggressive people tend to avoid doing whatever is expected of them, but without honestly refusing to do the particular task. Such a person will agree to take the responsibility for a job and then will proceed to fail. Tending to have difficulties at work and in intimate relationships, passive-aggressive individuals infuriate others with their lack of follow-through. They prefer to use procrastination and inefficiency to avoid their responsibilities, rather than openly expressing their frustrations or desires.

Schizoid Personality Disorder

Individuals with schizoid personalities prefer social isolation. They have a difficult time experiencing or expressing warmth or intimate feelings. These people may be quite successful in their careers, but they tend to be solitary and completely involved in their own world.

Schizotypal Personality Disorder

This group expresses schizophrenic symptoms in specific areas while appearing normal in other situations. For example, a person with a schizotypal personality might display strange mannerisms, speech patterns, or perceptions, but she will not be so out of touch with reality to be classified as a person who is schizophrenic.

Treatment: People suffering from personality disorders need the supportive counseling of experienced mental health professionals. The most common form of therapy is cognitive, but individual therapists may use a variety of methods. Many types of qualified therapists are available if you think you or someone you know needs counseling. Ask your physician for a referral, or call the local branch of the American Psychiatric Association for a list of professionals in your area. Help also may be obtained through community mental health clinics, family service centers, or from the referral services of a nearby hospital. Check your insurance coverage first, however; you may find that your policy has limitations on mental health coverage, and your insurance company may prefer that you use short-term therapy rather than traditional long-term psychotherapeutic treatment.

SCHIZOPHRENIA

Schizophrenia—literally "split mind"—is a psychotic condition that severely impairs a person's social and psychological functioning. Difficult to treat and often chronic, schizophrenia is characterized by social withdrawal, unusual speech patterns, bizarre thoughts, and eccentric behavior. The schizophrenic is unable to differentiate between reality and delusion, and auditory hallucinations are common. Unable to respond rationally to a situation, the schizophrenic may laugh when the appropriate response is to cry. The schizophrenic is indifferent to her physical surroundings, may dress or groom eccentrically, and often has a bewildered, disheveled appearance.

Current research indicates that schizophrenia is caused by neurobiologic defects. The abnormal brain chemistry and possibly, brain structure, that cause the disease can be inherited—but is not always. Equally common in both sexes, schizophrenia usually appears during adolescence and early adulthood and at times of great stress or loss. Onset is later in women, who also experience fewer hospitalizations, respond better to hospitalizations, and have better relationships with their families. Schizophrenia has some variations:

- People with *paranoid* schizophrenia have delusions of persecution, believing that they will be poisoned, attacked, or destroyed by others, or that people are stealing their ideas and using them for their own ends. They may hear voices and talk to voices in their minds which may tell them to commit certain actions.

- *Catatonic* schizophrenics usually alternate between bouts of extreme excitability and stupor. Often they remain mute and apparently unseeing for long periods of time, although they may be aware of what is going on around them.

- *Disorganized* schizophrenics are usually incoherent, displaying inappropriate and bizarre emotions and actions. At other times, they are expressionless and non-reactive.

People who suffer acute or severe eipsodes of schizophrenia must be treated in the hospital. Electroconvulsive therapy is used in some cases, but antipsychotic drugs are usually prescribed to reduce the person's agitation and lessen the psychotic symptoms. These drugs, called major tranquilizers, are used to treat patients suffering from a variety of psychoses, including schizophrenia, mania, medically caused disorders, and thought disorders caused by drug and alcohol abuse.

The antipsychotic drugs work by blocking the receptors in the brain that are linked by the nerve chemical dopamine. Chlorpromazine (Thorazine) and haloperidol (Haldol) are especially effective in treating people suffering from a psychotic episode. Side effects are numerous, however, including dry mouth, constipation, loss of bladder control, sexual difficulties, blurred vision, tremors, and an involuntary facial movement called tardive dyskinesia. These side effects are usually directly related to the dosage and the length of time the patient is on the drug. Altering the dosage frequently alleviates most of these problems. There are medications like benztropine mesylate (Cogentin) which can lessen some of these extrapyramidal symptoms. However, for tardive dyskinesia, you must discontinue the drug and wait—sometimes for several months—for the symptoms possibly to subside.

Some people will experience an episode of schizophrenia and later return to normal with the knowledge that they will relapse again with the same symptoms. In those instances, the most effective treatment is the administration of drugs to change the brain chemistry; this type of therapy usually lasts up to six months. Others, however, may suffer from severe chronic episodes of schizophrenia and require continued medication to maintain even a semblance of a normal life. In both cases, supportive psychotherapy can be used to help the patient and family and significant others understand and control the life stresses that may trigger an attack.

MENTAL DISORDERS DUE TO A GENERAL MEDICAL CONDITION

Mental confusion and disorientation can also be caused by a physical illness or infection that in turn influences brain function. Such medical disorders are best treated by dealing with the physical problem first, which can include cerebral infection, brain trauma, vascular accidents (stroke), brain tumors, degenerative disorders, nutritional deficiencies, endocrine disorders, and epilepsy. Although the cause of these mental disturbances tends to be an illness, the condition can also be the result of toxic chemicals and withdrawal from drugs and alcohol.

Symptoms and Diagnosis

The symptoms of these disorders are strikingly similar to those of psychogenic disorders, involving:

- impaired intellectual comprehension
- impaired speech patterns
- inability to calculate simple numbers
- faulty memory
- inappropriate decisions or judgment
- rapid mood swings
- general disorientation.

Endocrine disorders are a good example of how an organic disturbance in the brain can result in a loss of normal intellectual functioning and behavior. The endocrine glands—especially the thyroid and adrenal glands—are responsible for producing hormones in the body that affect energy level, growth and development, and sexual functioning. A hyperactive thyroid or hyperthyroidism (called Graves' disease) is characterized by agitation, hallucinations, sweating, and other symptoms of acute anxiety. An underactive thyroid, on the other hand, may lead to myxedema, which in turn can lead to episodes of severe depression. Hyperactivity of the adrenal glands

(Cushing's syndrome), is characterized by severe mood swings, general weakness, and obesity. Underactivity of the adrenal glands may cause Addison's disease, which can cause acute depression and/or anxiety. People with diabetes often experience depression. (See Chapter 29.)

SLEEP DISORDERS

Getting a good night's sleep is extremely important to our daily functioning and to our general mental and physical health. But a good night's sleep varies for different people—some require up to nine hours while others can do quite nicely with six. A middle-aged adult, however, usually needs at least 7½ hours of sleep a night to feel good the next day. If you don't get your required amount of sleep, you'll feel tired, less alert, and less efficient. A chronic lack of sleep—whether because of shift work, jet lag, or just watching too much television—can severely impair your judgment and lead to accidents at home, on the job, and on the road.

Insomnia

Occasionally you may experience difficulties falling asleep. Your wakefulness may be the result of a stressful day, sleeping in a strange bed, or apprehension before an exam or starting a new job. Short-term insomnia that lasts for a number of days may be caused by a death in the family, difficulties in a relationship, or worry over financial matters. Chronic or persistent insomnia may last for many weeks or months. It may stem from depression, overuse of alcohol and caffeine, or a reliance on sleep medications.

Treatment: If you have chronic difficulty falling asleep at night, the first step is to make certain changes in your bedtime routine that may help you fall asleep.

- Avoid strenuous exercise before bedtime. Regular exercise during the day is beneficial to sleep, but exercise right before going to bed has the opposite effect of too much stimulation instead of relaxation.

- Don't drink tea, coffee, or soft drinks containing caffeine for at least four to six hours before bedtime. Also avoid alcoholic drinks. The alcohol may make you fall asleep faster, but it can

CHANGING SLEEP PATTERNS

Sleep patterns vary considerably according to your age. Newborns sleep five or six times during the day, while the older child takes one or two daily naps in addition to sleeping through the night. Young adults, on the average, need at least seven to eight hours of sleep a night. Pregnancy can temporarily impair sleep because of hormonal changes. However, no medications must be used.

In later years—sometime after age 60—you may notice a tendency to return to frequent daytime naps and to less sleep at night. Instead of the continuous period of sleep you have become accustomed to, you may experience less deep sleep and more frequent awakenings. Your "insomnia," in that case, may simply be a normal adaptation to changing sleep patterns that occur with advancing years.

also disrupt normal sleeping patterns and result in awakening during the night.

- Refrain from napping during the day, if possible. Habitual napping can disrupt your need for sleep at night.

- Be cautious about your use of over-the-counter and prescription sleeping medications. It's all too easy to develop a dependence on these drugs, with a corresponding disruption in your normal sleeping patterns. And most of these medications lose their effectiveness after 4 to 6 weeks.

- Relax in the evening before you go to bed. Restrict your reading and TV watching to lighter fare, and avoid emotionally upsetting topics right before bedtime. Try not to worry about what you have to do the next day.

- Make sure your physical surroundings are conducive to sleep. The room should be sufficiently darkened, and the temperature of the room should be comfortable. People who work at home should avoid using their bedroom as an office; it may help if you can screen off that part of the room from the area around your bed.

- Don't force sleep. If you find yourself tossing and turning, get up and read or watch television until you feel sleepy. Try a glass of skim milk.

If all else fails, you may need the advice of a professional sleep expert to solve your chronic sleep problems. First, though, have a careful medical evaluation to determine if there is a physical component to your sleeplessness.

Sleep Apnea

A potentially serious disorder, apnea is characterized by recurrent halts in breathing, loud snoring, and deep gasps for breath. People suffering from this disorder often wake with a headache and feel tired and irritable during the day. More men than women suffer from sleep apnea, especially if they are overweight. At its worst, the lack of oxygen during the cessation of breathing could cause a heart arrhythmia or even a heart attack. Treatment may call for weight reduction, medication, or the use of a machine that delivers continuous air flow through a mask. Surgery to open the air passages is a last resort; this procedure has not been particularly successful in eliminating the apnea.

Restless Leg Syndrome

Sometimes, lying in bed at night, you may experience unpleasant creeping sensations deep inside your leg. This feeling forces you to move your legs in a jerking or kicking motion. You may have to get out of bed and walk around to relieve the symptoms. Sometimes your feet, thighs, and arms may also be affected. The causes of restless leg syndrome are not clear, although the syndrome often appears during times of stress. The disorder can stem from a neuropathy associated with diabetes, or from some mineral deficiency. Restless leg syndrome is not dangerous, but the sensations involved are uncomfortable and annoying, and can disrupt sleep. If your physician can't give you relief, you may want to consult a sleep specialist or a sleep clinic for diagnosis and treatment.

SLEEP CLINICS

Many large medical centers and hospitals have sleep clinics for the diagnosis of sleep disorders. You enter the clinic during the day and spend a few nights there for a complete sleep diagnosis and evaluation. A variety of tests are performed to measure your body movement during sleep, your brain waves, the level of oxygen in your blood, and your heart and breathing rates. The results of the tests will allow a specialist in sleep disorders to pinpoint the cause of your insomnia and to offer an appropriate treatment.

DUAL DIAGNOSES

Especialy in the last two decades, the incidence of dual diagnosis has gained in importance as a result of research. Dual diagnosis means that a woman is suffering from a substance abuse disorder and another major mental illness such as major depressive disorder, bipolar disorder, or schizophrenia. Treating one illness alone when two exist understandably leads to treatment failure. Therefore it is extremely important that without excessive shame and guilt, women patients tell their physicians, and other health professionals treating them, that they have an addiction problem as well as an emotional, psychological or psychiatric illness. Although the exact etiology is unknown, lesbians suffer from alcoholism to a greater extent than heterosexual women. Clearly societal pressures and discrimination can be involved. There are increasing numbers of treatment centers for people, and many specifically for women, with dual diagnoses. When properly recognized and treated, success rates are high and women recover to go on with better lives.

EATING DISORDERS

The act of eating has long been thought of as a crucial part of the psychological development of the human being. Many mental health professionals believe that a healthy attitude toward food symbolizes the security of feeling loved, while an abnormal anxiety about eating may reflect inner conflicts, a basic insecurity, and low self-esteem. There also may be physiological problems involved that are as yet poorly understood.

Obesity

Obesity is a controversial topic today, because severely overweight people are often made to feel responsible for their condition and suffer social stigma as a result. Recent research has shown that obesity—the state of exceeding ideal weight by more than 20 percent—is not always caused by excessive eating. Activity levels and the metabolic rate at which calories are burned are two factors affecting the creation of excessive fat in the body. Some people are more prone to gain weight than others because of their genetically determined metabolic rate.

Obesity is a health risk, however. Excess fat can affect the liver and increase the risk of diabetes. Extra fat may also be associated with higher triglyceride blood fat levels and increased risk of more heart disease and heart attacks. Hypertension, too, occurs three times more frequently in overweight people, and can lead to stroke. Cancers of the colon, rectum, gall bladder, ovary, cervix, and breast also tend to occur more frequently in women who are obese.

Many obese individuals could lose weight by implementing a more careful diet and by exercising more. However, dieting is not the final answer. Chronic dieting can cause repeated weight loss and gain—a phenomenon known as the yo-yo syndrome. This syndrome slows down metabolism and makes it harder to lose weight the next time around. The best solution is behavior modification. This means gradually changing your eating habits and increasing your physical activity. (See Chapters 3 and 4 for more details on how to lose weight safely and effectively.)

Anorexia Nervosa and Bulimia

Two common eating disorders—anorexia nervosa and bulimia—can be especially dangerous. Anorectics begin by showing an exaggerated interest in food—counting calories, baking for the family—but gradually eat less and less themselves. They diet excessively and often exercise to the point of near-exhaustion before someone else notices their emaciated physical condition and their abnormal fear of gaining weight. Bulimics, on the other hand, consume large amounts of food periodically—so-called binge eating—and then force themselves to vomit the food. Bulimics also have a great fear of getting fat, although most are in the normal weight range for their height.

In 85 to 95 percent of cases, anorexia and bulimia affect young women, often beginning in the teenage years. The specific causes of anorexia and bulimia are not known, although it is thought that several factors play a role in their development, including a biologic predisposition to the disease, social pressures to be slim, family disturbances and conflicts, and a fear of sexuality. Both anorexia and bulimia are serious diseases and call for immediate treatment. Severe and long-term anorexia can lead to extreme emaciation and even death. Bulimia can have serious health consequences by depleting the body of water and potassium and can also result in death from cardiac arrhythmia.

Treatment: Both disorders are difficult to treat, and relapses are common. In severe cases, hospitalization is necessary to control weight and to eliminate dangerous eating practices, such as vomiting and the abuse of laxatives and diuretics. In many cases, psychological counseling and diet counseling can help control the anorectic's abnormal eating habits. Bulimics usually respond to psychotherapy and behavioral therapy. Women suffering from eating disorders can also find sympathy and support in self-help groups and from group therapy.

DRUG AND ALCOHOL ABUSE

The symptoms of drug abuse vary, depending on the substance, but most chronic users experience a loss of appetite, a drop in efficiency, radical changes in mood, and a deterioration in relationships. Drug abuse usually begins with intermittent recreational use, when someone takes a drug to be social, to alter her state of mind, or to feel euphoric or less anxious. Other drug habits begin after drugs have been prescribed by a physician. Over time, the user develops a tolerance for the substance and it becomes necessary to take more to get the same high as before. Not everyone who takes a particular drug becomes addicted. Studies have shown that a person's susceptibility to drugs depends upon her state of mind, life circumstances, general lifestyle, and family predisposition to addiction.

Although almost all drugs change the body's chemistry, a drug is only classified as a dependency drug when the symptoms of withdrawal are severe. Such withdrawals can be dangerous—even fatal—and should be supervised by an attending physician. Heroin, morphine, and nicotine are the most addictive drugs because they are both physically and psychologically addictive—physically because they cause pain when discontinued, and psychologically because the pleasure they provide leads the addicts to believe they cannot function without the drug.

It is almost impossible to break a serious addiction without outside help. The best option is to go to a drug detoxification unit of a hospital, where the withdrawal process is carefully monitored. After the withdrawal process, patients are encouraged to end all interactions with other drug users, seek ongoing psychological help, and join alcohol and narcotic abuse support groups such as Alcoholics Anonymous (AA) and Narcotics Anonymous (NA).

Most alcoholics usually begin drinking to socialize or to reduce a feeling of stress. Gradually the amount of alcohol consumed increases until there is impaired control over alcohol intake. The actual number of drinks consumed can vary from person to person. Some people can tolerate very little alcohol before becoming intoxicated. Body size is also important—women, for example, generally can not drink as much as men. In fact their bodies can tolerate on average only one-third the amount of alcohol as can men. Women also develop cirrhosis and chronic hepatitis sooner than men and die more commonly and sooner than men from the hepatitis and cirrhosis. Again, severe alcoholism is difficult to control without the help of others. AA has been a great source of support and strength for many people suffering from an addiction to alcohol.

Women who drink alcohol during pregnancy put their unborn babies at great risk of developing birth defects and what is known as fetal alcohol syndrome. The FDA has stated that six drinks per day are enough to cause severe damage to the fetus. Even two drinks a day may interfere with fetal development. Most physicians advise women to abstain from alcohol altogether during the conception period and the first 12 weeks of pregnancy. After the first trimester, an occasional drink may be taken, although it is much wiser to abstain from alcohol completely to ensure the safety of the unborn child. (For more information on substance abuse, see Chapter 7.)

CHAPTER 9

Staying Healthy in Spite of Stress

Jeanne Spurlock, M.D., F.A.P.A.

How Stress Affects the Body
What the Hypothalamus Does
Why Women Are So
Vulnerable

How to Cope with Stress
How to Change Your Behavior
How to Turn Off the Physical
Symptoms of Stress

Listen to Your Body

Perhaps you already understand the familiar price that stress can exact: those butterflies in your stomach, the trouble concentrating, a feeling of being overwhelmed, pressured, or tense. It may start as something minor: You've worked all day in an office, behind a counter, or in a factory trying to please supervisors who don't understand the limitations of time. Finally, you are at home. The phone rings. You are trying to unpack eight bags of groceries. The children are hungry. Laundry baskets of unwashed clothes catch your eye. Your husband is calling to tell you that he will be late. At 6:00 P.M. in a messy kitchen, you feel your life is horribly disorganized and out of your control. You notice that you are breathing in short, uneven gasps. Your head starts throbbing. Your hands get cold. An imaginary band running across your shoulders tightens its grip on your muscles. Your tension is creating more tension. As a woman living in the 1990s, you may know these feelings only too well. This is clearly demonstrated in the following vignettes.

Eileen is a 38-year-old graphics designer for a major catalog company in New York City. Recently, at the end of a long, pressure-filled day, she excused herself from a meeting, walked to the ladies' room down the hall, and threw up. It wasn't the flu that upset her stomach.

At age 23, with no previous cardiac symptoms, Karen thought she was having a heart attack. Carrying 22 credits in graduate school, Karen was also playing in a concert band, working for the school newspaper, helping her sorority, and serving on the board of several honor societies. It was too much to do. "My chest got very heavy. I couldn't breathe," she recalls. "It was so painful. I got myself to the infirmary and the doctor there said, 'You are having a panic attack.'"

Dorothy, 44, feels as if she is in a pressure cooker with a busy ophthalmological practice, six children, and a husband. She races from office visits with patients to the supermarket for groceries and barely suppresses the daily rise of panic about carrying out her carpool assignments and meeting professional deadlines. Feeling guilty, exhausted, and continuously hassled, Dorothy wouldn't dare put herself first "no matter how pressed I am for time to unwind."

When she was 57, Josephine found herself sitting in her surgeon's office listening to her plans to operate on Josephine's wrists in order to relieve the pain of an arthritic condition. She had been working as a nurse in her state's sexually transmitted disease unit, and each day on the job brought more stress and less movement in her hands. "I couldn't even comb my hair without propping my elbows on a bureau," she recalls. Instead of surgery, however, Jo accepted early retirement. Within three months, her disabling symptoms disappeared.

Mary, a 55-year-old widow, has assumed the responsibility of caring for three grandchildren, ages 6, 4, and 14 months, in order to prevent their placement in foster care. Mary's daughter, a known substance abuser for nearly a year, was charged with neglect and abuse. Mary's anger about the situation was quickly replaced with guilt, and then the somatic symptoms surfaced.

Stress can make you sick. Doctors know this to be true, although patients don't always want to make such a mind-body connection. In study after study, the medical research in the last forty years has proven just how physically demanding and potentially life-threatening chronic stress really is, especially for women.

Stress is simply part of the human condition. In fact, a certain amount of daily pressure is absolutely normal and can make you more alert, more vibrant, and more motivated to reach your goals. Women often thrive in busy environments. For too many women today, however, this happily busy level of stress is exceeded every day. As emotional and physical caretakers for many people in their lives, some women insist on pushing themselves from morning until night filling a multitude of traditional roles while coping with a job and financial responsibilities that often conflict with parenting and home.

The link between your brain and body is very tangible and neither you nor your physician can afford to separate your physical complaints from your emotional equilibrium. Medicine has made dramatic advances in caring for and curing some of the problems of acute infectious diseases, but now we need to turn our attention to what appears to have become an epidemic of female stress-induced illness.

HOW STRESS AFFECTS THE BODY

Although individual physical and emotional reactions to stress vary, the results are similar. A stress overload activates areas of your brain that then send involuntary impulses to organs elsewhere in your body. You can blame your general adaptation reflex—an involuntary series of physical reactions—as well as your ancestors for your biological inability to handle excess stress without getting sick. When you become frightened, your body switches into its emergency "fight or flight" mode. This is a completely natural, normal response involving your endocrine system, your autonomic nervous system, the hypothalamus in your brain, and your limbic system.

What the Hypothalamus Does

The size of a grape, your hypothalamus takes care of a multitude of responsibilities. (See Fig. 9.1) Located in the center of your brain and linked to your pituitary gland, it stores hormones and reigns over your endocrine system, the network of glands all over your body. The hypothalamus sends messages to your nervous system and communicates directly with its neighbors in the brain. You can envision this structure as the ultimate link between your mind and body. The hypothalamus turns on the tap of your physical sensations when you respond to something emotional, whether in fear,

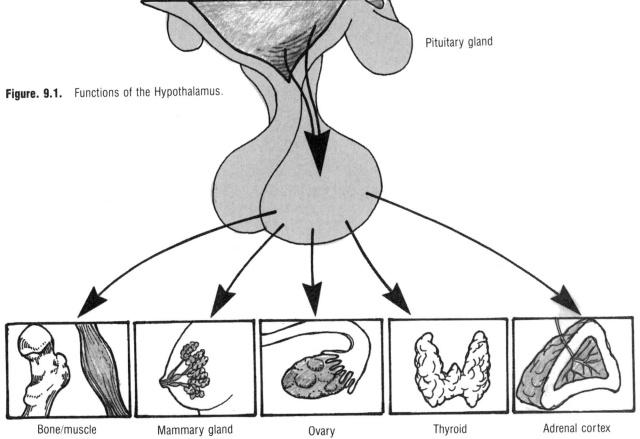

Figure. 9.1. Functions of the Hypothalamus.

Pituitary gland

Bone/muscle   Mammary gland   Ovary   Thyroid   Adrenal cortex

The hypothalamus is a part of the brain that is linked to the pituitary or "master" gland. The hypothalamus causes the release of hormones to the pituitary, which in turn triggers the release other hormones into the bloodstream. These hormones, produced by glands throughout the body, affect growth, metabolism, and all aspects of reproduction. The ovary, thyroid gland, and adrenal cortex are under the control of the pituitary gland. The hypothalamus and pituitary cause the mammary glands to begin producing milk after birth. Hormones also affect bone strength and can cause muscles to become tense during stressful situations.

love, anger, frustration, or anxiety. These intangible sensations soon become quite tangible as your body reacts.

Some researchers have called the hypothalamus "the master gland," because it produces at least nine different hormones triggering almost all of the other glands in your body to swing into action or quiet down. Extreme fear, for example, affects the body in many different ways. Your pupils will widen to let in more light. You will experience an increase in alertness because of more neurotransmitters in your brain. Your adrenal glands will begin to pump more adrenaline and other hormones into your bloodstream. Your heart races, your blood pressure rises, your muscles tense. Your liver starts converting starches to sugars for energy. Digestion slows. Experts have even determined that your blood's clotting powers will be enhanced during stressful situations. Sweat production increases and the hair on your body may feel prickly and actually stand on end. All these physical reactions were designed to save your life. Your body is getting ready to defend itself. But these reactions are no longer physiologically useful in modern life and can actually be harmful if you keep yourself in such an alert state for too many hours each day.

Not surprisingly, a daily regimen of racing heartbeat, pulsing blood, tensed muscles, undigested food stuck in your stomach, and elevated levels of hormones coursing through your circulatory system pose all kinds of potential health problems. Take the hormone cortisol, for instance. It is released under stress to inhibit inflammation at the site of any potential wounds, yet it is unlikely that you will need the assistance of cortisol. Your boss isn't really going to inflict bodily harm on you if you can't finish the paperwork on your desk. He or she may scream or fume or threaten disciplinary action, of course, but that cortisol coursing through your veins, getting ready to heal cuts, abrasions, or bruises from a real fight, isn't helping you at all. In fact, it's hurting you, because cortisol can boost your blood pressure and lead to hypertension.

Too much stress also affects your immune system, weakening it and making you more susceptible to colds, coughs, and infections. It has been traced as the culprit in flareups of arthritis and asthma. Your urinary tract can also be affected. There is a natural balance of friendly and unfriendly organisms that normally co-exist in our digestive and urinary systems. Constant anxiety can destroy this immunological balance, however, leading to an overgrowth of the harmful bacteria and an infection.

THE PSYCHOLOGICAL SIGNS OF STRESS

Ask yourself the following questions:

- Are you nervous, anxious?
- Do you feel depressed or sad?
- Are you irritable or moody?
- Do you often become frustrated?
- Are you forgetful?
- Do you have trouble thinking clearly?
- Can you make decisions without agonizing?
- Is it difficult to learn new information?
- Do you have insomnia?
- Are you plagued by negative thoughts?
- Are you fidgety?
- Are you accident-prone?
- Do you bite your fingernails or cuticles?

Why Women Are So Vulnerable

While it is true that men may face more immediate life-threatening occupational hazards, women appear to be more vulnerable to stress-induced illnesses, for a variety of reasons. First, they are socialized to being caretakers, and as such they almost automatically take on responsibilities that men might not even consider. This alone adds to the stress loads they carry. Second, women as a whole are less likely to be in positions of power and are not as able to control what's going on in their environment as most men. If you can't say no, the stress you feel can be doubly disastrous because you don't see any escape. The less power you have over the circumstances of your everyday existence, the heavier the stress load.

It may be obvious that what complicates a woman's stress is work. Men who are stretched thin at their work places often go home to relax. Women, on the other hand, go home and keep on working. In spite of the increasing number of women with careers and jobs, traditional roles in their homes still take precedence for many women. They can expect to be in charge of everything from child care to laundry, food preparation, social calendars, and runny noses. Delegating these duties to others in their households helps, but in the long run most women are still in charge. Given this situation, their minds as well as their bodies work overtime. When they become angry about too much to do in too little time with too little help, the anger only adds to their overstressed physical condition. Even women who sense their own need to slow down are programmed toward overcommitment because they feel guilty about not being able to be everything to everyone in their lives. Time spent alone or nurturing their own mental and physical well-being might be construed as selfish, so they push even harder on all fronts—home, work, and social. Sociologists speculate that many women today may be disadvantaged because they have incorporated a male standard for achievement in the work world with an old-fashioned female standard for perfection at home.

THE PHYSICAL SYMPTOMS OF STRESS

These symptoms, if chronic, may be signs of extreme anxiety and stress. They may also relate to a physical disorder. If they are sudden, severe, or persist, see your doctor.

- Back pain
- Muscle tension
- Headaches
- Shaking hands
- Diarrhea
- Constipation
- Pounding heart
- Chest pain
- Sweaty, cold hands
- Shortness of breath
- Indigestion or gas pains
- Burping
- A burning sensation in your chest
- Feeling faint or dizzy
- A lingering head cold
- Ringing in the ears
- Grinding your teeth
- Hives or skin rashes
- Loss of appetite
- Feeling nauseated, vomiting
- Pain in your stomach

HOW TO COPE WITH STRESS

To get some control into your life and tame the stress that could be making you sick, a two-way approach is recommended. First, it is necessary to change your behavior so you can slow the emotional pace of your life. Second, learn how to turn off your general adaptation reflex. You can do this by using exercise and relaxation techniques.

How to Change Your Behavior

Allow yourself regular leisure time. Leisure time is a necessity, not a reward for having completed all your tasks. Deep psychic benefits come from forgetting your chores and what time it is. For example, take a magazine into the bathroom, fill the tub, climb in, and relax.

The leisurely soak will give you the strength to do more later. Take an hour or half-hour to be by yourself each day. Many highly successful people have discovered that a key to keeping their minds sharp and their bodies healthy is to sit quietly and daydream a little each day. If sitting still makes you feel anxious or guilty, browse in a book store, walk around the block, or find some other undemanding yet pleasurable activity. A caution, however: Even leisure activities offer little refreshment if you run through them, squeezing in a quick bath, a little tennis, racing to the fast-food restaurant with kids, or are always considering what must be done next. The key is to plan—don't wait for free time to suddenly appear. The only way to create time for yourself is to take it away from some other activity. Personal time for refueling and staying healthy will never be available unless you plan for it purposefully.

Set goals for yourself. This may mean reordering your daily priorities. When you give a little of yourself to everything, you commit a great deal of yourself to nothing. Think back to the days when you have been most fragmented. Were you trying to complete an impossibly long list of things to do? If you work, try to take work breaks that remove you physically or mentally from the office. If possible, don't take office work home with you.

Insist on help with regular chores. Learn how to delegate without guilt. Basic changes aimed at lightening your load can ease your stress considerably. Pick something in your life that you find hard to ignore—unmade beds, dirty dishes—and ask for help. If something can be ignored, however, let it be until you have more leisure time to tackle that particular chore. Don't be a perfectionist.

When you start to delegate items on your "to do" list, decide on tasks (1) that you can give to someone else, (2) that others (especially kids) can do for themselves, (3) that you're doing out of habit, (4) that are low-priority and a waste of your energy, and (5) that you are only doing to please others or to make them feel guilty. In the meantime, when you feel pressed for time, ask yourself, What will happen if I don't do this project? You may be surprised to find out how many chores can easily be dropped without any repercussions or anyone even noticing.

Don't combine too many activities. Some women can't resist the urge to talk on the telephone, reshuffle the daily demands clipped to their desk or kitchen counters, and cook a meal all at the same time. They may be experts at combining activities, and most of the time this ability gives them a great sense of satisfaction. However, one of the reasons many women end up feeling stressed is because they feel fragmented, worn down, and weary from having to respond to too many people and situations. Occasionally slowing down to focus on one thing is essential to keeping your emotions and those of the people around you balanced. If you really want to enjoy a meal or a conversation with someone, it is important to concentrate on that activity to the exclusion of everything else.

Take advantage of your natural body rhythms. There may be 24 hours in a day, but your mood and energy level can't keep up with the clock all day. The sooner you figure out when your prime time is, the less overwhelmed you will feel. Most people are at their peak between 10:00 A.M. and 2:00 P.M., but you know your own body best. By adjusting your routine slightly you may be able to eliminate some of the stress from your life. For example, save routine tasks for periods when your energy is at its lowest point. Devote your peak hours to more demanding or enjoyable projects.

Stop running to answer every request. A ringing telephone, a doorbell, or the sudden demand of an impatient co-worker makes some women jump, no matter what else they have been doing. Even in mid-bite, midsentence, or midnap, you may feel obliged to answer all such calls for your immediate presence. Some experts believe that women who have trouble managing stress operate under the tyranny of believing that these demands on their life are always important. Often they are not. In fact, the really important matters in life don't always appear to be urgent. Prioritizing doesn't mean shirking your responsibilities. It does mean making a conscious effort to separate what's important from what's merely "urgent" at the time. Think first: Is this *really* important, or could it be done later? Then give your attention to the things that really count.

Learn how to say no. For many women, turning down someone who asks for a chunk of your time is never easy. It is nice to be needed, but adding extra burdens can wreak havoc on your day. These suggestions may help. (1) Say no fast, before they can anticipate a yes. Hedging with "I don't know" or "Let me think about it" only complicates your life, adding stress because you'll have to call back and beg off later. (2) Be as polite and pleasant as possible. (3) Offer a counterproposal. If you can't take on a complete responsibility for a new project, consider sharing with someone else or suggesting another person for the assignment.

Look at time as your life. When you stop trying to spend, save, and invest time, you'll feel less stressed out. Of course, your time is important. It's your life, after all. By looking at it from such a mercenary, rushed, overstressed viewpoint, you may be missing out on much that is truly enjoyable as well as the activities and people that make life worth living.

Locate the source of your stress. Sometimes women don't stop to focus on exactly why they feel overwhelmed. If you can analyze your day's load of stress, you may be able to pinpoint a particular problem and be able to deal with the stress more effectively. For instance, the next time someone in your office hands you several projects simultaneously and each one is dubbed an emergency, think before you panic. Instead of agonizing alone, go back to your boss and ask which one should be done first, second, and third. The more information you can gather and the more support you can pull together, the easier it will be to cope with the stress.

How to Turn Off the Physical Symptoms of Stress

You probably don't need medication or therapy to relieve the physical symptoms of stress. The first important step is simply to recognize the particular way you experience stress. The second step is to take any unwanted side effects seriously. Third, you need to learn how to turn off your body's "fight or flight" reflex by using breathing, exercise, or relaxation techniques. Use the following methods the next time you feel yourself being physically engulfed by stress.

Breathe deeply. Breathing is critical to dealing with stress effectively. A lack of oxygen restricts blood flow and causes muscles to tense. When you are panicked, you tend to take short, shallow gasps of air, hardly using your diaphragm at all. Your chest muscles and the accessory breathing muscles in your shoulders are overloaded and do all the work of respiration. The next time you are in a stressful situation, (1) sit up straight, (2) inhale through your nose with your mouth closed, (3) exhale through your mouth with your lips pursed (as if you were whistling or kissing), (4) make your exhalation twice as long as your inhalation (inhale for two seconds, exhale for four, for instance). Use your abdomen when you breathe, consciously pushing your belly out. Try putting one hand over your stomach, in fact, to see how it rises and falls. You are allowing more air to enter your body, and in the process you will slow down your heart rate, lower your blood pressure, and eventually break the stress cycle.

Practice progressive relaxation techniques. Sit in a quiet spot and take off your shoes or any uncomfortable clothing, including eyeglasses. Close your eyes, uncross your legs, place your hands in your lap palms up, and let your head rest easily. (You also can lie down.) Start by tightening the muscles in your feet and toes and then relaxing them. Gradually work this tightening and relaxing pattern up through your legs, back, chest, and head, including your face. Clench your jaws. Hold that tension. Then relax.

Another relaxation exercise is to picture yourself in a pleasant place. Perhaps it's a calm lake or a mountain view that puts your mind at rest. Visualize this scene in your mind as you slowly let each part of your body go limp. Breathe deeply. Aim for at least 10 minutes or more of progressive relaxation, if possible. To know if you are truly relaxed, feel the temperature of your hands. Warm hands mean a relaxed body. If your hands are still cool, you know you are still tense. (Put them on your neck to test the temperature.) Continue your relaxation until they warm up.

To get the most healthy benefit from any relaxation technique, you'll have to practice it often. Choose a time of day when you won't be interrupted. Turn off the radio, TV, and stereo. If you learn how to switch into this relaxation mode in private, you'll be better able to do it under stress.

Exercise your shoulders and neck muscles. We store stress in the muscles of the upper back, shoulders, and neck. Learn how to release this tension by gently moving that area of the body. The movements don't have to be complicated. To loosen up the tightness:

- *Shrug your shoulders.* Stand up or sit. Push your shoulders up around your ears and tighten the muscles as much as possible. Let them drop and relax. Repeat.

- *Stretch up and overhead.* While sitting in a chair, bring your arms overhead, holding them straight with fingertips pointing toward the ceiling. Elbows shouldn't be locked. Reach skyward with your right hand and then with your left hand. You should feel the stretch, but nothing should hurt. Breathe comfortably throughout.

- *Swing your arms.* Stand up. Let your arms stand loose at your sides. Lean forward slightly and swing your arms back and forth and from side to side across your chest. Relax. Stop swinging. Lift one arm up over your head, and look over your right shoulder. Hold that position. Relax and breathe deeply.

- *Walk.* Go out for a walk, but leave your pocketbook behind; if you carry a bag, you might throw your body off balance. Walk briskly and throw your shoulders back as you move. Don't race. Hurrying may make you slouch forward unconsciously, creating tension in the curve of your shoulders. Throw your shoulders back, expand your chest area, and breathe deeply.

LISTEN TO YOUR BODY

As our critical knowledge of the mind-body connection grows, it becomes even more apparent that you are your own best weapon in defending yourself against stress-related illness. Become a more active listener to the signals your own body may be sending. Don't deny or ignore symptoms of stress. A consultation with your doctor may be advisable. It may be that she will determine that the symptoms are indeed related to stress and reaffirm the importance of taking your leisure time seriously. If you aren't enjoying the responsibilities of your life, then you are probably overestimating your capacity to handle stress. It might be that the stress you experience at a particular time in your life is overwhelming. Don't be reticent about seeking professional help at those times. Such a move can be life-saving. So it was for Mary, the 55-year-old grandmother who was previously described. She arranged to see her doctor before her scheduled appointment. Her doctor found her blood pressure, previously controlled by medication, to be elevated to an alarming degree. Her medication was changed, and a referral was made to a mental health facility for an evaluation. This referral led to a therapeutic encounter that enabled her to resolve her anger and guilt about her daughter and to explore the possibility for assistance from social agencies. Mary accepted the therapist's admonition that she couldn't be all things to all people.

CHAPTER 10

Violence and Women

Marjorie Braude, M.D.

Stalking. Date Rape. These are frightening new words that have been coined to describe violent offenses against women. Violence in all of its forms has become woven into the everyday fabric of our lives.

- Every 6 minutes a woman is raped.
- Every 15 seconds a woman is punched, slapped, kicked, or otherwise physically abused by a man she knows.
- Every day, approximately four women are murdered by their husbands or boyfriends.

These horrifying statistics point out that half of all American women experience violence from men at some point in their lives—often at the hands of husbands and lovers. Even if you have managed to escape violence yourself, you more than likely know someone who is a survivor of rape, sexual abuse, or battery. Violence can strike anywhere: it affects women of every class, ethnicity, and level of education, in rural villages, the suburbs, and in urban settings.

As if real life isn't threatening enough, much of our popular culture seems to encourage this pervasive climate of violence. From the pages of pornographic magazines with their scenes of brutal bondage to films and television programs depicting women who are stalked, terrorized, and tortured, women are viewed more often than not as helpless victims and men as ruthless aggressors. Even today's popular music—particularly rap—continues to assault our ears with denigrating lyrics about women who need to be taught to stay in their place.

Whether we are aware of it or not, the fear engendered in us by both the real and fictionalized images of violence affects our daily lives. Consider how it has affected and limited your own life. Are you afraid to go out alone at night? Are you cautious to the point of isolation? Have you joined the growing ranks of women who own and carry a weapon?

Unfortunately, as careful as we may be outside our homes, often it is from those within our closest circle that we have the most to fear. According to a 1992 report by the National Crime Victim Center, nearly eight out of ten rape survivors knew their attacker. Childhood sexual abuse occurs most often between a father or stepfather and a daughter, not with some evil lurking stranger. Domestic battery—injury of a women at the hands of her husband or lover—is responsible for more injuries to adult women than from any other cause, including car accidents and muggings combined.

A GROWING CALL FOR ACTION

Despite the alarming statistics, there is some encouraging news. Clearly, no one simple antidote to violence against women exists, but people are working on all fronts to develop cures. Today more and more women are taking control of their own lives, as well as helping to work with others to stop the cycle of violence in their homes and on their streets. Crisis centers, shelters, and hotlines for rape and domestic abuse now exist all over the country. Classes in self-defense are increasingly being filled by women. Paradoxically, the media, besides being a contributor to glorifying violence, is also its "unmasker": By documenting the violence, the veil of secrecy and shame has been lifted from the faces of women who want to share their stories of surviving rape, child sexual abuse, and battery. Magazine articles, television shows, and documentaries are now covering gender-based violence, including how to recognize and protect against it and how to recover from it.

To some degree, the legal, political, and medical establishments have joined the media. Crimes against

A BATTLE BETWEEN THE SEXES?

Although the status of American women has risen dramatically within the past century, many men and women remain confused about their sexual and societal roles. Some experts claim that the rising number of violent crimes against women reflects men's intense anger over the political and economic power women appear to be gaining in modern America. As Susan Brownmiller theorized in her landmark book, *Against Our Will: Men, Women and Rape,* "It [rape] is nothing more or less than a conscious process of intimidation by which *all* men keep *all* women in a state of fear." Others see the rise in gender-based violence as stemming from long-held ideas about male aggression ("boys will be boys") and female subjection that are reinforced by a society obsessed with sex in its advertising, music, movies, and television.

women are being taken more seriously than ever before. For example, restraining orders designed to protect battery victims from their abusers have recently been issued more often and more strictly enforced. New laws have been passed to cover crimes against women. For example, a 1993 study conducted by the Centers for Disease Control and Prevention showed that the incidence of stalking—that is, repeated harassment and surveillance with threats of violence—has rapidly increased; 48 states now have some form of anti-stalking laws that call for prison terms and fines. These laws have given the police more authority in an area where they previously had none.

On still another front, those in mainstream medicine, specialty societies, nursing, and other health professions have been urged to increase their responsibilities to those patients who are the survivors of abuse. Until recently, too often physicians never saw past the broken ribs or lacerated eyes to the underlying problem of domestic abuse. They literally put a Band-Aid on the problem by focusing only on treating the injuries and sending the abused woman back to her abuser. Today that picture is changing as more and more medical schools, residencies, and ongoing medical education forums are training physicians to recognize and treat survivors of gender-based violence.

THE EFFECTS OF VIOLENCE ON WOMEN

All gender-based crime results in a special set of circumstances for its survivors. A common term that defines the effects of violence and trauma is post-traumatic stress disorder (PTSD). Short-term or one-time assault can result in PTSD, as well as long-term effects of victimization.

Some women react to the stress of violence by experiencing repeated mental flashbacks. They are hypersensitive to their surroundings and react strongly to any event or location that reminds them of the trauma. Other women, rather than recalling the event, try to deny the incidents ever happened. Associated memories may begin to trickle in after some coincidental event; however, many women so successfully block

the crime (particularly if they were victims of childhood sexual abuse) that it is only through long-term psychotherapy and/or judicious hypnosis that the event can be remembered at all. Perhaps worst of all, gender-based violence often results in the stripping of self-esteem and self-confidence. In fact, the survivor is often left blaming herself and not the perpetrator of the crime.

A woman who has experienced violence needs both immediate crisis support and intervention as well as long-term physical, psychological, legal, and social help. The particular challenges a woman faces depends to a large degree on the type of gender-based crime to which she is subjected.

RAPE

According to statistics collected by the National Victim Center, about 683,000 women were raped—forced against their will into sexual acts—in the United States in 1990. Altogether, more than 12 million American women, or one in every eight, have been raped at some time in their lives.

The word *rape* comes from the Latin *rapere,* "to take by force." The traditional legal definition of rape in the United States is carnal knowledge (vaginal penetration) of a female through the use of force or the threat of force and without her consent. Most states have revised, or are in the process of revising, that definition to include oral, rectal, and vaginal contact,

as well as penetration. Most importantly, we have come to understand that rape is an act of aggression, not a sexual act performed out of passion or lust. The need to humiliate and overpower, not sexual gratification, is the motivation for the attack.

The act of rape is one of the oldest forms of aggression against women. The Bible relates many tales of rape, as does the folklore of peoples throughout the world. The author Susan Brownmiller has noted that rape has often been considered as "an unfortunate but inevitable by-product of the necessary game called war." Japan, for example, has only recently admitted—and only because it was forced to by public opinion—

that during World War II thousands of Korean women were forced into brothels used by the Japanese military. In our own time, we have become aware that many women in war-torn Bosnia-Herzegovina have been raped by Serbian forces. Like rape in general, wartime rape is an act of violence that should be prosecuted as a war crime when it is a deliberate strategy or tactic in the war.

Date Rape

A commonly held misconception about rape is that it involves a surprise attack by a stranger. The truth is that 80 percent of rapes are committed by someone who was known to the survivor—including a husband, a father, an uncle, or other male relative and increasingly acquaintances and dates. In fact the term *date rape* has become all too common as more and more women come forward to relate their experiences of being forced to have sex with men whom they were casually dating.

One clue to the persistence and pervasiveness of rape in a supposedly enlightened society can by found in the results of a 1988 survey conducted on a Midwestern college campus. Both young men and women were asked: Is it all right if a male holds a female down and forces her to engage in sexual intercourse (1) if he spends a lot of money on her? (39% of men and 12% of women said yes); (2) if she has had intercourse with others? (39% men and 18% women answered yes); (3) if she says she will have sex and then changes her mind? (54% men and 31% women responded yes). With answers like these it should not be surprising that when 7,000 students were surveyed on 32 campuses, one of eight women said they were raped and one in four women were victims of an attempted rape.

Although rapes can occur any time of the day or night, according to FBI Uniform Crime Reports it is more likely to happen late evening or early morning on a Saturday or Sunday. Rapes occur on poorly lit side streets, in dormitory rooms on college campuses, and in living rooms after casual dates. (Almost half of all rapes occur in or around the victim's home.) Some rapists use knives, guns, or other weapons to intimidate their victims; others pose a threat by their physical strength alone.

PREVENTING RAPE

Unfortunately, there is no foolproof way to prevent rape, but there are commonsense steps you can take.

- Take normal precautions against rape: never walk alone late at night; always make sure your home is secured; never get into a stranger's car; never hitchhike; never allow anyone to follow you into a building.

- If you live alone, use only your first initial and last name on the mail box or tenant list.

- Teenage girls, who are particularly vulnerable, should understand that there is safety in numbers and whenever possible should travel in a group. They should be strongly warned against picking up strangers or bringing them back to their homes or dorms.

- If possible, take a self-defense course and learn how to resist an assailant.

- Be aware that any date could turn into a date rape.

- Know the name of every man you date and be somewhat reserved on a first date. (You might offer to pay for half of the date so you don't "owe" him.)

- If you are going to go home with a man you just met (which is never a good idea), tell someone and let the man know that you have done so.

- If any date begins to "cross the line," let him know immediately that you don't approve. Look for an escape route.

- Never allow yourself to be pressured into sexual intercourse. If you feel you are being pressured, extricate yourself from the situation and leave.

- Use alcohol and drugs with great caution.

The rape survivor often describes her experience as one in which every aspect of her awareness and being is attuned only to protecting herself and escaping with her life. Depending on her assessment for survival, one woman might physically fight her assailant, while another is unable to resist. If a woman survives a rape, it is testimony that she had made the right choice and why she is considered to be a survivor and not just a victim.

The Aftermath: Picking up the Pieces

The woman who has just survived a rape needs safety, comfort, and crisis intervention. Rape hotlines are available in many communities to give women advice, support, and information about their options throughout the rape aftermath. Often, however, the survivor feels too afraid, disoriented, ashamed, and defiled by the experience to report it to the authorities or to seek help at a hospital or clinic. Typically the rape survivor only wants to take a hot shower or bath; unfortunately, that also washes off the tangible evidence on her body that rape has taken place. The last thing she may want is an examination of the same intimate parts of her body that were just invaded and abused. And she may well be terrified of further violence from her assailant or be scared that she will receive an unsympathetic response from medical or legal professionals.

However, it is imperative that a rape survivor seek medical care as soon as possible, both to receive emergency medical treatment and to establish evidence that the rape took place. If the survivor goes to the hospital for a post-rape examination, she should be informed that hospitals are generally legally required to report rapes. These rules were established in response to criticism that some survivors—particularly when a wife who accused her husband of rape—were not taken seriously and evidence was not routinely gathered and preserved. (It should be noted that since 1975 more than 30 states have passed laws defining marital rape as a punishable crime.)

When the police are involved, they should make a careful documentation of all injuries. Specimens such as vaginal fluid (which might indicate the presence of semen), foreign bodies, pubic hair, blood, and saliva should be collected as evidence. Photographs of any injuries are especially important because most cuts and bruises are healed by the time the case goes to court.

Once severe injuries are treated, physicians usually offer medication to protect survivors from sexually transmitted diseases that may have been passed by the rapist. Although the reported incidence of gonorrhea following rape is only 3 percent and that of syphilis is 0.1 percent, medical attention can ensure that neither is contracted. If the patient desires, she will be tested for the AIDS virus. (Even if her attacker is caught, the rape survivor is not entitled to know his HIV status, and he cannot be forced to take an AIDS test.) A second test after six months will better determine whether AIDS was contracted. Pregnancy is another problem. Despite a low risk—only about 1 percent of survivors become pregnant following a rape—doctors usually administer medication to prevent conception if requested to do so by the survivor.

The psychological assessment and treatment of the rape survivor is crucial as soon as her medical condition has been stabilized. Indeed, in many ways the physical injuries are easy to treat compared with the longer-lasting emotional scars left by the rape.

The Psychological Approach

Rape has a profound effect upon a woman's life and her view of the world. Her self-esteem—her image as someone who can operate in the world with some degree of safety and success—may be shattered, and it may be very difficult to put the psychic pieces back together again.

Almost without exception, a survivor blames herself to some extent for the attack. She often bombards herself with accusations: "Why did I take that route home?" "Why did I say yes to the date?" "Why did I wear that dress?" Blaming the victim is part of the rape scenario: In New York one convicted serial rapist said boldly, "Women get raped because of the way they dress." Even friends and family often join in the chorus: "What were you wearing?" "How much did you drink?" "Why did you let him kiss you?" "Why did you go to his room?" The survivor may, in fact, become so obsessed with her role in the rape that she plays the scene over and over again to see if she might have changed the course of events.

When the assailant is someone the survivor knows, which is the case in a large majority of rapes, the guilt and blame is compounded and her judgment about all men may be thrown into question. In addition, her ideas about sex and her own sexuality may be distorted by the rape, especially if she, like many women, felt some sexual stimulation at any point during the rape. Becoming sexually active following a rape is difficult for most rape survivors. There are other traumas as well.

The Rape Trauma Syndrome

Rape survivors appear to pass through several stages of emotional reactions, similar in some ways to those experienced by the grief-stricken. The length of time needed to pass through each stage varies considerably, and many women find themselves returning to different stages during the course of recovery. The common reactions experienced by rape survivors have been described by nursing researchers Burgess and Holwstrum as rape trauma syndrome and are now included by the American Psychiatric Association in descriptions of post-traumatic stress disorder in the diagnostic manual. The physical reactions include pain, nausea, insomnia, changes in sleeping and eating patterns, and hot and cold flashes. Emotional reactions include self-doubt, guilt, mood swings, and anxiety.

Immediately following the rape, the survivor may also feel:

■ *Denial.* Numb and uncomprehending, she may deny the experience happened altogether or rationalize the event away, even if it means convincing herself that she consented.

■ *Anger and grief.* After the shock and the denial has worn off, a survivor often moves on to the reaction stage. At this point, the survivor admits to herself that she has in fact been viciously violated and allows herself to react emotionally to the event.

■ *Depression.* Faced with a loss of self-esteem, self-confidence ("How did I let that happen to me?"), and for some a loss of independence as they cling to those around them for support and protection, some survivors fall into a long-term depression. Psychotherapy and support groups can be important and helpful at this stage, as long as the therapist or group leader is trained in working with the consequences of trauma on women.

■ *Take action.* At some point, a woman may choose to transform her lifestyle to protect herself from another attack. Once they have gained some perspective—a process that may take from several days to several years—many survivors become mobilized to take some action relating directly to the rape. For some, this may mean simply telling someone close to them the details of the event; for others it may mean joining a support group or even starting a rape hotline in the community.

■ *Acceptance.* A survivor's sense of safety and view of the world is usually permanently altered by experiencing a rape.

Rape and the Legal System

For many survivors, the process of taking action against the rapist at some stage in the acceptance process can be a powerful healer. By all accounts, however, less than 15 percent of all rapes are reported. Women who are raped by men they know are often particularly reluctant to report it, because they know there is a chance they will not be taken seriously by the criminal justice system. The police investigation is often long and tedious, and the trial does not usually take place until months after the attack. If a woman decides to prosecute, she will need ongoing support from her family as well as from the police, prosecutors, and perhaps her medical team.

Even today, women who are raped feel overwhelmed by a legal system that often places the burden of proof on the victim rather than on the accused. Until only recently an eyewitness was required to prove that a rape occurred at all. Without question, convicting a rapist in the absence of corroborative evidence such as a serious injury, torn clothes, or blood stains is still difficult.

On the positive side, legislatures in 47 states have passed rape shield laws that limit the so-called loose woman argument—the defense can no longer focus on a women's sexual past. These laws, which vary by state, protect both the identity and past sexual history of rape survivors while describing the specific "exceptional circumstances" where it will be permitted.

Despite the rape shield laws, during the actual trial the behavior and personal history of the survivor still becomes as much of an issue as the facts surrounding the incident itself. Nevertheless, most women who decide to prosecute ultimately feel more empowered and

IF YOU ARE IN DANGER OF BEING RAPED

Rape is a crime of violence, in which injury or death may be threatened. Any clues that the rapist gives you about his person, motivations, or weaknesses may be useful in preventing the rape, or, if you cannot prevent it, surviving it. Possible strategies are:

- *Make a loud nose.* Many women now routinely carry a whistle that makes a piercing sound or scream "Police" to attract attention.

- *Run,* but only if there is a safe haven near you. Any attempt to flee that fails may make the situation worse by angering the rapist.

- *Stall* the attacker by speaking calmly and rationally to him. Try not to plead, cry, or otherwise show terror—that may be just the reaction he is hoping to elicit.

- *Urinate or vomit.* If nothing else works, try something that may repulse your attacker. Saying you have a sexually transmitted disease or AIDS may also scare him off, but it may enrage him, too.

- *Fight.* This strategy should be attempted only as a last resort, especially if he has a weapon. However, studies have shown that women who actively resist and who act quickly are more likely to avoid rape than those who are passive or show no resistance. (The optimum time to act is within the first 20 seconds when the body often releases chemicals into the blood system that help you to put up a fight.)

- *Do nothing.* Once you feel that you have no chance of avoiding the attack, try not to do anything that will anger the attacker. Some women have made the choice of asking the attacker to use a condom. Although this request could help avoid pregnancy or the spread of a sexually transmitted disease, it has sometimes later been turned against the rape survivor as proof that she consented.

- *Keep alert.* If you are raped, as difficult as it may be, pay attention to anything that might help you later identify the man: height, skin color, eye color, hair type and color, scars, language and accent, odors, and clothing. When you have the opportunity, write down or even tape facts about the rape.

- *Get help.* As soon as you can, call the police (911). You are the victim of a violent crime and most police now understand this and will help you. Keep in mind that, even if you do call the police, you are not obligated to press charges or take the matter to court. Such decisions can be made at a later date.

- *Collect evidence.* Do not shower, bathe, or douche; if you remove your clothes, put them in a plastic bag and seal it. Although your instinct may be to physically wash away every memory of the event, you will also be destroying evidence that can be used to identify and convict your assailant.

- *Tell someone.* If you do not want to call the police, call a rape crisis counselor—ask the telephone operator to connect you with the nearest center available. It is important that you tell someone—you are less likely to recover if the rape remains your secret.

For More Information and Help

National Organization for Victims Assistance
1757 Park Road N.W.
Washington, DC 20010
202-232-6682

Violence Against Women Act Task Force
NOW Legal Defense and Education Task Force
99 Hudson Street
New York, NY I0013
212-925-6635
Washington, D.C., office: 202-544-4470

---

in control than those who refuse to do so. Psychologically, too, it offers some form of closure to the event. One survivor who was raped by a former boyfriend clearly understood that it was going to be difficult to prove her charges. As she said, "I don't care if I don't win. When the police arrested him at work, at least I knew I had ruined his day."

Because of the difficulty in winning criminal cases,

some women take a different legal route and bring civil charges against the rapist in an attempt to collect damages. Also, a majority of states have passed some form of victim compensation legislation, and the survivor may be reimbursed for medical expenses and lost earnings. The survivor must meet eligibility requirements and may have to cooperate with criminal justice agencies.

CHILDHOOD SEXUAL ABUSE

A random survey of 769 college students indicated that 20 percent of girls and 9 percent of boys reported they had been sexually abused before they were 18. Other sources estimate that the number could be as high as one in every four girls and one in every seven boys.

The sexual abuse may take many forms, including sexually suggestive language, prolonged kissing and petting, vaginal and/or anal intercourse, and oral sex. It can be one or two incidents in a short period of time or continue over several years. Young girls are often abused by men they know: fathers, stepfathers, grandfathers, uncles, brothers, cousins, their mothers' or sisters' boyfriends. (A small percentage of children are abused by their mothers.) The abuser is typically someone who is welcomed into the victim's home. Some children are abused by people they come in contact with on a regular basis and whom they have been taught by their parents to trust, such as neighbors, coaches, clergymen, teachers, babysitters, doctors, dentists, and camp counselors.

SIGNS OF SEXUAL ABUSE

Sexual abuse is often achieved without physical force or battery, so the child may not show overt signs of abuse. For this reason, it is important to be aware of the subtle clues that may signal a child's distress. Physical signs include:

- lacerations, irritation, pain, or injury to the genital area;
- discharge from the genital area;
- pregnancy;
- a sexually transmitted disease;
- difficulty with urination.

Behavioral indications include:

- one child being treated in a significantly different way from other children in the family;
- aggressive, hostile, or disruptive behavior toward adults;
- provocative behavior (including flirting);
- sudden regressive behavior such as acting childishly and crying;
- inability to make friends.

Sometimes the clues come directly from the child; the adult needs to hear between the lines. Be suspicious if a child says, "He fooled around with me," "I don't like to be alone with . . . ," or "I'm afraid to go home." These signs are now taught to teachers, daycare workers, and other adults who come in regular contact with children. Most states have laws that require professionals who work with children to report suspected child abuse to a responsible agency.

To Report Abuse

National Child Abuse Hotline
1-800-422-4453

Parents Anonymous
1-800-423-0353

For More Information and Help

National Committee for Prevention of Child Abuse
332 South Michigan Avenue
Chicago, IL 60604
312-663-3520

A sexual relationship with an adult is, by its very nature, one over which the child has no control; because it often occurs within the family context or with a trusted family friend or teacher, the child may assume there is implied parental approval. Incest—sex with a member of one's family—and sexual abuse in general are never the child's fault. The law correctly insists that sexual abuse is always the fault of the adult. In father-daughter incest, for example, it is the father who chooses the relationship. Even if the rationale is that the daughter "asked for it," it is the adult's responsibility to say no.

The Aftermath of Child Abuse

The reactions of the child vary widely depending on the age of the child; her stage of development; the amount of fear, physical violence, and pain that the child experiences; the frequency and length of time over which the abuse occurs; and the reaction of non-abusing adults.

Because the experience of sexual abuse runs so counter to a child's need to love and relate to the adults in her life, it is frequently dissociated from the child's consciousness. Often the child visualizes herself out of her body, thereby losing perceptions, feelings, and whole blocks of memory. (An extreme form of dissociation may result in a child developing multiple personalities.) Although the psychological mechanisms of dissociation and denial of the experience help the child survive at the time of abuse, they often play havoc in her later life. The suppressed experience often manifests itself in fear, repression of emotions, and the inability to form lasting, healthy relationships.

Survivors of incest and sexual abuse know that the emotional and physical scars often last for a lifetime. The victim often blames herself long after the abuse has ended—for not saying no, for not fighting back, for not telling anyone about the abuse, for having trusted the abuser.

Some survivors feel the need to confront their abuser and to hear the person admit that the events actually took place. Those who decide to prosecute often face the same kind of difficulty faced by battered or raped women. The legal and medical professions are, however, becoming more sensitive in recognizing, treating, and taking action against child abuse.

DOMESTIC BATTERY

More than two million women a year are officially identified as abuse survivors. Since this number only reflects the reported cases, the true scope of the problem can only be estimated. It is estimated by some that an astounding 30 to 40 percent of the injuries that cause adult women to go to hospital emergency rooms have been inflicted by batterers. Most women who are battered by their husbands or lovers will suffer repeated injuries over several months and even years. Some will even die at the hands of their batterers. Battery first may take the form of implied threats ("If you ever talk to me that way again, I won't be responsible for the outcome") and then escalate to physical violence: shoving, punching, kicking, biting, scalding, choking, and marital rape. Most abusive injuries are inflicted on the head, neck, chest, abdomen, and breasts. Injuries may also occur on the arms, which are used to deflect blows. Physicians treating abused women report every kind of injury imaginable, from broken ribs to detached retinas to mutilated sexual organs. In addition to phys-

ical abuse, women may find themselves the victims of emotional abuse; their husbands or lovers so verbally humiliate and abase them that nothing is left of their self-esteem or self-confidence. Quite often, emotional abuse escalates into physical violence.

Like rape, battery has been around since the beginning of time. Popular culture abounds with examples of battery from the *Honeymooners* TV show (bus driver Ralph Cramden regularly threatened to send Alice "to the moon") to the Rolling Stones song "Under My Thumb." Rappers, too, regularly sing about "slapping my bitch."

The roots of the battery syndrome are as deep as those from which rape grows, and in many ways the patterns are similar. Battery is a pattern of behavior that results in a man establishing power over a woman through fear and intimidation. Battery usually occurs when men believe they are entitled to control their partners, and it continues because battered women usually end up believing it too. That is why it is believed to be such an unreported epidemic.

Like rapists, batterers come in all shapes, sizes, and ethnic backgrounds. But they do share several common characteristics: they are generally insecure, frustrated, jealous, possessive, and often display a Jekyll-and-Hyde personality, alternating periods of abuse with periods of affection. Almost all abusive husbands come from homes in which there was physical abuse between their fathers and mothers, and many battered wives also witnessed physical and emotional battery as they grew up. Because parents serve as powerful role models, children learn that violence is a useful and effective way to bring about desired behavior. The male child learns from watching his mother's reaction that she is afraid of the father, and he may apply this knowledge in adulthood by using violence or the threat of violence to achieve his own goals. A female child exposed to battery will learn passivity at all costs and, perhaps, that violence is a man's natural right. The pattern of abuse is a vicious circle that is hard to break.

The Abusive Relationship

Although there is a small percentage of women for whom violence is so much a part of the fabric of their lives that they enter a relationship knowing that there may be violence, most relationships are loving at the beginning. Indeed, for most women, violence inflicted by their mates comes as a surprise and at first may seem to be an aberration. However, a pattern emerges in which anger and tension build within the male partner until he explodes in a violent episode. After his rage is spent, he usually expresses deep remorse and promises that he will never do it again. Such a cycle is repeated over and over again until the woman no longer believes in herself or in the man to whom she is committed.

These relationships often reach a special intensity. The perpetrator of the violence is very attuned to the woman's every action, to her presence or absence, and to whether or not she is attending to his needs. Each episode of violence gives the man more coercive power over his victim, and as it continues, he may limit her access to food, sleep, and medical care. (He may even hide her car keys.) Indeed, isolation is a powerful weapon in the batterer's arsenal: a battering husband usually stops his victim from communicating with friends or relatives and swears her to secrecy, even

threatening to kill her if she tells anyone about the violence.

In turn, the battered woman becomes hypersensitive to the man in her life as he demands more and more of her attention. She often feels forced to obey his commands about her housekeeping, her meal preparation, and her behavior toward others. Freedom for the battered woman ends when her husband comes home, and it is replaced with submissive, often fearful behavior linked to the perpetrator's moods and desires. Because inadvertent actions may bring on his violence, battered women live in a constant state of terror. (Anything can tip the scale toward violence, but alcohol seems to be a trigger.) If children are part of the family,

PORTRAIT OF AN ABUSER

What kind of person would physically and emotionally abuse his wife? Researchers are still searching for answers, but studies have pointed out the following characteristics:

- Abusers have a need to control the environment around them, especially the people who are closest to them. Beating up their wives periodically is one way to ensure compliance.

- Men who have been brought up in a violent home are most likely to abuse their female partners. Other risk factors are unemployment, less education, and drug and alcohol use. One should not forget, however, that many well-educated professional men—doctors, lawyers, business executives—also beat their partners.

- Many abusers are dependent on their wives and jealous of them. Fearing abandonment, they minimize the attacks and blame the victim for any violence inflicted on her.

Unfortunately, abusive men often resist treatment. Court-ordered batterers' education and treatment groups (which address the battering as a criminal enforcement of power and control) have had reasonable success. A few men do come to such groups voluntarily. Conventional models of couples' or family therapy are absolutely contraindicated where one member of the couple is committing criminal assaults on the other. Most important, men must be confronted with the results of their battery and learn that if they don't change their behavior, they will go to jail.

they, too, become involved in the pattern of fear and violence.

Why do women stay in violent relationships? Often out of terror because of their partners' threats to kill them or take their children away. The less educated and able to earn money a women is, the more likely she is to stay in the relationship. Although the role of women in the workplace is changing, women still face fewer job opportunities and usually earn considerably less than men. If the woman has children, the challenge is compounded. She can't help but be aware that even a court award of child support is no guarantee of economic stability. And there is still strong societal pressure to "stand by your man." The victim is strongly (if figuratively) tied to her batterer—she is bound by a combination of threats, intimidation, manipulation, control, and coercion.

Battered women often feel too ashamed and full of self-blame and hatred to admit that they've let themselves be hit over and over again. Many women are so numb from repeated abuse and injury that they are barely able to function, and they sleepwalk through their lives. Battered women typically experience extreme anxiety and depression; in fact, 26 percent of all women who attempt suicide are survivors of violence. Battered women are 16 times as likely to abuse alcohol as the average adult woman, and many abuse drugs. Trapped by circumstances that seem to be beyond their control, battered women often suffer through years of physical and emotional torture at the hands of their mates before they reach out for help.

Myth: "He can't live without me."
Truth: You can't live with him.

Myth: "The kids need a father."
Truth: Kids do not need a father who is likely to beat them as well.

Myth: "It will get better."
Truth: It only gets worse.

Myth: "He'll kill me if I go."
Truth: He may well kill you if you stay.

Getting Out, Getting Help

Although doctors and nurses are often in a good position to recognize abuse and to intervene, research has shown that they often fail to report such incidents to the police or to explore the reason for the violence with the patient. Doctors are increasingly able to identify symptoms and then to help a battered woman recognize the serious, often life-threatening, circumstances in which she finds herself. Keeping the woman's safety and the safety of her children in mind, the physician may help her remove herself from the abusive situation.

Women who are beaten are twice as likely to be

IF YOU ARE BATTERED

- If your husband or lover hits you, try to defend yourself, paying particular attention to protecting your stomach and head.
- Call for help, scream, and if you can get away, run.
- Fight back only if you judge that it won't make him hurt you more. Retaliating with violence tends to cause escalation of the violence.
- Document the abuse by taking pictures or telling someone—a friend, a neighbor, or the police (call 911). If you do call the police, get a copy of the police report.
- Threatening to divorce or leave your partner *may* interrupt the violence.
- A personal safety plan is essential. A counselor or advocate from a domestic violence program may help you work one out. Plan possible destinations in an emergency with friends, relatives, or a shelter. Keep the money necessary to get there, and have a survival fund for yourself. Plan a means of transportation. Have some clothes and personal essentials packed or at a safe location. Plan for your children also.

For More Information

202-232-6682 is a national 24-hour hotline.

National Coalition Against Domestic Violence
P.O. Box 18749
Denve, CO 80218-0749
303-839-1852

National Clearinghouse for the Defense of Battered Women
137 S. 9th Street
Philadelphia, PA
215-351-0010

beaten when they are pregnant. Pregnant abused women suffer from emotional stress, have less prenatal care, often don't follow nutritional guidelines, and are more likely to abuse alcohol and drugs. Few studies have examined the effects of abuse on pregnant women, but it appears that physical abuse may cause injuries or aggravate chronic illnesses that lead to decreased fetal growth or premature birth.

When a battered woman seeks psychological help, it is critical that the therapist understand that her symptoms, no matter how severe, are a product of her terror, isolation, and inability to escape her situation and in most cases are not indicative of a long-term psychological disorder. The therapist cannot get an accurate view of the underlying problems until the source of terror is removed. The impact of many psychological diagnoses is to create or reinforce the idea that the problem of violence is her fault. Sometimes tranquilizers or antidepressants are prescribed to help a battered woman to function, but it is important for both physician and patient to keep medications to a minimum. If she is oversedated, she may not recognize danger or act on it in time to save herself or her children.

A particularly dangerous time for the battered woman is when she is planning, carrying out, or has recently achieved her escape. Most women who die at the hands of their abuser are killed at this time. It is also after the decision has been made to leave that a desperate woman may turn on the perpetrator during an attack and kill him. Most women who kill their abusers see no possibility of escape. Women who kill their batterers often report that those to whom they turned in the legal or medical professions could not or did not help.

Life after Battery

Since domestic violence emerged as a topic of discussion in the late 1970s, most communities across the country have opened hotlines and shelters to battered women. Some medical facilities have a social worker available. It is critical for a battered woman to find whatever resources and support are available in her community.

Shelters can be a lifesaver, providing a woman and her children a safe haven for an average stay of about four to six weeks. (About half of the children who are admitted to women's shelters have also been abused.) A shelter is a place where a woman can begin to heal her emotional and physical wounds while slowly regaining her self-confidence and ability to function. She can also learn about her legal options in terms of divorce, child support, and, if she wishes, criminal prosecution of her abuser.

In many states police and prosecutory practices are rapidly improving. Police are being trained to be more sensitive and many cities now have mandatory arrest policies for a batterer. In many cities prosecutors will pursue the case whether or not the victim presses charges.

Testimony from battered women in court cases and in interviews emphasizes that the first step to recovery is to admit that the abuse exists as a real problem. The next step is to stop hoping that the problem will go away. Once an abused woman recognizes that she (and her children) have every right to feel safe in her home she is on her way to finding the self-confidence she needs to rebuild her life. After a woman leaves the abusive situation behind her, she is often able to have healthier subsequent relationships.

Moving Toward Solutions

In recent years, the problem of violence against girls and women has been viewed as a public health crisis. We can all take small steps by walking with other women in "Take Back the Night" rallies, volunteering in shelters, and reporting child abuse if we suspect it. We can help break the cycle of violence by breaking the silence—by sharing our own experiences.

CHAPTER 11

Aging

Judith C. Ahronheim, M.D., F.A.C.P.

The population of the United States is aging rapidly. By the year 2030, nearly 22 percent of the population will be over the age of 65 years. Average life expectancy has been increasing steadily since the turn of the century. To a large extent this is due to the decrease in the death rate of infants. The average life expectancy of a woman is 7 years longer than that of a man. It is estimated that a woman who lives to age 65 can expect to live an additional 19 years.

The gain in years lived at midlife and beyond can be a mixed blessing. Chronic diseases occur more often in the elderly, and the years gained may not necessarily be ones of good health and function. There is some evidence that women can expect to live a smaller portion of their lives free of disability than men.

A healthy lifestyle, preventive care, and increased awareness of the special health needs of elderly women can help improve the quality of their lives. Many conditions that affect older women can be prevented or relieved through lifestyle modification and early medical care.

THE DEMOGRAPHICS OF AGING

As women age, they confront some difficult social issues. In comparison to men, older women are more likely to be unmarried, to live alone or in an institution, and to rely on others for support, both financial and otherwise.

Because women live longer than men, the ratio of women to men increases with age. This difference is most pronounced after the age of 85, when there are approximately two and one-half times more women than men. As a result, more women than men live alone for longer periods. The differences in living arrangements are related not only to the longer life span of women but also to the fact that men tend to marry younger women and that divorced or widowed men are more likely than women to remarry.

Among those living in an institution, the ratio of single (widowed, divorced, or never married) women to men is much higher than it is among the elderly who do not live in institutions. Approximately 90 percent of the oldest residents of nursing homes are women. An older woman is more likely to live in an institution if she has survived her spouse or her spouse is too sick to take care of her.

Caregivers of elderly people tend to be women. Of those who provide care to elders in their activities of daily living, 72 percent are women, mostly wives and daughters. These caregivers spend an average of 4 hours a day assisting their elders. Those employed outside the home frequently need to curtail their paid work time to perform these functions. Many spend far more than 4 hours a day in these activities, and some must rearrange work schedules or leave their work altogether.

Some older people who depend on the care of others are subjected to abuse by their caregivers. Such abuse is not necessarily active but may result from neglect.

The financial status of older women is substantially below that of older men. In 1992, the median income of older women was only 56 percent of that of older men. Approximately 16 percent of women 65 and older, compared with 9 percent of men the same age, live below the poverty level. The highest poverty rate is among elderly African-Americans, followed by Latinos. It is estimated that 63 percent of African-American women 75 years of age and older are poor.

In contrast to racial differences in economic status, older African-American women may be healthier than white women. Although average life expectancy at age 65 is approximately equal for African-American and white women, at older ages African-American women can expect to live 1 or 2 years longer. Education improves this advantage. An 85-year-old African American woman with more than 12 years of formal education can expect to live 3.6 years longer than her white counterpart.

Increasing age increases the risk of disability and the need for assistance in the activities of daily living, such as shopping, cleaning, grooming, cooking, bathing, and going to the bathroom. Among people age 65 and older, approximately 1 in 16 require such assistance, and as a person ages that figure increases to 1 in 2 by age 85. Chronic illness, such as arthritis, hearing impairment, visual impairment, and heart disease are common. Although these diseases do not necessarily impair function, they do increase the risk of disability. The disability rate seems to be declining slightly in recent years, however, and the decline is more pronounced among women than men. This may be related to improvements in recognizing and correcting disabilities, as well as increased use of devices that allow disabled people to be more independent.

THE BIOLOGY OF AGING

It is hard to define a normal aging process. Each person ages uniquely, depending on genetics, lifestyle, and exposure to agents in the environment. Because the prevalence of disease is high in later life, it can be difficult to distinguish a normal aging process from a disease process.

Some people view aging as a buildup of disease. Therefore death only can be avoided if disease could be completely eliminated. The control of some infectious diseases has prolonged survival into midlife and later, when survivors are more vulnerable to diseases of later life, such as cancer and atherosclerosis, a buildup of plaque that causes arteries to narrow and leads to strokes and heart attacks. As certain diseases are eliminated, however, new ones emerge.

The total absence of disease is more a theory than a reality. When certain human cells are allowed to grow in a laboratory, they divide only a finite number of times, and then the normal process of cell multiplication stops. This pattern of "pure aging" (senescence) has been seen in many species, although the precise number of cell divisions varies. It has been suggested that a biologic mechanism, a sort of programming built into cells before birth, determines life span. This program, in addition to other factors, may determine how long humans and members of other species live.

Some scientists believe that factors in the environment affect the aging process. Free radicals have been linked to aging; these excited molecules react readily with many substances including tissues in the body. Humans are constantly exposed to free radicals from the environment; they are by-products of most functions of the body as well. There is evidence that free radicals have a part in diseases such as arteriosclerosis (thickening of the walls of the arteries leading to heart attacks and strokes), cataracts, and cancer. Free radicals may damage the makeup of cells, causing the aging process to speed up. It is difficult to distinguish free radical damage leading to the degenerative diseases of aging from the pure process of aging. Although evidence suggests that free radicals damage cells in tissues, there is little evidence that this promotes senescence.

Certain enzymes, or antioxidants, produced by the body reduce the damage caused by free radicals. Other antioxidants include beta carotene (a member of the vitamin A family), vitamin E, and vitamin C. Current research focuses on how these and other components may affect heart disease, cancer, and visual disorders. Since women have been underrepresented in studies of antioxidants and heart disease, the effect of these and other nutrients remains unclear.

A great deal of attention has been devoted to research on antioxidants and other dietary modifications and their effect on the degenerative diseases of aging and longevity. The effectiveness of these or other strategies is controversial. Proving whether a certain approach prevents cancer is difficult because cancer can take up to several decades to develop. There also is evidence that deficiencies in antioxidants cause certain diseases.

It is premature to recommend specific strategies to prolong women's life span. However, lifestyle modifications, such as healthy diet, smoking cessation, regular exercise, and early cancer detection can help prevent premature death from disease in most people.

A HEALTHY LIFESTYLE

As women live out their later years, they must be able to enjoy their later years to the fullest extent. One way to do this is to lead a lifestyle that promotes health, lowers risks, and in general helps them feel better. Routine health care allows disorders to be detected in their early stages, when they are more easily treated. A healthy diet and exercise program can help prevent some health problems in older women and improve how they look and feel. Preventive health care and some simple adjustments in lifestyle can go a long way in improving women's quality of life.

Routine Care

Many older women do not regularly see a doctor, even though they had routine examinations when they were in their reproductive years. The risk of disease as a person ages makes it imperative that women over age 65 see their doctors for exams and screening tests on a regular basis.

During a routine visit the doctor performs a physical exam that includes a pelvic exam, and checks your blood pressure, height, and weight. The doctor or nurse should ask you about your general health status as well as other aspects of your mental and physical condition that could affect your health. On the basis of this discussion, certain tests are recommended and, if necessary, treatment and follow-up visits are planned.

Screening tests are done when a person isn't sick. They are often done in a general population to detect disease, and sometimes are done if a disease isn't present but the risk is higher. Mammography is very important for older women because the risk of breast cancer rises with age. Other screening tests are recommended at regular intervals as a woman ages. Certain tests are recommended for all women over 65 (see "Routine Care for Women 65 Years and Older"). Additional tests

may be suggested based on a woman's history ("Additional Evaluations Based on Risk Factors").

Diet, Nutrition, and Weight

Elderly people can have special nutritional requirements. It may be necessary for a woman to alter daily dietary intake based on her nutritional status, medical disorders, and the drugs she takes. In general, American women should strive to maintain a low-fat diet to lower the risk of cardiovascular disease and stroke and to include adequate amounts of calcium and fiber to meet their changing health needs. However, these rules do not apply to everyone.

Calcium may help prevent bone loss caused by a

ROUTINE CARE FOR WOMEN 65 YEARS AND OLDER

Screening Tests	Interval (may vary—ask physician)
Pap test to detect cervical cancer	Yearly
Blood glucose test for diabetes	Yearly
Mammography for breast cancer	Yearly
Total cholesterol and HDL cholesterol	Consult physician but at least once
Fecal test for occult blood to check for silent bleeding in digestive tract	Yearly
Flexible sigmoidoscopy to examine the colon and rectum for signs of cancer	Every 3–5 years
Thyroid-stimulating hormone test to check for thyroid disease	Every 3–5 years
Hemoglobin and ferritin level to check for iron deficiency	Consult physician but at least once
Immunizations	
Tetanus-diphtheria booster	Every 10 years
Influenza vaccine	Yearly
Pneumococcal vaccine	Once

ADDITIONAL EVALUATIONS BASED ON RISK FACTORS

Evaluation	Who Is at Risk
Urinalysis for protein	Women with diabetes
Skin exam	All women, expecially those often exposed to sun, with fair complexions, or previous skin cancer
Tuberculosis skin test	Women in close contact with someone who has TB; medically underserved, low-income populations; residents of long-term care facilities
Lipid profile	Women with coronary heart disease
Colonoscopy	Women who have bowel or colon disease or a family history of colorectal cancer
Fecal test for occult bleeding and hemoglobin and ferritin tests	Women regularly taking aspirin or NSAIDs for arthritis
Glaucoma	All women over 40, African-Americans, or those with a family history of glaucoma

condition called osteoporosis in older women. How much calcium you should take and for how long is still unclear. Even so, the National Institutes of Health has recommended that postmenopausal women consume 1,500 milligrams per day of calcium. Foods rich in calcium include dairy products, sardines, spinach, and vegetable greens. For example there are 302 milligrams of calcium in one 8 ounce cup of skim milk. Supplementation may be needed, but excess calcium intake should be avoided. Consult your physician about the type and amount of calcium to take (see Chapter 3).

Older women often complain of constipation. A diet high in fiber (the portion of plant food that the body eliminates without digesting) improves gastrointestinal function and may help to control weight and cholesterol if it replaces a high-fat diet. Foods rich in fiber include fruits, vegetables, and grains.

People often gain weight as they age. Their metabolism becomes slower and they need less food to maintain the same weight. Although modest weight gain is not thought to be harmful at older ages, being overweight (20 percent or more than usual of optimal weight) can pose health risks for women with high blood pressure and diabetes. An exercise program, combined with a healthy diet, can help burn off more calories as well as prevent problems linked to being overweight. Unplanned weight loss late in life is usually a sign of a serious problem. Weight loss also can occur in people unable to obtain food, such as those with memory loss, physical disabilities, or limited financial resources.

Loss of appetite is not a part of normal aging, but there may be a delay in recognizing and managing nutritional deficiencies in older people. Many nutritional deficiencies that occur in older women are related to their poor health. Feeding disorders may be temporary. For example, frail patients may stop eating when they are ill but gradually their appetites return as they gain strength.

Patients may stop eating or need to be fed at a very slow rate at frequent times throughout the day; to satisfy their nutritional needs, tube feeding is sometimes suggested. Fluids and nutrients, or pureed foods, are supplied through a tube inserted into the stomach via the nasal passages or through the wall of the abdomen. Patients have the right to refuse tube feeding, either on their own, through written instructions like a living will, or through someone designated to act for them, just as they have the right to refuse any other form of medical

treatment.

Exercise

Exercise continues to be important in later life. It improves cardiovascular fitness, may help slow the bone loss that occurs with osteoporosis, helps lower blood sugar in people with diabetes, and helps control cholesterol. In addition, exercise promotes weight loss, muscle strength, and a general feeling of well-being. Studies suggest that lack of exercise contributes to frailness and weakness in elderly people.

Exercise can promote cardiovascular illness by increasing the efficiency of the heart's function. As the body works, it requires more oxygen and the heart beats faster. Exercise increases the body's ability to use oxygen, which enables a person to exercise more without feeling tired. Exercise must reach a certain level to provide this benefit. The target heart rate can be a guide to reaching a level of exercise that provides cardiovascular fitness. However, this guide should be used cautiously late in life, when silent heart disease may exist (see Chapter 4).

Some forms of exercise strengthen the back muscles making them less prone to injury and strain. Other types of exercise help prevent bone loss by strengthening the bones and keeping them from becoming brittle. To provide bone strength, weight-bearing exercises are best. For instance, walking and lifting weights are forms of exercise that are weight bearing, whereas swimming and cycling, although they are good forms of cardiovascular conditioning, are much less likely to prevent bone loss.

An older woman who has not been exercising should consult her physician before beginning an exercise program. She must begin a new exercise program slowly and carefully. Physical changes may increase the risk of injury, and heart disease may be present but not apparent.

Older women should choose a form of exercise that is safe and comfortably within their physical capabilities. Jogging and high-impact aerobics can cause injury at any age but such exercises pose additional risk of injury to older people. Better options for cardiovascular fitness include walking, low-impact aerobics, and swimming.

People with severe physical impairments may still improve their level of fitness by doing limited exercise in the sitting position. Elderly patients who become ill and need to be hospitalized or confined to bed for even a few days suffer rapid deterioration of their physical condition because they canot move around. This can be avoided by maintaining some level of physical activity during and after illness, which also lowers the risk of bed sores (pressure ulcers), pneumonia, and blood clots.

Hormone Replacement Therapy

On average, at around age 51 or 52 a woman goes through menopause, although for many women it occurs a decade earlier or several years later. At the time of menopause, a woman's ovaries stop producing the hormone estrogen and she stops having menstrual periods. When this occurs, certain changes take place in a woman's body. She may experience hot flashes, night sweats, or difficulty sleeping. While these symptoms are temporary, other changes are taking place that have more long-term, less obvious effects. They include osteoporosis, bone loss that occurs with reduced estrogen levels, and cardiovascular disease. A lack of estrogen also can cause dryness of the vagina, which is noticeable during sex, as well as increase the risk of bladder infections and urinary tract problems.

To prevent these changes and the problems they can pose, therapy can replace the estrogen no longer produced in the body. However, although estrogen may be highly effective in suppressing hot flashes, its use for other conditions is less certain, particularly late in life. Because giving estrogen alone increases the risk of cancer of the lining of the uterus, it is given with another hormone, progestin, which protects against this cancer. The protective effect of progestin may make the estrogen less effective in preventing cardiovascular disease, but most studies indicate a benefit to combined hormone replacement therapy (see Chapter 30).

It is not clear how long a woman should take hormone replacement therapy or how long there is a benefit. Estrogen may be unsafe for women with a previous cancer of the breast or lining of the uterus, liver disease, or a history of blood clots in the lung related to hormone treatment (such as birth control pills) or pregnancy. For most women in their 50s or 60s, hormone replacement therapy offers benefits that they should seriously consider, but later in life the benefits may be outweighed by potential risks.

Sexuality

Women over the age of 70 years can and often do remain sexually active. The major cause of lack of sexual activity in older women is the lack of a male partner. Older women are able to experience sexual feelings and orgasm. Sexual responsiveness and desire may be affected in both sexes by depression, medical illness, or medications.

After menopause there is less lubrication in the vagina and the walls of the vagina become thinner and dryer. This can cause pain during intercourse. Estrogen can be effective in alleviating this problem whether it is taken by mouth in pill form or placed in the vagina as a cream or suppository.

Older couples should feel free to express their sexuality in ways that bring them pleasure. This may involve trying new positions that are less physically demanding or forms of sexual expression other than intercourse.

Substance Use

Tobacco and alcohol pose a risk to everyone. It is never too late to benefit from ending smoking or excess alcohol intake.

Among persons age 65–74, about 18 percent of women smoke. While this figure seems relatively low, it should be interpreted with caution. Because smoking increases the rate of death from coronary heart disease, stroke, and cancer, many people who smoke do not live long. Smoking is also a major contributor to lung disorders, such as emphysema and pneumonia, which can have devastating effects on the elderly.

Alcoholism is underrecognized late in life. The problem can arise after someone has suffered a loss or may have become established over years. The aged brain is more sensitive to alcohol, which in excess can cause confusion, falls, and injury. As it interacts with other drugs, alcohol can either interfere with their action or increase its own or the drugs' effects. This can pose a particular problem in the elderly because their rate of metablish is slowed, making it more difficult to process the drugs in their systems (see Chapter 7).

Medications

Elderly people not only take more medications than any other age group, but also experience more adverse side effects. This is related to several factors, including exposure to a larger number of medications, drug interactions, errors in taking medication, delayed elimination of medications from the body, and a higher sensitivity to the medications themselves.

Because of changes that take place with age, ordinary doses of drugs remain within the body for longer periods than expected and can build up to high levels over time. In all age groups, the organs most responsible for removing drugs from the system are the kidney and liver.

Kidney function declines on the average with advancing age. When drugs are given that depend on the kidneys for processing, repeated use of the drug causes it to build up and become toxic. Commonly prescribed drugs in this category include digoxin, a heart medication; certain antibiotics; cimetidine (Tagamet), a drug given for peptic ulcer; and lithium, a drug given for certain psychiatric illnesses. Whenever these and other drugs are given to the elderly the doses must be carefully adjusted and monitored.

With advancing age the liver may be less able to process certain drugs. Examples of drugs processed by the liver include diazepam (Valium); flurazepam (Dalmane), a sleeping pill; and theophylline, an antiasthma medication.

In addition to a lowered ability to remove drugs from their bodies, elderly people may be more sensitive to normal doses because the drug itself behaves differently. This effect is related to changes in various organs that occur with advancing age or with actual disease, which is more common in late life. Because disease often is not obvious in the elderly, the patient may have no symptoms until the stress of a medication is introduced.

The effects of a drug may be exaggerated in the elderly. For example, a normal dose of a sedative, intended to reduce anxiety or to have a calming effect, may produce sluggishness or confusion. Confusion is a side effect that can be produced in older people by a large number of drugs, probably because of the high prevalence of Alzheimer's and other forms of brain disease. In addition to sedatives, other medications that may produce confusion in elderly patients include sleeping pills, corticosteroids, arthritis medications, certain antidepressants, and some drugs given to lower blood pressure.

Although it is not always possible to predict the body's ability to process medication, cautious prescribing can help avoid overdose. Tests can be done to measure the amount of drug in the blood. These tests are available for many medications and are generally reliable. It is helpful to keep a list of *all* medications taken and their dosages, especially if they have been prescribed by more than one doctor, so the list can be reviewed by a doctor if there are problems (see Chapter 39).

HEALTH CONCERNS OF AGING

Early recognition and treatment of diseases that often occur in the elderly can help manage these disorders and keep them from progressing in some cases. The leading causes of death in women 65 years of age and older are cardiovascular disease, stroke, cancer, and pneumonia. Major causes of illness and disability include osteoporosis and arthritis, heart disease, falls, and hearing and vision impairment.

Cardiovascular System

The number one cause of death in both women and men is cardiovascular disease. This includes coronary heart disease, which causes the deaths of 236,000 women annually, as well as stroke and congestive heart failure—all of which increase dramatically with age. Coronary heart disease is the leading cause of death in women and outnumbers deaths in women caused by all cancers combined.

Coronary heart disease occurs in women about 10 years later than it does in men. Some believe this delay is due to the protection that estrogen provides against heart disease. Once a woman passes menopause, her risk begins to approach that of a man.

Coronary heart disease often is unrecognized in women. Women are diagnosed at later stages of disease than men are and are less often referred for diagnostic procedures. Women also tend to have surgical treatment, such as coronary artery bypass surgery, later in the course of the disease, which results in a higher rate of complications and death from the procedure. Women also have a greater degree of disability after heart attacks compared with men and are less likely to be referred for exercise and rehabilitation. The reasons for these differences are unclear.

The risk factors for coronary heart disease include diabetes, hypertension, cigarette smoking, abnormal cholesterol (see below), and family history. With the exception of family history, all of these factors can be controlled to lower the risk. Women with diabetes have a three-fold increased risk of heart attack, and it is a stronger factor for women than men. Diabetes can be controlled through a combination of diet, exercise, and medication to normalize blood sugar (glucose) level.

Hypertension, or high blood pressure greater than about 160 (millimeters of mercury) systolic pressure and 90 (millimeters of mercury) diastolic pressure, increases the risk of heart attack and stroke. The main form of hypertension affecting the elderly involves elevated systolic pressure with normal diastolic pressure. Although hypertension cn have side effects and must be carefully monitored in the elderly, newer medications are very well tolerated.

PREVENTING CARDIOVASCULAR DISEASE

The following guidelines can help protect you against cardiovascular disease:

- Quit smoking
- Have your blood pressure checked even if you feel well, and take medication if it is too high. Weight loss and reduction of salt intake are sometimes helpful.
- Be tested for diabetes if you have risk factors or symptoms and follow your doctor's recommendations regarding diet, exercise, and medication.
- Eat a low-fat, low-cholesterol diet and have your cholesterol levels checked.
- Exercise to increase cardiovascular fitness and help control hypertension and diabetes.
- Consider hormone replacement therapy.

There is no safe level of cigarette smoking. As few as one to four cigarettes per day increases the risk of heart attack. Smoking also affects other aspects of body function that increase the risk of stroke.

In women, high-density lipoprotein (HDL) cholesterol protects against heart attack, whereas low-density lipoprotein (LDL) cholesterol increases the risk. Estrogen increases HDL and decreases LDL. After menopause the ratio of LDL to HDL (or the ratio of total to HDL) cholesterol increases. Hormone replacement therapy appears to have a beneficial effect on cholesterol ratios and thus on the risk of heart disease. Women also can often control cholesterol levels through diet.

A woman with a family member who had a heart attack before age 60 has a high risk of coronary heart disease. That relative could be a mother, father, or other first-degree relative. Women with this history should receive special attention in screening for coronary heart disease.

Heart attacks in women are often fatal. Prevention, early recognition, and treatment of coronary heart disease can prevent debility and premature death and are important aspects of a woman's general health care (see Chapter 27).

Musculoskeletal System

Approximately 50 percent of people aged 65 or older have arthritis or rheumatism (pain and stiffness in some portion of the musculoskeletal system). They can be a source of discomfort and disability, representing common daily problems for many elderly (see Chapter 34).

Arthritis

Arthritis is the most common inflammatory disease of joints, and 70 percent of those who have arthritis are women.

The most common cause of arthritis among the elderly is osteoarthritis, also known as degenerative joint disease. At least 40 million people in the United States have some evidence of the disease. Whereas osteoarthritis affects the knees or hands of older women, it more often affects the hips in older men. Both sexes may have pain in the spine (see Chapter 22). Osteoarthritis can be relieved with rest, muscle-strengthening

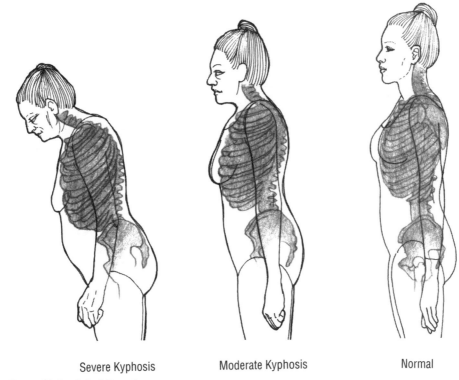

Severe Kyphosis   Moderate Kyphosis   Normal

Figure 11.1 Spinal Curvature
Progressive forward curvature ("kyphosis") occurs in women at high risk of developing spinal osteoporosis.

exercise, medication, and use of an assistive device, such as a cane. In severe cases, surgery is an option. Hip and knee replacement surgery may be highly effective late in life. Advanced age alone is not a reason to avoid such surgery, and many very elderly people have benefited from surgery.

Two other forms of arthritis, gout and pseudogout, are more common with advancing age. Gout is caused by a buildup of uric acid crystals in the joints, most commonly the big toe or the knees. It causes redness, swelling, and pain in the affected joint. In post-menopausal women, gout is usually related to the use of diuretic medications that increase the level of uric acid in the blood. Stopping the diuretics or switching to different medication can reduce or stop the attacks. Pseudogout is not caused by uric acid crystals and is unrelated to diuretic use. It has symptoms similar to gout and is treated with medications used for arthritis.

Polymyalgia rheumatica (PMR) is a syndrome that includes achiness and severe stiffness that are worse in the morning. It affects people over age 50, two-thirds of whom are women. The disorder is diagnosed by a blood test and treated with corticosteroids, usually for about a year.

Temporal arteritis may accompany PMR but is a more serious form of the disease. It is an inflamation of the arteries that lie on the forehead, and the symptoms are headaches, dizziness, and blurred or suddenly lost vision. If treatment with corticosteroids is not begun right away, permanent loss of visiton may occur.

Osteoporosis

Bone loss, which can result in osteoporosis, occurs as a normal part of aging. Rate of bone loss accelerates in women for a few years after menopause, when fractures linked to bone loss begin to increase dramatically. Among people over age 65, eight times as many women as men have spinal fractures due to bone loss. By age 90, at least 30 percent of women have had fractured hips, the most severe form of osteoporotic fracture, which often results in disability and serious health problems. Osteoporosis also leads to weakening and collapse of the spinal bones, resulting in forward curving of the spine (see Figure 11.1). The best treatment of osteoporosis is early prevention through diet, exercise, and hormone replacement therapy.

Osteomalacia

A condition that also causes bone fragility in the elderly, osteomalacia often coexists with osteoporosis and has similar symptoms. Osteomalacia is reversible, however, and osteoporosis is not. Osteomalacia is usually caused by vitamin D deficiency. Vitamin D controls the body's use of calcium and is found in certain foods, such as deep sea fish and fortified milk products. Elderly men and women who lack exposure to sunlight are at risk of vitamin D deficiency. This problem can occur in cold climates or when people are housebound or reside in nursing homes. Even though the condition is treated with vitamin D, excessive doses may cause illness and should be avoided.

Accidents

Although spinal fractures can occur without trauma, most fractures in the elderly occur as the result of a fall. As many as one-third of older adults fall at least once a year, and these falls often result in fractures. Falls can be caused by a number of preventable problems, such as being distracted, slipping, or stumbling. Among the elderly, most falls occur indoors. Falls also occur due to medical problems, such as overmedication, strokes, TIAs (a type of stroke), heart rhythm disturbances, or general weakness or illness. An elderly person should be carefully evaluated after a fall to detect any problems. People with physical disabilities should receive physical therapy and training in the use of devices such as canes, walkers, or leg braces. The home should be evaluated for potential hazards, such as slippery rugs or shaky handrails, and made as safe as possible (see Chapters 5 and 34).

Memory Loss

With increasing age, there is increasing risk of developing problems with memory. When memory loss is severe enough to interfere with work or social functioning, and when there is an accompanying impairment in intellectual function, the condition is known as dementia. The most common form of dementia is Alzheimer's disease, a condition that is more common in women than in men. The higher prevalence in women may be due to the fact that the disease usually appears late in life, when there are more women than men.

Alzheimer's disease is not an epidemic. Recent publicity reflects scientific scrutiny of a condition that once was once called "senility" and was thought to be due to "hardening of the arteries." With increasing

awareness of the true causes of "senility," more cases of Alzheimer's disease have been correctly diagnosed. In addition, as more and more people survive into old age, more cases of Alzheimer's disease, as well as other forms of dementia, will be identified.

Older men and women without signs of dementia commonly complain of memory loss. For example, people often complain of walking into a room but forgetting the reason they are there. This problem occurs at all ages, however, and can be due to trivial factors like distraction. This sort of memory lapse is less likely to create anxiety in a younger individual than it is in an elderly one, who might be concerned that it is a sign of Alzheimer's disease. Certain changes are common with age that may be quite normal, including slower speed in processing visual, auditory, and sensory information and difficulty finding words, especially proper nouns. True dementia, however, is common only among people who survive into their eighties and beyond.

Most people who seek medical attention on their own because of memory loss are functioning normally and may not be at high risk of developing Alzheimer's disease. People brought to the attention of physicians by concerned family or friends, however, often have already developed a significant problem.

Memory loss always should be evaluated because it can be linked with a number of disorders. If a significant change in a person's memory and mental abilities has taken place within hours, days, or weeks, medical attention is required right away. Rapid changes in memory are usually due to overmedication or serious medical illness.

When memory loss slowly progresses over a year or more, a reversible cause rarely exists. In all cases, a careful medical evaluation and regular follow-up are required.

People with dementia have a higher risk of being injured. They also may have other medical problems, such as an infection, that makes the condition worse. A wide variety of medical illnesses may have the symptoms of sudden worsening of dementia, lethargy, incontinence, and lowered intake of food and fluid. Such situations require immediate medical attention.

The Immune System

People in later life are more prone to certain infections. This may be partly related to changes in the immune system that protects the body from disease. The function of these cells combating disease declines with age. Some elderly may be less able to produce antibodies in response to vaccines for pneumonia or influenza, which protect them from these diseases. Despite this, vaccinations are very effective in most elderly people and we strongly urge receiving them as recommended (see "Routine Care for Women 65 Years and Older"). Two important infections that occur among the elderly are pneumonia and urinary tract infections.

Pneumonia

Pneumonia that is not acquired in an institution is most often due to the bacterium pneumococcus, which can be prevented with a vaccine. Chronically ill or disabled elderly, especially those in institutions or who have just undergone surgery, are also at increased risk for pneumonia caused by other bacteria. Although the vaccine does not protect them, the infection can be treated with antibiotics. If treatment is given, usually the patient's underlying health rather than a specific type of bacterium determines whether she will recover.

Immunizations

Vaccines make people immune to a disease. Immunization with pneumococcal vaccine is recommended for all people age 65 and older. Since a variety of bacterial pneumonias can occur as a complication of influenza, and since death due to pneumonia increases with age, all persons over the age of 65 should receive an annual influenza vaccine shot. It must be given every year because the virus that causes influenza is constantly changing. This vaccine only prevents infection caused by influenza virus, which is why immunized people can still get flulike illnesses not due to the virus.

Diphtheria and tetanus are potentially serious illnesses that can be prevented by immunization. Although these diseases do not occur frequently today, most deaths caused by them occur among the elderly, who are the least protected for several reasons. Most of today's elderly did not receive standard immunizations because such programs did not exist during their school years. Women are the group at highest risk because most women did not receive immunizations given through the military. Even if a person did receive the vaccine, its effectiveness is reduced over time. Elderly people uncertain of their immunization histories should have a series of three shots in six months.

Blood

Iron deficiency can be a cause of anemia in older adults of both sexes. In the United States, many foods are fortified with iron, so iron deficiency usually does not result from lack of iron in the diet. Instead, iron deficiency in the United States is almost always due to blood loss. Among the elderly, blood loss can be silent and may result from either a peptic ulcer (an ulcer of the stomach or upper intestine) or colon cancer.

Because there may be no signs or symptoms of blood loss, and only small amounts can be lost over time, iron deficiency may be the first sign of a serious disease. Iron deficiency usually can be detected by a blood test; and other tests may confirm the results. Older people who are taking vitamin supplements should select products that do not contain iron because supplemental iron might mask an iron deficiency due to silent blood loss.

A stomach condition called atrophic gastritis that occurs with aging can interfere with the body's ability to absorb B–12. Vitamin B–12 deficiency can produce anemia and neurologic problems, but it is uncertain how often this occurs in the elderly today. There are some simple and very sensitive tests to measure vitamin B–12 in the blood. Use of these tests has led to the detection of low levels in many elderly, but the link with disease is not clear. In theory, vitamin B–12 deficiency can produce disease of the nervous system, including psychiatric syndromes, memory loss, and spinal degeneration, even before anemia occurs. A number of healthy older people have low vitamin B–12 levels, and low levels do occur more commonly in patients with dementia, but B–12 supplementation rarely restores memory. Low B–12 levels should be treated with B–12 injections, or in some cases pills, as determined by a physician. (See Chapter 33).

Atrophic gastritis is a condition that is often treated with B–12 injections, but consult your physician.

People with chronic illness often have what is called anemia of chronic disease. Thus form of relatively mild anemia usually requires no specific treatment.

The Urinary System

Urinary tract disorders often occur in older women and can be related to a problem in the system or in an underlying disorder. Symptoms can be caused by urinary incontinence, infection of urine, or structural problems. Urinary incontinence can have a major impact on women and their families and be a source of embarrassment, loss of mobility, and low self-esteem. Available treatments can be very effective even in women in very late life.

Urinary Tract Infections

Although these infections are very common in women of all ages, a large number of elderly women have recurrent bladder infections. This may have to do with changes in the bladder and surrounding tissues that are exposed to bacteria. While as many as one-half of older woman have signs of bacteria in their urine, the condition should not be treated unless symptoms are present because overtreatment with antibiotics can lead to the development of antibiotic-resistant strains of bacteria. Vaginal estrogen cream can help prevent urinary tract infection in postmenopausal women.

Urinary Incontinence

Urinary incontinence often occurs in older women. The inability to control one's urine can be a source of embarrassment and low self-esteem. Treatments are available, however, and may be effective in women in very late life.

Urinary incontinence is the involuntary loss of urine. The most common causes are "unstable blad-

der" and "stress incontinence," which often coexist. In unstable bladder, symptoms may include urgency, which is the strong desire to void (or urinate), accompanied by the fear of leakage, and frequency, which is defined as voiding more than seven times in 24 hours or every two hours. Another symptom is nocturia, which is being awakened from sleep by the urge to void two or more time per night. Symptoms can be related to another medical problem or to the use of medications.

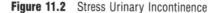

KEGEL EXERCISES

These exercises can strengthen the muscles of the pelvic floor surrounding the urethra, vagina, and anus. A doctor or nurse should show you how to do them. The muscles should be contracted and held for about 3 seconds, then released for 3 seconds, 12–15 times in a row, five or six times a day. As an alternate method, you can perform 10–12 contractions each for 10 seconds three times a day. The exercises should not be done while voiding. At least 40 exercises per day must be done to benefit from the program.

Figure 11.2 Stress Urinary Incontinence

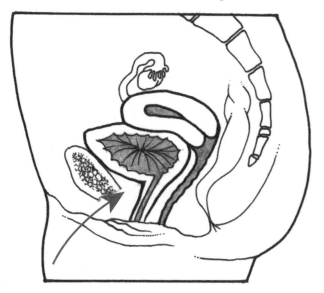

Normal anatomy—no urine leakage under pressure.

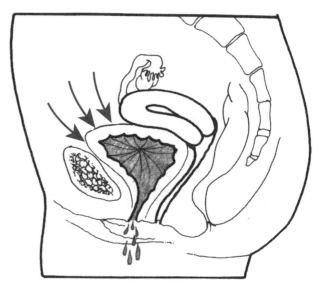

Abnormal anatomy:— patulous urethra and loss of sharp bladder angle lead to urine leakage under pressure.

Stress incontinence consists of leakage of small amounts of urine after a cough, sneeze, or any maneuver that increases the abdminal pressure exerted on the bladder. Most often stress incontinence results from the relaxation of the supporting tissues of the urethra, bladder, and other pelvic organs. These changes are thought to be related to childbirth, but many older women who never have given birth are affected probably because of age-related changes in supporting tissues. After menopause, these tissues become stretched and weakened because of a lack of estrogen. (See Figure 11.2).

Other Causes of Incontinence

Hospitalized woman may experience temporary urinary incontinence after surgery or if they are chronically bedridden. Mild incontinence may be brought on or preexisting incontinence may temporarily worsen as a result of an acute bladder infection, which causes irritation to the bladder or urethra; however, older women often have bladder infections when symptoms are not present. The sudden onset of urinary incontinence may result from a state of confusion, which should receive immediate medical attention because it could be a sign of serious medical illness.

Patients with dementia often have urinary incontinence. It is uncertain if the incontinence is directly related to a specific problem in the brain or due to confusion about the location or method of toileting, or both. Standard incontinence therapy does not work in these patients. Toileting on schedule—for example, every 2–4 hours, depending on the woman's needs—may help keep her dry. Incontinence garments, or diapers, can be used, although they are not acceptable to some women. Adult diapers must be changed frequently and special attention should be given to hygiene. A catheter, a tube placed and left in the bladder to drain the urine into a bag, should be avoided because it invariably leads to bladder infection.

Incontinence can be caused by medicine, especially in older women who may already have abnormal function of the bladder or urethra. The most common offenders are diuretics, especially potent ones such as furosemide. If this drug must be taken, it is often helpful to take it during the time of the day that best suits the woman; for instance, she could take it when she is at home and has easy access to a bathroom. Other medications that can produce incontinence include prazosin (Minipress) or terazosin (Hytrin), which are used to control blood pressure but which weaken the urethra and allow urine to leak.

Medications can also cause retention of urine and "overflow incontinence." Because the bladder is not completely emptied, the woman has feelings of urgency and frequency. Medications that cause urinary retention include some antidepressants, some older antihistamines, and narcotics. Urinary retention can also be caused by severe constipation, which can compress the outlet of the bladder. Urine retention can be related to bladder malfunction, which can be caused by neurologic problems or underlying disease. Persistent urinary retention is very rare in older women.

Treatment

Some bladder disorders can be corrected with surgery or medication, and they can be eased with exercises and devices that help retain urine. Advanced age should not prevent a woman from receiving care. Unstable bladder may be eased by medication to relax the bladder and by self-training to "hold the urge" for longer intervals. Stress incontinence may respond to estrogen or to Kegel exercises that strengthen the muscles controlling urine (see "Kegel Exercises"). These exercises can improve bladder control in many women but are less effective in later life, when other bladder problems coexist.

The Digestive System

Constipation and ulcers are common problems of the digestive system in the elderly but not necessarily a part of normal aging. Older people tend to use laxatives more than younger adults, although this may have to do with traditional beliefs about regularity. The definition of what constitutes constipation varies from person to person. As with any age group, a change in bowel habits should be evaluated by a doctor.

Constipation

Constipation often occurs in elderly people who are immobilized, such as those who are homebound or live in nursing homes. These people tend to get constipated because of lack of exercise, decreased intake of fiber and fluids, medical problems that can interfere with bowel function, and certain medications. Medications that cause constipation include calcium channel-blocking agents, calcium supplements, aluminum-containing antacids, narcotics, and certain antidepressants or related compounds.

Treatment of constipation consists of physical exercise, increasing the intake of fluid, changing medications if possible, and eating food high in fiber. Excess fiber intake (as found in fiber containing cookies) should be avoided, however, especially in bedbound patients, because it may worsen the problem. Laxative abuse, longstanding daily use of laxatives, may damage the nerve supply in the bowel and make constipation worse. Laxatives should be used, however, in patients with physical limitations who are prone to fecal impaction. In this extreme form of constipation there may be little or no bowel movement.

Ulcers

Ulcers can occur in the duodenum (upper small intestine) or the stomach (gastric ulcers). Ulcers in the duodenum are more common, but the risk of gastric ulcers increases with age. Older people are at a higher risk of gastric ulcer because of thinning of the inner lining of the stomach. They also use aspirinlike medications more frequently, particularly nonsteroidal anti-inflammatory agents (NSAIDs), such as ibuprofen. Although these medications relieve arthritis and other painful conditions, they may disrupt the stomach lining and produce an array of ulcer and ulcerlike conditions.

Occasional use of NSAIDs is usually not a problem, and some products are available without a prescription. Repeated use of even moderate doses can pose a major risk among the elderly, however. It is best to treat painful conditions with other medications, such as acetaminophen (Tylenol and other brands) or, if pain is severe, narcotic-containing preparations. When prolonged use of NSAIDS is required, the woman should be monitored closely by a physician with periodic checks of stool and blood samples, including iron levels. Ulcer disease is more likely to be silent in the elderly and may produce painless bleeding. Blood loss can be slow and steady, which can be detected on a routine stool exam or blood test, or it can be massive. Certain patients may benefit from antiulcer medications. It is now known that bacteria play a role in ulcer disease, but they appear to play little or no role in NSAID-induced stomach ulcers.

Duodenal ulcers are almost always benign and heal readily with proper treatment. Approximately 5 percent of gastric ulcers are cancers, and this rate is somewhat higher among older people. It is essential, therefore, that gastric ulcers be biopsied initially and then reevaluated after a course of treatment to be sure they have healed (see Chapter 33).

Skin

Some changes in skin occur with aging, while others are due to damage from the sun and other environmental factors. With normal aging, changes occur in collagen, an important protein in the skin. Sun damage is usually confined to exposed areas and can be shown by comparing these areas (forehead, neck, hands, and forearms) with skin protected from the sun (lower back, abdomen, and buttocks.) These differences are most pronounced in light-skinned individuals, especially those who have had a great deal of exposure to the sun throughout their lives. The differences are least obvious in people with deeply pigmented skin. Solar damage causes wrinkles, freckles, precancerous lesions called actinic keratoses, and skin cancer.

Normal aging results in skin sagging but not wrinkling or developing other problems caused by environmental skin damage. Normal aging causes a loss of elastic tissue, changes in an important protein in skin called collagen, and thinning of the upper layers of the skin. Body fat is redistributed from the layer immediately beneath the skin to the deeper layers, and from the extremities, face, and neck to the trunk. This redistribution gives the appearance of skin sagging and wrinkling.

Tretinoin (Retin-A) is a medication used for acne that is available as a cream and appears to reverse some of the effects of environmental skin damage. There is no evidence, however, that it reverses age-related skin changes.

Use of sun blocks and reducing sunlight exposure can prevent premature aging of the skin and can reduce the risk of skin cancer. Sunlight is important to the production of vitamin D, however, so exposure should not be avoided entirely. Sunlight also may have an effect on mood, and its role in causing seasonal affective disorder, a condition in which depression is linked to lack of exposure to daylight, is being explored.

Skin cancer occurs more often with increasing age. The most common form in late life is basal cell carcinoma. Unlike other forms of skin cancer, basal cell carcinoma rarely spreads to distant sites. It grows very slowly and is almost always curable. The tumor can affect adjoining areas, however, and should be removed without delay (see Chapter 35).

CHAPTER 12

Sexuality

Maj-Britt Rosenbaum, M.D., F.A.P.A., and
Kathleen O'Hanlan, M.D., F.A.C.O.G., F.A.C.S.

Sexuality is an aspect of an individual's personality that is shaped by biologic, psychologic, and social factors. Extending far beyond sexual function, sexuality is a personal set of experiences and values that encompasses a person's sexual identity, her feelings about sexual expression, and how she relates to others sexually. It involves a complex set of interactions that evolve and change throughout a person's life.

Women are increasingly becoming aware of their sexuality and less repressed about their own sexual needs and choices. Because sexuality is highly personal and individualized, there is great variety within a normal range of sexual expression. Women differ in their sexual interest and response, and a woman's feelings about her sexuality may change based on her circumstances and the time of her life. Women's sexual satisfaction often does not occur spontaneously but must be developed. For many women, exploring and learning about sex is a lifelong process. Women should take an active role in this process to ensure that they derive the most enjoyment from it.

Sexuality can be a source of gratification that brings personal contentment, good mental health, and intimacy with a partner. It can also result in anxiety and disappointment when the needs of either or both partners are not met. Sexual problems are common in adults and can be caused by mental and/or physical factors that have a bearing on the delicate and highly subjective balance of what constitutes a satisfying sexual experience. Fortunately, most sexual problems are amenable to treatment.

SEXUAL DEVELOPMENT

The continual process of sexual development begins at the time of conception. It is influenced early in life by identification with a specific gender and is shaped by parents' perceptions, religious values, and cultural aspects. In some cases this can lead to mixed or conflicting messages, which can create confusion in establishing a set of personal values about sex. As a woman matures and discovers her own sexual identity, she can explore methods of expression that are pleasurable and acceptable to her.

A person's biologic sex is established at the time of conception. The genes from the mother and father join to determine whether the baby will be a boy or a girl, and sex organs develop accordingly. At around age 2, a child exhibits characteristics that relate to his or her gender—masculine or feminine. This is the first step in developing a sexual identity.

Gender identity involves an individual's acceptance of his or her biologic sex and demonstration of behavior that can be considered masculine or feminine. There is not always a clear distinction, however, between male and female or masculine and feminine behavior. Usually, in formulating a sexual identity, traits of both sexes are present.

Another aspect of sexual identity is orientation. This relates to whether a person is attracted to the same or the opposite sex. A person's sexual orientation begins to develop during childhood and usually is fixed in the teenage years. A woman may be attracted to men or to other women or to both. Because many cultures provide models only of heterosexuality, however, some lesbians and gay men do not allow themselves honest expression until a few years later.

Physical aspects of sexual development begin to occur during puberty. Changes are triggered by rising levels of hormones and begin between the ages of 9 and 14. Girls begin to develop about 2 years earlier than boys.

During puberty, girls have an increase in height and weight, and their body shape changes to the contours of a woman. First breast buds begin to develop, then armpit and pubic hair sprouts, and then last, menstruation begins. Boys also develop hair on their bodies during puberty. A boy's voice becomes deeper, and his penis and testes grow larger. The new hormones that initiate puberty also create new sexual desires in adolescents.

Both men and women are capable of having full and satisfying sexual function throughout their lives. This cannot always be accomplished without some effort, however. A woman reaches her peak of sexual responsiveness in her late 30s and early 40s, whereas a man reaches his peak in his late teens or early 20s. Women can help ensure their sexual gratification by being aware of what can promote as well as interfere with it. Sexual response follows a natural pattern and anything that interrupts that pattern can create sexual difficulties.

SEXUAL RESPONSE CYCLE

Sexual response follows a cycle that begins with desire, moves through arousal and into plateau, and culminates in orgasm and a return to normal (see "Anatomy of the Sexual Response, below"). It is not necessary to go through every step of the complete cycle to achieve sexual satisfaction, and women may differ in their experience of sexual response. Sexual response is both emotional and physical. Emotionally, numerous factors can enhance and diminish response. Physically, sexual response follows a pattern that centers around the swelling of the labia and clitoris caused by the congestion of blood and the building of muscle tension throughout the body. The sexual response cycle is not a step-by-step pattern but rather a slow process by which one stage gradually merges into the next.

Desire

Sexual desire precedes and accompanies sexual arousal. It is the excitement of body and mind that makes a person interested in and receptive to sexual stimulation.

Arousal

Sexual arousal begins in women with vaginal lubrication. The amount of lubrication may vary with the

ANATOMY OF THE SEXUAL RESPONSE

A number of organs play a role in the sexual response cycle:

- *Labia:* Flaps of skin, or "lips," that surround the vulva.
- *Vulva:* The external female genital area and the opening to the internal organs.
- *Vagina:* A canal that leads from the external genital organs to the uterus.
- *Uterus:* A muscular organ found in a woman's pelvic region that holds the fetus during pregnancy.

amount of stimulation, a woman's previous sexual history, her age, or hormonal status. Parasympathetic nerves, the "relaxation" nerves, cause the blood vessels serving the genital organs to increase the blood supply and cause congestion. The labia—"lips" surrounding the vulva (the opening to the vagina)—swell from the congestion of blood. The clitoris, a small organ located above the opening to the vagina that is the highly sensitive source of sexual excitement, also swells from congestion. The same congestion is the source of the fluid of sexual excitement, which flows from the vessels into the vagina during sexual stimulation. The nipples of the breasts also may swell and become erect.

As a woman becomes more stimulated, the labia become thicker and redder. The clitoris becomes erect and moves under its hood, or the fold of skin that partly surrounds it. Direct contact of the clitoris may be too intense at this point, but stimulation of the clitoral shaft through the hood can heighten pleasurable sensations.

Plateau

Heart rate, blood pressure, and breathing rates increase as stimulation increases. The vagina expands as the surrounding tissue congests with blood. This is the beginning of the plateau phase, which can last from a few minutes to an hour. Women frequently try to hurry through this essential phase but should, rather, be encouraged to take their time and enjoy it.

Orgasm

The peak of sexual excitement occurs with a series of rhythmic muscle spasms. This pleasurable sensation on the vulva and in the vagina can extend to the uterus and anus and sometimes the whole body. It is a reflex sensation that in women can last 20 to 60 seconds. Orgasm can vary in intensity. Some women can have more than one orgasm, whereas others have one orgasm and find further stimulation of the clitoris to be unappealing. (See Fig. 12.1)

Resolution

After orgasm, breathing, heart rate, and blood pressure return to normal levels. Genital and pelvic organs are

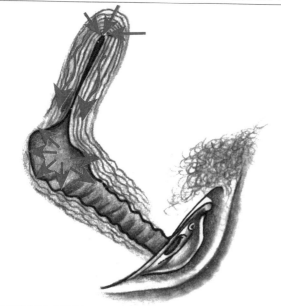

no longer engorged with blood and return to their unaroused state. Orgasm is typically followed by a feeling of calmness. Males usually fall into a refractory period, during which they cannot have an erection. A woman does not experience this refractory period, however, and is physically able to achieve multiple orgasms if she is stimulated to do so.

Figure. 12.1 Orgasm
During the orgasmic stage, muscular tension is released in contractions that for most women are extremely pleasurable. The arrows show the direction of enlargement of the upper vagina and contractions of the uterus. Orgasm varies greatly in length and intensity for each woman and often feels different at different times for the same woman.

SEXUAL EXPRESSION

Most women feel they must achieve orgasm to be sexually satisfied and that the best way to do this is through direct stimulation of the clitoris. Only about 25 percent of women have orgasm with intercourse according to most surveys of women's sexuality. Women usually need other forms of direct or indirect clitoral stimulation to reach orgasm. This may come in the form of breast stimulation, whole body contact, or most often, by either the woman or her partner directly stimulating the clitoral area.

Women must learn what types of stimulation their bodies need during sex so that they can reach an orgasm. Some women learn what brings them pleasure by experimenting with manual masturbation or using sexual devices, such as vibrators. During heterosexual intercourse, certain positions, such as the woman on top or thrusting hip movements, may provide more direct clitoral stimulation. Although some women respond to various forms of stimulation, most show a preference for one form. The usual means of attaining orgasm include (in order of preference) manual or oral stimulation of the clitoris, intercourse with the woman on top, intercourse with the man on top, vibrator stimulation, and the woman stimulating herself to orgasm in front of her partner. For lesbians, the most common method of attaining orgasm is by oral or manual stimulation of the clitoris and vagina.

An adequate level and duration of stimulation is required for a woman to be aroused. Stimulation can be mental as well as physical. Sexual fantasy, combined with physical stimulation, is much more effective than physical stimulation alone.

Most women are biologically able to have an orgasm. If a woman tries too hard, however, she can become the victim of performance anxiety, which inhibits her ability to achieve orgasm. Instead of focusing only on the end result, a woman will find it more satisfying to experience the full range of sexual pleasure that comes with closeness and intimacy. An orgasm is not always essential to having a satisfactory sexual experience.

Most women need a nurturing environment in their relationship to be sexually responsive. Although men desire a nurturing relationship and find their sexual responsiveness enhanced by it, they are not as affected as women are by its absence. The positive emotional tone of a relationship and the resultant feelings of trust and mutual respect are important factors in a woman's sexual expression and response.

Between 5 and 10 percent of women prefer other women as sexual and life partners. Homosexuality has been observed in most animal species and should be regarded as one of the many natural expressions of human sexuality. Sexual orientation appears to be influenced by both the environment and genetics but bears no correlation with any psychological or physiologic disease traits. The unfortunate disdain that some cultures have for their homosexual members is without any basis in scientific fact and is a cause for distress among lesbian and gay individuals. Bisexual relationships, when a person has sexual experiences with both men and women, are more common among women than men. Partners in these relationships are often chosen more on the basis of their personal traits rather than their gender.

In some cases, a woman may choose not to have

any sexual partners for a given time. She may wish to be celibate for a number of reasons, such as recovering from the loss of a spouse or a broken relationship or wanting to devote attention to another part of her life.

Sexuality and sexual needs are key parts of most people's lives, yet many women are reluctant to talk about them. Understanding personal sexual values is essential to understanding sexual needs, desires, and preferences. These preferences should be communicated to sexual partners so an open attitude toward meeting each other's needs can be maintained.

FACTORS THAT AFFECT SEXUAL FUNCTION

Sexual satisfaction involves a complex interplay of biologic and emotional factors, social conditioning, personal expectations, and physical aspects. It should not be surprising, therefore, that these factors, singly and in combination, can have an impact on sexual function. Stress, performance anxiety, misconceptions about human sexual response, problems in a relationship, a reaction to illness, and specific medical or surgical treatments can lead to sexual difficulties. Some of these influences are temporary, whereas others may require major adjustments or adaptations.

Stress and Anxiety

Stress, emotional problems, fear, and anxiety can interfere with a person's desire to have sex. Daily stresses, such as the demands of children, insufficient time alone with a partner, or the inability to relax can lead to decreased desire. Concerns about work or finances, family problems, or a personal crisis decrease a person's sexual interest and responsiveness.

Anxiety can often cause sexual problems. It can stem from focusing too much on technique or performance and from evaluating the experience only in terms of performance. Another source of anxiety is concern about the partner's expectations and whether they will be met. This can lead to what is called *spectatoring*, in which a person becomes so absorbed in monitoring what is happening that she is unable to experience it.

One of the most common causes of sexual problems in women is a lack of knowledge about sexuality by their male partners. Men were not born with the specific knowledge or skill to stimulate a woman to orgasm. Most partners need to be taught which methods of stimulation work best for each woman. This can create anxiety when a woman does not know how her body can respond sexually or a partner who doesn't listen to her. She may also become anxious if her partner wants to perform a sexual act that she is uncomfortable with. Anxiety can also stem from guilt that has its roots in childhood conditioning.

A woman may avoid sex because of fear of pain, of what will happen, of pregnancy, of getting a sexually transmitted disease, or of dealing with issues of unexpressed lesbianism. Other forms of fear are the loss of self and fear of intimacy.

Relationships

Interpersonal relationships with sexual partners can have a strong influence on sexual function and the satisfaction that can be derived from it. An interpersonal problem with a woman's partner is often the cause of a sexual difficulty. It is usually only a matter of time before a problem in a relationship includes a sexual problem. Sometimes the problem in the relationship is caused by a sexual problem. In this case, a woman should communicate her sexual needs to her partner. If the partner doesn't respond or rejects her requests, the problem centers on the relationship and is not sexual.

Sexual problems in relationships often center around communication. A woman may feel shy or embarrassed when talking about sex and may be reluctant to discuss her preferences in case her partner thinks she is criticizing. She also may assume that her partner knows what she wants. This lack of communication goes both ways. It is important for a couple to talk openly about what pleases them as well as what they find troubling.

In the presence of performance anxiety and spectatoring, the partner may feel tension that makes it difficult to talk openly and freely. This often takes the form of not talking about the problem at all, having discussions that lead to angry exchanges, blaming each other, or rationalizing one's behavior. This type of communication often takes nonverbal forms, with partners indicating to each other in various ways their unhappiness in the sexual relationship. Eventually, the couple may cease to have sex and refuse to discuss it.

Couples should try to keep lines of communication open. Partners need to talk to each other and to acknowledge their fears and concerns so they can discuss their sexual problems.

Sexual Abuse

Sexual trauma or abuse as a child can inhibit sexual response in an adult. Some women who have been victims of sexual abuse feel that their sense of trust has been violated and may have difficulty relating to their partners in an intimate and sensual way. Other women respond by completely losing their sexual desire. Another lesser known and rare effect of sexual abuse is relentless sexual seeking and compulsive behavior.

Drugs and Illness

Serious illness is a major personal event that concerns the person who has the illness as well as those around him or her. It often reduces the frequency and quality of sexual activity. Chronic disease can have a negative impact on a woman's ability to feel and be sexual. The effect of illness depends on the disease itself, the age and attitude of the person affected, and the impact on the partner. All serious disease can affect a person's sex life through fatigue, limited energy, and reduced sexual drive. A sexual problem can stem from the disorder or the treatment or both (see "Effects of Drugs on Sexual Function").

Certain disorders affect sexual activity through damage to nerves that control sexual response. Others are caused by lack of adequate blood circulation. For still others, the cause is not known but can involve a complex interaction of factors, both physical and mental. In many cases, the effects are more obvious in men because they cause impotence. In women, sexual function may be preserved but there may be difficulty with vaginal lubrication. One of the most important aspects of a medical disorder's effect on sexual activity is the amount of pain associated with it. Pain may prevent couples from engaging in sexual activities known to be

pleasurable. Although medical disorders can cause physical and psychologic problems that may affect sexual adjustment, in many cases interest in sex is not lessened, and patients with such problems can enjoy satisfying sexual experiences (see "Medical Conditions That Can Affect Sexual Function").

Illness can interfere with sex, just as it interferes with other activities. For an illness that comes on suddenly and is treated, the effect on sexuality may be

EFFECTS OF DRUGS ON SEXUAL FUNCTION

Medications that interfere with sexual function in women do so by decreasing desire or inhibiting orgasm. The most common of such medications are antihypertensive agents, antipsychotic drugs, and antidepressants. Tamoxifen, a drug used to treat women with breast cancer, can cause vaginal dryness in premenopausal women. Chemotherapy for cancer employs powerful drugs that affect many aspects of a person's bodily function, including sexual drive and ability to become aroused. Similarly, there are numerous drugs that cause sexual problems in men. They include antihypertensive agents, anticonvulsants, tranquilizers and antidepressants, and drugs for treating ulcers and heart disease.

Intoxication with alcoholic beverages diminishes both men's and women's arousal states and inhibits orgasm. Chronic alcohol use also lowers sexual drive. Alcoholics are thus prone to have sexual problems, and these problems are often worsened by concurrent drug abuse. Substance abuse of drugs such as morphine, codeine, and heroin can seriously impair sexual function. Users have lowered sex drive and less sexual activity.

temporary. For chronic illness, however, the interference can result in a quality-of-life problem. Women must not hesitate to report changes in sexual response associated with disease to their doctor. Women should expect to receive help or referral to a knowledgeable therapist; they should be able to pursue a satisfying sex life despite their illness.

MEDICAL CONDITIONS THAT CAN AFFECT SEXUAL FUNCTION

Arthritis

Painful joints can inhibit sexual activity and the partner may be concerned about causing pain. Arthritis also limits mobility and thus can have an effect on the forms of sexual expression. A woman's membranes may be dry with some forms of arthritis, resulting in a lack of vaginal lubrication. Sexual comfort can be enhanced by using positions that avoid prolonged pressure on affected joints, using vaginal lubricants, and taking pain medication and applying heat to joints before having sex.

Cardiovascular Disease

People with a heart condition may have pain with exercise and lack circulation to the extremities. Although sexual activity may be physically and emotionally stressful, it rarely leads to severe complications in patients with a cardiac disease. The amount of energy expended during normal sexual activity is about the same as climbing a single flight of steps. A person's ability to tolerate exercise can be tested to determine the safety of sexual activity.

Diabetes

Nerve damages, which occurs with diabetes, can lead to difficulty having orgasms in women and impotence in men. In women, this can result in less vaginal lubrication and contraction of the muscles of orgasm. In men, the problem is compounded by lack of blood circulation and hypertension, which also contribute to impotence. Control of diabetes may result in an improvement in sexual function.

Epilepsy

Epilepsy causes an electrical "short circuit" in the messages sent by nerves to the brain. It can result in loss of sex drive, decreased sexual responsiveness, and partial or complete impotence.

Kidney Disease

Complications of kidney disorders can cause loss of sex drive and, in men, impotence. The effects are related to hormone imbalances often associated with this condition as well as nerve damage and other medical problems that are often present. In women, careful attention should be given to possible vaginal infections that could cause discomfort during sexual activity.

Spinal Cord Injury

Any damage to the spinal cord can interfere with sexual function, depending on the location of the injury. It can cause paralysis and loss of sensation, resulting in lack of lubrication in women and impotence in men. Both women and men can often continue to have orgasms, however. With special preparation and devices, women and men with spinal cord injuries can maintain sexual activity.

Stroke

A blockage in the vessels that supply blood to the brain can result in paralysis of part of the body, muscle weakness, and less ability to move around. This can have an effect on sexual activity. Because the nerves are usually not damaged, however, sex is possible with some adjustments.

Thyroid Disease

Any hormone imbalance can affect sexuality. In thyroid disease, changes in hormone levels can cause menstrual problems in women, impotence in men, and loss of sex drive in both. The decrease in energy and other complications can also be a factor. Sexual problems caused by the disease go away when it is treated.

SPECIAL CONCERNS FOR WOMEN

Any change in a woman's life that relates to her reproductive system can raise concerns about her sexuality. These can be normal changes, such as those that come with pregnancy or menopause, or they can be medical problems, such as cancer of the breast or reproductive organs. Having a sexually transmitted disease or an abnormal Pap smear may also cause a woman to experience uneasiness about her sexuality. These conditions can all affect sexual function, especially if the woman is worried about them. A woman should seek advice from her doctor about these conditions and their impact on her sexual life and health.

Pregnancy

There are different patterns of sexual activity during pregnancy. Some women have a decrease in sexual activity during the first three months of pregnancy, an increase in the middle of pregnancy, and a decrease again at the end. In other women, sexual activity decreases steadily during pregnancy, as do sexual interest and the ability to have an orgasm. This variation in activity could be related to a number of factors, including emotional and physical ones. In the beginning of pregnancy, physical discomfort can lead to a decreased desire for sex. In the second trimester, however, women often feel less uncomfortable. Near the end of pregnancy, the discomfort can return. Most women have expressed an increased desire to be held while they are pregnant.

Some couples mistakenly think that making love will hurt the baby, so they avoid having sex. Most women can continue to have sexual relations with their partners all through pregnancy without harming the baby. For the sake of comfort and ease, they may wish to experiment with different positions and techniques that create less pressure on the uterus. If there is a problem in the pregnancy, such as a risk of preterm birth, the doctor may suggest that a couple stop or limit sexual activity.

After pregnancy, women who breast-feed may notice a lack of vaginal lubrication during sexual activity. This is caused by changes in hormone levels and can be relieved with the use of vaginal lubricants or hormones.

Hormone levels return to normal at about 10 weeks after delivery, although there is wide variation among women. Some begin to have menstrual periods as early as 1 month after delivery. Women who breast-feed return to normal more gradually and may not begin having menstrual periods until 36 weeks after delivery. Even though they are not having periods, however, they can become pregnant. Most doctors agree that a woman can begin having sex after pregnancy as soon as she feels comfortable.

Menopause

During menopause, a woman's ovaries stop producing the hormone estrogen. This can lead to changes that affect her sexual function. The main change is vaginal dryness. Lack of vaginal lubrication can make sex painful. Low levels of estrogen may also cause the walls of the vagina to thin and be more prone to sexual discomfort and injury. This can be corrected through estrogen-replacement therapy. The hormone is taken as a pill or absorbed through a patch. Locally applied vaginal cream can also be used.

Women do not lose their sexual drive during or after menopause. Most women continue to enjoy a sexually fulfilling life throughout their later years. Factors that could interfere with this include health and relationship problems, availability of partners, and emotional concerns that may accompany menopause.

The nature of a woman's sexual activity may change as she ages. She may take longer to become aroused and may need more stimulation to have an orgasm. Some older women have fewer vaginal contractions during orgasm. Older men may have difficulty getting or keeping an erection. As their sexual needs change with age, couples may move their focus away from the traditional genital-focused approach to other forms of sexual pleasure. These may include manual stimulation, oral-genital stimulation, and rubbing the external genitals against each other. For many couples, although the physical form of their lovemaking may change, the intensity, satisfaction and frequency remain unchanged.

Older couples who are not comfortable with creating diverse experiences of sexual behavior may find their sexual activity limited. At some point, couples may be content to stop having sex. If both partners are comfortable with this situation, it does not have a negative effect on their relationship.

Sexually Transmitted Disease

Certain diseases are sexually transmitted by both heterosexual activity and possibly also by lesbian sexual activity (see Chapter 19). Herpes causes painful blisters in the genital area. Pelvic inflammatory disease is an infection of the internal pelvic organs that can cause deep vaginal and pelvic pain. Condyloma (venereal warts) are transmitted sexually and can grow to be quite large and uncomfortable. Some sexually transmitted diseases don't cause pain but permanently damage reproductive organs and cause infertility. Sexual activity is the most common way of transmitting the fatal illness AIDS. To avoid contracting a sexually transmitted disease, a woman should practice safe sex: She should always use a condom or rubber dam, with spermicide when she has a sexual relationship with anyone. A woman may elect at some point in the relationship to be monogamous, but there is always some risk of a partner's prior history or future infidelity. Furthermore, the partner may be an intravenous drug user, an AIDS risk.

Cancer

Cancer and its treatment can affect a woman's sexuality. In addition to the anxiety produced by the diagnosis, a woman may have concerns about its effect on her future sexual capability. Cancer can also affect a woman's appearance and self-esteem, particularly if it involves loss of an organ. Emotionally, a woman is faced with the possibility of death, disfigurement, and the possible rejection by her partner, and physically, she must confront the rigors of surgery, radiation or chemotherapy.

Radiation therapy is often used in the treatment of cancer of the cervix, vagina, and uterus. It causes the vagina to lose its elasticity and decrease in size and length. After radiation treatment, a woman may need to use a vaginal dilator coated with estrogen cream to keep her vagina open. It should be used daily, and sexual activity can be resumed as soon as clearance is given by the oncologist.

Surgical treatment of gynecologic cancer may involve hysterectomy, or removal of the uterus. The ovaries and part of the vagina also may be removed. There is some controversy over the role of the uterus in orgasm, but a few women report a difference in the nature of their orgasm after their uterus has been removed. Women who equate the loss of their uterus with the loss of their femininity are more apt to have difficulties postoperatively.

Cancer of the vulva may require removal or reconfiguration of the external genital organs. This will affect appearance and may narrow the opening to the vagina. Conservative surgery that retains nearly normal appearance and function has cure rates similar to radical surgery and is used in most cases.

Colorectal cancer is the third leading cause of death from cancer in the United States. If the rectum and part of the colon are removed surgically, the nerves in the area may be damaged and affect sexual response. The presence of a colostomy (an opening in the abdominal wall to drain the colon after the rectum is removed) may inhibit sexual activity initially.

Breast cancer, and in particular mastectomy, can have a major psychologic effect on a woman as well as on her partner. The woman may feel deformed or mutilated, resulting in low self-esteem and an inability to function sexually. She may also experience rejection by her partner.

About 33 percent of women who have had mastectomies have not resumed sexual activity 6 months after discharge from the hospital. This may be related to factors in the woman or her partner or both. Counseling a woman and her partner in advance of surgery may help them cope better. Group therapy for the cancer survivor and the spouse and family can help restore and maintain the relationships and may have beneficial effects on survival probability.

SEXUAL PROBLEMS

Sexual problems can arise at any stage of the sexual response cycle. They can occur at any time in a woman's life, and they can appear after a woman has enjoyed a long-term satisfying relationship. Sexual problems can occur in four basic areas: lack of desire, lack of arousal, lack of orgasm, and pain during intercourse.

Lack of Desire

Some women lack interest in sex. They may avoid initiating sex or participating in it and be slow or unable to achieve arousal. If they do have sex, they often do not find it very satisfying.

Lack of desire is most often caused by a problem in

the couple's relationship. There may be feelings of anger or resentment, which may stem from previous sexual failures or from other problems in the relationship, such as conflicts in attitudes or values. A woman who has difficulty having an orgasm may become conditioned to failure, eventually losing her ability to become aroused and then losing her desire to have sex.

Lack of desire can also be affected by all of the other factors that influence sexual response. It can occur in response to a temporary situation, such as stress or illness, or it can develop into a long-term problem. It can also have a physical basis, such as a reaction to drugs, but it more often results from an emotional response to anxiety, depression, and guilt. Lack of desire for members of the opposite sex can occur at any age if a woman begins dealing with repressed awareness of her lesbianism.

Counseling can be effective in treating sexual problems involving low desire or a lack of desire. These problems are more complex and difficult to treat than other sexual problems, and psychotherapy is often needed to help the woman explore the underlying conflict.

Lack of Arousal

Some women have an interest in sex but are unable to become aroused. Such woman may have difficulty achieving adequate vaginal lubrication for intercourse. This is often the result of a lack of stimulation. The woman and her partner may not know how to help her become aroused. Frequently, lack of arousal is related to lack of holding, kissing, and caressing or may be caused by a lack of technical skills. The woman may feel uncomfortable communicating her likes and dislikes to her partner. Her partner may not understand or be able to follow her instructions. Exercises have been developed to help couples overcome this problem (see "Therapy"). They are designed to teach individuals how to better relate to their partners physically and how to minimize peformance pressure or anxiety.

Lack of arousal also may occur if a woman is having feelings of fear, anger, or guilt about sex. These feelings can arise from negative or constricting messages about sex as a child. Such lessons need to be unlearned as an adult.

Lack of Orgasm

As many as 20 percent of women have never had or rarely ever have an orgasm with sexual activity. Surveys show that only about 45 percent of heterosexual women but 95 percent of lesbians have orgasms regularly. Almost all women are physiologically capable of having an orgasm, either through self-stimulation or partner stimulation—manually, orally, or with a vibrator. Most heterosexual women require some form of direct clitoral stimulation in addition to intercourse to have an orgasm. It is possible that orgasms are more frequent among lesbians because their most frequent form of sexual activity involves direct clitoral stimulation.

Some women don't have an orgasm because they have not been adequately aroused. Orgasm cannot occur without a high level of arousal, something some women may fail to recognize. They may feel that heterosexual intercourse is the only "acceptable" way to be stimulated and refuse other forms of more direct stimulation, possibly cutting short arousal.

A woman may try so hard to achieve an orgasm that she becomes a spectator rather than a participant. She may be so eager and so anxious to have an orgasm that her body becomes too tense and is unable to respond.

In general, problems that cause lack of orgasm are the same as those that cause other sexual problems. Treatment focuses on exercises to learn how the female body responds and on how to provide adequate stimulation. It can also involve learning new approaches to sexual expression.

Pain During Intercourse

Two conditions, called *dyspareunia* and *vaginismus,* are characterized by pain during vaginal penetration. They can be caused by a physical or emotional factor or a combination of both.

Dyspareunia may involve pain with initial vaginal penetration, with deep thrusting, or following sexual activity. It can occur if there is a lack of estrogen to allow vaginal lubrication, with a pelvic infection, in the presence of a tumor or cyst, or with a condition called endometriosis (in which cells similar to the lining of the uterus grow outside the uterus and cause inflammation).

Vaginismus is a spasm of the pubic muscles of the lower vagina that makes penetration by the penis or by any object into the vagina painful, difficult, or at times impossible. Some women are unable to even have a gynecologic examination, whereas others experience vaginismus only during sex.

Vaginismus may be related to a previous painful experience, such as childhood sexual abuse or rape as an adult. It can be caused by a number of medical conditions, such as infections, vaginal irritations, or pelvic or anal skin problems. It can also be a response to fear.

With dyspareunia, once the cause of the symptoms is treated the problem usually goes away. With vaginismus, some form of psychotherapy is essential. It may be necessary for a woman to perform exercises with either her finger or a dilator to condition herself to the sensation of something being inserted into her vagina.

Male Sexual Dysfunction

Impotence is the common term for male inability to achieve the arousal state and to maintain an erection. Other forms of male sexual dysfunction include premature or retarded ejaculation and lack of sexual desire.

Because of the differences in their sexual development, men and women of the same age often differ in their sexual interest and responsiveness. As a natural part of aging, an older man's erection is not as strong and it doesn't last as long. Erectile dysfunction can also be caused by alcohol and drug abuse, medications, medical conditions, and surgery.

Emotional factors such as stress, depression, fear, and hostility often contribute to male sexual dysfunction. For example, men often experience impotence after divorce or death of a spouse.

If the impotence occurs suddenly and reappears off and on, it is usually considered psychological in nature. If it appears gradually and becomes progressively worse, it is likely to have a physical cause. If a man has firm erections while asleep at night he is usually physically able to have an erection during intercourse. The cause of the problem then tends to be psychological.

Erectile dysfunction that has a psychological basis is treated through counseling. If the cause is physical, the choices involve creating other satisfying methods of sexual expression, having a device surgically implanted to enlarge the penis to its erect size, or giving up sex.

If a man cannot have an erection, he cannot have vaginal intercourse, although other forms of sexual expression may be just as satisfying. If treatment or removal of the agent that is causing impotence doesn't work, a couple may use other forms of manual-oral stimulation. A man can have an orgasm without having an erection.

THERAPY

If a woman or her partner has a problem that cannot be resolved through communication and exploring new ways of expressing sexuality, the couple may find it helpful to seek professional advice and counseling. Most therapists do not view sexual problems as individual and prefer to treat couples. Treatment involves a series of steps in behavior modification aimed at reducing the demand for performance, identifying and modifying emotions that interfere with sexual responses, and teaching the couple physical and emotional behaviors that promote responsiveness.

Sex therapy is based on the principle that sexual problems are learned behavior patterns. Therapists help the couple identify barriers to sexual responsiveness that may arise from learned behavior such as lack of knowledge, guilt, fear, and cultural attitudes. The therapist then helps the couple remove these barriers through a process of relearning. The couple also explores aspects of its relationship that may be causing sexual problems.

Sex therapy often includes exercises called sensate focus. These exercises help the couple relate to each other physically without performance pressure or anxiety. Each partner takes turns caressing each other's body, slowly progressing to genital stimulation then, if desired, to sexual activity. Sensate focus is designed to help couples develop nonverbal means of communicating to each other how they like to be stimulated.

A woman who suffers from lack of arousal may benefit from a series of self-stimulation exercises designed to help her become more acquainted with her body and with what stimulates her sexually. It involves a step-by-step approach to manual stimulation to orgasm by the woman herself, then in front of her partner, then with her partner.

Sex therapists can come from different fields and levels of education. In seeking a qualified one, the following criteria should be met:

- Advanced degree in the profession: M.D. (psychiatrist), Ph.D. (psychologist), M.S.W. (social worker), M.A. or M.S. (marital and family therapist or nurse), or M.F.C. (marriage and family counselor).

- Competence in working with couples with marital problems.
- Training in human sexuality and the treatment of sexual dysfunction.
- Certification by the American Association of Sex Educators, Counselors, and Therapists (AASECT).

Sources of information on sex therapists include clinics sponsored by a university, medical school, or social agency. A university department of psychology or medical school department of psychiatry may also be able to provide a referral. Do not accept referrals from a doctor, clergymember, family member, or friend without checking thoroughly the credentials of the therapist and asking about his or her qualifications.

Most people will have a transient sexual problem at some point in their lives. This is certainly normal. Sexuality is an important part of living, and it should be experienced to its fullest potential. That can be achieved through self-awareness, communication, and professional support as needed.

PART III

REPRODUCTIVE HEALTH

CHAPTER 13

Genetics

Linda M. Brzustowicz, M.D.

Genetics is the study of heredity, or characteristics that are biologically passed from parents to children. It is important to distinguish between genetic traits, which are inherited, and familial traits, which may be passed on through rearing practices or other factors in the environment. Eye color is a genetic trait, while the language one speaks is a familial trait. Both are passed from parents to children, but only one is biologically determined.

Unlike some of the other fields of medicine, genetics is not a specialized study of one particular part of the human body. Genetic diseases can affect any parts, functions, or behaviors of the body. This is because genetic material is present within every cell of our bodies. From the moment of conception, our genes provide the blueprint of our development from fetus to infant to child to adult. They contain the instructions for building a human from a simple sperm and egg cell, and for running all of our complex systems smoothly. Any errors in this set of instructions can lead to some kind of defect or disease.

Genetics plays an increasingly important role in health care. Thousands of characteristics and diseases are known to be inherited. Recent advances in biotechnology allow for the identification of the specific genetic defects responsible for some of these disorders, and have provided the possibility of prenatal testing for these disorders and many others. The rapidly growing number of new technologies for genetic testing and potential therapy has made this a particularly difficult field for the consumer to keep informed about.

Understanding some of the basic concepts of genetics will make much of the detailed information more understandable. Two critical concepts in human genetics are how our genetic information is organized and how it is passed from one generation to the next during reproduction. Almost all of our genetic material occurs in duplicate. It might be useful to think of it as having two copies of an encyclopedia set. The two copies are not quite identical, but about 99.9 percent the same. Let's say they represent two slightly different editions. Having two different copies can be useful, particularly if there are some typographical errors in one copy or if one somehow gets damaged during use. We can turn to the second copy as a backup for important information.

During reproduction, we need to package our genetic material into our egg cells in such a way that it can combine with the genetic material in a sperm cell to make a human. To provide the child with the right amount of genetic material, the mother and father each donate one copy of the encyclopedia. The child receives half of her genetic material from her mother and half from her father. But the encyclopedias are not necessarily passed down as the original sets; as each volume is packaged into the egg, there is an equal chance that it may be that volume from Edition 1 or Edition 2. The egg cell has a single full set, but with different volumes from different editions. A similar process occurs in the packaging of the sets into the sperm cells, but the two sets that the father has are different editions from the two sets of the mother. If we call the mother's sets Editions 1 and 2, and the father's sets Editions 3 and 4, we can see that there are four possible combinations that can exist in a new child for any particular volume of the encyclopedia: Editions 1 and 3, Editions 1 and 4, Editions 2 and 3, or Editions 2 and 4 (See Fig. 13.1). In each case, one copy was inherited from the mother and one from the father.

It is easy to see that, when you consider the entire two sets of encyclopedias that are inherited by the child, there will be quite a few possible combinations. Two siblings could inherit substantially different encyclopedia sets. It is this mechanism, taken over many individuals and many generations, that allows for the enormous amount of diversity that we see among different people.

MENDELIAN AND NON-MENDELIAN INHERITANCE

Mendelian Inheritance

Much of our understanding of patterns of inheritance stems from the work Gregor Mendel presented in 1865. Mendel conducted breeding experiments with garden peas and followed the expression of physical characteristics through generations of offspring. For example, Mendel observed that when he crossed two strains that differed in seed color, one producing green peas and one producing yellow peas, all of the hybrid offspring produced yellow peas. Based on this result, yellow color is called the dominant trait, while green is considered recessive. But even though these hybrid offspring produced peas that were the same yellow color

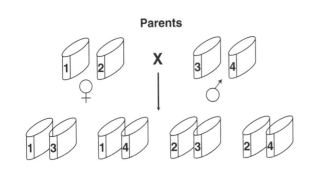

Parents

Figure 13.1 Inheritance
The inheritance of chromosomes from one's parents can be understood by using the analogy of an encyclopedia set. Each set has 23 volumes (chromosomes), making a total of 46 volumes (chromosomes) per person. A child inherits one set (in this illustration, either set 1 or set 2) from her mother and another set (3 or 4) from her father. Thus there are four possible combinations of the two sets that are passed down to the parents' offspring.

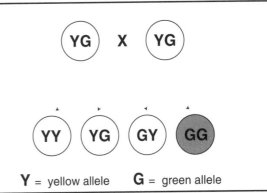

Y = yellow allele **G** = green allele

Figure 13.2 Mendel
In Mendel's experiments, yellow peas (YG, top row) were produced when yellow and green peas were crossed because yellow was a dominant trait. This means that a pea that inherited at least one yellow allele would be yellow, but one that inherited only green alleles would be green. When these yellow peas were crossed with themselves, however, the combinations of their chromosomes (bottom row) produced three-quarters yellow peas (YY, YG, and GY) and one-quarter green peas (GG). This is because the YG peas in the top row each contained a recessive allele for the color green, which was passed on from both parents 25% of the time.

as one of their parents, they were genetically different. When the yellow-producing parent plants were crossed with themselves, all of the offspring produced yellow peas. When plants from the yellow peas of the green-yellow cross were crossed with each other, a very different picture emerged. While 75 percent of these offspring still produced yellow peas, 25 percent produced green peas. The ability to produce green peas, even though not expressed in the offspring of the original cross, was preserved and passed on to the next generation. This ability of two traits, such as yellow and green color, to pass through generations and retain their ability to produce the original physical characteristics is called Mendel's first law, the law of independent segregation.

We now understand the biological mechanisms that underlie this process. Many "higher forms" of life (including both garden peas and humans) have two copies of most of their genes, and are referred to as diploid organisms. The two copies of a particular gene may be identical or they may be different. The different forms, or alleles, of a particular gene may produce differences in a particular physical feature. In the above example of peas, we examined the effects of a single gene that controls p . color, and followed the interaction of two different forms of the gene: one allele that produces green peas, and one allele that produces yellow peas. Since each pea plant has two copies of this color gene, there are three possible genetic situations, or genotypes: two green alleles, two yellow alleles, or

one green and one yellow allele. Since yellow is dominant to green, only two physical appearances, or phenotypes, exist: yellow or green. Pea plants that have two yellow or two green alleles are called homozygous and will produce peas of that color. The heterozygous plants, those with one yellow and one green allele, will produce peas of the dominant color: yellow. Note that plants with the same phenotype (yellow peas) may actually have different genotypes (homozygous for yellow or heterozygous for yellow and green). This will explain why peas that look alike may not reproduce alike.

In sexual reproduction, diploid organisms inherit a haploid genome (containing one copy of each gene) from each parent. Haploid gametes (sperm and egg) are produced through the process of meiosis. During meiosis, the two copies of each gene are lined up through the precise arrangement of the chromosomes. The two copies are then segregated into different gametes. Returning to Mendel's pea experiment, the original parents are homozygous for the yellow allele and homozygous for the green allele. All the offspring of this cross will inherit one yellow allele from one parent and one green allele from the other parent. So while they will produce yellow peas, they will all be yellow-green heterozygotes. What will happen when we cross two of these heterozygotes? Each parent may produce gametes that contain either a yellow or a green allele.

Four types of combinations are possible. Listing the contribution from the first parent first and the second parent next, the four possible genotypes of the offspring would be yellow-yellow, yellow-green, green-yellow, and green-green. The corresponding phenotypes of these plants would be yellow peas, yellow peas, yellow peas, and green peas, or 75 percent yellow and 25 percent green, the result originally described by Mendel (See Fig. 13.2).

Turning from benign color variations to disease states, we realize the very different patterns that can exist if a disease-producing allele is dominant or recessive to the normal allele. Diseases that can be caused by a defect in only one copy of a gene will follow a dominant pattern of inheritance, while those requiring defects in both copies will show a recessive pattern. Humans have approximately 100,000 genes, arranged on 23 chromosome pairs. The first 22 are called autosomes, while the last pair are called the sex chromosomes, due to their role in sex determination. Women have two copies of an X chromosome, while men have one X and one Y chromosome. If a disease allele is located on a sex chromosome, the pattern of inheritance will be related to the sex of the individual. The commonly described patterns of inheritance are autosomal dominant; autosomal recessive; X-linked dominant; and X-linked recessive; and are detailed in the next section.

Mendelian Patterns of Inheritance

Autosomal Dominant

In autosomal dominant inheritance, the gene causing the trait in question is located on one of the autosomal chromosomes. The trait is dominant, meaning that only one of the two copies of the gene is responsible for the manifestation of the trait or disease. Autosomal dominant disease alleles are often quite rare; one parent is usually heterozygous for the disease-producing allele, while the other parent is homozygous for normal alleles. An example is Huntington's disease, a neurological condition characterized by progressive uncontrollable movements and dementia. The gene involved in this disease is located on autosomal chromosome number four. If a person inherits one defective copy of this gene, they will develop Huntington's disease. It does not matter if the other copy of that gene is normal or defective, the disease will develop in either case. Au-

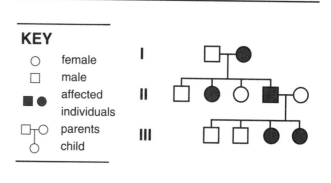

KEY
○ female
□ male
■ ● affected individuals
□⊤○ parents
○ child

Figure 13.3 Autosomal Dominant Inheritance
Autosomal dominant traits can be passed on to offspring who inherit the dominant trait from only one parent. In this diagram the affected parent is heterozygous for the trait, meaning that he has one dominant and one unaffected gene. The dominant gene is passed on to his children 50% of the time, and the affected children also have a 50% chance of passing it on to their children (assuming that their partners are unaffected).

tosomal dominant traits and diseases demonstrate typical patterns of inheritance in families. Individuals in multiple generations are affected. For disorders with full penetrance affected individuals always have an affected parent. (See the section on complicating factors for definition.) On average, half of the children of an affected parent will be affected, without relation to the sex of the children. A family demonstrating a typical autosomal dominant pattern is shown in Figure 13.3.

Autosomal Recessive

In autosomal recessive inheritance, the gene causing the trait in question is again located on one of the autosomal chromosomes. The trait is recessive, meaning that both of the copies of the gene must cause the trait for it to manifest itself. Alleles that produce autosomal recessive disorders tend to appear more frequently in the population. An example is cystic fibrosis, a disease of ion transport that manifests with respiratory and digestive difficulty. The gene involved in this disease is located on autosomal chromosome 7. A woman must inherit a defective copy of this gene from each of her parents to develop cystic fibrosis. If she inherits only one defective copy, she will be healthy, but she will be a carrier of the disease. Autosomal recessive traits and diseases demonstrate typical patterns of inheritance in families. There is usually no family history for the disease, and while affected individuals do not have an affected parent, both of their parents are carriers. On

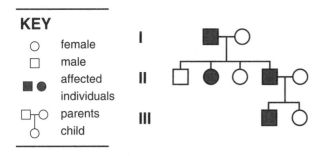

KEY
- ○ female
- □ male
- ■ ● affected individuals
- □─○ parents
  ○ child

Figure 13.4 Recessive Inheritance

For an autosomal recessive trait to be manifested, a person must carry two copies of the recessive gene. In this diagram neither parent is affected, but each carries one copy of the defective gene. On average, three out of every four (75%) of their children will be unaffected, and two of these three will be carriers. One out of four children will have the disease.

average, one quarter of the children of two carriers will be affected, half will be carriers like their parents, and the last quarter will inherit two normal copies of the gene in question, all regardless of the sex of the children. If the affected individuals have children with a non-carrier normal individual, all of their children will be carriers, but phenotypically normal. If they have children with a carrier, half their children will be carriers and half will be affected. If two individuals affected by the same recessive disorder have children, all of their children will be affected. A family demonstrating a typical autosomal recessive pattern is shown in Figure 13.4.

X-Linked Dominant

In X-linked dominant inheritance, the gene causing the trait in question is located on the X chromosome. The trait is dominant; only one copy of the gene causing the trait or disease is needed for it to manifest itself. X-linked dominant traits and diseases demonstrate typical patterns of inheritance in families. Individuals in multiple generations are affected. For disorders with full penetrance (see the complicating factors section), affected individuals always have an affected parent. Because the X chromosome is involved in sex determination, X-linked dominant disorders will show particular patterns with regard to sex. Since a man transmits his only X chromosome to his daughters, but not to his sons, all of an affected man's daughters will

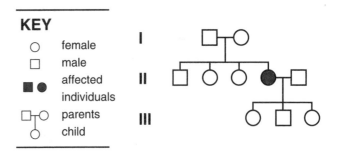

KEY
- ○ female
- □ male
- ■ ● affected individuals
- □─○ parents
  ○ child

Figure 13.5 X-Linked Dominant

An X-linked trait is one carried on the X chromosome of either a male or a female parent. In the case of an X-linked dominant trait, only one copy of the defective gene is needed for the disease or condition to manifest itself. In this diagram the gene is located on one of the grandmother's X chromosomes. She thus passes on the gene to half of her children, on average, whether they are boys or girls. Each affected son in turn will pass on the disease to half of his offspring.

be affected, but none of his sons will be affected. Since a woman may transmit either of her two X chromosomes to her daughters and sons, half of all her children, on average, will inherit the defective gene and be affected. A family demonstrating a typical X-linked dominant pattern is shown in Figure 13.5.

X-Linked Recessive

In X-linked recessive inheritance, the gene causing the trait in question is located on the X chromosome. The fact that the trait is recessive has different implications for men and women. Since women have two X chromosomes and therefore two copies of the involved gene, both copies of the gene have to cause the trait or disease for it to manifest itself. If a woman has only one defective copy, she will be healthy, but be a carrier of the trait or disease. Men have only one X chromosome, with most of the genes carried on the X chromosome present in only one copy (a small region of the Y chromosome, called the pseudoautosomal region, does carry a second copy of a small number of X chromosome genes). If a man inherits even a single defective copy of an X-linked gene, he will manifest the disease. Men cannot be carriers of X-linked traits or disorders. An example of an X-linked recessive disease is Duchenne muscular dystrophy, a disease that produces muscle degeneration. To be affected, a woman would usually need to have defective genes on both her X chromosomes, while a man would only need to inherit

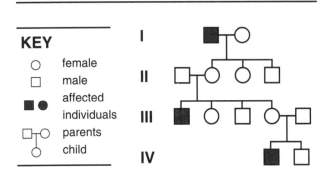

KEY

○ female
□ male
■● affected
   individuals
□⊤○ parents
   ○ child

Figure 13.6 X-Linked Recessive

An X-linked recessive trait manifests itself under different conditions for male and female offspring. Because the gene is recessive, two copies, one on each X chromosome, have to be present in a female child for her to have the disease or condition. If the gene is present on only one of her X chromosomes, a normal gene on the other X chromosome would suppress it. In that case she would then be free of the disease herself but would be a carrier. In male offspring only one copy of the gene is necessary for the disease to be present because males necessarily inherit a Y chromosome from their fathers, meaning that the X chromosome must come from their mothers. If a male's X chromosome carries the gene, he will have the disease because he has no other X chromosome carrying a dominant gene to suppress the trait. Males, therefore, cannot be carriers of an X-linked recessive disease; they either have the disease, and the gene that causes it, or they have neither the disease nor the gene. In this diagram the father is affected, with the defective gene present on his X chromosome. None of his children will have the disease, but all of his daughters will be carriers. (None of his male children will carry the gene or have the disease.) If the mother were a carrier, on the other hand, half of her sons would have the disease, and half of her daughters would be carriers. Half of all of her children would be free of both the disease and the gene.

one defective copy. Since a man inherits his single X chromosome from his mother, he would have to inherit a defective copy from her. The mother usually is a carrier, with only one X chromosome carrying a defective gene, and so half of her sons, on average, are affected. Assuming that her daughters inherited a normal gene from their father, half of the daughters, on average, of a carrier woman will be carriers. If the mother is a carrier and father is affected, half of the daughters will be carriers, while the other half will be affected. If both of the mother's copies were defective, she and all of her sons would be affected, and all of her daughters would be carriers. Since a man never transmits his X chromosome to his sons, an affected male never produces affected sons. An affected man will, however, pass his X chromosome to all his daughters.

Assuming that they have inherited an X chromosome with a normal gene from their mother, they will all be carriers, but not affected. Their sons will have a 50 percent chance of having the disease. The typical pattern of X–recessive inheritance is shown in Figure 13.6. Only males are affected and there are skips in the generations affected, with links through carrier daughters.

Genetic Recombination

The above examples illustrate the patterns that are seen when the inheritance of one trait is followed. What can we observe when we follow the inheritance of two different traits in the same family? Mendel's second law, independent assortment, states that the genes for different traits are independently transmitted to the gamete. Under this law, the inheritance of each gene is an independent, random event, with the outcome of the segregation of one gene pair having no influence on the segregation of any other gene pair. Returning to the garden pea, let us now consider pea color and a second trait, pea shape. Mendel worked with peas that had two types of shapes, round and wrinkled. In the same way that yellow was dominant over green for pea color, round is dominant over wrinkled for pea shape. If two true-breeding (i.e. homozygous) strains of peas are crossed, one with round yellow peas and one with wrinkled green peas, the expected hybrid offspring will produce round yellow peas, but will be heterozygous in both shape and color genes. What result will we expect if we cross two of these hybrid offspring? (See Fig. 13.7) These hybrids can produce four types of gametes: round-yellow, round-green, wrinkled-yellow, and wrinkled-green. This cross produces the following results: 9/16 round-yellow, 3/16 round-green, 3/16 wrinkled-yellow, and 1/16 wrinkled-green producing plants. If we closely examine these numbers, we can see that the genes for color and shape are independently assorting. If we consider only the round peas (12/16), we can see that 75 percent are yellow (9/12) and 25 percent (3/12) are green. Likewise, among the wrinkled peas (4/16), 75 percent (3/4) are yellow and 25 percent (1/4) are green. The 75 percent yellow peas and 25 percent green peas ratio we found from the original cross is unaffected by the characteristics of pea shape, demonstrating independent assortment.

Sometimes genes do not follow this law, but demonstrate a tendency to segregate particular combinations together. Let us assume that, instead of the above results, we found something very different when we

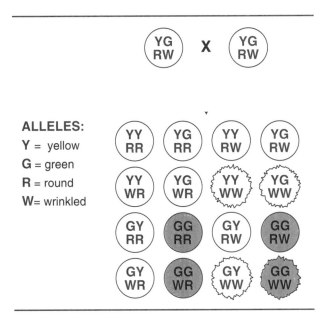

ALLELES:

Y = yellow

G = green

R = round

W= wrinkled

Figure 13.7 Cross-Breeding

Gametes resulting in crossed hybrids of peas. The parents each have a dominant gene for yellow color (Y) and a recessive one for green (G), along with a dominant gene for round shape (R) and a recessive one for wrinkled (W). Shown are the 16 possible combinations of these genes that could be inherited by the offspring. In each case a dominant allele (Y or R) will suppress its recessive counterpart (G or W), so that a pea with, for example, the genotype YGRW would be yellow and round like the parents, whereas one with the genotype GGWW would be green and wrinkled.

crossed the round yellow pea producing hybrid plants with themselves. Suppose we found that 3/4 of the offspring produced round yellow peas, and 1/4 of the offspring produced wrinkled green peas. If we were to consider only the round peas, we would find that 100 percent of them are yellow. Likewise, if we examined only the wrinkled peas, we would find that 100 percent of them are green. In this cross, the genes for yellow color and round shape seem to be transmitted together, while the genes for green color and wrinkled shape also seem to be transmitted together. When we observe this type of violation of the law of independent assortment, we say that the genes for color and shape are linked.

Linkage occurs when genes are located close to one another on a particular chromosome. When chromosome pairs separate to create the haploid gametes, the copies of the diferent genes situated together on a particular chromosome are carried off as a unit. The closer two genes are physically to one another, the more frequently they will segregate together, and the tighter they are linked. However, even tightly linked genes may be separated by the normal process of chromosome break-

age and exchange. The probability that such a genetic recombination, or crossover, will occur between two genes is proportional to the physical distance between them. While genes may vary greatly among individuals, there is extreme consistency in the order in which the genes are located on the chromosomes. If two genes are tightly linked in a certain group of individuals, they will ordinarily be tightly linked in all individuals. Maps of chromosomes which reflect the probability that neighboring genes will co-segregate, called linkage maps, can thus be generated from a specific set of individuals and generally applied to the population as a whole.

Complicating Genetic Factors

Sometimes not all individuals inheriting a disease gene show signs of the illness. A variety of genetic mechanisms can complicate the inheritance pattern, even among disorders that are caused by a defect in a single gene, or that clearly show a classical Mendelian pattern of inheritance. This is called reduced penetrance, and is suggested when a disorder appears to be genetic, but manifests itself in fewer than expected family members, such as only one of two identical twins. Split-hand deformity, also known as lobster-claw malformation, is an autosomal dominant disorder of hand and foot formation. It is estimated that only 70 percent of individuals inheriting the gene for this disorder will actually exhibit a deformity. Reduced penetrance can disguise the true mode of inheritance of the responsible gene by producing a pedigree with apparent skipped generations, when non-penetrant individuals who have the defective gene produce children with the deformity.

Sometimes a single gene defect can produce a variety of different symptoms, so that even within the same family, affected members do not seem to have quite the same disease. This is called variable expressivity, and requires thorough diagnostic criteria that will consider all possible different forms. Marfan syndrome, an autosomal dominant disorder of fibrous connective tissue, illustrates this point. People with Marfan syndrome typically have abnormalities in skeletal, ocular, and cardiovascular systems, but specific individuals may have abnormalities limited to only one or two of these systems, and the severity of symptoms can vary widely.

Non-genetic diseases that appear to be an inherited illnesses are called phenocopies. Returning to the example of split-hand deformity, similar-looking defects may be caused by intrauterine trauma due to amniotic bands. The presence of many phenocopies in the population can, again, disguise the mode of inheritance of the genetic cases of illness.

Sometimes different defects in the same gene exist within a population. These different defects may produce similar but non-identical diseases that seem to "breed true" within any specific family: allelic genetic heterogeneity. In two different forms of muscular dystrophy, Duchenne and Becker, the same gene coding for the protein dystrophin is involved. In Becker muscular dystrophy, the damaged gene produces a partially functional product and so the disease is relatively mild. In Duchenne muscular dystrophy, the gene product is badly damaged or totally absent and the resulting disease is very severe.

Multiple genes may be involved in causing a single disease, with the defects working in isolation or together. Sometimes defects in entirely separate genes can produce clinically identical diseases, called non-allelic genetic heterogeneity. Retinitis pigmentosa refers to a group of inherited diseases which cause loss of vision by retinal degeneration. Defects in any of several genes, located on different chromosomes, can cause this disorder. Diseases can also be produced by the interaction of defects in more than one gene, producing more complex patterns of inheritance.

Carriers

Carriers may pass on a genetic defect without suffering from the disorder caused by it. There are several different ways a person may be a carrier. For autosomal recessive disorders, two defective copies of the gene are needed to produce disease. Individuals with only one defective copy are carriers. When two carriers produce children, 25 percent will inherit two defective gene copies and be affected. The situation is slightly different for X-linked recessive disorders. Since women have two X chromosomes, they may be carriers if one of their X chromosomes carries a defective gene. However, as men only have one X chromosome, inheriting only one defective gene on the X chromosome will produce a disease in them. Therefore, a woman who is a carrier for an X-linked disease can have affected sons, regardless of the genetic status of the boys' father. Half of her sons, on average, will be expected to inherit her X chromosome carrying the defective gene and have the disease. Finally, individuals may be carriers for dominant disorders under special circumstances. Some genetic disorders exhibit reduced penetrance, so that

not all individuals with the genetic defect actually display symptoms of the disease. Half of the children of such an individual, however, would be expected to inherit the same genetic defect. Their chance of exhibiting the actual disease would again depend on the penetrance of the disorder.

Non-Mendelian Modes of Inheritance

While the Mendelian modes of inheritance explain the pattern of many inherited disorders, they do not explain them all. In recent years, a number of very different genetic mechanisms have been uncovered which explain some of these other patterns. Under Mendelian inheritance, a defective gene, regardless of whether or not it is inherited from one's mother or father, will cause the same problem. However, it sometimes does matter who passes on a disease gene. In the case of Prader-Willi and Angelman syndromes, two very distinct genetic disorders, deletions in the same small region of chromosome 15 can cause Prader-Willi syndrome when the defective chromosome is inherited from the father, but causes Angelman syndrome when inherited from the mother. Cases of diseases like this, along with a large amount of experimental data using mice, suggest that some genes function differently depending on whether they are inherited from a mother or from a father. While many of our genes apparently function identically despite their sources, certain genes seem to be "imprinted" with the parent of origin and have variable functioning.

To produce a healthy individual we need more than just a specific amount of DNA; we need to have the proper balance of maternally-derived and paternally-derived genetic material. During reproduction, a problem may arise that produces just this sort of imbalance. Sometimes, when the chromosomes pairs are splitting-up and individual chromosomes are segregating into individual egg or sperm cells, an error may occur. A pair may not split properly, so that the sperm or egg ends up with not just the usual one copy, but two copies of a particular chromosome. After fertilization, the early embryo would have three copies of that chromosome, which would be a very harmful situation. One of that set of three chromosomes may be lost at a very early stage of cell division in the embryo, so that only two copies remain. Sometimes it happens that the chromosome that is lost originated from the parent who had initially contributed only one copy. The result is an embryo with the right total number of chromosomes, but with both copies of a certain chromosome inherited from a single parent. This is called uniparental disomy, and can happen with chromosomes inherited from either the mother or the father. If, for example, a child has two copies of chromosome 5, both of which come from her mother, we would say this child has maternal uniparental disomy for chromosome 5. Now even that can occur in two variations. When the same maternal chromosome is duplicate, we call this isodisomy. If there is one copy of each of the mother's two different chromosome 5, it is called heterodisomy. This type of condition can cause problems in two different ways. In isodisomy, the child would be affected by any recessive disorders that are carried on the chromosome that is present in two copies. This mechanism is rare, and explains how a child can be affected by a recessive disorder when only one parent is a carrier. And since this rare event is the basis of a child being affected, the risk for subsequent children to also be affected is very small, as compared to 25 percent risk for the case where both parents are carriers. The other way that isodisomy can cause problems is if the involved chromosome carries any imprinted genes. As explained at the start of this section, imprinted genes function differently depending on whether they are inherited from the mother or from the father. For these genes it is important to have one copy from each parent to assure proper health. While not all of our chromosomes carry imprinted genes, some do, and isodisomy for those chromosomes can cause a variety of abnormalities, usually generalized problems of growth and development.

Uniparental disomy occurs when the extra chromosome is lost early, so that all cells in the embryo have the right total chromosome number. What happens if this correction occurs somewhat later? The situation can arise where some of the cells in the embryo have the correct number of chromosomes while some of the cells still have three copies. This will produce an individual who is mosaic for the two cell types. Depending on the proportion of cells of each type, and which particular body parts are composed of which type of cells, very different clinical manifestations of illness may be present.

Mosaicism is actually very common, as all women are mosaic. While we each have two copies of the X chromosome, only one copy is active in any particular cell. The other copy is inactivated, and exists as a genetic remnant called a Barr body. X-inactivation is normally a random process that occurs when the embryo has only 16 to 64 cells (although damaged X chromosomes may be preferentially inactivated). In a female embryo that has inherited one normal X chromosome and one X chromosome carrying a gene with a recessive mutation, it may happen by chance that the normal X is inactivated in more cells that the defective X. If the percentage of cells with the normal X chromosome inactivated is great enough, the woman may not just be a carrier for this X-linked disorder, but may actually be affected with it. There is also unequal X-inactivation in female identical twins, with preferential inactivation of the paternal X chromosome in one twin and preferential inactivation of the maternal X chromosome in the other twin. This may also produce a situation where one of the twins actually suffers from an X-linked recessive disorder, while the other is only a carrier.

Another non-Mendelian pattern of inheritance may be caused by the small amount of our DNA that is present in our mitochondria rather than in our chromosomes. These small organelles within our cells are responsible for energy production. Mitochondria reproduce very much like bacteria, by simple division, with the production of two daughter mitochondria that are genetically identical to the original mitochondria. During sexual reproduction, very few mitochondria are present in the sperm cell, with virtually all of the embryo's mitochondria inherited from the mother via the egg. There are a number of genetic defects that can occur within the mitochondria and lead to illness. These diseases exhibit a pattern of transmittal by every affected mother to all of her children; the father never transmits the disease to any of his children or their descendants.

The frequency or severity of a disease sometimes progresses in a family with each passing generation. This phenomenon is called anticipation, and was originally thought to be due to increased awareness and vigilance on the part of the family and doctors, with ill individuals known to be at risk noticed and diagnosed at an earlier age than ill family members from earlier generations. Sometimes this may be the case, but we also now know that certain genetic diseases, such as Huntington's disease, myotonic dystrophy, and fragile-X mental retardation, can actually become more severe in subsequent generations. This is because the genetic defect that causes these illness is unstable (a repeated pattern of three bases of DNA, called an expanded trinucleotide repeat) and may actually become larger when the gene is passed from parent to child. Depending on the disorder, there may also be preferential expansion of the defect when it is inherited from the mother or from the father.

CELLULAR AND MOLECULAR GENETICS

Genetic Material

Genetic material is passed from parents to children through egg and sperm cells. It is present in every cell of our bodies and can be isolated from any tissue, including blood, skin, and muscle. Many different names are used to refer to this material and its different levels of organization. Language serves as a good analogy for this organization. The alphabet, words, sentences, and paragraphs represent more and more complex structures of a language, each constructed by stringing together simpler units. Likewise, DNA, genes, and chromosomes represent increasingly complex genetic structures.

DNA is deoxyribonucleic acid, the chemical that makes up our genetic material. it occurs in four slightly different forms or bases: adenine, thymine, guanine, and cytosine (often abbreviated A, T, G, and C), which are the "letters" of the genetic alphabet. The human genome is estimated to consist of approximately three billion bases of DNA, arranges one after another into 23 strings, or chromosomes. "Typos" cause a point mutation, also called a single base mutation, that may result in disease.

RNA is ribonucleic acid, a chemical messenger closely related to DNA. Through the process of transcription, genes are copied, base for base, into RNA. This copy (called messenger RNA or mRNA) is then transported to the site in the cell where proteins are actually manufactured (ribosomes). Through the process of translation the genetic code is read by the cell and the protein is assembled.

Genes are strings of DNA bases that specify the construction of particular proteins. Proteins are the basic elements of our cellular functioning; everything in our body either is a protein or was made or regulated by a protein. Humans have approximately 100,000 different genes. The DNA in genes is organized into three base "words" called codons. Each codon will instruct the cell to add a particular amino acid (the building blocks of proteins) to a growing protein chain. Mutations, or errors, in the codons can result in the addition of the wrong amino acid, which may alter the functioning of the final protein. Certain codons tell the cell when the gene is finished, and the protein chain should be terminated (stop codons). A mutation may result in a premature stop codon. The resulting partial product may be nonfunctional, or may be unstable and rapidly degenerate.

Chromosomes are long threads of DNA that contain thousands of genes. Each individual of a particular species normally has the same number of chromosomes. Normal human cells have 46 chromosomes, including the two determining a person's gender. Chromosomes are normally present in pairs; one of each pair inherited from the individual's mother and one from her father. The non-sex determining chromosomes are called autosomes, and are numbered 1–22, based on size. The distribution of genes on the chromosomes is not random: Chromosome 1 will normally contain the same genes, in the same order, in all different people, similar to the way one would expect different copies of the first volume of an encyclopedia to always contain the same entries. The sex chromosomes, X and Y, determine an individual's sex. Women have two X chromosomes, while men have one X and one Y. Women normally pass one X chromosome to their children, while men may pass either an X or a Y, thus determining the sex of the child.

Cytogenetics is the branch of genetics dedicated to the study of chromosomes and the diseases caused by chromosomal abnormalities. Cytogeneticists can examine an individual's chromosomes under a microscope to look for certain types of defects. A karyotype is an ordered arrangement of the chromosomes from a single cell of an individual and may provide evidence of a defect. Karyotypes may be examined in children and adults and also prenatally by amniocentesis or CVS samples (See Chapter 14.) A karyotype can reveal extra chromosomes (such as three chromosome 21s, or trisomy 21, the cause of Down's syndrome); missing chromosomes; chromosomes containing deletions (a piece of the chromosome, but not the entire chromosome, is absent); or abnormal combinations (such as a piece of chromosome 5 stuck, or translocated, into chromosome 1). Many of these chromosomal defects produce very serious illnesses, and may often result in a miscarriage.

Genome refers to all of the genetic material of an organism. A haploid genome is the material contained in an egg or sperm cell, which together combine at conception to form a diploid genome: the amount of material contained in the somatic (non-reproductive) cells of our bodies.

Mutations are changes in a person's genetic material. They can caused by exposure to radiation (such as sunlight or X-rays), exposure to toxic materials (such as cigarette smoke or asbestos), or by a chance error of the cell's reproductive machinery. Mutations occur in two general types. Somatic mutations occur in one of our body's cells, and while the mutation is passed on to all descendent cells, it is not passed on to our children. Cancers often arise from somatic mutations, with the growing tumor representing the descendent cells of a single, very harmful, mutated, ancestor cell. Germline mutations occur in the genetic material of the egg or sperm cells, and are passed on to the next generation, and to all generations to follow. Some inherited forms of cancer seem to occur through a combination of somatic and germline mutations. A mutation in one copy of a gene may be inherited through the germline, with cells that acquire a somatic mutation in the other copy of that same gene then becoming cancerous. In this situation, the susceptibility to cancer is inherited in an autosomal dominant fashion.

Changes in our genetic material occur often. Fortunately our bodies have repair mechanisms that catch and correct most of these changes. Of the changes that do slip by, many are not harmful because they do not affect our genes. It is estimated that only 2–5 percent of our DNA actually represents genes. Mutations in the remaining 95–98 percent of our genetic material are unlikely to cause any serious problems.

Gene therapy refers to procedures and technology that correct genetic defects in individuals with genetic disorders. The exact procedure necessary to make this correction varies according to the disease. In autosomal or X-linked recessive disorders, the disease usually results from a lack of a functioning copy of a particular gene. The goal of gene therapy is to introduce a good copy of the gene back into some cells of the body. This has been done by removing cells from sick individuals, inserting a healthy copy of the gene into these cells in a laboratory, and then returning the cells to the patient's body. The cells then can grow in the body, producing the missing gene product. There are some limitations to this method, however. While it is relatively easy to do this procedure in blood cells, which freely circulate in the body, or even in some muscle cells, which could be returned to major muscle groups by multiple injections, it is very difficult to remove and replace brain cells, for example. So this type of gene therapy would not be very helpful for brain diseases. A variation on this method would be to use a modified virus to deliver the good copies of the genes into the desired part of the body. An infection with this virus could modify the cells without the need to remove and re-inject them. Such a virus would obviously need to be developed and used very carefully.

With dominantly inherited disorders, gene therapy poses more difficult problems. Here, the difficulty may be that the defective gene is producing a harmful product. It would not be enough to add a good copy of the gene; the defective copy must somehow be fixed or neutralized. While we may one day be able to correct all defective copies in all cells where they are causing problems, again, perhaps with custom-made viruses, it is likely that this will occur far in the future. A different strategy involves inserting a new gene that produces a product interfering with the defective gene, and neutralizing it. While this approach may be somewhat easier, it still presents a challenge to deliver the new gene to the necessary parts of the body.

GENES IN POPULATIONS

The Frequency of Genetic Diseases Vary in Different Populations

Despite the fact that the DNA sequences of any two humans would be overwhelmingly identical, it is clear by simply looking at different people that there are differences in our genomes. Some individuals, however, look more similar to each other than others. Members of the same family may have many features in common, while members of the same ethnic group may still have some, but fewer, common features. Members of the same race will have still fewer features in common. These differences reflect the fact that certain genetic elements may be shared by members of a certain population but that the genetic composition of different races and ethnic groups are somewhat different. Just as genes that govern physical features differ in their distribution within different populations, genes responsible for certain diseases are unevenly distributed. For example, about one in twenty-two U.S. Caucasians have one copy of the genetic defect causing cystic fibrosis, while that gene defect is very rare among the African-American population and the Caucasian population in Finland. Among U.S. Caucasians, about one in thirty Americans of Ashkenazi ancestry are carriers for Tay-Sachs disease, while only one in 170 are carriers among the rest of the

Caucasian population. Thus when calculating genetic risk for certain disorders, it becomes important to take into account a person's race and ethnicity. The differences in the frequencies of certain genetic disorders is usually most pronounced between populations that historically have been separated. If two populations meet and inter-marry, the differences disappear as the two gene pools are blended together.

Consanguinity

Consanguineous marriages, or marriages between blood relatives, are fairly common within certain cultures. Unfortunately, children from these types of marriages may be at a very elevated risk for genetic illness. For a child to inherit a recessive disease, both parents must be carriers. For a rare recessive disorder, where the chance of any individual being a carrier is one in 1000, the odds of both parents being carriers would be 1 in 1,000,000 (1/1000 x 1/1000). The chance that any given fetus will inherit defective genes from both parents is 1 in 4,000,000 (1/4 x 1/1,000,000). Let's instead consider two parents that are first cousins. The most likely way that they would both be carriers would be if one of their grandparents were a carrier, and had passed the disease gene to both of their parents. Since there are two great-grandparents at the top of the consanguinity loop, the chance that one would be a carrier would be 2/1000 (2 x 1/1000). There is a 1/2 chance that any given child will inherit the defective gene, so the odds that both the grandparents would be carriers would be 1/4 (1/2 x 1/2), assuming that one great-grandparent were a carrier (remember there is a 2/1000 chance of that). The odds that both parents would be carriers, again assuming that their parents were carriers, is again 1/4 (1/2 x 1/2). Finally, the chance that any child of theirs would be affected is 1/4, assuming they are both carriers. When we multiply out the probabilities of each of these people being carriers and a child being affected, we get 1/32,000 (2/1,000 x 1/4 x 1/4 x 1/4). While this is quite a low number, compared to the risk for a child from a non-consanguineous marriage (1/4,000,000), the risk to the child from the consanguineous marriage is increased by 125-fold.

Fitness and New Mutations

Why mutations that cause disease seem to persist in the population sometimes appears to be a bit of a mystery. If these mutations are so harmful, why don't they just die out? There are several factors that influence the persistence of a disease mutation. First of all, it is important to consider whether the mutation is always harmful. Sometimes mutations that cause disease may be helpful under other circumstances. A good example of this is sickle cell anemia. This is a recessive disorder, caused when an individual inherits two copies of the sickle form of hemoglobin (the protein responsible for the transport of oxygen within our red blood cells). Individuals with two copies of sickle hemoglobin are often quite ill, while individuals with only one copy are said to have sickle-trait and usually have only relatively minor symptoms. So why is this mutation so common in some populations? While sickle cell disease is clearly a liability, under certain circumstances sickle-trait may be a benefit. Specifically, individuals with sickle-trait have an enhanced resistance to malarial infection. So while sickle-trait may not be helpful for individuals living in urban America, it is clearly helpful in malaria-endemic regions of the world. To the population as a whole, the benefits of having many individuals with sickle-trait outweighs the losses due to those individuals who die early because they have sickle cell disease. This situation is called a balanced polymorphism, as there is selective pressure to retain the mutation in the heterozygous (carrier) state at the same time that there is selective pressure to lose the mutation when it is in a homozygous (disease) state. Some equilibrium is reached between these two forces, which determines the level of the mutation within the population. If the pressure to retain the mutation is removed, such as, in the sickle cell example, by migration to a non-malarial area, the mutation would be expected to die out. Selection is greatest against individuals with two copies of the disease gene. However, as most copies of the gene within the population reside within only mildly affected carriers, it may take many generations until a significant decrease in the disease frequency is noticed.

What about diseases that never offer any selective advantage? How do they persist within the population? There are two ways for this to happen. First, the disease may have no impact on the individual's genetic fitness. Genetic fitness is simply a measure of how many offspring an individual with a particular illness has, compared to the general population. It is clearly very different from general health, but in evolutionary terms, it is the most important measure of an organism's success. Certain illnesses may be quite devastating, but if they attack after the childbearing years, they may have little or no impact on genetic fitness. Huntington's disease is an example of this. With its onset typically in a person's 40s, individuals usually have already had their children and passed on the mutation before they are afflicted with this devastating illness.

The other way severe illnesses may stay in the population is through the production of new mutations. As in the case of the balanced polymorphism, opposing forces will work to establish an equilibrium level of mutant genes in the population. The decreased fitness of the gene works to eliminate it from the population, while the occurrence of new mutations serves to increase the disease frequency. Where these forces balance determines the rate in the population. For some severe illnesses, new mutations represent a very significant source of diseased genes. In Duchenne muscular dystrophy, approximately one-third of all affected males born into families without a known history of this illness represent new mutations.

METHODS OF GENETIC STUDY

While certain molecular genetic techniques are quite new, other methods of genetic study have been in use for many years. The first step in determining if a disorder is genetic is usually to determine if it is familial. Family studies compare the rates of illness in relatives of an affected individual (the proband) to rates of illness in the general population. An increased rate in the relatives of a proband suggests that the disorder is familial. While genetic disorders are familial, familial problems may not be genetic, but due instead to environmental factors such as rearing practices. So while certain families may have an unusually high concentration of doctors or lawyers, it is unlikely that this is due to genetic factors. And while genetics may play a role in language development, which language one first learns to speak would also seem to be a familial trait, and not a genetic trait.

If a disease appears familial, the next step is to determine if it is actually genetic. Two classic approaches to this question are adoption studies and twin studies. In adoption studies, children who might be at high genetic risk on the basis of being born into a family with elevated rates for a disorder are examined after being raised in a family with no elevated rate. Likewise, children at low genetic risk who are raised in families with a high rate of disease can be examined. If the disorder is genetic, the adopted children would be expected to show disease at a rate consistent with their family of origin. If the disorder is only familial, their rate of disease should instead reflect that of the family in which they were raised. In twin studies, rates of disease are compared between identical and fraternal twins. Since identical twins are identical genetically, they would be expected to be more similar to each other (i.e. either both have the disease or neither have the disease) than fraternal twins, who are genetically no more similar than any two siblings. If the disorder is familial but not genetic, the identical twins would be expected to be no more similar than fraternal twins or any other sibling pair.

Segregation analysis and pedigree analysis are methods used to investigate the specific mode of inheritance. In segregation analysis, the patterns of disease in many families are compared to what would be expected under different models of inheritance, with the goal of identifying the most likely pattern. Segregation analysis is limited by the assumption that the same mode of inheritance will be operating in all families. Pedigree analysis also seeks to identify a pattern, but using only a single, large, multi-generation family. While the risk of multiple modes of inheritance is greatly reduced by this approach, it is limited by the possibility that the identified pattern will be applicable only to the studied family.

Linkage studies are ordinarily undertaken once it has been firmly established that a disorder is genetic, and usually when something is known about the mode of inheritance. The goal of linkage studies is to identify a chromosomal region or regions related to an inherited disease, with the aim of isolating the responsible genes, identifying the causative mutations, and ultimately understanding function in both the normal and pathologic state. While linkage studies are most commonly used to study diseases, any inherited characteristic that can be observed or measured may be studied. The general method of these studies is to compare, within families, the presence or absence of the characteristic with the pattern of inheritance of different chromosomal regions. This is done by isolating DNA from the blood of family members, and following the inheritance of multiple, naturally occurring variations in the DNA (called markers) through the different members. The location of these markers are known (i.e. what region of what chromosome), and so by comparing the inheritance of these markers with the disease under study, it can be determined what markers the disease is linked to, or physically close to, on the chromosome (see genetic recombination in Mendelian and Non-Mendelian Inheritance). By observing the patterns of coinheritance of the disease with number markers from the same region, the disease gene can be localized to a very small region of DNA.

DNA-BASED GENETIC TESTING

Genetic tests based on the direct analysis of an individual's DNA have become commonplace. They are frequently used to make predictions about the chance that a fetus has inherited a genetic illness (prenatal testing), for determining if a currently healthy individual is likely to develop a late-onset illness (presymptomatic testing), and to check if someone has a single copy of a defective gene for a recessive disorder (carrier testing). While these tests represent a major advance in the field of human genetics, they do have their limitations. Utilizing the background first presented, we will examine some of the more frequently available types of tests and analyze their differences.

The first major distinction between tests is between those based on an analysis of the actual mutations responsible for disease and those based on genetic linkage. The concept of gene linkage was discussed in the genetic recombination section of this chapter. Gene linkage, or the localization of the genetic region where a disease-causing mutation resides, usually precedes the isolation of the actual genetic defect involved in the disease. Therefore, linkage-based tests are usually possible sooner, anywhere from months to years before a direct mutation test. Linkage-based tests are limited by several factors. The main limitations result from the fact that they infer an individual's disease status from other information, and so there are several potential sources of error. Some of the information must come from other family members, as linkage follows the inheritance of traits through families. It is important to have another affected family member to compare with the individual in question. If the only other affected person in a family is unavailable, then the usefulness of linkage tests is minimal. (Actually, all that is needed is DNA from the affected person. This can sometimes be isolated from things like stored tissue biopsies. DNA banking services are also available, both commercially and through some universities, for families that wish to store DNA for possible future use in linkage-based tests.)

DNA markers that are known to be linked to, or located close to, the disease in question are typed in the family, and the pattern of inheritance of these markers is used to infer the inheritance of the disease. The problem is, however, that *close to* the gene is not the same *as* the gene. Remember that even closely linked locations on the chromosome can be separated through recombination, potentially causing an incorrect test result if a recombination occurs between the marker and the disease gene. Usually, the markers being used are very close to the disease gene, so that the chance of this happening is less than one percent. The most accurate tests check markers on both sides of the disease gene. That way, if a recombination occurs between the gene and the marker on one side, it should be detected by looking at the marker on the other side. If the flanking markers are very far apart, however, it is possible for two recombination events (a "double recombination") to occur between them without being detected. For most tests with tightly-linked markers, the chance of an incorrect answer due to a double recombination event is very small (less then one in 10,000). Another problem is that, even though close markers may be used, key individuals in the family may be "uninformative" for those markers, limiting the usefulness of the test for that family. Again, the best tests will use several markers available on each side of the disease gene, so that if one marker is uninformative, another may be studied. Finally, for a test to be accurate, it is important that the disease in question be caused by a gene at the location being tested. Remember that same-looking diseases can be caused by defects in genes on entirely different chromosomes. *All a linkage test determines is whether two people have inherited a certain region of DNA in common.* It is possible for a test to be 99.99 percent accurate in making that determination, but if 40 percent of cases of the disease are caused by defects in genes from other locations, then the test will be accurate for predicting disease only 60 percent of the time. When evaluating the reported accuracy of a linkage-based test, it is important to inquire if the disease in question is known to have any non-allelic genetic heterogeneity (i.e. can be caused by genes at other locations), and if it does, if that has been figured into the reported accuracy.

As already mentioned, direct mutation tests usually

become possible sometime after linkage-based tests. They look directly at the gene involved in causing the illness, and focus on searching for specific, known defects. A major advantage is that they do not require the participation of an entire family. Linkage studies require another affected individual, but one may not be available for a variety of reasons. There is also a cost difference between analyzing the DNA from one person or a whole family. The major draw-back of direct-mutation tests is that they only search for known defects. It is possible for the test to miss a new or unusual mutation. Positive answers, for example, when a mutation is found, are usually highly reliable. Negative results do not mean that there is no mutation, but rather that none of the mutations tested for was found. For certain disorders where the exact mutation is always the same, such as sickle cell disease, the negative results are very reliable. But some diseases are caused by many different mutations. Numerous mutations have already been identified as causing cystic fibrosis, with a typical direct-mutation test checking for about thirty of them. Mutations are not selected at random for testing; only the most common are singled out. For some diseases the few most common may be responsible for 80–90 percent of actual cases of illness. However, it is important to remember that the frequency of particular mutations may vary from one population to another. The sensitivity (what percentage of true cases they actually detect) of these tests should be reported for a particular population, and it is important to know how that population was defined when evaluating the test. In U.S. Caucasian populations, a test for 32 mutations will be about 90 percent sensitive. This same test detects only about 40 percent of mutations in African-Americans. A test of only six mutations can detect about 97 percent of mutations among people of Ashkenazi ancestry. If the sensitivity of a direct-mutation test has not been checked against your ethnic group, it will be very difficult to interpret a negative result. In that type of situation, a linkage-based test may actually give a more accurate result.

With all the available DNA tests, people sometimes wonder if there is any value to being tested for something when there is no known family history or ethnic predisposition to that particular illness. Most genetic disorders are rare and the tests are still fairly expensive, so the value of randomly testing healthy individuals is probably limited. As an example we can again consider cystic fibrosis, the most common serious recessive illness in the U.S. Caucasian population, with approximately one in 22 individuals being a carrier. While this may seem like a high number, remember that for any affected children to be born, both parents must be carriers. The odds of both parents being carriers is 1 in 484 (1/22 x 1/22). The chance for a particular child to be affected by cystic fibrosis is only 1 in 1936 (1/484 x 1/4). For something even just a little less common, such as a disorder where 1 in 100 people are carriers, the chance for a particular child to be affected would be only 1 in 40,000.

A final consideration about testing is research laboratories versus hospital or commercial laboratories. Research and diagnostic labs are organized in very different ways. While a research lab may be developing the most advanced test, they typically are not set-up to handle clinical samples as carefully as a diagnostic lab. Diagnostic labs are very, very careful to assure that there are no mix-ups between samples. Research labs typically don't have the money or personnel to maintain such careful tracking of samples. Unless there is something unusual about your situation that requires the most advanced test, it is generally a better idea to go to a reputable diagnostic lab for clinical testing. The best situation is using a diagnostic lab that works closely with a research lab investigating that particular illness. The diagnostic lab will then have access to the most up to date tests, but will still provide the careful sample handling they are best designed to do.

CHAPTER 14

Genetic Counseling

Karen L. David, M.D., M.S., F.A.A.P. and Penny Steiner-Grossman, ED.D., M.P.H

No field of medical knowledge is exploding more rapidly and with more potential impact upon women—and the reproductive choices they make—than the field of genetics. Once almost an afterthought in the training of physicians, genetics and its relationship to human health and disease now make front-page news with regularity. The news is both exhilarating and daunting.

Scientists are rapidly learning which of the estimated 100,000 genes located on chromosomes in each of our body's cells could be the cause of any of nearly 5,000 inherited disorders. With this new knowledge, genetic tests are being developed to look for specific disease genes, a step that could ultimately lead to better treatments and eventual cure of the conditions altogether. Moreover, prenatal tests of fetal health before birth can now predict earlier and with even greater accuracy whether there is a likelihood of an inherited disorder or birth defect.

Nevertheless, it is not always easy to decide when to use this technology, how to interpret the results, and what course of action to take. Families dealing with the possibility of an inherited disorder or birth defect in an unborn baby, or confronting the reality of a child or adult who is already affected, need the help of trained individuals—medical geneticists and genetic counselors—to establish a diagnosis and to guide them through the process of understanding the facts about the disorder, appreciating the potential risks to other family members, choosing a course of action, and coming to terms with their decision. This process is called genetic counseling.

Although this chapter is presented as a guide for those contemplating using genetic services, it is far

WHEN GENETIC COUNSELING HELPS

Genetic counseling can be helpful to any woman, either before or during pregnancy, who is concerned about the risk to her unborn baby posed by a number of situations. These may include:

- a family history of genetic disease or birth defects,

- a chromosome problem associated with advanced maternal age such as Down syndrome,

- exposures to potentially harmful substances,

- two or more unexplained miscarriages or a previous baby with a birth defect,

Likewise, families searching for explanations of the appearance of a genetic condition or birth defect in a family member can seek genetic counseling and testing to predict the likelihood that other family members will be affected. Far more than just testing, the genetic counseling process offers education about human inheritance and knowledge about specific disorders of concern to a family.

from encyclopedic; the field of genetics is moving too rapidly for that. Those seeking more detailed information about genetic testing should make contact with a medical geneticist or hospital genetics unit, or contact one of the agencies listed at the end of this chapter.

THE GENETIC CONSULTATION

Testing and counseling go hand in hand in a genetic consultation. Counseling is needed to help the geneticist and the client decide mutually whether testing is appropriate and which tests may be needed; information from test results, including a possible diagnosis, is essential for counseling to be effective. From the start, the emphasis in genetic counseling is on educating you and the members of your family about the actual or suspected condition that has prompted the consultation so that you may become experts. If you or a member of your family is referred for a genetic consultation

because of the existence or perception of some increased risk, a member of the genetic counseling team will discuss the reason for the referral with you and ask you some basic questions, including your date of birth, length of gestation if you are pregnant, information about any prenatal exposures (such as medications, smoking, alcohol or drug use, or chemicals at work), ethnicity, and details about your and your family's medical history. One result of this consultation is a diagram called a pedigree.

Sometimes, as part of this initial visit, you or your

family member may be offered a physical examination by a medical geneticist, a physician trained in the specialty of genetics. During the examination, the medical geneticist can often observe certain physical characteristics that may speed the process of making the diagnosis or lead to the recommendation of appropriate tests. The benefits and risks as well as the limitations of each test will be explained so that you can arrive at a decision about whether or not to undergo the test. The counselor may give you brochures or offer to show you a videotape explaining the procedure. If you decide in favor of the test, you will be asked to sign an informed consent form, depending on the nature of the test. (Later in this chapter, we describe some tests that may be recommended.)

The results of the various tests will require study and interpretation. The next phase of the genetic counseling process is to put this information into perspective as a prelude to independent decision-making on your part. A member of the genetics team will discuss the cause of the condition, its variability, any available treatments, the likelihood that it may affect other family members, and its potential impact on family planning. The concept of risk is usually presented in terms of numerical probability (fractions or percentages), with the understanding that what seems a high risk to one person may not seem so to another.

Finally, the counselor will present the options, reproductive and otherwise, open to you and your family in a manner that does not favor one option over another. This non-directive approach respects the fact that decisions involving genetics are often difficult to make, take time, and must be made independently by the family in the context of their moral and cultural values, religious principles, reproductive goals, and perceptions of risk. Often, the social concerns of parents—the cost of caring for a child with a birth defect or genetic condition, the presence or absence of family support, the availability of appropriate schooling, and access to support groups to alleviate stress—weigh heavily in the decision-making process. The most productive genetic counseling sessions allow enough time for these concerns to be addressed.

THE IMPORTANCE OF FAMILY HISTORY

Knowing the details of your family's medical history is an important component of the genetic counseling process.

Traditionally, women in the family are often the keepers of this information. The records and documents they accumulate may provide the first clues that an inherited condition in one or more family members could affect a prospective pregnancy, an unborn baby, or a living relative. Not all inherited disorders can be detected by testing, but many can. The test results can provide the basis for decisions about whether to continue a pregnancy, how to prepare for the birth of an infant with special needs, or how to anticipate or ameliorate an adult-onset genetic disease. Even if a family member is adopted, it may be possible to find out medical information about the birth family, depending on state laws governing the release of such information.

Constructing a diagram of your family's health history, called a pedigree or family tree, is not difficult, but you must follow certain basic rules:

- Begin the pedigree with yourself and work backwards to include at least three generations if possible.

- Squares represent males and circles represent females.

- Parents are connected to each other with horizontal lines and to their children, left to right in birth order, with vertical lines.

- Smaller symbols indicate stillbirths and miscarriages.

- Generations are numbered using Roman numerals.

The diagram below shows a pedigree of a family with several members who have Huntington's disease. (See Fig. 14.1). (Although it is generally the task of the genetics professional to prepare a formal pedigree such as this one, it is useful to put together a rough diagram yourself containing the important facts before speaking with a geneticist or genetic counselor.) A pedigree takes into account not only any genetic or familial disorders that run in the family, but also the ethnic and geographic origins of family members. This information is important, as we shall see later, in the inheritance of such conditions as sickle cell disease (mostly in African-Americans, Caribbeans, and Latinos), Tay-

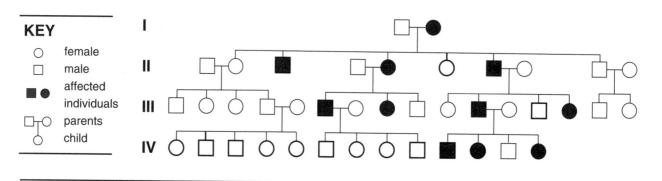

Figure 14.1 Family Tree
A family tree, or pedigree, will generally be constructed by your genetic counselor. This pedigree shows a family in which Huntington's disease, an inherited condition, appears in several generations.

Sachs disease (mostly in Jews of Eastern European ancestry), and thalassemia (mostly in those from Mediterranean countries and much of Asia). It is also important to know about any consanguineous marriages (marriages between relatives) and about any spontaneous abortions, stillbirths, neonatal deaths, chromosome abnormalities such as Down syndrome, birth defects such as cleft palate and congenital heart defects, or mental retardation. In the case of birth defects or mental retardation, it is helpful to have photographs of the affected family member(s) as well as any available medical records. When possible, a physical examination of the relative is very important. Any of this information may supply the clues needed to learn about an actual or potential inherited disorder or birth defect.

While a family history of an inherited disorder or birth defect is certainly not the only reason for seeking genetic counseling, the pedigree often forms the foundation upon which the counseling process can build.

GENETIC COUNSELING AND PREGNANCY

Most women seek or are referred for genetic counseling because they are pregnant or intend to become pregnant and have some questions or concerns about the health of their unborn baby. These concerns can be broken down further into two categories: family history indicators (such as ethnic predispositions to inherited disorders, or a history of known genetic disorders, birth defects, or chromosomal abnormalities) and other indicators (such as advanced maternal age, abnormal test results in pregnancy, or exposure to potentially harmful substances during pregnancy).

Family History Indicators

Ethnic Predisposition

Ethnic predisposition to a particular genetic disorder is an important reason for obtaining genetic testing and counseling during pregnancy, if not before. The following conditions are all autosomal recessive, which means they require two genes—one from each healthy parent—for the condition to occur in a child.

- *Sickle Cell Disease.* In sickle cell disease, the normally flexible and round red blood cells become rigid and crescent-shaped. The disease causes anemia, bouts of pain caused by blocked blood vessels, and increased susceptibility to serious infections such as pneumonia. About 1 in 10 African-Americans carries one recessive gene for sickle cell disease; this is called sickle cell trait. More than 50,000 Americans have two copies of the gene and have sickle cell disease. People of Caribbean origin and many Latinos also have sickle cell trait, as do smaller numbers of Greeks, Italians, Asian Indians, and Saudi Arabians. When both partners have sickle cell trait, they have a one in four chance with each pregnancy of having a child with the disease. This can be determined during pregnancy by prenatal diagnosis or at birth by newborn screening.

■ *Thalassemia.* Individuals of Asian and Mediterranean origin (including Greeks and Italians) are at risk of inheriting thalassemia when both parents carry a single recessive gene (called thalassemia trait). Some forms of thalassemia are very serious and may result in stillbirth or cause severe anemia, requiring a continuous program of blood transfusions for the child or even bone marrow transplantation. Prenatal diagnosis is also available for thalassemia.

■ *Tay-Sachs and Gaucher Disease.* Couples of Eastern European (Ashkenazi) Jewish descent need to be aware that they might be carriers of the recessive genes for a number of disorders, of which Tay-Sachs disease is the best known. Babies with Tay-Sachs disease are born deficient in an enzyme, hexosaminidase A, that is essential for proper nerve cell functioning. These children gradually lose mental and physical functioning and generally die before the age of five. Approximately 1 in 25–30 Ashkenazi Jews is a Tay-Sachs carrier; the rate for Sephardic Jews (those originally from Spain, Portugal, and North Africa) is about 1 in 100. Screening with a simple blood test before or during pregnancy is a routine practice, and prenatal testing is also available.

Another recessive genetic disease caused by an enzyme deficiency, Gaucher disease, is even more common than Tay-Sachs disease, with a gene carrier rate of approximately 1 in 12 Ashkenazi Jews. Gaucher disease causes the build-up of fatty deposits in the liver and spleen, resulting in the enlargement of these organs. It can vary from mild to severe. Carrier testing and prenatal diagnosis are available to those with a family history of the disease. Routine testing is not currently offered.

■ *Cystic fibrosis.* Caucasians are at increased risk for cystic fibrosis (CF), a generally severe disease characterized by thick mucus secretions in the lungs and other parts of the body. There are approximately 30,000 Americans with CF and as many as 1 Caucasian American in 20 may carry one of the many forms of the gene for CF. CF is less frequent in Latinos, infrequent in African-Americans, and very rare among Asians. When both members of a couple carry such a gene, they have a one-in-four chance with each pregnancy of having a child with CF. At present, a DNA-based test for the cystic fibrosis gene is available especially to people with a family history of the disease (see below), but the test is not yet able to identify all carriers in all ethnic groups. In most cases, a fetus at risk for CF because of family history can be identified through prenatal diagnosis. In the future, testing for the CF gene may be available for population screening.

The diseases mentioned above are only a few of the numerous genetic conditions for which specific ethnic groups are at special risk. Less often, these conditions may also affect members of other ethnic or racial groups. However, the frequency of the gene in the particular group combined with the severity of the disease may suggest the need for targeted screening to identify asymptomatic carriers of the specific gene, a process called genetic screening. In any case, it is prudent to remind the obstetrician and the genetic counselor of your and your partner's ethnic background so that you can be offered the appropriate testing.

Known Inherited Disorders

Many people are aware that one or more members of their family has a condition that seems to be inherited. Naturally, they may be concerned that a future child of theirs will develop the same condition. Some examples of these inherited diseases are cystic fibrosis; neurofibromatosis, a condition causing a wide range of symptoms including darkened patches of skin ("cafe au lait" spots) and multiple benign tumors of nerve and fibrous tissue; hemophilia, a disorder of the clotting mechanism in the blood; the fragile-X syndrome, the most common inherited form of mental retardation in males; and muscular dystrophy, a group of muscle-wasting diseases. Each of these diseases is inherited in a different pattern, and each has different recurrence risks: cystic fibrosis is an autosomal recessive disorder, neurofibromatosis is an autosomal dominant disorder, hemophilia is X-linked recessive (transmitted on the X chromosome), and the fragile-X syndrome is inherited in a manner that does not fit neatly into any of these categories. There are many varieties of muscular dystrophy, each inherited in a specific pattern (see Chapter 13).

What many of these and other inherited disorders have in common, however, is the increasing availability of tests predicting whether an individual or a fetus carries the gene for the condition. Couples aware of a family history of these or other inherited diseases can now seek genetic counseling, either to test for the presence of the altered gene or genetic marker in their blood or to undergo prenatal testing for the disorder. The information they obtain through testing and counseling helps the couple decide about the pregnancy and about care of the infant after birth. For example, in the case of cystic fibrosis (CF), the gene causing the disease has been traced to the long arm of chromosome 7, and specific carrier tests using DNA analysis can now identify the majority of mutations of this gene. In fact, about 90 percent of Caucasian-American CF carriers can now be identified by DNA testing for over 30 mutations, a process called mutation analysis or direct gene detection. (Carrier identification is more direct if the particular mutations in the family member with CF are identified. Unfortunately, failure to detect a mutation does not ensure that a person is not a carrier, since approximately 10 percent of Caucasian-American carriers will not be detected by current methods. The percentage varies depending on the ethnic group.)

Since those affected by CF can now live well into their twenties and even longer, a woman with CF may seek genetic counseling to ascertain the risk that a child of hers will have the disease. If testing of her partner by mutation analysis is negative, the chance for CF in a child of theirs is much reduced but not eliminated. If her partner does have a CF mutation, prenatal diagnosis can determine whether the baby will be affected.

Birth Defects

There are many types of birth defects, all with their own causes. A family history of problems such as neural tube defect, congenital hip dislocation, cleft lip, and cleft palate is a good reason to seek out the help of a geneticist when you are pregnant or planning a pregnancy. Let's choose one of the more common birth defects, congenital heart defects (CHD), to illustrate.

There are numerous types of CHD that affect the various structures of the heart with varying degrees of severity. The prevalence of these defects in liveborn infants is about 4–8 for every 1,000 births. Sometimes congenital heart defects are associated with particular physical features, called extracardiac malformations, that make specific inherited disorders or chromosomal problems easy to identify. Many of these defects once caused death in infancy. Today, because of medical and surgical intervention, increasing numbers of individuals with CHD are surviving to adulthood, thus increasing the need for genetic counseling of the families of affected individuals.

Most congenital heart defects are probably the result of combined genetic and environmental factors (multifactorial inheritance). Virtually all forms of CHD show some familial pattern of occurrence: Recent studies have demonstrated rates of familial occurrence for obstructive defects involving the left side of the heart that are four to six times higher than for other types of defects. For example, in siblings there is about a 14 percent rate for hypoplastic left heart syndrome, an 11 percent rate for bicuspid aortic valve, and an 8 percent rate for coarctation of the aorta. The risk to children when one parent has CHD is generally between 2 and 4 percent. Higher rates have been reported in some forms of CHD if the parent with CHD is the mother.

Genetic counseling can be of enormous help to the family concerned about the recurrence of a congenital heart defect. The interpretation of recurrence risks varies depending on the specific anatomic defect or genetic syndrome and the presence of other affected relatives. A complete family history taken during genetic counseling can also reveal any exposures to harmful substances that may have contributed to the defect in question. Prenatal diagnosis, specifically fetal echocardiography (sonography of the fetal heart), is available at many centers beginning at about the twentieth week of pregnancy, sometimes in conjunction with amniocentesis and chromosome analysis. If tests reveal the presence of a congenital heart defect, the genetics professional and a pediatric cardiologist can prepare the parents for the extent of the disability so that they may make a decision about the pregnancy and/or prepare in advance for the delivery and early nursery care.

Mental Retardation

Mental retardation in a family is another important reason for seeking genetic counseling. The condition has many genetic as well as nongenetic causes. Using one example, fragile-X syndrome is the most common inherited form of mental retardation in males. Only recently described, fragile-X syndrome is caused by an abnormally expanded gene associated with a so-called fragile site on the X chromosome transmitted by one of the parents. The presence of fragile-X syndrome in a family is often suspected when there are one or more retarded members, usually boys, who may have elongated faces, prominent ears, and unusually large testes after puberty. Girls with fragile-X are affected less often but may have learning disabilities or mild mental retardation. In affected boys, the expression of fragile-X syndrome is variable and mental retardation may be mild or severe. Because fragile-X carriers, both male and female, may not show any symptoms of mental retardation at all, carrier testing is recommended to help the family determine the risk to prospective children. In addition to chromosome analysis, direct DNA testing for the fragile-X gene is now available. Prenatal diagnosis can even predict to some extent the severity of the mental retardation.

Stillbirths, Unexplained Miscarriages, or Infants with Multiple Congenital Malformations

A personal or family history of stillbirths, multiple unexplained miscarriages, or chromosomal problems such as Down syndrome is another reason for pursuing genetic testing and counseling. Miscarriages, also called spontaneous abortions, are quite common and occur in about 15 percent of pregnancies. Chromosomal abnormalities in the fetus, usually extra or missing chromosomes, account for approximately half of all first-trimester miscarriages. (About 7 percent of stillbirths have a chromosome abnormality, and one of every 200 liveborn infants has a chromosome abnormality such as Down syndrome.) In searching for the cause of a miscarriage or stillbirth, the physician can order a chromosome analysis of the fetal cells; if the results are abnormal, this will provide an explanation for the loss of the pregnancy. In most cases of missing or extra chromosomes, no chromosome problem is found in the parents. However, when there is a liveborn infant with Down syndrome, there may be an increased risk for recurrence in future pregnancies.

Two or more miscarriages, an unexplained stillborn, or a liveborn with physical abnormalities may also be the result of a different kind of chromosome imbalance. One of the parents, for example, may have a chromosome "rearrangement." An example of such a rearrangement is a so-called balanced translocation, in which material normally found on one chromosome has been exchanged with material from another. This transfer causes no health problems for the parent who carries the rearrangement but may result in chromosomally abnormal egg or sperm cells (germ cells) that lead to a chromosomal imbalance in the fetus. A miscarriage, a stillbirth, or a liveborn with multiple congenital malformations may be the result.

In another type of rearrangement, a part of one chromosome can break and rejoin to itself in an inverted position, reversing the gene order on that chromosome. While not all inversions lead to problems, sometimes an inversion in the chromosomes of a parent can cause the formation of abnormal germ cells.

Approximately 1 in 20 couples with multiple miscarriages has some kind of chromosome rearrangement in one parent. Knowing about such chromosome rearrangements can help to explain the loss of repeated pregnancies and assist the couple in doing some advance planning for the next pregnancy.

Other Indicators for Genetic Counseling in Pregnancy

Maternal Age

The most common reason today that women seek genetic testing and counseling during pregnancy is advanced maternal age. Most doctors currently consider advanced maternal age as 35 years or older at delivery because the chance that a baby will be born with Down syndrome rises markedly with increasing age. It is about 1 in 350 at age 35, 1 in 100 at age 40, and 1 in 30 at age 45. Down syndrome, also known as trisomy 21, is the most common chromosomal abnormality among live-born infants and is due to an extra chromosome number 21 (trisomy 21), resulting in a total of 47 chromosomes instead of the usual 46. The reason for this is usually the failure of separation of the two paired 21 chromosomes during germ cell formation, resulting in a sperm or more often egg cell with 24 instead of the usual 23 chromosomes. Children with Down syndrome have characteristic facial features, including skin folds at the inner eyelids and upslanting eyes. They have some degree of mental retardation and may have congenital heart defects. While these children can learn to read and write and participate in family life, adults with Down syndrome continue to need supportive services.

Other much rarer chromosomal abnormalities also become more prevalent as maternal age increases. These include trisomy 18 and trisomy 13, both of which result in severe physical and mental defects. Infants born with either of these syndromes rarely survive more than a few months.

Because the risk for these and certain other chromosomal abnormalities increases with maternal age, it is customary for physicians to offer prenatal testing for their pregnant patients who will be 35 or older at the time of delivery, regardless of the number of prior pregnancies they may have had. Prenatal diagnosis of Down syndrome and other chromosome problems is made using the techniques of amniocentesis, chorionic villus sampling (CVS), and chromosome analysis, all of which are covered later in this chapter.

ALPHA-FETOPROTEIN AND OTHER SCREENING TESTS

Alpha-fetoprotein (AFP) is a protein produced by the developing fetus that is excreted into the amniotic fluid in small amounts. Normal levels of amniotic fluid AFP vary with gestational age. Minute quantities also find their way into the maternal bloodstream. Excessive amounts, however, suggest the possibility of a neural tube defect, a structural problem in the formation of the brain and spinal cord. Neural tube defects can range from a failure of brain development (anencephaly) to a structural defect in the spinal cord and the bone, muscle, and skin that normally cover it (spina bifida or meningomyelocele). Because a fetus with an open spine defect will leak additional amounts of AFP into the amniotic fluid, AFP levels in the mother's bloodstream, called maternal serum AFP (MSAFP), will also usually be higher, suggesting that her fetus may have a neural tube defect. However, MSAFP may also be elevated for other reasons, such as the fetus having kidney disease, a defect of the abdominal wall (omphalocele or gastrochisis), the existence of a twin pregnancy, or incorrect gestational dating. Low levels of MSAFP have been associated with an increased risk of Down syndrome, making the test a useful screen for Down syndrome pregnancies in women under age 35. Other serum markers in maternal blood—human chorionic gonadotropin (hCG) and perhaps estriol—are also useful screening tools in combination with MSAFP for Down syndrome and most likely trisomy 18. Maternal serum screening using a combination of two or three serum markers is abnormal in the majority of pregnancies wth Down Syndrome.

Since virtually all obstetricians are now offering their pregnant patients maternal serum screening at about 16 weeks gestation, it is important to understand the test for what it is—a screening test. Such a test may suggest an increased risk but does not prove conclusively the existence of some condition in the fetus. Many factors may influence levels of MSAFP, among them the age of the fetus, a twin pregnancy, race, the weight of the mother, and maternal insulin-dependent diabetes. If, after considering these factors, MSAFP levels are still abnormal, further testing by ultrasound and amniocentesis is recommended. Even then, results are usually normal, with a normal outcome of the pregnancy. Maternal serum screening tests for use in the first trimester are being developed.

Exposures during Pregnancy

Many pregnant women seek genetic counseling because they have been exposed—or fear they may have been exposed—to substances or situations that are potentially harmful to the fetus. Environmental agents that can cause birth defects in the fetus are called teratogens, and they include certain medications, maternal diseases, infections, X-ray exposures, alcohol, and drugs. Exposure to chemicals and other agents in the workplace is another potential cause of birth defects (see Chapter 6). As might be expected, there is often a dose-response relationship between the degree and timing of exposure to a teratogen and the potential for birth defects, although for most teratogens the level of safe exposure is not known.

Most teratogens cause damage during the first trimester of pregnancy when the embryo is undergoing rapid development and cellular differentiation. However, even within the first trimester there is an especially critical window of opportunity—usually between the eighteenth and the fortieth day after conception when most organ systems are developing—where the potential for harm is greatest. However, organ systems such as the nervous system continue to develop throughout pregnancy and remain vulnerable to birth defects caused by teratogens. To complicate matters, maternal and fetal genetic differences make some fetuses more susceptible than others to teratogenic exposures during pregnancy. For some exposures, however, there are methods to estimate the level of risk to which the fetus has been exposed and to evaluate fetal health. The following exposures are a partial listing of those with the potential to cause harm during pregnancy.

Rubella: When maternal rubella (German measles) occurs during the first eight weeks of pregnancy, the chance for birth defects in the newborn is about 85 percent. However, the potential for harm still exists into the second trimester. The infection in the mother may be mild or even go unnoticed, but the effects on the fetus can be numerous and may include growth deficiency, hearing loss, eye problems such as cataracts or glaucoma, heart defects, and mental retardation. Fortunately, there is an effective vaccine against rubella infection routinely given to all children in the United States. For women who have not been vaccinated in childhood, there is a simple blood test available to determine their immunity to rubella. When rubella immunization is done before planning a pregnancy, the vaccine poses no danger to the fetus. Even if inadvertently given during pregnancy, it appears to pose minimal, if any, risk.

Cytomegalovirus: One in every 100 infants born in the United States has cytomegalovirus (CMV), a virus that causes a mild, flu-like illness in the mother or no symptoms at all. Severe problems to the fetus can result when the mother has the virus for the first time during her pregnancy (primary infection). Although the majority of these babies are asymptomatic at birth, the 10 percent of babies who do develop early symptoms have small heads (microcephaly), mental impairment, problems with the retina of the eye, hearing loss, jaundice, and enlargement of the liver and spleen. Mortality is relatively high among this group of infants, about 20 to 30 percent. However, even babies who are asymptomatic at birth may go on to develop problems such as microcephaly or a progressive hearing loss. In addition, there is evidence that women who have had CMV in the past (recurrent maternal infection) may also have babies at some risk for hearing impairment. Again, a simple blood test can tell you about your immunity to CMV.

Toxoplasmosis: Toxoplasmosis is caused by an intracellular parasite sometimes present in uncooked or poorly cooked meat and in cat feces. It can result in a mild, flu-like illness that causes swollen glands and fatigue or has no symptoms at all. If the infection occurs in the woman during pregnancy, transmission to the fetus is quite possible, potentially causing a wide range of problems, regardless of when the mother was infected during pregnancy. These problems include mental retardation, convulsions, inflammation of the choroid and retina of the eye, hydrocephaly or microcephaly, and hearing loss. Other problems in these infants are anemia and jaundice. While many babies with toxoplasmosis are asymptomatic at birth, they may go on to develop problems in infancy and childhood, such as deafness, impaired vision, and mental retardation. However, once a woman has developed immunity to toxoplasmosis, the chance for problems in future babies is very low. Blood tests to determine immunity to toxoplasmosis are available.

Chickenpox: Varicella infection (chickenpox) in the mother causes few problems with fetal development in most instances. When it does cause problems (in less than 5 percent of cases and mainly during the first trimester of pregnancy), it can result in prematurity and growth deficiency, as well as a characteristic scarring of the skin overlying the affected sensory nerves. Mental retardation, seizures, malformation of the limbs, and eye problems may also occur. Again, the risk in the first trimester is greater than in the second trimester. A test for immunity to varicella infection is available and a new vaccine is currently under consideration for general use.

There are other infections in the mother, such as herpes, hepatitis, syphilis, HIV infection, and so on, that can be transmitted to the fetus during pregnancy.

Maternal Diabetes: Poorly controlled diabetes in the mother can result in a wide range of infant birth defects, including central nervous system defects, neural tube defects (anencephaly and meningomyelocele), congenital heart defects, vertebral malformations, and malformations of the skeletal, genitourinary, and gastrointestinal systems. The period of greatest risk to the fetus is the first eight weeks of pregnancy. Most of the defects appear to be related to elevated blood sugar in the mother, so optimal control of sugar metabolism in the mother, both before conception and in pregnancy, can reduce the likelihood of birth defects. Good control of sugar can also decrease the chance that a baby will be larger than normal at birth (macrosomia) or will develop low blood sugar or low calcium levels soon after birth. Prenatal monitoring and delivery of the baby in a well-equipped facility can minimize complications. (See Chapter 30 for more information on diabetes.)

Alcohol: The effects of alcohol on the fetus, called fetal alcohol syndrome (FAS), include a spectrum of problems, such as growth deficiency and developmental delay, characteristic facial features, and congenital heart defects. The most serious effects involve the nervous system and can result in mental retardation, poor motor development, and hyperactivity. In fact, FAS is now the leading cause of mental retardation in the United States. Because some effects on the fetus can occur in women consuming even moderate amounts of alcohol (at any time in pregnancy but especially during the first trimester), the best advice to pregnant women is to avoid alcohol altogether.

Cocaine: Cocaine is currently used by more women of childbearing age than any other drug. Its effects on the fetus can be wide-ranging and severe: spontaneous abortion and stillbirth, placental abruption (separation), prematurity, low birth weight, brain hemorrhage, neurological and behavioral abnormalities, and possibly gastrointestinal and genitourinary malformations. Cocaine causes constriction of blood vessels, and this suggests that disruption of optimal blood supply to the fetus may lead to many of the problems associated with its use. Because cocaine in all its forms can harm the fetus at any point during the pregnancy, its use should be strictly avoided.

Medications: About 5 to 10 percent of pregnant women taking Dilantin (phenytoin), one of the most commonly prescribed drugs to control epileptic seizures, give birth to an infant with a recognizable pattern of facial features, underdeveloped nails, congenital heart defects, and occasionally learning difficulties. Other babies exposed to Dilantin may show only very mild effects. Most show no effects at all. Tegretol (carbamazepine) and Depakene (valproic acid) are sometimes associated with malformations in the fetus, especially neural tube defects such as meningomyelocele (about 1 in 100). Women with seizures who are considering a pregnancy will benefit from consultation with their treating physician or a medical geneticist to consider both the type of medication and the dose for optimal control of seizures during pregnancy.

Accutane, an anti-acne medication, may cause numerous severe fetal problems, including neurological, heart, and facial defects. Lithium, prescribed for bipolar disorder (formerly called manic-depressive illness), can cause a specific type of congenital heart disease in infants exposed to it during the first trimester of pregnancy. Examples of other medications known to cause birth defects when taken during pregnancy include diethylstilbestrol or DES (structural changes in the cervix and vagina and, rarely, adenocarcinoma of the vagina), tetracycline taken in the second and third trimester (staining of the teeth), and Coumadin, an anticoagulant (multiple neurological and skeletal anomalies). If you are planning a pregnancy, be sure to ask your physician to check on any risks associated with both your old and newer medications.

EXPOSURES OF THE FATHER

There is some preliminary evidence that exposure of the father to certain environmental agents may also cause damage to the sperm and possibly to the developing fetus. A recent study of cocaine-using fathers found evidence that the drug can bind to sperm and, if present at conception, may cause damage to the embryo. In addition, a father's social drinking may have an indirect effect on fetal health: it may make it more difficult for his partner to avoid drinking alcohol altogether during her pregnancy. In the future, there is likely to be a great deal more research in this important area.

Exposure to X-Rays and Other Imaging Techniques: Although very large doses of radiation have been associated with fetal loss and microcephaly, the lower doses of radiation delivered during diagnostic X-ray examination are believed to pose little danger to the fetus. Nevertheless, as a general rule, X-ray examinations should be performed before a pregnancy or delayed until after delivery, unless medically necessary. If you need to have X-rays performed on another part of your body during pregnancy, be sure to ask the radiologist to shield your pelvis and abdomen. You should also ask about the safety to the fetus of the radio-opaque dyes sometimes used during X-rays.

Nuclear scans use radioactive substances in small amounts to diagnose certain medical conditions. Some of these substances have the potential to cause harm to the fetus. If you are pregnant or planning to become pregnant, alert your physician.

Magnetic resonance imaging (MRI) does not use ionizing radiation to visualize structures in the body. While the safety of MRI in early pregnancy is still under investigation, it is wise to consult your doctor about the latest research developments.

Sonography is a commonly used imaging technique, employing sound waves, that is safe for the fetus.

Investigation into the risk of maternal-fetal exposure to potential teratogens continues. For example, chronic use of megadoses of vitamin A, not generally thought of as harmful in the past, are now considered a potential cause of malformations in the fetus. Consultation with your doctor before pregnancy will help you to avoid potentially harmful exposures.

Other Reasons for Genetic Counseling and Testing

Once again, family history is a major motivating factor for consultation with genetics professionals, even when a specific pregnancy is not the immediate concern. For example, a family might want to ascertain the risk, based on family history, that one or more of them might develop a genetic disease of adult onset, such as adult polycystic kidney disease, Huntington's disease, or a hereditary form of cancer. Another family may simply wish to gain an understanding of the origin of a condition, such as genetic deafness, that appears in some family members.

As with genetic counseling during pregnancy, the

GENETIC DEAFNESS

More than half of all childhood deafness can be traced to genetic causes. Close to 200 types of genetic deafness exist, about a third of which occur with other physical symptoms, such as changes in the eyes, the ear shape, the heart, bones, kidneys, or other parts of the body. These combinations of symptoms are called genetic deafness syndromes. Not all types of genetic deafness are apparent from birth; it is posible for a child to be born hearing and for genetic deafness to manifest itself later in childhood or even in adulthood.

Genetic deafness must be differentiated from environmental deafness resulting from maternal infections such as rubella or cytomegalovirus (CMV), from certain diseases such as meningitis, or loud noises later in life. Environmental deafness has no effect on the genes of the person who is deaf, and such a person is likely to have children with normal hearing.

Genetic deafness can be inherited in a variety of ways. The most common mode of inheritance, accounting for 80 to 85 percent of all genetic deafness, is autosomal recessive, in which two genes are needed—one from each hearing parent—for deafness to occur. About 15 to 20 percent of genetic deafness is autosomal dominant, or caused by a single dominant gene. In this form, there is a 50 percent chance with each pregnancy that a child will inherit the gene for deafness from the deaf parent. X-linked deafness, in which the gene for deafness is carried on the X chromosome, is very rare, causing only about 1 to 2 percent of genetic deafness.

Genetic counseling can be very beneficial, both for hearing adults who have a deaf child or another family member who is deaf and for deaf adults themselves. In the case of hearing parents, the geneticist or genetic counselor may be able to identify the type of deafness in the family member, help the family to anticipate the likelihood that future children will be deaf or hearing, and recommend hearing tests soon after birth. Genetic counseling also may provide the first opportunity for a deaf individual to understand the cause of his or her deafness, and may answer questions about childbearing. When deafness is part of a syndrome including other physical problems, genetic services can offer help in coordinating access to other medical specialists. In recent years, the genetics community has become increasingly sensitive to the unique cultural, linguistic, and communication issues that are shared by deaf people.

importance of gathering your family's health history cannot be overemphasized. The conditions discussed below represent only a few of those that may be of concern to families and individuals.

Some Adult-Onset Genetic Diseases: Adult Polycystic Kidney Disease, Familial Hypercholesterolemia, and Hereditary Cancers

The dilemma facing all those at risk for adult-onset genetic diseases is that symptoms may not appear until well into middle age or later, long after families have been completed and disease-causing genes passed on to children.

■ The prototype for this kind of condition is adult polycystic kidney disease (APKD), easily the most common genetic disease with approximately 500,000 Americans of all races and both sexes affected. Most often caused by an altered gene on chromosome 16, dominantly inherited APKD leads to the development of hundreds, perhaps thousands, of renal cysts that disrupt kidney function and may lead ultimately to renal failure and the need for a kidney transplant. The liver, spleen, and pancreas also may develop cysts, and in some families there may be an increased risk of cerebral aneurysm. Screening with sonography can reveal cysts in the kidney before symptoms appear. A DNA test is available to tell whether an individual has a high probability of carrying the gene and may develop the disease later in life. However, this test is only useful in families in which there are known cases of APKD and DNA of these individuals can also be studied. Not surprisingly, this kind of predictive testing imposes a burden of information on individuals that may cause considerable emotional discomfort. Recently the gene on chromosome 16 causing APKD was identified. This may soon allow for direct testing for the gene without the need to study family members.

■ Familial hypercholesterolemia (FH) is another common inherited adult-onset disease, causing high blood cholesterol levels and precipitating a heart attack as early as age 35. This disorder is caused by a single dominant gene found in approximately 1 of every 500 Americans. FH is due to an abnormality in the uptake of cholesterol into the body's cells, trapping it in the bloodstream, where it accumulates and causes atherosclerotic plaques. A family history of early heart attacks certainly suggests the need for cholesterol screening. Although the first heart attack may not occur until the fourth decade or later, high blood cholesterol levels can be detected in childhood, alerting primary care physicians and geneticists to the possible presence of FH in the family. There are specific genetic tests that can confirm that diagnosis. Control of cholesterol levels can then be achieved, in most cases with a combination of dietary and lifestyle changes and medications.

■ Five to ten percent of all cancers are dominantly inherited, among them hereditary breast and ovarian cancers, familial adenomatous polyposis (a form of hereditary colon cancer), and hereditary nonpolyposis colon cancer. In each of these cancers, an accurate family history alone may be sufficient to identify individuals who are at risk for the disease and should be offered surveillance and/or genetic testing. In some cases, DNA testing can even identify gene carriers for specific cancers. At this early stage, some form of intervention can often reduce the risk or minimize disability.

■ A gene for hereditary breast cancer, transmitted in an autosomal dominant fashion, has just been identified on the long arm of chromosome 17. This will soon allow for direct testing of women at risk for alterations in the gene. Even now, DNA testing is useful in selected families. A second gene for hereditary breast cancer has been located on the long arm of chromosome 13. Early onset of breast cancer (in the thirties or even younger), the increased risk to the other breast, and the occurrence of early breast cancer in relatives help to differentiate hereditary breast cancer from nonhereditary forms. Women at risk for hereditary breast cancer—constituting 5 to 9 percent of all breast cancers—are currently offered earlier mammograms, more frequent breast examinations, and in selected cases preventive mastectomy.

Similarly, family members at high risk for hereditary ovarian cancer can be identified by their position in the pedigree. In both these cancers, close female relatives, usually daughters, sisters, and mothers of the affected person, face a nearly 50 percent risk over time of developing the cancer. In some families, predisposition to both ovarian and breast cancer appears to be governed by a single gene, found on the long arm of chromosome 17 (BRCA1).

■ Familial adenomatous polyposis (FAP) is an autosomal dominant condition, traced to a gene on chromosome 5, in which dense carpets of precancerous polyps blanket the colon. In FAP, physicians can detect asymptomatic gene carriers by early adulthood by examining the retina of the eye for certain nonpathologic changes and the colon for polyps. Since colon cancer usually develops in these individuals in early to middle adulthood, screening with colonoscopy and surgical intervention are also offered early. Preventive proctocolectomy (removal of the colon and rectum) eliminates the risk to the individual who carries the gene for this trait. (A DNA test to identify gene carriers has recently been developed.)

■ Another autosomal dominant condition, hereditary nonpolyposis colon cancer, accounts for as much as 13 percent of all colon cancers. Gene carriers of this disorder are at increased risk for cancers of other parts of the body as well. Recent identification of several genes responsible should soon allow recognition of presymptomatic family members.

In the examples above, genetic testing and counseling, while often generating anxiety, can also provide relief from uncertainty and the hope for prevention or amelioration through new surveillance techniques and improved medical and surgical treatments. Unfortunately, there are other adult-onset diseases for which advances in knowledge on the contribution of hereditary factors have not yet resulted in specific genetic tests. Just a few examples of these are lupus, rheumatoid arthritis, alcoholism, schizophrenia, and most forms of diabetes and Alzheimer's disease.

GENETIC TESTS AND WHAT THEY INDICATE

Ultrasound Examination (Sonography)

A routine part of prenatal care for many women, sonography or ultrasound examination is a valuable tool for the estimation of gestational age, placental and fetal position, and twin pregnancies (level I or obstetric sonography). Sometimes other problems are discovered during a routine examination; because it shows some of the physical features of the fetus on a screen, ultrasound can detect certain structural birth defects. Fetal or level II sonography is performed if there is a suspicion that a structural birth defect may be present. For example, some neural tube defects such as anencephaly or meningomyelocele, congenital heart and kidney malformations, and skeletal defects can be confirmed with this test.

An abdominal sonogram for fetal anatomy is performed in a doctor's office or outpatient facility as early as 15 weeks, when certain fetal structures are relatively easy to visualize. The test can be performed earlier or later, depending on the anomaly that is suspected; a vaginal version of ultrasound can also be performed even earlier in pregnancy. Sonography is considered safe and causes no discomfort for mother or fetus. A technician glides an instrument repeatedly over the mother's abdomen, generating a sound wave picture of the shape of the fetus and its internal structures, the placenta, and the umbilical cord. Although a sonogram is useful in diagnosing a wide range of fetal malformations, it cannot detect all such defects prenatally.

Amniocentesis

One of the most commonly performed prenatal tests, amniocentesis is the withdrawal of a small sample of the amniotic fluid surrounding the fetus. In addition to cushioning the fetus, amniotic fluid contains fetal cells normally sloughed off during the process of growth as well as other substances, such as alpha-fetoproptein (AFP), that provide important information about fetal health before birth. For example, analysis of the chromosomes in fetal cells collected during amniocentesis may reveal a chromosome abnormality such as trisomy 21 (Down syndrome) or other chromosome defects.

Amniocentesis is currently offered to all pregnant women 35 and older at the time of delivery and to women with a personal or family history in themselves or their partners of a chromosome problem or neural tube defect, and to women at risk for a fetus with a genetic disorder, such as Tay-Sachs disease or thalassemia major, detectable by biochemical or DNA studies. Amniocentesis is also offered to women with abnormal maternal serum alpha fetoprotein (MSAFP).

Amniocentesis is usually performed between the fifteenth and twentieth weeks (or sometimes earlier, depending on the physician) in an outpatient facility or physician's office. On occasion, the test will be performed later in pregnancy if a problem is suspected. Guided by ultrasound, the physician first locates the position of the fetus and placenta; he or she then inserts a thin hollow needle through the woman's abdomen into her uterus, well away from the fetus. About a tablespoon of amniotic fluid is withdrawn for analysis. Results generally take about 10 to 14 days. The test causes only slight discomfort, much like that experienced during blood drawing, and poses about 0.5 percent (1 in 200) risk of miscarriage. Women taking the test are advised to avoid strenuous physical activity for the remainder of the day on which the test is performed. Amniocentesis is also available to women with twin and triplet pregnancies. (For more information on amniocentesis, see Chapter 17.)

Chorionic Villus Sampling (CVS)

Because the results from amniocentesis testing are not available until the second trimester of pregnancy, there was an impetus for the development of a test that could detect genetic disorders early in pregnancy. CVS testing is generally performed about the tenth week of pregnancy. The physician inserts a thin needle through the abdominal wall (transabdominal CVS) or uses a narrow tube placed in the vagina for insertion through the cervix into the uterus (transcervical CVS). Instead of sampling amniotic fluid—which is of low volume this early in pregnancy—the syringe draws out a few of the tiny hair-like projections, or villi, that are part of the developing placenta. These villi contain fetal cells that can be analyzed for the presence of many genetic abnormalities, including chromosome problems. Results are usually available within 10 days. Rarely, amniocentesis may be required later to verify the results of CVS testing. CVS will not provide results for some conditions, such as neural tube defects. In the case of neural tube defect, MSAFP with sonography and/or amniocentesis are generally recommended.

CVS testing has certain advantages: If the test finds a chromosome problem or hereditary disorder and if the woman and her partner elect not to continue the pregnancy, she can have an abortion during the first trimester when it is safer and easier to obtain. In the future, a disorder discovered early in pregnancy by CVS testing may be treated in utero with medications, surgery, or even with gene replacement. Even today there are isolated situations in which early interventions can improve health of the fetus. The risk of miscarriage with CVS may be slightly greater than that of amniocentesis, but it is still quite low. A few studies have suggested a causal relationship between CVS done earlier than 10 weeks and a rare malformation of the fingers and toes in newborns. The magnitude of this risk, if any, is quite small.

CVS testing is not as widely available as amniocentesis, although it is available in many major medical centers. Women with twin pregnancies can have CVS testing, but confirming amniocentesis may be required. Transcervical CVS testing generally is not advisable for women with a recent history of vaginal infection.

Techniques are now being developed to isolate fetal cells from the maternal circulation. In this way, fetal cells would be available for prenatal diagnosis without the need for amniocentesis or chorionic villus sampling. Prenatal diagnosis of the pre-implantation embryo is possible in special circumstances as part of in vitro fertilization.

Chromosome Analysis

Chromosome analysis is the examination of body tissues and/or blood samples under the microscope so that individual cells may be isolated and their chromosomes counted, specially stained (banded), and examined to investigate the possibility of a chromosome abnormality. About 1 in 200 newborns has some kind of chromosome alteration, although not all lead to problems. Many types of tissue may be used for chromosome analysis, including blood samples, skin cells, cells from amniotic fluid or chorionic villi, and fetal tissue from a miscarriage. Cells are cultured for a period of hours or days, depending on the type of tissue. They may be first stimulated by the addition of special chemicals to synthesize DNA and divide. Other chemicals are added to arrest the cells in a stage of cell division called metaphase and enhance the identification of the chromosomes. Cells are then photographed through the microscope, prints are made, and the individual chromosomes cut out and arranged in pairs, a process called karyotyping (See Fig. 14.2). Generally about 20 cells are counted and several karyotypes are done on the tissue sample in order to observe a consistent pattern in the number and configuration of the chromosomes.

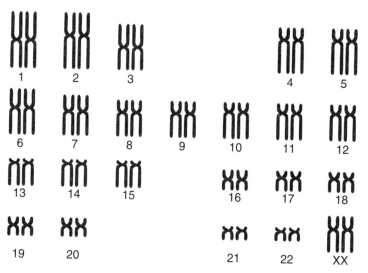

Figure 14.2. Karyotype

Shown here is a representation of a normal female karyotype, illustrating all 23 pairs of chromosomes including two X chromosomes.

DNA Testing

The identification of genes associated with diseases, as well as the discovery of DNA markers in the vicinity of those genes, has made available new diagnostic tests for a wide variety of genetic disorders. When the specific gene and its mutations are known at a DNA level, the gene can be detected using a specific test. Such a test has recently been developed for Huntington's disease, for example. This method is known as direct DNA analysis or direct gene detection, and examples of its use are the detection of sickle cell disease, the thalassemias, and cystic fibrosis. On the other hand, when the gene has not been isolated and analyzed for alterations, genetic markers alongside the suspected gene must be identified, a process known as indirect detection or linkage analysis. A current example of linkage analysis is the DNA test for adult polycystic kidney disease. It is usually necessary to test several members of a family to trace the presence of the linked marker and to identify susceptible individuals. With the recent identification of the gene on chromosome 16, however, direct gene detection may be possible soon.

DNA testing can be performed using any tissue sample containing DNA, for example, white blood cells, skin cells, amniotic fluid cells, or chorionic villi. There are numerous commercial, university, and hospital-based laboratories specializing in DNA testing. Confidentiality of test results is safeguarded. DNA banking, the storage of DNA from tissue samples, may aid in later diagnosis of a genetic condition in a family member when the gene for a particular disorder is identified or new mutations are discovered, often long after the affected individual has died.

Newborn Screening

A genetic screening test is one that is performed on an entire population, or subset of a population, for the purpose of identifying individuals at risk for certain genetic disorders. An example already mentioned is MSAFP screening in pregnancy. In the United States, newborn screening is now conducted in every state in order to identify babies with certain genetic or metabolic disorders that can be treated shortly after birth, even before symptoms appear.

The list of conditions screened depends upon the populations at risk and other public health considerations. For example, all states screen newborns for phenylketonuria (PKU), a recessively inherited disorder of metabolism characterized by elevated levels of the amino acid phenylalanine and resulting in mental retardation if untreated. Fortunately, a phenylalanine-restricted diet beginning soon after birth can insure normal development. Sickle cell disease is another condition included in newborn screening protocols in many states. As with PKU, early identification of babies who have sickle cell disease can allow for early treatment, such as daily penicillin to decrease the threat of bacterial infection, education of the parents, and amelioration of complications of the disease. Newborn screening also identifies infants who carry the sickle cell trait, enabling parents, with the help of genetic testing and counseling, to understand their chances of having future children with sickle cell disease.

A third example is newborn screening for congenital hypothyroidism, a problem with the normal development of the thyroid gland affecting about 1 in every 3,000 newborns (see Chapter 29). Timely treatment with thyroid hormone can prevent the onset of mental retardation that may result from this condition. In newborn screening, a few drops of blood are taken from the baby's heel within several days after birth. Results are sent to the physician or hospital caring for the family. Any infant with an abnormal result is retested to confirm the initial result. If the abnormal result is confirmed, the baby will be referred by the hospital or pediatrician for special care soon after birth. In some states, only abnormal results are reported to the parents; those parents wishing to know the outcome of newborn screening, even if results are normal, may have to contact their physician or the hospital where the baby was born.

CONFRONTING DIFFICULT DECISIONS IN GENETICS

As new medical technologies become available to provide additional information on which to base decision-making about health, studies have shown that people tend to make use of them. This does not always hold true for new technologies in the field of genetics, however. Choosing new knowledge in this field may open

NEW TREATMENT OPTIONS FOR GENETIC DISORDERS

While new possibilities for treatment raise the hopes of families already living with a genetic disorder, they may also generate some concern about whether or not to try them, how successful they are likely to be, and what risks they may entail. A recent national survey conducted by the March of Dimes Birth Defects Foundation (1992) revealed that many Americans felt somewhat uneasy about the idea of gene therapy and even misunderstood its basic purpose: to help people overcome genetic disease rather than to change physical characteristics of normal individuals. Nearly three-quarters of those surveyed favored strict government regulation of the practice.

Trials for some of these new treatments, such as gene therapy, are just beginning. Gene therapy affects only the health of the individual being treated and does not prevent future generations from inheriting the condition. For example, not long ago, a patient with familial hypercholesterolemia was injected with cells—taken from her own liver—that had been supplied in the laboratory with a normal gene she lacked. The gene is responsible for directing the production of a receptor protein that acts as a sponge for harmful cholesterol in the body. Researchers hope that the genetically altered cells will multiply in her liver and result in a dramatic lowering of cholesterol levels. Similarly, in cystic fibrosis, scientists have devised a way to deliver the normal gene for a protein that controls salt balance in the body. (In people with cystic fibrosis, the abnormal gene causes the build-up of thick mucus in the lungs.) Researchers have packaged this gene in a specially treated cold virus delivered through a patient's airways. In a manner similar to the previous example, they are hoping that the normal gene will replicate in just enough airway tissue to prevent mucus build-up and reduce symptoms.

Although gene therapy may still be in the experimental stages, other treatments for genetic conditions are already reporting successes. For example, in some people with type I Gaucher disease, intravenous replacement of the missing enzyme, glucocerebrosidase, has resulted in a significant lowering of fatty deposits stored in the liver. Enzyme replacement also results in a reduction of the size of the liver and spleen, sometimes greatly enlarged in this disease. There is still more to be learned about how much enzyme should be given and how long treatment should go on. Nevertheless, it is not likely that enzyme replacement therapy will be tried in other inherited metabolic disorders. Other therapies, such as bone marrow or organ transplantation, can be life-saving in certain genetic conditions.

Some genetic disorders can even be treated in utero. For example, congenital adrenal hyperplasia (CAH), an autosomal recessive condition resulting in masculinization of the external genitalia of female fetuses during gestation, can be treated successfully by giving oral corticosteroids to the mother during pregnancy. This preventive treatment decreases the need for surgery on the infant after birth. Women with phenylketonuria (PKU) who were treated successfully with dietary restriction of phenylalanine during infancy and childhood to prevent mental retardation still have a high incidence of mental retardation and other birth defects in their own newborns, who are not affected by PKU. However, continuing restriction of phenylalanine in the diets of these women before and during pregnancy to lower fetal exposure to phenylalanine can actually reduce the frequency of these problems.

Other treatments hold out the promise of primary prevention of some genetic conditions. A prime example is the use of folic acid (one of the eight B vitamins) before conception and very early in pregnancy to prevent neural tube defects such as meningomyelocele and anencephaly. Prior studies showed that folic acid substantially lowers the risk of neural tube defects recurring in a family where one child has already been born with such a defect. In a recent controlled study of the use of a vitamin supplement containing folic acid compared with a trace element supplement taken before conception and early in pregnancy, folic acid dramatically reduced the incidence of these defects in families with no prior history. As a result of these and other studies, the U.S. government is actively considering whether to fortify flour and other foods with folic acid. The current recommendation is that all women during childbearing years take a daily supplement containing at least the recommended allowance of 0.4 mg of folic acid per day, in addition to the folic acid contained in leafy green vegetables, dried beans, liver, and some citrus fruits. For women who have already had a child with a neural tube defect, higher amounts of folic acid are recommended when considering a pregnancy. See your doctor for advice.

the way for even more difficult choices, such as whether to undergo prenatal testing and whether to continue a pregnancy with an affected fetus. Another difficult choice may be deciding whether to be tested for certain genetic conditions before they are symptomatic, especially if the outcome of the disorder may be severe or fatal.

Deciding For or Against Prenatal Testing

For some women, especially those from certain religious or cultural backgrounds, accepting prenatal testing may suggest the possibility of abortion. Under these circumstances, some women and their partners may decline prenatal testing and simply accept whatever risks are likely. Women who decline prenatal testing, for whatever reason, may still worry about the outcome of the pregnancy and will benefit from the support of family members and the genetic counselor while they wait.

For many other women, however, the choice is not so simple: They may choose prenatal testing and then be faced with deciding whether or not to continue the pregnancy based on the information revealed by the tests. More often than not, results are normal and they experience relief after learning that the condition tested for is not likely to occur.

A decade ago, prenatal tests such as amniocentesis offered little hope for treatment of a genetic condition in utero or shortly after birth. Increasingly, prenatal testing can diagnose conditions that are treatable and, in some cases, even curable. The science of genetics is moving so rapidly that gene therapy and other treatments for many genetic conditions are likely to be available within the next few years, making abortion only one of a range of available options.

Even when genetic conditions diagnosed prenatally cannot be treated, parents often gain valuable time to prepare themselves emotionally and practically for the birth of a child with special needs. Prenatal diagnosis may also provide information that can alter the management of the rest of the pregnancy, the mode of delivery, and the care of the baby in the first few days of life.

Deciding Whether to End a Pregnancy

When prenatal diagnosis reveals an abnormality in the fetus, both parents experience feelings of grief for the loss of the healthy baby they had hoped for. While some couples may have the support of their families during this crisis, others may feel distanced from family members who may have their own feelings about the abnormal fetus, as well as about a possible abortion. The couple may even decide to keep the news from family members and friends. This tends to further isolate the parents who may then rely on the obstetrician or nurse-midwife, the genetic counselor, and/or a member of the clergy for emotional support while they move toward a decision about the pregnancy.

It is important to recognize that deciding to end a pregnancy after prenatal diagnosis of a serious fetal anomaly or genetic condition can be agonizing for parents. For one thing, having conceived a child with a serious health problem can deal a severe blow to any parent's sense of self-esteem, especially if one parent feels responsible for having caused the birth defect by transmitting the gene causing the problem. The couple may not even agree between themselves on whether to end the pregnancy. Moreover, a decision to abort, while sometimes in conflict with the parents' moral values or religious beliefs, may be influenced by the wish to spare the family the heartbreak or the expense of raising a child with a serious genetic disease or birth defect. This can engender further guilt. Most difficult of all is the fact that for many couples, this pregnancy has been planned and its potential loss represents the loss of a desired child.

Willingness to abort an affected fetus seems to vary with the perceived seriousness of the problem. Parents may need to gather information on treatment and prognosis of the condition and to meet a child or family with this condition to help them arrive at a decision. Several studies have shown that more women would consider aborting a fetus with severe mental retardation, while fewer would abort for a serious physical disability. Other studies show that when parents already have a child with the disorder, they are less likely to decide to abort an affected fetus.

It is also difficult to decide not to end the pregnancy. Some women may not believe the results of prenatal diagnosis, may fear the abortion procedure itself, or may be opposed to abortion altogether. Continued support from the medical team and the availability of information and support groups can help women and their partners to prepare for the delivery and the care of their infant after birth.

Women and their partners who must make these decisions need the kind of supportive, nondirective guidance that genetic counseling can provide. This kind of supportive approach should begin at the first meeting and well before the diagnosis is made known to the parents. One recent study from the University of Rochester Genetic Counseling Center encouraged women participants to describe their experiences and needs and to allow these descriptions to be recorded on tape. Most of the women stressed the need for a counselor to be present with the couple when they received the news, to provide both emotional support and information to help them begin to deal with the reality and urgency of the situation. Even those women who were not opposed to abortion per se required a great deal of time to make what for some may have been the most difficult decision of their lives.

Once the decision for or against abortion has been made, the Rochester study found, women and their partners who worked with supportive counselors, such as genetics professionals, members of the clergy, or social workers, needed to continue that relationship through the delivery or termination and beyond. In the case of a second trimester abortion, this support was particularly crucial. Some of the women reported experiencing difficulty dealing with hospital personnel whom they perceived as critical of their decision. Yet, while many women initially experienced ambivalence and loss after ending the pregnancy, with time most felt they had made the correct choice. Many are eased through this period of adjustment by continued contact with the counselor and by participation in pregnancy loss support groups. These groups help women and their partners come to terms with their loss and look toward the future, hopefully to the birth of a healthy baby.

For women who choose to deliver a child known by prenatal testing to have a genetic condition or birth defect, groups made up of parents dealing with a similar problem can provide invaluable emotional support and enable the sharing of coping strategies. While not all parents are ready to join a support group, those who do join report experiencing the relief of expressing feelings they could not share with family members and friends. They also experience the added benefit of being able to listen with empathy and provide practical help to others confronting the same diagnosis. Many are also active in raising funds for research and raising awareness through public and professional education campaigns. There are more than 150 support organizations for specific genetic diseases and birth defects;

names and addresses can be obtained by contacting the Alliance of Genetic Support Groups or one of the other organizations listed at the end of this chapter.

Deciding Whether to Be Tested for Genetic Conditions Before They Are Symptomatic

Genetic tests that can predict whether we will develop certain diseases in adulthood are quite different from prenatal tests because they forecast our own genetic futures and those of our relatives, sometimes without the ameliorating effect of available treatment or cure. Choosing to be tested for Huntington's disease, for example, an uncommon but fatal degenerative neurological disease inherited in an autosomal dominant pattern, means the person being tested has to choose between profound relief if the gene is not found and knowledge of eventual decline and death from the disease if it is found. This is not a choice easily made, because the burden of knowing may be very great and may cause considerable psychological distress in those who receive an unfavorable report. Huntington's disease appears in middle age, often after families have been formed. Any child of a person with the gene is at a 50 percent risk of inheriting it. To date, few families where the Huntington's gene appears have taken advantage of presymptomatic testing. Nevertheless, a recent Canadian study found that when a group of participants at risk for Huntington's disease was counseled, both before and after testing, just getting a result—either favorable or unfavorable—gave them some relief from the agony of uncertainty and increased their psychological well-being. Another choice faces families affected by diseases such as adult polycystic kidney disease or familial hypercholesterolemia, in which presymptomatic diagnosis allows for close medical follow-up and early treatment. With the availability of new DNA tests for single-gene disorders, more individuals and families will be asked to choose whether to get tested. Although it is hard to know how many will decide that knowing is better than not knowing, the results of these tests can often lead to preventive strategies to reduce the effects of the disease and to prolong healthy life.

LOOKING TO THE FUTURE: ETHICAL ISSUES IN GENETICS

As new discoveries in genetics continue to stimulate hopes for the future treatment and prevention of a host of hereditary disorders, they also raise troubling questions about who should have access to genetic information about individuals who are tested for those disorders. The 1992 March of Dimes Birth Defects Foundation study cited earlier in this chapter found that 57 percent of the 1,000 Americans polled thought that others besides the person tested had a right to know whether a genetic defect had been found. Of these, 58 percent said insurers had a right to the information and 33 percent thought employers should also have the information.

The results of this survey have troubled experts in medical ethics because they seem inconsistent with experience. Two decades ago the availability of a hemoglobin test for sickle cell was followed by widespread misuse of the information—by employers, the insurance industry, and the military—to the detriment of people with the disease as well as carriers of sickle cell trait, most of whom were African-Americans. More recently, the experience with AIDS has shown that the potential for abuse of information made available through testing is still with us: Many Americans have had their coverage reduced, their claims denied, or their policies eliminated altogether when insurers learned of their HIV status. The situation is similar for millions more Americans with other chronic conditions, and a number of cases of discrimination based solely on genetic makeup have already been reported. In the workplace, despite the recent enactment of the Americans with Disabilities Act, there is concern about whether companies will begin to use genetic testing as a way to avoid hiring employees with the potential for costly hereditary illnesses. Although laws have been enacted in a number of states barring discrimination based on the results of genetic tests, many of these laws apply only to carriers of specific conditions, such as sickle cell disease, Tay-Sachs disease, or cystic fibrosis. Several states have already shown interest in drafting legislation to offer wide protection to Americans who choose genetic testing.

WHERE TO FIND HELP

Alliance of Genetic Support Groups
35 Wisconsin Circle, Suite 440
Chevy Chase, MD 20815
800-336-GENE or 301-652-5553

March of Dimes Birth Defects Foundation
1275 Mamaroneck Avenue
White Plains, NY 10605
914-428-7100

Metabolic Information Network
P. O. Box 670847
Dallas, TX 75367-08547
214-696-2188 or 945-2188

National Center for Education in Maternal & Child
  Health
2000 15th Street North, Suite 701
Arlington, VA 22201-2617
703-524-7802

National Organization of Rare Disorders (NORD)
P. O. Box 8923
New Fairfield, CT 06812-1783
203-746-6518 or 800-999-NORD

National Society of Genetic Counselors
233 Canterbury Drive
Wallingford, PA 19086
215-872-7608

The availability of DNA tests to identify carriers of common diseases such as cystic fibrosis and their potential use in population screening poses another kind of concern. In an economy characterized by shrinking resources for social welfare, will pressure be applied to families at risk for an inherited disease to undergo prenatal testing and selective abortion should the fetus be affected? We already know that some couples may consider ending a pregnancy after an abnormal prenatal test not because they do not want the child, but because of concern that the societal supports for raising such a child—adequate schooling, health insurance, future employment opportunities—may not be available to them.

Underlying the solutions to these and other ethical concerns is the need for acceptance of the idea of genetic variability, the notion that each of us has among our estimated 100,000 genes a certain number that predispose us to one condition or another. But our genes are not necessarily our destiny: Those of us who are born with certain defects or develop certain conditions may be only mildly affected; those severely affected may lead exemplary lives, accomplish much, and may ultimately benefit from improved treatments. In the end, the considerable advances in genetics we are witnessing may lead us to an appreciation of the contributions made by all of us—regardless of the genes we carry—to the variety of the human experience.

CHAPTER 15

The Reproductive System

Katherine A. O'Hanlan, M.D., F.A.C.O.G., F.A.C.S., and Jean L. Fourcroy, M.D., PH.D.

The organs that form the reproductive system allow humans to reproduce. Men and women have different reproductive systems that work in unison to create new life. If something goes awry with the components of the female or male reproductive system, it can affect not only the ability to have children but may also cause serious disorders warranting early detection and treatment.

STRUCTURE AND FUNCTION

The reproductive and genital organs of a fetus form during the fourth week of pregnancy. At that time, nerve, blood vessel, and tissue bundles form in patterns that distinguish males from females when they are fully developed. Development of these organs in the fetus ends during the first trimester. (See Fig. 15.1).

Many of the anatomic structures in one sex correspond to those in the other. For instance, The female clitoris and the male penis are derived from the same structures, contain the same number of nerves, and are the site of intense sensitivity during sexual activity.

A child is born with male or female reproductive organs, but these organs remain undeveloped until puberty. Then a spurt of hormones causes rapid growth and development of reproductive organs, changing body structure and function and making a person capable of reproduction.

Females usually mature sexually between the ages of 10 and 14, when the ovaries begin producing the hormone estrogen. This causes the hips to widen, breasts to develop, and body hair to grow. It also triggers menstruation, the monthly cycle of bleeding that is a key part of a woman's fertility. Women continue to produce estrogen and menstruate until about age 50. The amount of estrogen produced by her ovaries slowly decreases until a woman reaches menopause, when her periods stop and she is no longer able to become pregnant naturally.

Males develop sexually a little later than females. At puberty, the hormone testosterone causes an increase in height, muscle development, and the growth of the sex organs, which then produce sperm. Boys may have nocturnal emissions of semen, or wet dreams, at puberty. Around age 50, the production of

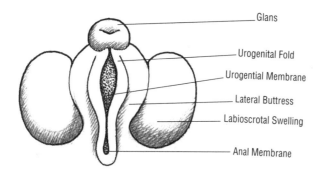

Figure 15.1 Fetal Genitalia
The fetus's external genitalia develop during early pregnancy. Both male and female genitalia arise from the same structure (top), which has begun to form by about 4-7 weeks of gestation. The *glans* gives rise to either the male glans of the penis (bottom left) or the female clitoris (bottom right). The *urogenital membrane* will eventually develop into the urethra, and the *labioscrotal swelling* will form either the male scrotum or the female labia

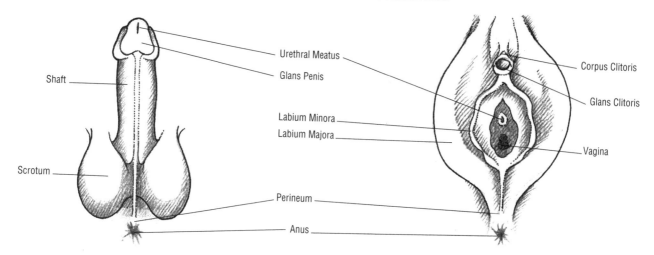

testosterone in men may decrease. Although lowered levels of testosterone do not seem to affect the ability to have an erection, it may result in a decrease in sexual desire.

The Female Reproductive System

A woman's external genital area is called the vulva. It is made up of the labia minora—the inner lips enclosing the opening to the vagina—and the labia majora—the outer, hair-bearing lips surrounding the opening of the vagina and the urethra, the opening to the bladder. The clitoris is a small bud-shaped organ, located just above the urethra. It is the most sensitive area of the external female genitals. Bartholin's glands are located on either side of the vaginal opening.

The vagina is a muscular tube leading from the external genital organs to the uterus. The opening of the uterus, the cervix, projects into the upper end of the vagina. (See Fig. 15.2). It varies in shape and size depending on whether a woman has had children. The cervix can be felt by inserting a finger into the vagina.

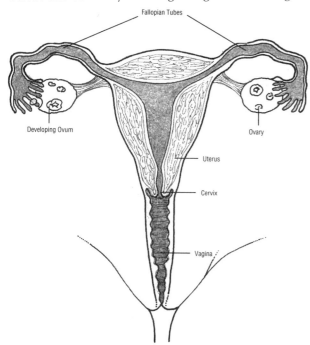

Figure 15.2 Female Reproductive System
A woman's reproductive organs are located in the lower abdomen. Each month, an egg released from an *ovary* moves through a *fallopian tube* to the *uterus*. If an egg is fertilized, it is embedded in the inner wall of the uterus, where it develops into a fetus. The fetus passes through the *cervix* and *vagina* during delivery.

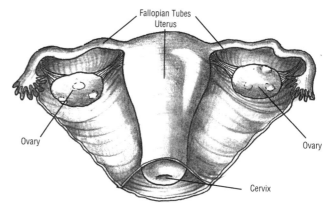

Figure 15.3 The Uterus
The uterus (seen here from the back) is a hollow, muscular organ that varies in size and shape. In women who have not had children, it usually measures about two and a half to a little over three inches long. In women who have had children, it ranges from about three and a half to four inches long.

It cannot be penetrated by a penis, a tampon, or a finger.

The uterus is a hollow, muscular organ, about the size of a pear, in which the fetus grows during pregnancy. (See Fig. 15.3) The lining of the uterus, the endometrium, changes in thickness depending on a woman's menstrual cycle. The fallopian tubes extend from either side of the upper end of the uterus. They are about 4 inches in length and reach outward toward the ovaries. (See Fig. 15.4) The ovaries are the female sex organs that produce eggs and female hormones.

A woman is born with 2 million undeveloped eggs in her ovaries—more than enough to last during her reproductive life. Each month, an egg matures in the

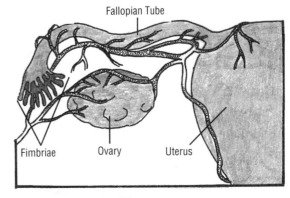

Figure 15.4 The Fallopian Tubes
The fallopian tubes extend outward from either side of the uterus. At the end of each tube, fingerlike projections called *fimbriae* are situated close to the surface of the ovary. During ovulation, the egg released by one of the ovaries enters the tube through the fimbriae.

ovaries and is released into the fallopian tubes. This process is called ovulation. If a man and a woman have sex at that time and the man's sperm unites with the woman's egg, fertilization occurs. The fertilized egg then moves into the woman's uterus where it becomes attached to the endometrium and begins to grow into a fetus. (See Fig. 15.5) If the egg is not fertilized, it dissolves in her body. The endometrium, which thickens before ovulation to prepare for the fertilized egg, begins to break down and menstruation, or bleeding occurs. The hormones estrogen and progesterone, produced in the ovaries, regulate the menstrual cycle (see "Hormones of the Reproductive System").

Estrogen is secreted by the ovaries throughout a woman's reproductive years, affecting all the cells of the body. Special estrogen receptors are located in the breasts, the lining of the uterus, the cervix, and the upper vagina. Cells with estrogen receptors grow when estrogen is in the blood, whether it is secreted from the ovaries or taken in pill form. The lining of the uterus has the greatest number of receptors, and it thickens on a monthly basis. Each month, when estrogen levels decline, the lining is broken down and results in a menstrual period.

Progesterone is a hormone secreted by the ovaries after ovulation. It causes the uterine lining cells to stop growing and to simply prepare to nourish an egg should it be fertilized and become implanted in the uterus. At menopause, when ovulation ceases, no more progesterone can be made by the ovaries.

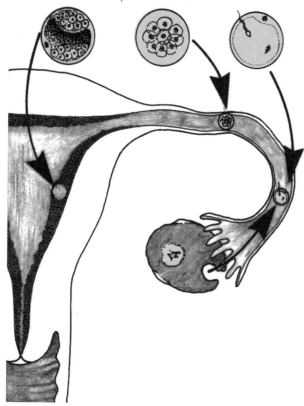

HORMONES OF THE REPRODUCTIVE SYSTEM

The reproductive systems of both women and men are regulated by hormones produced by glands that are part of the endocrine system. At the onset of puberty, the hypothalamus gland sends a signal to the pituitary gland to secrete hormones that cause the development of sexual organs.

The hypothalamus cells in the brain secrete peptides to signal the pituitary. This area regulates eating, drinking, sleeping, waking, body temperature, chemical balances, heart rate, hormones, sex, and emotions.

The pituitary, a small, gray, rounded gland attached to the base of the brain, is an endocrine gland secreting a number of hormones. The pituitary is often referred to as the master gland of the body.

Gonads (sex glands) are the testes in the male and the ovaries in the female. These glands produce the male and female hormones that regulate reproduction:

- Estrogen is the female hormone produced by the ovaries that is responsible for ovulation.

- Progesterone is a female hormone produced by the ovaries after ovulation. It triggers the menstrual period. It prepares the uterine lining for the fertilized egg.

- Testosterone is the gonadal steroid secreted by the male. After puberty, the normal male secretes testosterone daily. It is responsible for the growth of the prostate and the penis during puberty.

The menstrual cycle is an average of 28 days, although some women have longer or shorter cycles. Ovulation occurs at around day 14 of the cycle (counting from the first day of the previous menstrual period), and it is at this time that a woman can become pregnant. Once released, the egg remains fertile for up to 48 hours. (See Figure 15.6)

Figure 15.5 Fertilization

The process of fertilization begins with the release of an egg from one of the ovaries. Normally, penetration of an egg by a sperm occurs in the far end of a fallopian tube (A) anywhere from 12 to 24 hours after ovulation. By the time the fertilized egg has reached the near end of the tube (B), it has already begun to divide. Implantation in the wall of the uterus (C) usually occurs 3-4 days after ovulation.

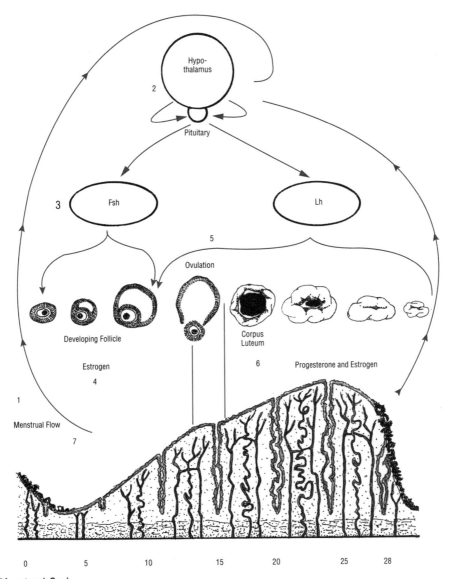

Figure 15.6 The Menstrual Cycle
During the menstrual cycle, an egg is produced, released into a fallopian tube, and eventually, the uterine lining is shed if fertilization does not occur. The average menstrual cycle typically lasts 28 days, but it may vary from 23 to 35 days.

1. The cycle begins on day 1 of menstruation, when the lining of the uterus (the *endometrium*) is shed as menstrual blood. Menstruation occurs in response to a decline in the hormones estrogen and progesterone, which occurs when an egg is not fertilized.
2. The decrease in estrogen and progesterone causes the *hypothalamus* to send a message to the *pituitary*.
3. The pituitary in turn releases *follicle-stimulating hormone* (FSH). Follicles are the structures inside the ovaries that produce eggs for fertilization. Each month, one follicle will produce the egg for that cycle.
4. FSH continues to be produced during days 1-13 of the menstrual cycle. Under its influence, the developing follicle begins to produce estrogen. This hormone stimulates the endometrium to grow and thicken in preparation for a fertilized egg. At this time, the mucus normally produced by the cervix becomes thin, clear, and watery.
5. As the developing follicle continues to produce estrogen, the hormone triggers the pituitary to release *luteinizing hormone* (LH). LH stimulates the follicle to release an egg into a fallopian tube. This event, called *ovulation*, typically occurs on day 14 of the cycle.
6. After releasing the egg, the follicle begins to change into a structure known as the *corpus luteum*. This structure then begins to produce the hormone progesterone, which causes the lining of the uterus to continue to thicken in preparation for a fertilized egg.
7. If the egg is not fertilized, a sharp drop occurs in the production of estrogen and progesterone. This triggers the shedding of the endometrium, which marks the start of another menstrual cycle.

ANABOLIC STEROIDS

Androgens are male sex hormones, one of which is testosterone. Anabolic steroids are synthetic androgens that have been designed to enhance the growth-promoting effects of androgens. Anabolic steriods are occasionally used, under a doctor's supervision, to treat skeletal and growth disorders and certain types of anemia. Steroids are also used illegally, mainly by athletes who want to quickly build muscle tissue. They have many potentially serious side effects: reduced sperm production, decreased size of the testes, and reduced natural sex hormone production, resulting in a diminished sex drive. Steroids can also lead to liver damage and cardiovascular disease and, if taken in early puberty, result in short stature.

The Male Reproductive System

Like that of females, the reproductive system of males is regulated by hormones, which have an effect through birth, puberty, maturity, and aging (see "Hormones of the Reproductive System"). The male genital organs (testes) produce sperm cells and transport them through a series of ducts to the female reproductive system. (See Fig. 15.7)

Each day a male produces about 50 million sperm, the smallest living cells of the body. When a man ejaculates during sexual intercourse, he releases millions of sperm, but only one joins with a woman's egg to fer-

tilize it. Sperm cells can live up to 5 days inside a woman. If a sperm cell joins with a woman's egg released at ovulation, fertilization occurs and a woman becomes pregnant.

The penis, a rod-shaped organ, also transports urine (see Fig. 15.8). Within the penis is the urethra, which carries the urine from the bladder. The penis also holds many blood vessels, which become engorged with blood during sexual excitement, causing an erection (tumescence).

The testes are two egg-shaped organs contained in a pouch of skin called the scrotum that hangs behind the penis. In each of the testicles there is a tightly packed mass of tubes surrounded by a protective capsule. Leydig cells in the testes produce the hormone testosterone, and the tubes in the testes produce sperm. The production of sperm requires a temperature that is lower than the body's internal temperature. Spermatic cords suspend the testicles within the scrotum and help to maintain the correct temperature for sperm production. When the outside temperature is low, the cords draw the testicles upward, nearer to the warm body.

The epididymis is a cordlike structure beside and behind the testes that transports sperm cells from the testicles to the seminal vesicles. Lying behind the bladder, the seminal vesicles store sperm. The sperm are mingled in a fluid that forms part of the semen that is released during ejaculation.

The vas deferens is a thick muscular tube, which is about 1/4 inch in diameter and about 18 inches long. It assists in the transportation and propulsion of sperm and fluid from the testicle in ejaculation. Vasectomy is a method of male sterilization by blocking or cutting the vas deferens.

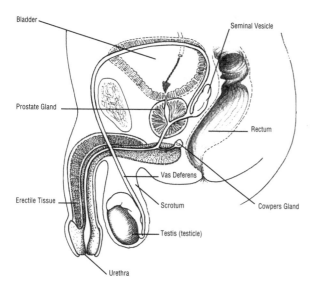

Figure 15.7 The Male Reproductive System
Sperm cells are produced in the *testes*, two roundish organs located within the *scrotum*. To develop normally, sperm cells need a temperature that is slightly lower (about 95°F) than normal body temperature. The scrotum's location outside the warmer body cavity provides the right conditions for sperm production. After being stored in the *epididymis*, a structure lying next to the testes, sperm cells move through the *vas deferens* and enter the *urethra*. There they are bathed in secretions from the *prostate gland* and the *seminal vesicles*, from which semen is formed. With sexual stimulation, secretions from the *bulbourethral glands* help to luricate the inside of the urethra, and the penis becomes erect. During ejaculation, the sperm-containing semen passes through the urethra to the outside of the body. Shown here is a penis with the *foreskin*, a sheath of tisue covering the head (*glans*) of the penis, intact; in many males, the foreskin is removed shortly after birth.

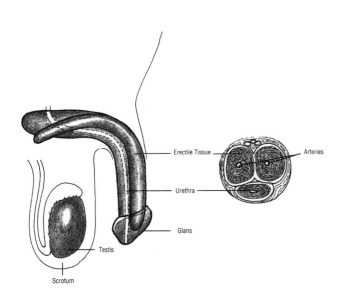

Figure 15.8 Internal Anatomy of the Penis
The shaft of the penis (left) consists of spongy erectile tissue through which two large arteries and the urethra run lengthwise (right). During sexual arousal, blood flow through these arteries increases, and the small veins that normally drain the tissue are temporarily pressed shut. Blood cannot drain, and the penis becomes enlarged and rigid.

The prostate is a walnut-shaped gland located below the bladder, surrounding the urethra. Its main function is to produce a fluid that nourishes sperm and helps transport sperm through the urethra during ejaculation.

Cowper's glands, also known as bulbourethral glands, are two teardrop-shaped structures each the size of a pea. They are situated on either side of the urethra and provide mucus and chemicals during sexual excitement. The mucus washes the urethra in preparation for ejaculation and serves as a lubricant.

Semen is the fluid that is ejaculated during the male sexual act. An ejaculation may contain as many as 120,000,000 sperm (see Fig. 15.9). Semen is milky white fluid containing not only sperm but also secretions from the seminal vesicles, prostate gland, and bulbourethral glands. These fluids combine to create the best possible conditions for the survival and function of the sperm. The mucus furnishes lubrication, but initially makes the sperm somewhat immobile. Within about a half hour after ejaculation, however, the fluid dissolves the mucus and the sperm become highly mobile.

Erection of the penis is provoked by sexual stimulation. Impulses are transmitted from the brain down the spinal cord to the penis by parasympathetic nerves. The messages signal the corpora cavernosa, two rod-shaped bundles of muscle in the penis on either side, to relax and fill with blood. As they fill, the corpora cavernosa expand and press against the veins that would normally drain blood from the penis. The penis becomes firm and erect, allowing penetration into the female vagina during sexual intercourse.

Sensations on the skin of the penis that occur during intercourse stimulate the organ's numerous nerve endings. These impulses are carried back to the brain. The sexual stimulation gradually builds in intensity until it causes a reflex action. Impulses travel down the nerves, passing through the genital organs, and trigger ejaculation, the rhythmic contractions of the smooth muscle of the testicles which expel their contents, the semen, into the urethra. The bulbourethral glands discharge additional amounts of mucus at this time. The act of ejaculation, and the feelings of intense pleasure associated with it, are the male orgasm or climax.

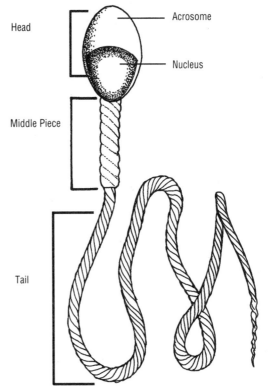

Figure 15.9 Sperm
The head, or *nucleus*, of a sperm cell contains 23 chromosomes. At the tip is the *acrosome*, which contains enzymes that break down barriers surrounding the female ovum. The *middle piece* consists of structures that power cell movement. The rapid movements of the *tail* propel the sperm cell through the female reproductive tract.

KEEPING THE SYSTEM HEALTHY

Understanding and monitoring your own reproductive system is key to keeping it healthy. Health maintenance involves routine self-examinations, regular checkups, prevention of problems, and being alert to signs of problems so they can be treated early. A number of practitioners treat the reproductive system (see "Health Care Practitioners").

HEALTH CARE PRACTITIONERS

Women can receive care for the reproductive system from any of the following health care professionals:

■ Obstetrician-gynecologist: A specialist who has completed 4 years of residency beyond medical school in the field of women's health. This physician may be the woman's primary care doctor or may be consulted for problems relating to the female reproductive system. An obstetrician-gynecologist may receive further training for 2–3 years in a subspecialty: maternal-fetal medicine (high-risk pregnancy and delivery), reproductive endocrinology (hormone and infertility issues), or gynecologic oncology (cancers of the female reproductive organs). Subspecialists are usually located in major medical centers and see patients on referral.

■ Internist: A specialist who has completed at least 3 years of internal medicine training beyond medical school. Some internists do gynecological exams (pelvics and Paps) and some do not.

■ Family physician: A physician who has completed at least 3 years of specialty training in family practice beyond medical school. Family physicians routinely do gynecological exams.

■ Nurse practitioner: A registered nurse who has received additional training and is licensed to perform certain procedures independently.

■ Nurse-midwife: A registered nurse who has additional training in providing obstetrical care to women.

For routine examinations, men can see an internal medicine specialist or a family practitioner. A man having a problem with his prostate or infertility may be referred to a urologist for evaluation.

The reproductive systems of both women and men are vulnerable to sexually transmitted diseases (STDs), such as syphilis, gonorrhea, herpes, chlamydia, human

SEXUALLY TRANSMITTED DISEASES

Diseases that are sexually transmitted (STDs) can affect both women and men. Often there are no symptoms; when they occur, immediate treatment should be obtained. Both sexual partners must be treated to avoid spreading the disease.

To protect against STDs, women and men should limit their sexual partners. Mutually monogamous relationships and using a condom each time they have sex are the best protection. Spermicides can provide additional protection from STDs. Some of the more common STDs include the following:

■ *Chlamydia* is a bacterial infection that can cause urethritis (inflammation of the urethra causing pain, burning, and discharge) in men and pelvic inflammatory disease in women, which can lead to infertility. It is treated with antibiotics.

■ *Gonorrhea* is a bacterial infection that can cause urethritis in men and pelvic inflammatory disease in women. It is treated with antibiotics.

■ *Herpes* is a viral infection that causes painful blisters on the lips or the genitals. When they are present, the virus can be spread to others. There is no cure but symptoms can be treated.

■ *Human papillomavirus* is a viral infection that can cause warts on the external and internal genital area. In women, it can cause abnormal Pap test results and lead to cancer of the cervix. The warts can be removed but there is no real cure for the virus.

■ *Syphilis* is an infection whose first sign is a sore on the genitals that may go away, although the infection does not; it can lead to long-term disability. Syphilis is treated with antibiotics.

■ *Trichomonas* is an infection caused by overgrowth of an organism in the vagina, causing a frothy discharge and itching. It is treated with a drug called metronidazole.

papillomavirus (HPV), and AIDS. To protect against STDs, you should limit your sexual partners and always use a condom during sexual intercourse. A woman having sex with another woman should be careful not to have contact with her partner's genital fluids or with any open sores on her partner's body. (The use of a dental dam or cellophane wrap has been advocated but has not been shown to be as clearly of value as the condom is for heterosexuals.) In men, certain STDs can appear as an inflammation of the urethra or a discharge, but also can occur without symptoms. In women, there can be no symptoms. Both women and men should be alert to the early signs of STDs, get treatment immediately, and avoid spreading the disease to others (see "Sexually Transmitted Diseases").

For Women

Every woman's genitals are shaped individually, with different sizes for inner lips, outer lips, and clitoris. Women of all ages should be familiar with the appearance of their genitals and be aware of what is normal for them. In this way, changes that may be the only signs of certain infections or precancerous conditions can be detected early. Early diagnosis means conditions can be diagnosed and treated before they have advanced to later stages. Small sores, ulcers, raw areas, or pigmented areas can be the first and earliest signs of cancer of the vulva. Use a mirror to inspect your vulva monthly to look for these signs.

Women should protect themselves from unwanted pregnancy by using some method of birth control. Ideally, the birth control method should also protect against infections; a barrier method, such as a condom, is ideal. Of course not all methods are perfect, and failures of contraception do occur. Early diagnosis of a missed period allows your maximum choice in expression of your reproductive desires. If you have had sex without birth control or your birth control has failed, ask your doctor about postcoital, or emergency, contraception.

You should have a pelvic examination and a Pap test annually to detect changes in the cervix that could be early signs of cancer (see "The Pap Test"). (See Fig. 15.10A-B.) Depending on your situation, your doctor

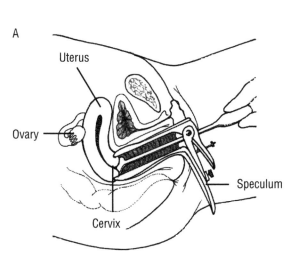

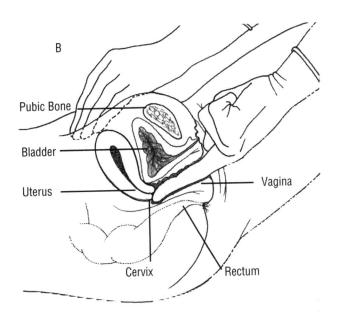

Figure 15.10 Tests
A woman should have a gynecologic exam, including a Pap smear, at least once a year or more if her doctor advises it. The Pap test (A) is performed by inserting an instrument called a *speculum* into the vagina to hold the walls of the vagina apart. A small spatula or brush is then used to collect a sample of cells from the cervix. The cell sample is then smeared onto a glass slide, which is examined under a microscope. A biannual pelvic exam (B) is recommended for every woman on a regular basis. For this exam, the doctor feels the shape, size, and position of the internal reproductive organs by inserting two fingers into the vagina and pressing down on the abdomen with the other hand. Many doctors also perform a rectal exam afterward.

may suggest you have this done more or less often. Any unusual bleeding, pain, or discharge should be brought to the attention of a doctor.

For Men

Recognition and treatment of problems that can arise in the reproductive system as a man ages are essential for a healthy life. Men should have regular checkups to watch for early signs of problems. For example, signs of prostate enlargement include changes or problems with urination such as more frequent urination, a feeling of a need to urinate, and a weak stream of urine. The checkup should include a thorough history and a physical examination. The history should include a family history as well as an occupational and medical history, past genitourinary surgery, or trauma to the reproductive organs. Men should ask their doctors questions regarding any illnesses, changes in sex drive, or drugs that may interfere with reproductive health.

Prostate gland enlargement does not increase the risk of prostate cancer, but cancer could be present at the same time or develop later. Many older men have some symptoms of prostate enlargement. All men over age 50 should have digital rectal examinations once a year to detect prostate cancer. The digital rectal exam involves the insertion of a finger into the rectum to feel the prostate. This important part of total health care can detect enlargement, abnormal texture, or hard areas of the prostate that could be signs of cancer.

Men of all ages should perform testicular self-examination monthly to detect problems that could be a sign of cancer of the testes. It only takes a few minutes and can be done easily and painlessly, preferably after a warm bath or shower or in a warm room when the scrotum is relaxed. To perform the exam, roll each

THE PAP TEST

The Pap test was named after Dr. George Papanicolaou, the physician who developed it. A Pap test can detect changes in the cells on the cervix that could be early signs of cancer. For the test, a women lies on an examining table with her feet in stirrups. An instrument called a speculum is inserted into her vagina to hold it open. With a small brush or scraper, a sample of cells is removed from the cervix and placed on a glass slide so it can be studied under a microscope.

If menstruation starts and is heavy at the time of an appointment, the appointment should be rescheduled. Also, a woman should not douche before the test.

Test results are reported in categories according to the Bethesda system. A negative result means that there are no abnormal cells present in the sample of cells. A positive result means that some abnormal cells are present and may require further testing. As with any test, however, the results depend on the quality of the lab work and the person evaluating the cells.

The Pap test has greatly reduced the number of deaths from cancer of the cervix, and is used to prevent cervical cancer. The test should be performed annually, with a pelvic exam, for women who have been sexually active or who have reached the age of 18. If results are normal for three consecutive years, the woman is in a monogamous relationship or is celibate, and has no risk factors such as infection with human papillomavirus or smoking, she may then have a Pap test every three years. Many physicians feel that a yearly Pap test will better detect abnormal cells that can develop into cancer.

testicle between the thumbs and forefingers of both hands. Any hard lumps or nodules should be brought to the attention of a physician.

SYMPTOMS

Any signs or symptoms of problems in the reproductive system warrant medical attention. In women, problems that can signal a disorder include abnormal bleeding or discharge, pain, or a change in the appearance of the genital organs. In men, changes in their urination or pain can signal prostate enlargement or cancer. In both women and men, any unusual lump or growth that can be felt or seen should receive medical attention.

In Women

In young women, any irregular bleeding may be linked to problems with the hormones secreted by the ovaries. In older women, changes in their menstrual periods could signal menopause. Some women may have irregular, unpredictable, and sometimes heavy bleeding during menopause. They have a slightly higher chance of developing precancerous or cancerous changes of the endometrium and should be monitored by a physician. An endometrial biopsy can determine whether precancerous changes are taking place. In this technique, a sample of the tissue lining the uterus is obtained and studied. After menopause, when a woman has stopped having menstrual periods for 12 months, any bleeding should be evaluated.

It is normal for women to have a clear vaginal discharge. This discharge cleans the vagina, maintains its normal state, and keeps it free of organisms. A discharge that is white or yellow, thick or frothy, or has an odor could be a sign of an infection. Itching also may occur. These symptoms could signal a major or minor problem; have them checked so the cause can be identified and treated.

Pain in the pelvic area can occur for many reasons, although it is usually due to either a cramping of the uterus or conditions affecting the ovaries. Pain in the pelvic region also can be related to any of the anatomic structures in this area, including the ureters, bladder, and rectum. If the pain is sudden, severe, and long lasting, or interferes with daily activities, consult your physician.

A pain in your right or left side can be a sign of ovulation. This pain, called *mittelschmerz* (literally, middle pain), is caused by the release of the egg. It may be accompanied by a clear vaginal discharge and increased sex drive. On rare occasions, there may be slight bleeding.

In Men

Certain symptoms can signal problems with the prostate in men. Many older men have enlarged prostate glands, but this condition does not lead to cancer. Prostate cancer is common in older men, however, so it should be considered when symptoms such as the following are present:

- Hesitant, interrupted, or weak stream of urination
- A sense of urgency, leaking, or dribbling of urine
- More frequent need to urinate, especially at night
- Difficulty starting or holding back urination
- Inability to urinate
- Weak flow of urine
- Painful urination or bloody urine
- Painful ejaculation
- Pain in the lower back, hips, upper thighs

Any of these symptoms requires further evaluation by a primary care physician or, if necessary, a urologist.

CONDITIONS AND DISORDERS IN WOMEN

The female reproductive system is a fairly complicated mechanism that sustains the monthly cycles that are part of fertility as well as pregnancy and childbirth. Because of the complexity of the reproductive organs and the functions needed to maintain it, some normal conditions as well as disorders may require regular medical attention.

BIRTH CONTROL

Many methods of birth control, or contraception, are available that have a very high degree of safety and effectiveness (see "Contraceptive Failure Rates"). These methods allow you to choose if and when you wish to have children and to plan your family just as you plan other aspects of your life. Without such methods, up to 85 percent of sexually active women using no contraception would be expected to become pregnant in a year. Some methods, such as condoms and spermicides, also provide protection against STDs and cancer of the cervix. All of them allow you control over your reproduction (see "Women's Choice About Contraception").

Hormonal Methods

Pregnancy can be prevented by using hormones to regulate fertility. The hormone estrogen prevents ovulation, the release of an egg. The hormone progesterone blocks the release of the egg during ovulation, although not as well as estrogen, and creates an environment in the uterine lining that makes pregnancy unlikely. These hormones may be used alone or in combination, depending on the technique.

Hormones are used for postcoital, or emergency, contraception, also known as the morning after pill. A doctor or family planning clinic can prescribe the pill, which is usually a combination of birth control pills taken at specific intervals. This technique can be used if a woman has had unprotected intercourse because her method failed or she was sexually assaulted or for any number of reasons. The morning after pill must be administered within hours of intercourse to be effective.

Oral Contraceptives

Birth control pills, or oral contraceptives, are very effective when used properly. There are two types of birth control pills: combination pills, containing the

ABORTION

The medical term for termination of a pregnancy by any cause is *abortion*. The term *spontaneous abortion* describes a natural end of the pregnancy, also called a miscarriage, before the fetus is able to live outside the uterus (about the first 6 months of pregnancy). If a spontaneous abortion is incomplete—if some tissue is retained in the uterus—a medical procedure may be required to be sure the uterus has been emptied and there is no risk of infection. An *elective abortion* refers to the surgical or medical termination of a pregnancy. When a woman is ill and cannot withstand the strain of the pregnancy, termination may be called therapeutic abortion.

With any form of abortion, the initial step is confirming the pregnancy. Most commercially available pregnancy tests inform you of your pregnancy status at the time of the first missed menstrual period. Although this usually occurs about 2 weeks after conception, some women have a lighter period and are unaware they are pregnant until they miss the next period, approximately 6 weeks after the date of conception.

Elective abortions can be performed in a physician's office as early as 1–2 weeks after a missed menstrual period. Using the menstrual extraction technique, the contents of the uterus are removed with a syringe. After 7 weeks of pregnancy, doctors use a procedure called vacuum curettage, the most common method of abortion in the United States. Beyond 13 weeks of pregnancy, more involved procedures are required.

Before the procedure, a woman has her blood type checked and a pregnancy test repeated. She is counseled by health care workers about the procedure and given a chance to ask questions. Consent forms must be signed by the patient and may be required from others, depending on state law. In most cases, the patient is also examined to confirm the length of the pregnancy so the physician can determine the best way to perform the procedure.

Vacuum curettage is performed with a local anesthetic, injected into and around the cervix. The cervix is then dilated, or opened, using a series of gradually larger metal rods or a synthetic material that swells. The contents of the uterus are then removed with a suction device. As the uterus contracts to its previous size, some cramping may result. The amount of blood lost is usually small. In most clinics, only about 1 percent of women have complications, such as infection, perforation of the uterus, or bleeding.

Abortions in later stages have a higher risk of complications and should be performed in a hospital or a specialized clinic. They can be done with suction or by administering agents that bring on labor. In some extreme cases, surgery may be required.

A drug called mifepristone can induce abortion; it is also known as the French pill, or RU–486 and is not currently available in this country. Efforts are ongoing to have this drug available so it can be offered as a safer, nonsurgical approach to abortion.

In the days when abortions were outlawed, women sought abortions from unlicensed providers who frequently did not use sterile techniques and who did not monitor women for complications. As a result, women developed advanced infections that spread from the uterus to the bloodstream and the abdominal cavity. Such infections could result in permanent sterility or death. Today, abortions are extremely safe when performed in a proper medical setting by a licensed practitioner. An abortion has no effect on a woman's ability to have children in the future.

CONTRACEPTIVE FAILURE RATES*

Method	Percentage of Average Use†
Contraceptive implants	0.05%
Vasectomy	0.2
Contraceptive injections	0.4
Tubal sterilization	0.5
IUD	4.0
Pill	6.0
Condom (male)‡	16.0
Cervical cap	18.0
Diaphragm	18.0
Periodic abstinence	19.0
Sponge	24.0
Withdrawal	24.0
Condom (female)‡	26.0
Spermicides	30.0
No method (chance)	85.0

* The failure rate is the estimated percentage of all women using the method who will have an unplanned pregnancy in the first year of use.

†Using a method consistently and correctly—the right way, all the time—makes birth control more effective than these rates show.

‡These methods are most effective against sexually transmitted diseases.

WOMEN'S CHOICES ABOUT CONTRACEPTION

A woman's choice about which method of birth control to use is largely affected by whether she wishes to have children in the future. Women who do wish to have children choose oral contraceptives most often (49 percent), whereas those who do not plan to have children or who have completed their families choose sterilization (61 percent). About 10 percent of women do not use any form of birth control. These women account for approximately 53 percent of all unintended pregnancies in the United States, half of which end in abortion. Women who are sexually active and not planning to become pregnant should exercise their options of birth control to avoid unintended pregnancy.

Among all women, these are the percentages of women who select specific methods:

Oral contraceptives	27.7%
Tubal sterilization	24.8
Condom	13.1
Periodic abstinence	2.1
IUD	1.8
Spermicides	1.7
Sponge	1

hormones estrogen and progestin, and mini-pills containing only progestin. Progestin is a synthetic version of the natural female hormone progesterone. Women use the combination pills most often; those women who cannot take estrogen use the mini-pill.

To be effective, the pill must be taken regularly. Some pills are taken daily during a 28-day cycle, whereas others are taken for 21 days, with no pills taken for 7 days before the next pack is started. Missing one pill can result in pregnancy. Birth control pills are generally safe for women in good health who do not smoke. There is no reason to have rest periods from oral contraceptives after they are taken for a number of years.

Aside from preventing pregnancy, birth control pills have other benefits. Oral contraceptives protect against cancer of the ovary and the endometrium. The longer a woman takes the pill, the greater the protective effect. Women who take the pill have a lower risk of ovarian cysts, ovarian and endometrial cancer, uterine fibroids,

noncancerous breast disease, and ectopic pregnancies. They also tend to have more regular periods with less monthly flow and fewer premenstrual symptoms. The estrogen in oral contraceptives also appears to increase bone density, reducing the risk of bone loss that occurs during menopause.

On the other hand, oral contraceptives have been linked to certain types of cardiovascular disease and cancer of the breast. These effects were observed when higher dose formulations were in use and other factors linked to disease, such as smoking, were not taken into consideration. In general, today's low-dose pills do not seem to pose the same risk. There is, however, an increased risk of thromboembolism (blood clots) in women who smoke and take the pill. Although one study has shown a link between breast cancer and oral contraceptives, others have not been able to confirm that finding.

Oral contraceptives can be used by most healthy women. Do not take birth control pills, however, if any of the following factors apply to you:

- Age over 35 and smoke
- History of vascular disease (including stroke and thromboembolism)
- Uncontrolled high blood pressure, diabetes with vascular disease, high cholesterol
- Active liver disease
- Cancer of the endometrium or breast

Women over age 35 who do not smoke can continue to take a low-dose pill with safety until menopause. Some women may develop bloating, spotting, severe mood swings, or breast tenderness. These problems, or a tendency toward them, require that the woman and her physician work together to find the right formula for her.

Implants

Implants involve a new technique of inserting small plastic tubes containing a progestin or levonorgestrel just under the skin of the arm (see Fig. 15.11). After an injection of local anesthetic to numb the area, the small tubes are imbedded under the skin in the upper arm during an office visit. The hormone is slowly released over a 5-year period. This method of contraception is very effective, but it can cause irregular bleeding and spotting. Other side effects include weight gain, head-

ache, acne, depression, abnormal hair growth, anxiety, and ovarian cysts. The implants need to be surgically removed, and there have been reports that this sometimes can be difficult.

Injections

The injection technique involves injecting a long-acting type of progesterone into the body every 3 months; the failure rate is low. The side effects with this technique include abdominal discomfort, nervousness, dizziness, decreased sex drive, depression, and acne. Some women have weight gain. This method can disrupt menstrual cycles and cause episodes of bleeding and spotting.

Barrier Methods

Some, but not all, barrier methods provide protection against STDs. They can be used in combination to offer extra protection against pregnancy and STDs.

Diaphragm

The diaphragm is a reusable round rubber disk with a flexible rim that fits inside the vagina to cover the cervix (see Fig. 15.12). It should be coated with a spermicide before it is inserted into the vagina. The success of the diaphragm depends partly on spermicidal cream

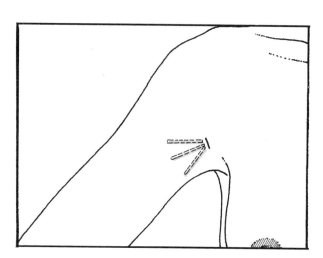

Figure 15.11 Implants
One of the newer methods of birth control is hormonal implants. These small, matchstick-sized tubes are inserted just beneath the surface of the skin, usually on the inner part of a woman's upper arm. The implants contain progestin, a synthetic form of the hormone progesterone, which is slowly released into the bloodstream to prevent pregnancy. Insertion can be done during an office visit, and the implants are effective for up to 5 years.

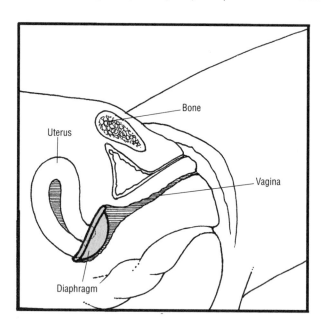

Figure 15.12 Diaphragm
One of the so-called barrier methods of contraception is the diaphragm, a rubber, dome-shaped device that is used with spermicide. It is inserted into the vagina to hold the spermicide in place against the cervix. The flexible rim of the diaphragm helps to hold it in place behind the pubic bone.

or jelly and partly on its function as a barrier to block entry of the sperm into the cervix. It must be fitted to the shape of the woman's vagina by a doctor or nurse.

The diaphragm should be inserted 1 hour before intercourse and should be left in place at least 6 hours after having sex. If intercourse is repeated, additional spermicide should be inserted into the vagina. When irritation occurs, it may be due to either the rubber or the spermicide. Changing brands of spermicide may solve this problem.

Cervical Cap

The cervical cap is similar to the diaphragm, although it is smaller. Fitting snugly over the cervix, it is held in place by suction (see Fig. 15.13). The cervical cap comes in four sizes to fit a woman's cervix. The cervical cap can be difficult to insert, and it doesn't fit all women. It can be left in a longer time than a diaphragm and can be used to contain menstrual fluid.

Condom

Condoms, for use by both men and women, are all available without prescription. They offer good protection against STDs, including the HIV infection that causes AIDS, as well as pregnancy when used properly. Condoms protect against both viral and bacterial infections, and their use lowers the risk of cancer of the cervix. With new sexual partners of unknown risk for STD, use condoms regardless of other contraceptive methods you may be using. Condoms are disposable. Use one time only and then discard.

The male condom is a sheath that fits over the erect penis and collects the sperm when a man ejaculates. Most condoms are made of latex rubber, although they can be made of animal intestines. Only latex rubber condoms protect against disease, however. Some condoms contain a spermicide (e.g., nonoynol) that immobilizes and kills the sperm, providing additional contraception. You can get extra protection by using a foam that contains spermicide, along with the condom.

The *male condom* should be applied just before intercourse, when the man's penis is erect, before he touches the sexual partner's genitals. When the penis is being withdrawn, the condom should always be held at the base so that there is less risk of spillage, leakage, or tears (see Fig. 15.14 A and B). Effectiveness is reduced if the condom tears during intercourse. If a leak or tear occurs, use a spermicidal jelly or foam as soon as possible.

The *female condom* is made of polyurethane, a thin but strong material that resists tearing during use. It consists of two flexible rings connected by a loose-fitting sheath. One of the rings is used to insert the condom and hold it inside the vagina. The other ring remains outside and covers the woman's labia and the

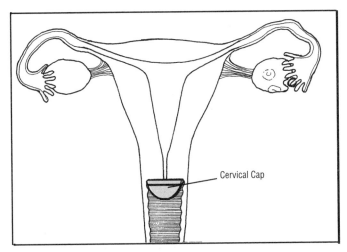

Figure 15.13 Cervical Cap
Similar to the diaphragm, the cervical cap is a small, cup-shaped, rubber device. Also used with spermicide, it is inserted into the vagina and pushed onto the cervix, where it is held in place by suction. The cap is somewhat more difficult to learn to place correctly than the diaphragm, but many women like it because it can be left in place longer and, for some, may be more comfortable.

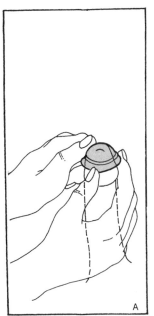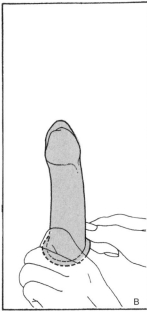

Figure 15.14 Male Condom
The male condom is one of the most widely used forms of contraception. It also offers protection against sexually transmitted diseases, including HIV, the virus that causes AIDS. The rolled-up condom is placed over the man's erect penis (A) and then unrolled downward (B). A small space is left at the tip of the condom to catch the man's semen during ejaculation.

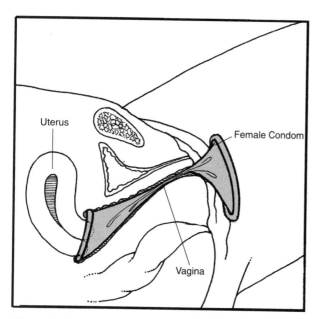

Figure 15.15 Female Condom
The newest form of barrier contraception, the female condom, also offers women protection against sexually transmitted diseases. It consists of a long rubber sheath with a closed ring at one end and a slightly larger, open ring at the other. The closed end is inserted into the vagina and fits over the cervix, like the diaphragm. The open end hangs outside the vagina, so that the interior of the vagina and the cervix are covered.

base of the penis during intercourse. The female condom is prelubricated and lines the vagina after insertion (see Fig. 15.15). It is designed for one-time use only. One advantage of the female condom is that it can be inserted several hours before sex. Its fairly high failure rate is often due to incorrect use. Used properly, the female condom is nearly as effective as other techniques.

Sponge

The sponge is available without a prescription; it is made of polyurethane and contains a spermicide. Before intercourse, the sponge is inserted into the vagina to cover the cervix, forming both a physical shield and chemical barrier to sperm. It should be left in place for at least 6 hours after intercourse. The sponge may be left in place up to 24 hours, and it is effective if intercourse is repeated during that time. As with diaphragms or condoms that contain spermicide, a small percentage of users may experience irritation or allergic reactions.

Intrauterine Devices

There are currently two types of intrauterine devices (IUD) available. One is a plastic device shaped like the letter *T* that is wound with copper, and the other is a device that releases the hormone progesterone. When placed inside the uterus, the IUD causes an inflammatory reaction in the uterine lining that prevents pregnancy.

The IUD device must be put in place by a trained physician or nurse. It is inserted through the cervix into the uterus. Threads hang through the cervix and must be checked monthly after each period to be sure the IUD is still in place (see Fig. 15.16). The IUD containing progesterone should be replaced every year, while the copper-containing IUD can be used for 8 years.

Some women have uncomfortable short-term side effects, including cramping and dizziness at the time of insertion; bleeding, cramps, and backache that may continue for a few days after insertion; spotting between periods; and longer and heavier periods during the first few cycles after insertion. Use of a copper IUD increases the amount of blood lost each month, while use of the hormone IUD decreases it. The device can migrate into the muscular wall of the uterus and sometimes tear it, although this is rare.

The copper-releasing IUD increases the risk of developing pelvic inflammatory disease (PID), which can result in infertility, especially in those at risk of PID. These people are not good candidates for an IUD; they include women with multiple sexual partners, those

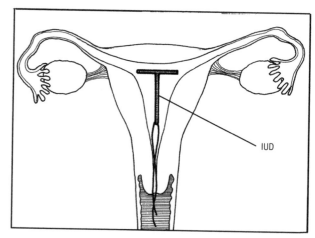

Figure 15.16 IUD
The intrauterine device (IUD) is a small, plastic device that is inserted into the uterus and left in place to prevent pregnancy. The two forms of IUD currently available are a T-shaped device wound with fine copper wire (shown here) and one containing the hormone progesterone.

with a history of PID, and women under 25 years of age who have not had children. An IUD is a good choice for women who have completed their families and are in monogamous sexual relationships.

Periodic Abstinence

Also known as natural family planning or the rhythm method, periodic abstinence relies on close observation of a woman's cycle to detect when ovulation occurs. Women using this method note the temperature increase that occurs just before ovulation and the change in cervical mucus from dry to wet and slippery that occurs around the same time. It takes into account the fact that sperm live an average of 5 days in the uterus and that the lifespan of the egg after ovulation is 1–3 days. In general, a couple should not have sexual intercourse 7 days before and 3 days after ovulation. Couples who use this method should obtain detailed instructions about it and follow the plan carefully. If used perfectly, this method can be very effective. It is less effective than other forms of birth control, however, because of the difficulty in predicting exactly when ovulation will occur.

Sterilization

Men and women who no longer wish to have children may choose to undergo sterilization. The technique for women is known as tubal ligation, and the one for men is called vasectomy. The procedure for male sterilization is less risky and less expensive than female sterilization (see "Conditions and Disorders in Men"). Sterilization should be considered a permanent form of birth control, although in some cases it can be reversed.

Sterilization in women is usually done by laparoscopy. Laparoscopic surgery has been nicknamed Band-Aid surgery because of the small size of the incision near or through the navel.

For the procedure, gas is introduced into the abdominal cavity; the gas pushes the intestine away from the uterus and fallopian tubes. A lighted tube called a laparoscope is inserted through the same incision to allow the surgeon to view the internal area. Operating instruments can either be inserted through the laparoscope or through a second small incision at the pubic hair line. The fallopian tubes are then sealed with electric current that also stops bleeding. In some cases, a ring or clip can be inserted over the tubes through the laparoscope to seal them (see Fig. 15.17). Other reversible means of sealing the tubes are being explored.

The procedure is very effective in preventing pregnancy. Complications are rare but include injuries to the bowel or blood vessels and infection.

Cancer Detection

When cancer develops in a woman's reproductive organs, it is rarely accompanied by symptoms. See Fig. 15.18). In some cases, cancer can be prevented by

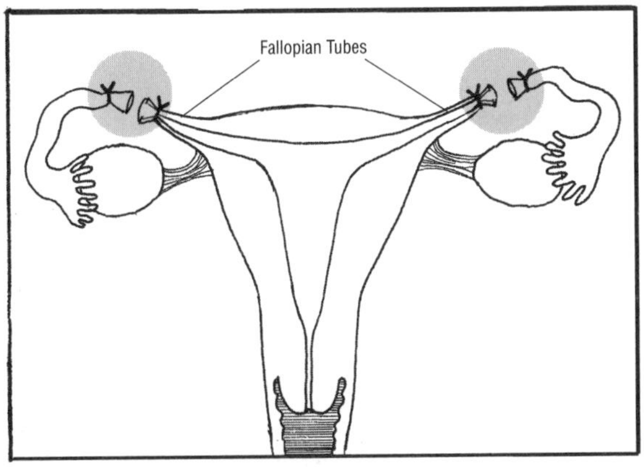

Figure 15.17 Tubal Ligation
Sterilization is a permanent form of birth control. In women, it is done by a procedure called tubal ligation, in which both fallopian tubes are cut and sealed by tying, banding, or clipping the cut ends. The egg released each month by one of the ovaries thus cannot be reached by the man's sperm.

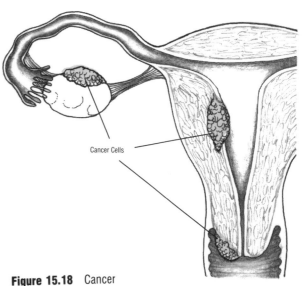

Figure 15.18 Cancer
Possible sites of cancer in women include the ovary, uterus, and cervix.

detecting precancerous changes in the cells. In others, noncancerous conditions can cause symptoms that must be explored to rule out cancer. Although the initial evaluation can be done by a gynecologist, a gynecologic oncologist, who specializes in cancer of the reproductive organs, should provide care once cancer is diagnosed. The earlier cancer is detected and treated, the better the chance for cure.

Cervix

The Pap test can detect changes in the cells of the cervix that are not cancer but may warn that cancer could develop (see Fig. 15.10). Some of these changes return to normal on their own, whereas for others, treatment can keep cancer from developing. The Pap test can allow almost all cases of cervical cancer to be prevented, which is why it is so important that you have one regularly.

There are virtually no symptoms during the earliest stage of cervical cancer. The most common early warning signs of cervical cancer are spotting or irregular bleeding or bleeding after intercourse. These signs should prompt an immediate visit to a gynecologist.

Risk factors for cervical cancer include early age at first intercourse, having multiple sexual partners, smoking, and infection with humanpapillomavirus (HPV). Because HPV is spread through sexual contact, the risk factors for contracting this virus include having multiple male sexual partners, who themselves have had multiple sexual partners. Women are most at risk during the teenage years when cervical cells are maturing.

In the Pap test, cells of the cervix are examined under a microscope to detect abnormalities (see Fig. 15.19). The results are reported in categories developed by the National Cancer Institute, called the Bethesda System, and treated accordingly:

- Normal: No abnormal cells are present.
- Atypical Squamous Cells of Undetermined Significance (ASCUS): These cells appear abnormal, but it is not clear exactly what that may mean. Although some doctors may believe that further testing is needed, in most cases these changes can be assessed by a repeat Pap test at a 3–6 month interval, preferably not during menstruation. If results are normal in two consecutive tests, annual Pap tests can be resumed and no further treatment is needed. About 70 percent of patients with results in this category need no further treatment.
- Low-Grade Squamous Intraepithelial Lesions: Includes changes seen with HPV infection as well as early precancerous changes, also called mild dysplasia or cervical intraepithelial neoplasia grade 1 (CIN 1). About 60 percent of these changes go away on their own, and about 15 percent go on to a more advanced stage. Follow-up may involve monitoring the condition with Pap tests at 3–6-month intervals and performing a procedure called colposcopy (see ''Procedures'') if the condition persists.
- High-Grade Squamous Intraepithelial Lesions: Includes moderate and severe dysplasia (CIN 2 and 3) as well as carcinoma in situ, which is a severe form of precancer. A sample of the tissue is obtained by biopsying the most severe area to confirm the types of abnormalities seen through the colposcope. The affected areas are then removed with local surgery using various techniques: loop electrosurgical excision procedure (LEEP), laser, freezing techniques, or electrosurgery (see ''Procedures''). A procedure called cervical conization may be performed to remove a cone-shaped wedge from the cervix.

A   B   C

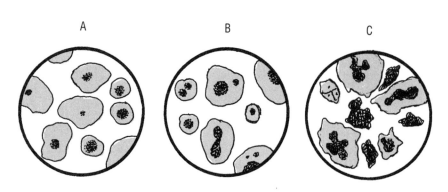

Figure 15.19 Pap Test
In the Pap test, cells collected from the cervix are examined under a microscope to detect abnormalities. Shown here are normal cervical cells (A), cells showing cervical dysplasia (B), and typical cancer cells (C).

■ Invasive Cancer: Early stage invasive cancer can be treated with either radical hysterectomy (removal of the uterus) or radiation therapy. In later stages, especially when the lymph nodes are involved, a combination of surgery, radiation, and possibly chemotherapy may be used.

There is a 90 percent likelihood that the treatment for early precancerous changes will completely remove any abnormal tissue. About 10 percent of women have an abnormal Pap smear during that first year after treatment. Treatment of this persistent area has a cure rate of about 90 percent. Thus, there is about a 99 percent cure rate with two treatments. Women who have been treated should continue to have yearly Pap tests, however, even after menopause or hysterectomy.

Uterus

Cancer of the lining of the uterus, the endometrium, is the most common gynecologic cancer. About 31,000 cases occur annually. The survival rate for this cancer is high if the cancer is diagnosed in a very early stage.

The most frequent symptom of endometrial cancer is spotting or irregular bleeding, which should alert a woman to seek treatment. Women in the menopausal years should consult their physicians immediately if they develop spotting after their regular periods have stopped for 1 year or more.

The greatest risk factor for endometrial cancer appears to be excess amounts of the hormone estrogen. Estrogen stimulates the uterine lining to grow, causing a condition called endometrial hyperplasia, a form of precancer. The excess estrogen can come from a variety of sources:

■ Hormone replacement therapy taken during and after menopause includes estrogen and progesterone. If estrogen is taken alone, a woman's risk of developing endometrial cancer is increased. By taking both estrogen and progesterone pills, however, a woman's risk of cancer is even lower than those who take no therapy.

■ Fat cells are the most abundant source of excess estrogen production. Some fat cells normally convert inactive adrenal hormones into very active estrogenlike hormones. These hormones overstimulate the uterine lining to grow, possibly out of control, into cancer. Women who are slightly overweight have a 3-fold risk of developing endometrial cancer and those who are nearly twice their recommended weight have a 10-fold risk of developing endometrial cancer.

The diagnosis is confirmed by performing a uterine biopsy to obtain a sample of the lining to study. This procedure can be performed in a physician's office, without any anesthesia. The "D&C," or dilation and curettage, is rarely needed now that suction biopsies can be done in the office.

Treatment usually consists of a hysterectomy. The ovaries are usually removed (oophorectomy), along with the lymph nodes. A careful search is made for any sign of further spread (see "Staging of Endometrial Cancer"). A general gynecologist can perform the surgery in early stage cancer but a gynecologic oncologist should always be available if advanced disease is found during the surgery. If advanced disease is diagnosed preoperatively, the gynecologic oncologist should perform the surgery. After surgery and complete pathological evaluation of the uterus, the ovaries, and the lymph nodes, further treatment may be recommended in the form of either radiation or chemotherapy.

Ovarian Cancer

Ovarian cancer is the most malignant of all of the gynecologic cancers. Approximately 24,000 women develop ovarian cancer each year, and unfortunately many are not diagnosed until the cancer is in advanced stages. The risk factors for ovarian cancer include advanced age, not having children or having them late in life, and a family history of ovarian cancer or other cancers such as breast or colon cancers.

Ovarian cancer gives only vague early warning signs, such as a change in bowel pattern, a feeling of

STAGING OF ENDOMETRIAL CANCER

Stage I	Cancer confined to the body of the uterus.
Stage II	Cancer extended from the body of the uterus to the cervix.
Stage III	Cancer spread out to lymph nodes or onto the ovaries.
Stage IV	Distant spread to the lung or into the bladder or rectum.

bloating, or simply pelvic discomfort. These symptoms may be due to pressure from a pelvic mass or tumor implants on the bowel wall.

When ovarian cancer grows, some women think they are only getting fat and don't investigate the cause of the swelling. The cancer can cause fluid to accumulate within the abdominal cavity, causing the abdomen to swell. This fluid contains cancer cells and can spread even into the lung cavity, where more fluid can accumulate.

Since there are so few warning signs in the early stages, this cancer is usually diagnosed later, when tumor nodules from the ovaries extend to the surface of the liver, the bowel, the stomach, or inside the abdominal wall. Cancer is often suspected by pelvic exam and confirmed by ultrasound. A blood test also can be performed to measure a substance called CA–125 that circulates in the blood. CA–125 is used as a tumor marker because levels are increased when tumors are present. Because levels are increased by the presence of many other benign disorders, this test is not used to screen healthy women.

Therapy usually begins with surgery to remove all the tumor, followed by chemotherapy. The chemotherapy is fairly effective at removing any tumor cells left after surgery. While a complete cure of this cancer occurs in only about 20–30 percent of women, chemotherapy usually prolongs life very significantly.

Ovarian Cysts

Often a cyst may develop on an ovary. This fluid-filled growth is not cancerous in most cases. Some may be the earliest sign that a cancer has formed, however, so all ovarian cysts should be taken seriously and evaluated. Ovarian cysts may have no symptoms; large cysts can cause a feeling of pelvic pressure or fullness. Diagnosis is usually by vaginal ultrasound: A small probe is passed into the vagina that reveals details of the ovaries and uterus. The CA-125 blood test can also be performed to assess the likelihood of ovarian cancer. Treatment of ovarian cysts range from careful monitoring of simple small cysts to surgical removal of any ovarian cysts that may suggest a malignancy. Oral contraceptives do not make an ovarian cyst disappear any faster. If you have an ovarian cyst that is under observation, your doctor should check it again within three months to make sure it has not changed or grown larger. Always get a second opinion before having surgery for an ovarian cyst.

Vagina

Cancer of the vagina that does not involve the vulva or the cervix is rare. One form is caused by exposure to a drug called diethylstilbestrol, or DES, in women whose mothers took the drug while they were pregnant. In the early 1950s DES was prescribed to women who were at risk of losing their pregnancies. Now, their daughters are at risk for some cancers of the vagina. A registry has been created to keep track of these women so they can receive careful monitoring. The cancer usually develops around age 19; treatment is by hysterectomy, and it has a 90 percent cure rate if identified in the earliest stage of growth.

Vulva

Vulvar cancer is a rare gynecologic malignancy. It almost always strikes women who are in the menopausal years and appears to be linked to infection with HPV. The cancer appears as a small sore or small lump on one of the outer lips of the vulva. Sometimes it can itch, but it usually does not cause any pain. Many women delay seeing their gynecologists, hoping the sore will disappear; however, this delay allows for continued tumor growth. If you have a small sore, lump, or ulcer on any area of the vulva that is new and does not go away within a week, see your physician.

The diagnosis is based on the results of a biopsy, in which the area is numbed and a small amount of tissue is removed to be studied. If the cancer is found in early stages, surgery is performed. Usually, the area of cancer must be removed with a rim of normal tissue of approximately 1 inch in diameter all the way around the cancer. This is called a radical partial vulvectomy. In most stages of disease, lymph nodes in the groin should also be removed. If cancer has spread to the lymph nodes, radiation therapy is usually required.

Ectopic Pregnancy

Normally, once the egg is fertilized in the fallopian tubes, it travels to the uterus and becomes implanted there. When, for any reason, the fertilized egg implants anywhere else along the route, the pregnancy is said to be ectopic, or in the wrong place (see Fig. 15.20).

Ectopic pregnancy occurs when the opening of the fallopian tube is twisted or narrowed, due to scar tissue formed by infection or surgery. The passage of the fer-

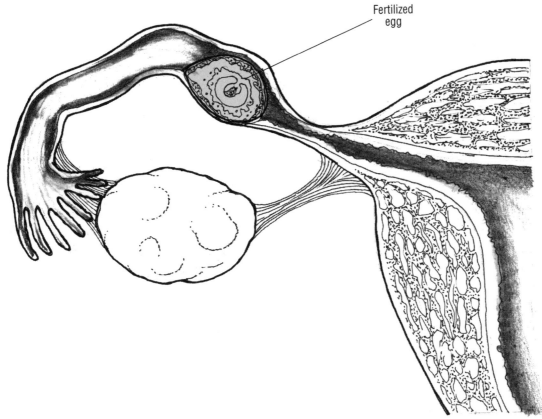

Fertilized
egg

Figure 15.20 Ectopic Pregnancy
In an ectopic pregnancy, the fertilized ovum becomes attached in a place other than inside the uterus. Most ectopic pregnancies occur in a fallopian tube.

tilized egg to the uterus is blocked, and the egg begins to develop within the fallopian tube lining, on the surface of the ovary, or within the abdominal or pelvic cavity. The egg can only develop for a few weeks before its growth is hindered by the size of the fallopian tube.

In an ectopic pregnancy, symptoms of early pregnancy, an abnormally light period, and pelvic pain can occur. Many women have no symptoms until the pregnancy causes a rupture of the fallopian tube or there is bleeding from a nearby blood vessel. This causes severe abdominal pain, shock, and collapse—a medical emergency of the first order.

If you have a history of tubal infections or previous ectopic pregnancy and suspect you are pregnant, you should be carefully monitored by your physician to be sure that the pregnancy is within the uterus. Ectopic pregnancy is diagnosed by doing tests to measure hormone levels that indicate pregnancy. Once pregnancy has been confirmed, ultrasound can determine its location and size.

If the fallopian tube has ruptured, ectopic pregnancy is an emergency that requires surgery to remove the pregnancy and control bleeding. In some cases, the tube can then be rejoined. Many surgeons are now performing this procedure through the laparoscope. Conservative surgery in which the fallopian tube is simply opened and the pregnancy lifted out is frequently possible and conserves the tube, and thus your ability to have children. Another procedure for small, early ectopic pregnancies involves the intramuscular injection of chemotherapy; the usual result is loss of the pregnancy in about 7 days.

Endometriosis

The tissue that lines the inside of the uterus responds to hormones that cause it to thicken and bleed each month. This tissue can also grow outside the uterus, on the pelvic organs. When this occurs, these areas can become inflamed and sometimes painful, and scar tissue develops.

Some women with endometriosis, even severe endometriosis, have no symptoms. Others can have intense pain, especially when the endometrial tissue is shed into the pelvic area during the menstrual period. The pain can be felt throughout the entire area or may be confined to the uterus. Pain usually appears only during the menstrual period, but can start just before and gradually increase until bleeding starts, usually easing after up to 72 hours. In addition to pelvic pain, endometriosis is a common cause of infertility because it causes the fallopian tubes to malfunction.

Researchers have not been able to pinpoint causes of endometriosis. One theory is that endometrial tissue travels through the fallopian tubes and becomes implanted on surrounding structures (see Fig. 15.21). Delay of pregnancy to beyond age 30 or later is associated with a higher risk of endometriosis. Women who have never had a pregnancy are at highest risk.

Laparoscopy is used for both definitive diagnosis and treatment of endometriosis. The treatment of endometriosis depends largely on the patient's needs and desires. If relief of pain is of most importance and childbearing has been completed, a hysterectomy with removal of the ovaries, followed by hormone replacement therapy, is often recommended. When fertility is desired, the spots of endometriosis can be removed by laparoscopy with laser therapy. Unfortunately, the condition recurs in about one-third of women treated.

Synthetic hormones can be used to shrink the endometriosis implants, but the effect is temporary. The implants usually return to their premedication level within a few months after treatment ends. Treatment can be given for only 6 months because it decreases the estrogen level. This brief remission of the disease can be time enough to allow conception soon after, if that is desired. Because prevention of ovulation can reduce the discomfort, many women take oral contraceptives. However, some still have pain and require surgery for relief.

Fibroids

Benign fibrous growths of the uterine wall are called fibroids. Some fibroids bulge outward from the wall; others extend from the uterine surface on a stalk. A fibroid can also extend into the uterine lining, compressing the endometrium or forming a growth on a stem within the endometrial cavity. About 20 percent of women of reproductive age have fibroids, and for most of them the fibroids pose no problem.

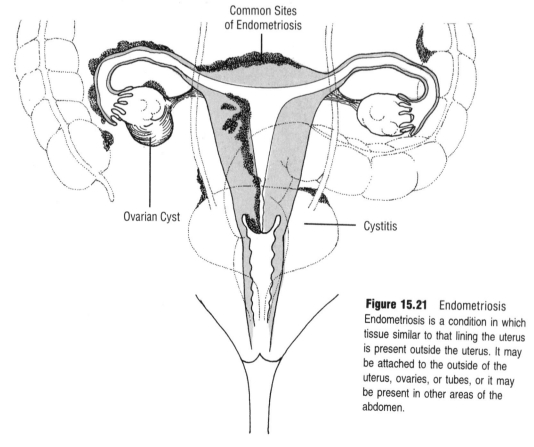

Common Sites of Endometriosis

Ovarian Cyst

Cystitis

Figure 15.21 Endometriosis Endometriosis is a condition in which tissue similar to that lining the uterus is present outside the uterus. It may be attached to the outside of the uterus, ovaries, or tubes, or it may be present in other areas of the abdomen.

Fibroids enlarge the uterus and can cause pressure and discomfort in the pelvis, however. Internal uterine fibroids can also compress the endometrial lining and cause excessive bleeding during and occasionally between menstrual periods. Younger women rarely have fibroids, but when they do, the fibroids can press against the lining of the uterus causing infertility. The most serious complication is pressure and blockage of the ureters, the tubes draining the kidneys. On rare occasions, a fibroid can develop into a malignant tumor. Fibroids have been the most common reason for hysterectomy in the past, as well as currently. The only reason for removing the fibroids or for doing a hysterectomy for fibroids is if they cause symptoms like bladder or pelvic pressure, excessive bleeding, infertility, or pain.

Ultrasound is used to determine the size and location of fibroids. Two types of surgery, if needed, are used to remove the growths:

■ Hysterectomy to remove the uterus and with it, the fibroids

■ Myomectomy to remove the fibroids only, leaving the uterus intact

The selection of the type of surgery used rests with the woman and her surgeon. For a woman who wants to maintain her fertility, a myomectomy is the treatment of choice. It might also be preferred by the woman who wishes to have her uterus and ovaries left intact.

Myomectomy usually involves more blood loss than a hysterectomy, because the fibroid can have a rich blood supply. During a hysterectomy, the location of each blood vessel that feeds the uterus is well known and can be clamped off so that little bleeding occurs. During myomectomy, the blood supply to the fibroid is less clearly defined and blood loss can be heavy. Many gynecologists recommend that women who do not want to retain fertility simply have the top half or the entire uterus removed in what is called a partial hysterectomy.

Sometimes this procedure can be made easier by shrinking the fibroid prior to surgery. This is done by prescribing hormones that mimic menopause and decrease the amount of estrogens, resulting in shrinkage of the fibroid by as much as 50 percent.

Women can usually become pregnant after removal of a fibroid and carry the pregnancy to full term, although they may occasionally require a caesarean delivery.

Menopause

At menopause, a woman stops menstruating and her ovaries no longer produce estrogen. The average age at the last menstrual period is 51. This natural process begins several years before, as a woman's ovaries produce less and less estrogen. The lack of estrogen can produce a number of effects:

■ Hot flashes or flushes can occur. These are sudden feelings of heat that spread over the body, often accompanied by a flushed face and sweating. They appear at any time without warning and are most troublesome at night when they can interfere with sleep.

■ Vaginal tissues may become dryer, thinner, and less flexible. This can result in painful intercourse, urinary tract problems, or sagging of pelvic organs because the tissues that support them lose their elasticity.

■ Osteoporosis, or bone loss can cause bones to become thin and brittle. Supplemental estrogen can help guard against it, as can a diet high in calcium, regular exercise, and stopping smoking.

■ Cardiovascular disease becomes more of a risk for women after menopause because estrogen no longer gives them natural protection from heart attack and stroke.

■ Emotional changes, such as mood swings, irritability, and depression can accompany menopause, but these symptoms are more likely related to insomnia caused by hot flashes at night than to the lack of estrogen.

Not all women have all of these symptoms and they are not always long lasting. You can continue to have a full and healthy life for many years beyond menopause. Some of the symptoms of menopause can be eased through diet and exercise. Others can be relieved by replacing the estrogen no longer produced by the ovaries. Hormone replacement therapy can relieve the symptoms of menopause, in addition to lowering the risk of heart disease and osteoporosis.

Estrogen is given along with the hormone progestin (a synthetic version of the natural hormone progesterone) to protect against endometrial cancer, a risk when estrogen is taken alone. Estrogen by itself causes the lining of the uterus to overgrow and increases the risk of cancer of the endometrium. Progestin is taken with estrogen to oppose it and keep the lining of the endometrium in check. In fact, taking progestin with estrogen actually lowers the risk of cancer to less than that of a woman not taking hormone therapy.

Estrogen is processed through the liver and affects the levels of cholesterol. Estrogen increases high-density cholesterol (the good cholesterol) and lowers low-density cholesterol (the bad cholesterol), thus reducing the risk of heart disease. Without estrogen, a woman's risk of heart disease approaches that of a man by age 65.

Women are at higher risk of osteoporosis because they have less bone mass than men to begin with and because they tend to have less calcium stored in their bones. Thus, when they lose the protective effect of estrogen, the natural process of bone loss speeds up so they are losing bone faster than it is being replaced.

Osteoporosis and cardiovascular disease do not have symptoms in their early stages as they are conditions that develop over time. Hormone replacement therapy to prevent symptoms of menopause also helps prevent these conditions. To provide long-term protection, the therapy must be taken long term.

Hormone replacement therapy is not for everyone. It is not recommended for women who have had breast cancer, endometrial cancer, or liver cancer. The link between breast cancer and hormone replacement therapy is still not clear. There may be a slight increase in a woman's chance of developing breast cancer if she has been taking hormones for more than 15 years.

Hormone replacement therapy can have other side effects. The progestin causes monthly bleeding or spotting, which can be unexpected and bothersome. Other side effects include breast tenderness, fluid retention, swelling, mood changes, and pelvic cramping. Because of the side effects, some women choose to take estrogen alone. These women should be monitored carefully for abnormal bleeding. Their doctors may suggest that an endometrial biopsy be performed so a small amount of tissue can be examined.

Women who prefer not to take hormone replacement therapy can obtain relief of symptoms and help prevent bone loss and heart disease in other ways. To facilitate decisions about hormones, women should have a fasting cholesterol and a bone density test. Estrogen cream, used in the vagina, can treat vaginal dryness. A balanced diet rich in calcium and low in fat, regular exercise, and avoiding alcohol and tobacco can help reduce the rate of bone loss and protect against heart disease. Regardless of age or whether they are taking hormone replacement therapy, women should

continue to have regular pelvic exams, mammograms, and Pap tests after they reach menopause.

Menstrual Problems

Most women experience some discomfort with their menstrual periods. Certain conditions, such as endometriosis or fibroids, can increase pain during menstrual periods. Any severe pain, unusual spotting or bleeding, or missed menstrual periods could be a sign of a problem that requires medical attention.

Amenorrhea

Amenorrhea is the absence of menstruation. This absence is normal before puberty, after menopause, and during pregnancy. Primary amenorrhea occurs when a woman reaches the age of 18 and has never had a period. It is usually caused by a problem in the endocrine system that regulates hormones. Secondary amenorrhea is present when a woman has had regular periods that stop for longer than 12 months. Amenorrhea may be triggered by a wide range of events:

Primary amenorrhea

- Ovarian failure
- Problems in the nervous system or the pituitary gland in the endocrine system that affect maturation at puberty
- Birth defects in which the reproductive structures do not develop properly

Secondary amenorrhea

- Problems that affect estrogen levels, such as stress, weight loss, exercise, or illness
- Problems affecting the pituitary, thyroid, or adrenal gland
- Ovarian tumors or surgical removal of the ovaries

To diagnose and treat amenorrhea it may be necessary to consult a reproductive endocrinologist. Treatment is based on the problem diagnosed. Blood tests are usually performed and many patients are asked to keep a record of their early morning temperatures to detect the rise in temperature that occurs with ovulation.

Cramps

The sensation of spasmodic cramping or a feeling of chronic achy fullness can occur with a normal menstrual cycle and a normal anatomy. The pain is due to uterine contractions, caused by substances called prostaglandins.

Prostaglandins circulate within the blood. They can cause diarrhea by speeding up the contractions of the intestinal tract and lower blood pressure by relaxing the muscles of blood vessels. Thus many women frequently notice that severe menstrual pain is associated with mild diarrhea and occasionally an overall sensation of faintness in which they become pale, sweaty, and sometimes nauseated. Some women actually have fainting spells because of the low blood pressure resulting from the action of prostaglandins.

To relieve cramps, your doctor may recommend drugs called prostaglandin inhibitors or nonsteroidal anti-inflammatory drugs (NSAIDs), which are available without a prescription. Taking medication immediately at the onset of any symptoms usually results in dramatic improvement or complete relief. Taking these drugs even before symptoms begin may help, too. Relief also may be obtained by applications of heat and mild exercise.

Excessive Bleeding

Some women experience a menopause characterized by irregular, unpredictable, often heavy bleeding. If you develop severe irregular bleeding as you approach menopause, or experience new bleeding a year after your final period, your doctor should do a biopsy to confirm that no precancerous changes have taken place. This biopsy does not need to be the traditional dilation and curettage (D&C) that is performed in a hospital under general anesthesia. Rather, the biopsy is a simple procedure that takes place in the doctor's office. A slender, soft, plastic canula is inserted through the cervix and a small sample of uterine tissue is obtained. The cost of this biopsy is about 10 percent of the cost of a regular D&C and provides the same information. These tests are 99.5 percent reliable in diagnosing a precancerous condition or cancer, if present. If there is no sign of cancer, excessive bleeding can be treated with hormone therapy or surgery on the lining of the uterus.

Pelvic Inflammatory Disease

Infection with the STDs chlamydia and gonorrhea can lead to pelvic inflammatory disease (PID). In PID, infection spreads upward through the cervix, the uterus, and the fallopian tubes into the pelvic cavity. White blood cells battling the infection cause a puslike discharge to surround the ovaries. The body tries to wall off this infection by creating filmy adhesions (a fibrous wall) from organ to organ to limit the spread of the infection. The adhesions can distort the fallopian tubes and result in infertility.

Early symptoms of PID include pelvic pain associated with fever and weakness; there also may be a vaginal discharge. If the infection continues, an abscess can form within the pelvis. The typical PID attack strikes after a menstrual period and begins with pelvic pain. Motion, even walking, can be painful. If the abscess develops, it can send bacteria into the blood stream, causing high fever, chills, joint infections, and even death.

Diagnosis usually is based on the symptoms and presence of the abscess. In some cases, a sample of the discharge from the abscess can be used to identify the organism causing the infection. Antibiotics can stop the infection before an abscess has formed, if treatment is started early. If the infection is severe, some patients may require intravenous antibiotics in a hospital setting. Surgery may be necessary to drain an abscess, but it is usually not necessary to remove the uterus, tubes, and ovaries.

Premenstrual Syndrome

The regular, recurring symptoms that occur just prior to menstruation are called premenstrual syndrome (PMS). PMS is not a disease but rather a collection of symptoms that disappear once the menstrual period has begun.

Nearly all menstruating women experience a set of symptoms that tell them their periods are coming. For some women, these symptoms can be quite severe, involving a combination of emotional and physical changes. Emotional changes may include anger, anxiety, confusion, mood swings, tension, crying, depression, and an inability to concentrate. Physical symptoms include bloating, swollen breasts, fatigue, constipation, headache, and clumsiness.

The diagnosis rests on confirming the cyclic nature of these symptoms and ruling out any underlying psychological or physical dysfunction. Many women are asked to chart their symptoms so they can be related to the menstrual cycle to detect a pattern. The symptoms usually occur about 7 days before a menstrual period and go away once it begins.

The cause of PMS is unknown, despite extensive research into abnormal types of hormones that are secreted at this time, unusual ratios of one hormone to another, and imbalance between sodium and body water retention. Many theories have been studied, but none has been shown to be the primary cause. As a result, the condition is difficult to treat.

Treatment is generally aimed at relieving symptoms. Keeping a calendar and being aware of when symptoms occur helps most women; simply knowing their distressing symptoms are related to the onset of their periods can have a calming effect. There are other things you can try to ease symptoms of PMS:

- Dietary changes provide relief for some women: Decreasing sodium, sugar, caffeine, and alcohol; increasing complex carbohydrates; and eating smaller, more frequent meals.

- Dietary supplementation of calcium, magnesium, and vitamins B_6 and E may reduce symptoms.

- Exercise has been shown to help in depression and, theoretically, may be of some benefit for PMS.

- Diuretics can relieve the feeling of bloating and swelling caused by fluid retention.

- Pain can be relieved with nonsteroidal anti-inflammatory drugs (NSAIDs).

- Oral contraceptives are helpful in relieving symptoms in some women.

- Severe breast tenderness can be relieved by taking bromocriptine, a drug that stops the production of certain hormones, but this drug does not help other PMS symptoms.

Many medications have been tried with limited success. Some of them are expensive and most have side effects. It may be necessary to combine some remedies on a trial and error basis, along with modifications in diet and exercise.

Rape

Rape is sexual intercourse by force; it is epidemic in our country. This violent crime has both psychological (see Chapter 10) as well as medical aspects that affect women's health.

A rape should be reported within 48 hours of its occurrence, as crucial evidence of it is more difficult to obtain after that time. Women should not wash, bathe, urinate, defecate, drink, or take any medication prior to reporting a rape. A practitioner experienced in this area should perform a thorough exam so there is evidence available if charges are brought against the accused rapist.

A physician first asks the women to describe what happened, and then examines her clothing for damage, taking particular note if there are any materials such as soil or stains such as body fluids sticking to the clothing. The physician next asks if any drugs or alcohol were taken by the woman or the rapist, because this may become an important issue during court procedures.

The physical exam consists of looking for evidence on the whole body, even though not every woman who has been raped has been physically injured. The physician measures and charts all injuries and may photograph them, looking carefully for bite marks, bruises, grip marks, and scratches. Samples are taken of the vaginal fluid to check for infection or sperm. Mouth swabs and saliva samples are obtained to look for bacteria and semen and possibly to perform DNA studies of the sample. Urine samples may be obtained to determine whether drugs were involved. Blood samples are obtained to test for HIV as well as hepatitis. If the HIV test is negative, another HIV test should be done in 6 months to determine whether the virus was contracted during the rape. A woman may be given treatment against possible STDs, and she should be offered emergency contraception if there is a chance pregnancy could result from the assault.

After the exam, comfort, support, and counseling are key to complete recovery. There are many groups available to counsel women who are recovering from previous molestation or rape.

Vaginitis

The internal environment of the vagina consists of a delicate balance of organisms that, along with normal vaginal secretions, keep it healthy and clean. When that balance is disrupted by either an infection, a health problem, or some type of irritation, vaginitis can occur. Bacteria or yeast that grows normally in the vagina can overgrow and cause itching, redness, and pain in the vaginal area. Infections from other organisms, as well as allergic reactions, can also cause vaginitis.

Any new discharge accompanied by an odor, or abnormal itching, could be a sign of a vaginal infection. The characteristics of the discharge—its color, odor, and amount—can be a clue to the cause. Yeast is the most common cause of vaginitis, but bacteria and parasites can also cause it. The cause of vaginitis must be identified for treatment to be effective.

Bacterial Vaginosis

Among the more common vaginal infections, bacterial vaginosis is caused by the *Gardnerella, Bacteriodes,* and *Peptostreptococcus* bacteria. The primary symptom is a foul-smelling, profuse, watery vaginal discharge.

The diagnosis is confirmed by microscopic examination of the discharge. Treatment for this infection is the antibiotic metronidazole. Often, the infection recurs; longer treatment may be needed to prevent recurrences.

Yeast Infection

Some women are unusually susceptible to this most common of all vaginal infections. The cause may be a recent course of antibiotics that can decrease the normal vaginal bacteria and allow for an overgrowth of yeast. Other conditions, like diabetes and HIV infection, are also associated with recurrent yeast infections.

Your doctor will want to confirm that yeast is the cause by examining the vaginal discharge under a microscope. Discuss multiple recurrent yeast infections with your physician, because other problems such as diabetes should be ruled out.

Once you can recognize the symptoms of yeast vaginitis, you can treat yourself by purchasing any one of the over-the-counter antifungal creams or suppository preparations. Treatment is also available in pill form by prescription.

PROCEDURES FOR WOMEN

Cryotherapy

Cryotherapy involves freezing cells on the cervix to remove abnormal cells. Freezing kills cells but does not remove them from the vagina. The dead cells dissolve into the vaginal fluid and are washed away in the normal secretions. This can cause an increased vaginal discharge for about 2 weeks after the procedure.

Colposcopy

In colposcopy, the cervix, vagina, and vulva skin are examined systematically under microscopic magnification. When abnormal areas are detected, a sample is taken for further examination (a biopsy).

During the procedure, a speculum is inserted in the vagina to spread the vaginal walls, and a vinegar solution is sprayed into the cervix. The abnormal surface cells appear white, and normal cells remain pink. The entire area is examined, and a biopsy of any white area is performed.

Most women have a slight cramp for a minute or so during the biopsy. Otherwise, this procedure requires no anesthesia and is well tolerated. If a woman has severe cramps with her menstrual cycle, medication can be given before the exam to reduce discomfort.

Occasionally a scraping of tissue is obtained from the inner lining of the cervix beyond the limits of the area that can be seen. This scraping provides extra assurance that the entire abnormality has been identified. Once the biopsy results are available, therapy can be started.

Dilation and Curettage

Often referred to as a D&C, dilation and curettage removes the lining and contents of the uterus. Once the

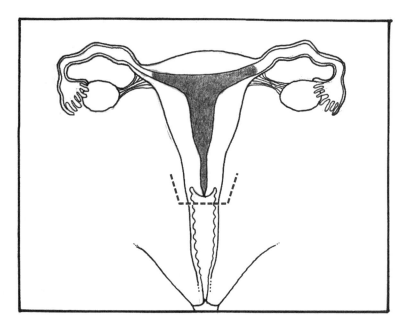

Figure 15.22 Dilation and Curettage

Dilation and curettage (D&C) is a procedure used to remove the endometrium (the lining of the uterus) and the contents of the uterus. A speculum is inserted into the vagina, the cervix is grasped with a small tonguelike instrument, and the inside of the uterus is gently scraped out with another instrument.

cervix is widened by dilators, the uterine lining is scraped out with a curette, a spoonlike instrument. A D&C is used to perform abortions, remove the lining of the uterus in cases of severe bleeding, or test for uterine cancer (see Fig. 15.22). A D&C is performed in a hospital or an ambulatory surgery center using general anesthetic. Rapid recovery with minimal spotting for 1 to 2 days can be expected. It has largely been replaced by the office biopsy.

Hysterectomy

A complete or total hysterectomy is removal of the entire uterus with the cervix. A partial (see Fig. 15.23A)

hysterectomy involves removing only a portion of the uterus (see Fig. 15.23B). A radical hysterectomy involves the removal of the uterus, cervix, lymph nodes, and other support structures around the cervix and uterus. (see Fig. 15.23C) A hysterectomy can be performed through the vagina or through a cut in the abdomen, depending on the reasons for the surgery.

Reasons for performing a hysterectomy should be clearly understood prior to the procedure. Following are the most common reasons for a hysterectomy:

- Fibroids
- Endometriosis
- Cancer

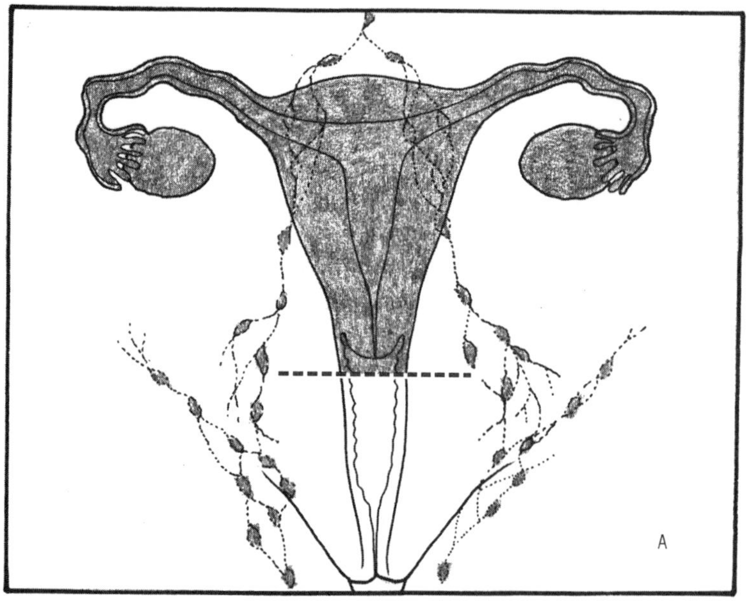

Figure 15.23 Hysterectomy

Hysterectomy, the surgical removal of the uterus, may be done in a number of ways, depending on the problem being treated. A total hysterectomy (A) involves the removal of the entire uterus, along with the ovaries and fallopian tubes. In a partial hysterectomy (B), the uterus and tubes are removed, but the ovaries and cervix are left in place. A radical hysterectomy (C) entails removal of the entire uterus, the tubes, and the ovaries, along with the lymph nodes and the support structures surrounding these organs.

A

A

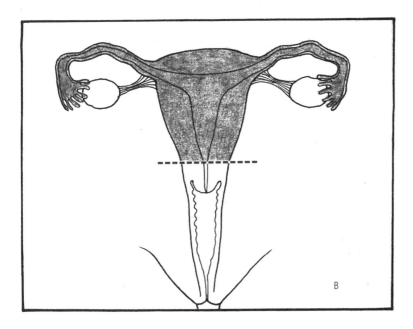

B

- Endometrial hyperplasia
- Menstrual/menopausal symptoms
- Cervical dysplasia
- Pain

A vertical incision in the lower abdomen is used for abdominal hysterectomy or for cancer or a very large fibroid. For other conditions, a horizontal incision is placed just above the pubic bone, which can be hidden in the pubic hair (see Fig. 15.24). This location results in less postoperative pain.

A vaginal hysterectomy involves less discomfort than an abdominal hysterectomy because no abdominal incision must be made. Vaginal hysterectomies are seldom performed on women who have had no children because the ligaments are tighter and the vaginal passage is small. It is indicated when there is a small uterus, and the patient has had children, because the vagina and the connecting structures of the uterus are more pliable.

Vaginal hysterectomy is now available to more women because it can be done with a laparoscope. When the laparoscope is used, it is placed into the abdomen through a small incision in the abdominal wall. The laparoscope is a telescopelike probe that can identify the structures and cut away problems outside the uterus, such as adhesions. The uterus can then be

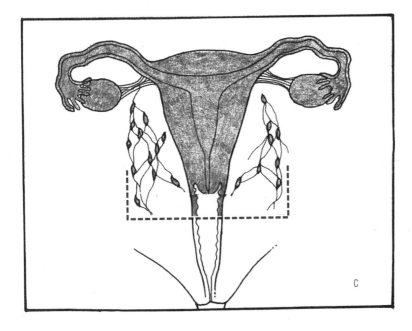

C

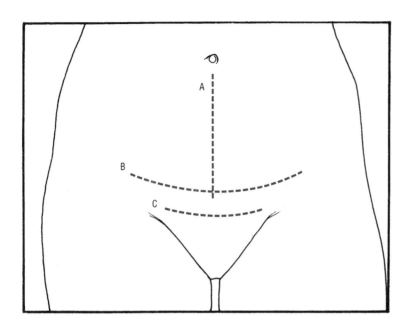

Figure 15.24 Hysterectomy Incisions
The type of incision used for a hysterectomy depends on the reason for and nature of the problem for which it is being performed. A vertical incision (A) may be used for uterine cancer or a very large fibroid. Other conditions may necessitate the use of a transverse, or horizontal, incision (B). The location and size of a transverse incision also depends on the problem being treated; a low transverse incision (C) often can be hidden in the pubic hair.

removed through the vagina with less postoperative pain and scarring.

Recovery time varies depending on the procedure. Usually, normal activities, including sex, can be resumed in about 4–6 weeks. Until then, activities such as driving, sports, and light physical work may be increased gradually. Adhesions, or scar tissue, can develop after any surgery. They can cause pain during bowel function, intercourse, or exercise. If adhesions are particularly troublesome, laparoscopic surgery can be used to relieve them, although they may return in the future.

Very few women notice a change in their sexual sensations after hysterectomy that could be related to the functions of the uterus during sexual activity or to their own sense of loss of their uterus. For most women, however, hysterectomy has no effect on sexual satisfaction. Many women have a sense of freedom from symptoms of the condition corrected, as well as from the concern of monthly periods and potential pregnancy. If you have any doubts about having a hysterectomy, always get a second opinion.

Hysteroscopy

Hysteroscopy allows the inside of the uterus and the openings of the fallopian tubes to be viewed on a video camera or a monitor. The hysteroscope is a telescope that is inserted to look at the walls of the uterus for signs of disease or other problems (such as an IUD that has slipped out of place). It can be guided to the fallopian tubes to find any obstruction and, in some cases, remove it. Some surgical procedures can also be performed with hysteroscopy. The procedure may be performed in a doctor's office using local anesthetic.

Laparoscopy

In laparoscopy, a lighted tube with a magnifying lens on the end allows the operator to see inside the body. Laparoscopy can be used to diagnose a condition, such as endometriosis; it also can be used to perform surgery.

Laparoscopic surgery uses small holes or punctures rather than one large incision. These small incisions result in less postoperative pain and shorter recovery, as compared with an abdominal incision. Women usually return to work within 3 or 4 days after laparoscopy in comparison to 4 to 6 weeks after more extensive surgery.

Many procedures can now be done through a laparoscope:

- Hysterectomy
- Removal of the gallbladder
- Removal of segments of colon

- Assisting vaginal hysterectomy
- Removal of fibroids
- Removal of the fallopian tubes
- Sterilization
- Removal of ovarian cysts

Laser

Laser therapy uses a beam of very intense and focused light to perform surgery. It is used to remove abnormal tissue from the cervix that could be a sign of early cancer. The laser also can remove warts that result from HPV infection. To increase the likelihood of complete cure, a small margin of normal tissue may also be removed. An anesthetic is given before surgery, and recovery is usually very rapid.

Loop Electrosurgical Excision Procedure

For a loop electrosurgical excision procedure, known as LEEP, a high-intensity electrical current passes through a wire used to cut a thin slice of tissue from the cervix. This tissue can be examined under a microscope. In addition to obtaining samples of tissue for diagnosis, LEEP also can be used for treatment by removing abnormal tissue. A local anesthetic is administered before the procedure, and pain medication may be given to ease postoperative discomfort. A minimal discharge is experienced after this procedure.

Ultrasound

In ultrasound, inaudible super-swift sound waves are projected into the body. The reflected echoes are captured to create an image of the internal structures of the body; this is transferred to a black and white image on a monitor screen. From this image the physician or diagnostic expert can tell the size and shape of the ovaries, the uterus, and other pelvic structures. It can determine the age and exact location of the fetus within the uterus. In some situations physical details of a fetus can be identified; it is especially helpful in confirming a possible multiple birth.

CONDITIONS AND DISORDERS IN MEN

When there is a disorder in the reproductive system of men, it can affect several functions, including urination and sexual function.

Benign Prostatic Hyperplasia

The prostate gland continues to grow during most of a man's life. It is common for the prostate gland to become enlarged as a man ages. This growth is called benign prostatic hyperplasia, or BPH. Over half of all men over age 60 and about 90 percent of all men in their 70s and 80s have some symptoms of BPH. Symptoms include a weaker urinary stream and a need to urinate more often, especially at night.

Symptoms are caused by pressure from the prostate growth around the urethra, which obstructs the bladder. The bladder cannot fully empty, leaving urine behind. Eventually this can lead to urinary tract infections, bladder or kidney damage, bladder stones, and incontinence. The cause of BPH is not clear, but is dependent on aging and androgens. Although some of the signs of BPH and prostate cancer are similar, having BPH does not seem to increase the chances of getting prostate cancer.

When BPH causes a partial obstruction of the urethra, certain factors can bring on symptoms. Some over-the-counter cold or allergy medicines can prevent the bladder from allowing urine to pass. Other conditions that can bring on urinary retention include alcohol, cold temperatures, or a long period of immobility.

Treatment may not be required in the early stages. If problems develop, however, medical or surgical treatment may be required. Some medications used to treat BPH shrink the prostate cells or relax the smooth muscle of the prostate. The blood pressure drugs terazosin (Hytrin) and doxazosin can be used to relax smooth muscle in the prostate.

Sometimes, surgery to remove the enlarged part of the prostate is recommended. In most cases, surgery is performed through the urethra with a light-transmitting instrument that has an electrical loop at the end to cut tissue. Surgery can also be performed through an open incision. Most men recover completely within 6 weeks. Sexual function may take a while to return but usually is not affected. After surgery, most men experience retrograde ejaculation, in which they achieve orgasm during sex but the semen travels backwards to the bladder rather than forward out the penis.

Cancer

Prostate Cancer

One of the most common cancers in the United States, close to 200,000 new cases of prostate cancer are diagnosed each year. The prevalence of prostate cancer increases rapidly with age, reaching about 50 percent in men over 70. The cancer incidence is higher in African-American than in white men. In the early stages there are no symptoms.

The cancer is usually discovered by digital rectal examination (DRE), in which a hard lump or growth in the prostate gland can be detected before symptoms develop. Tests are then performed to confirm the diagnosis. In addition to imaging studies, blood tests to measure a chemical called prostate-specific antigen (PSA) are performed to detect the high levels that occur in the presence of cancer. Biopsies are done to obtain a piece of tissue for further study and, if cancer cells are present, the stage of disease is determined (see "Stages of Prostate Cancer").

Treatment can include surgery, radiation therapy, hormone therapy, or a combination of these treatments. Because prostate cancer cells use the male hormones to grow, blocking production of these hormones with gonadotropin androgens and antiandrogens may control the disease. All of these treatments have side effects. The chance of complete cure is good when the disease is detected in its early stages.

Testicular Cancers

Cancer of the testis is the most common type of cancer in men between the ages of 18 and 35. Two to three new cases per 100,000 males occur in the United States each year. White men are four times more likely than African-American men to develop testicular cancer. Seminoma, the most common type of testicular cancer, has a high cure rate when treated early.

Any unusual lump on the testis, or any new lump, even if it is not painful, should be evaluated by a physician. When a tumor is found in one testis, surgical removal is required; the remaining testis maintains the

STAGES OF PROSTATE CANCER

Stage I	Cancer, confined within the prostate, is not felt or detected but found incidentally after surgery.
Stage II	Cancer, within the prostate, is usually felt on digital rectal exam.
Stage III	Cancer found outside the prostate in adjacent tissues.
Stage IV	Cancer has spread outside the gland and has metastasized to distant tissues.

body's normal functions. The loss of both testes results in loss of hormone production, and testosterone therapy will be necessary to maintain sexual function.

Cryptorchidism

Cryptorchidism is also known as hidden testis or undescended testis, because the testis has not reached its normal position in the scrotum. A physician can confirm the absence of the testis by feeling the scrotum, and all young boys should be checked early for this condition. The undescended testis must be removed if it cannot be put in the normal scrotal position because it carrries increased risk of testicular cancer.

Epididymitis

Infection of the epididymis, the coiled tube that transports sperm to the vas deferens, is caused either by the STDs, including chlamydia and gonorrhea, or by the E. coli bacteria. This condition is easily transmitted and can be very painful. The infecting organism can sometimes be identified in samples of urine. Antibiotics are usually prescribed. Ice packs applied to the scrotum reduce swelling and pain. It is important to distinguish epididymitis from torsion of the testis, which should be treated immediately.

Gynecomastia

Enlargement of the male breasts, know as gynecomastia, can occur on one or both sides. It is usually triggered by an imbalance in the normal ratio of androgen to estrogen in the blood supply—either androgen production is decreased or estrogen levels are increased. Gynecomastia can occur normally in newborns, at adolescence, or with aging. It also can result from several endocrine disorders and some medications; gynecomastia should be evaluated.

Erectile Dysfunction (Impotence)

The inability to have or keep an erection sufficient to permit intercourse or masturbation is called impotence or erectile dysfunction. Nearly every man experiences temporary impotence related to fatigue, stress, or illness. More than 10 million men in the United States are chronically impotent. The problem increases with age; 30 percent of men age 65 have recurrent episodes of impotence.

Many factors can affect the complex interaction of vascular, neurologic, and endocrine systems that allow normal erectile function. Although sexual function and desire may decrease with age, age is not necessarily a cause of impotence. Medication side effects, stress, smoking, and alcoholism can be risk factors. Inadequate testosterone, anxiety, premature ejaculation, and Peyronie's disease are some of the treatable causes of the problem. Diabetes is the most common disease associated with erectile problems.

Treatment requires a medical history and physical examination; this should include an evaluation of testis size, shape, and consistency and palpation of the shaft of the penis. A testoterone level and a nocturnal penile tumescence test can be used to detect whether a man is having an erection at night while he sleeps. If a man is physically able to have an erection, his impotence could be caused by psychological reasons, and he may benefit from counseling.

Some of the methods of treatment include the use of penile or intracavernous injections, vacuum devices, and penile implants. Support groups, changes in lifestyle, or medications can be helpful.

Infertility

Defined as the inability of a couple to conceive after 12 months of unprotected intercourse, infertility is thought to affect 10–15 percent of married couples in the United States. Some of the known causes of male infertility include chromosomal abnormalities, loss of germ cells that produce sperm (which can occur dur-

ing treatment for cancer), deficient hormones, or physical abnormalities. Infertility can be caused by an inadequate number of sperm, or the sperm may be present but not strong enough to penetrate the egg.

A physician's examination should include palpation of the testes and the epididymis to look for possible obstructions that could prevent sperm from traveling out the penis. A rectal examination should be performed to evaluate the prostate and possible abnormalities of the structures involved in ejaculation. Two or more semen analyses should be done. Additional tests may include evaluation of the hormone testosterone. Treatments are directed at the specific causes identified by the couple's history, the physical exams, and testing. (See Chapter 16).

Peyronie's Disease

In Peyronie's disease a firm plaque or growth occurs on the connective tissue of the penis. This plaque can cause pain during an erection and make vaginal penetration difficult. This growth is not malignant and can go away on its own. If it lasts more than one year, surgery may be helpful.

Premature Ejaculation

Ejaculation that occurs just before or shortly after penetration of the woman is considered premature. Often associated with problems in a relationship, it may also be due to inadequate control over the ejaculatory process and does not have a physical cause.

In the past, treatment included efforts to decrease anxiety by concentrating on nonsexual fantasies, use of cerebral depressants or sedatives, and distractive maneuvers such as compressing the glans of the penis. To decrease penile sensation, anesthetic ointments were applied, condoms were used, and penile movement in the vagina was minimized. Today it is recognized that this is a psychological problem that requires behavioral therapy. Such therapy is usually successful when both partners participate.

Priapism

Priapism is a prolonged, often painful penile erection that lasts for more than 4 to 6 hours. It is not associated with sexual desire. Causes are often unclear but include leukemia or sickle cell anemia. Prolonged erections also can result from the use of drugs and injections into the penis to correct erectile problems. The condition must be treated right away by a urologist to prevent permanent damage to the penis.

Prostatitis

An inflammation of the prostate, prostatitis may arise suddenly or be longlasting or recurring. Symptoms include difficulty urinating; pain in the lower back, muscles, joints, or the area between the scrotum and anus; or painful ejaculation. If untreated, prostatitis can cause abscesses, spread of infection, and urinary retention. Prostatitis is diagnosed by a careful digital rectal examination and urinalysis to identify any bacterial infection. When the condition is caused by bacteria, it is treated with antibiotics; hot baths sometimes provide relief from the symptoms.

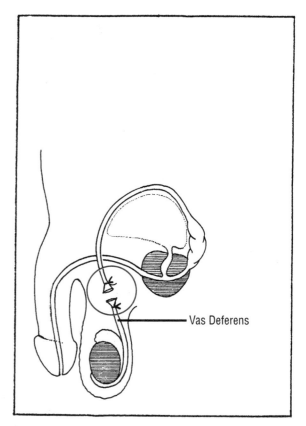

Figure 15.25 Vasectomy
Vasectomy, a form of sterilization for men, is a relatively simple procedure that is very effective for the prevention of pregnancy. A small incision is made in the scrotum, and the vas deferens, the tube through which sperm move from the testes to the urethra, is cut and the ends tied off. Reversal of the procedure has a high success rate.

Retrograde Ejaculation

In retrograde ejaculation, orgasm occurs, but no ejaculate leaves the penis. This condition usually arises after surgery to remove an enlarged prostate, when the muscles around the bladder neck are removed. Instead of being expelled through the penis, sperm enters the urethra near the opening of the bladder and is flushed out with urine. Although a man may be unable to have children, without special assisted techniques, he retains his libido, potency, and ability to have an erection and orgasm.

Testicular Failure

Testicular failure is rare. It is caused by both chromosomal abnormalities as well as damage to the mature testes due to disease or injury. The loss of sex drive

typical with this condition often can be restored through a program of androgen replacement. Fertility cannot be restored.

Varicocele

A swelling in the scrotum caused by enlarged veins, varicocele is common in otherwise healthy men. It is caused by problems with the valves located in the veins leading from the testes. The blockage causes blood to back up, resulting in swelling and infertility. When varicocele causes infertility, surgery is necessary.

PROCEDURES FOR MEN

Nocturnal Penile Tumescence Test

Sleep-associated erections can be monitored with the nocturnal penile tumescence test to evaluate impotence. Normal males have three to five erections per night's sleep. Both intrapenile injections and the penile tumescence test may be used in a complete diagnostic evaluation.

Semen Analysis

Semen is collected from a male after 2 or more days of abstinence. Ideally, two or more samples are taken over a 75–90 day period. A normal sperm count is at least 20 million sperm per milliliter. At least 50 percent of the sperm should be moving, with a significant number moving rapidly forward, and at least 50 percent of the sperm should appear normal on microscopic examina-

tion. This test should be performed as a part of an infertility evaluation.

Vasectomy

About a half million men in the United States have vasectomies each year. A vasectomy is a disruption of the vas deferens. It often is performed through a small puncture in the scrotum through which the vas (tubes that carry sperm from the testes to the urethra) are tied (see Fig. 15.25). No stitching is required, and the operation takes no more than 10 minutes. Recovery takes about 1 week. A semen analysis must be done to make sure the disruption is complete.

Vasectomies are usually reversible. A vasovasectomy is the rejoining of the two ends of the vas; this procedure has a high success rate, and a pregnancy rate of up to 60 percent can result.

CHAPTER 16

Understanding Your Fertility

Satty Gill Keswani, M.D., F.A.C.O.G.

The meeting of a female egg and a male sperm to form a new life is a delicate process that the average woman takes for granted. Yet, a woman can become pregnant only a few days in each menstrual cycle. If intercourse doesn't occur during this fertile period, pregnancy is not likely to happen. And, a woman can become pregnant for only part of her life—between when her periods start and when they end at menopause. As a woman ages, she becomes less fertile. This is true—on a smaller scale—for men as well.

Normal couples have about a 20 percent chance of conceiving with each menstrual cycle if no birth control is used. After 6 months of unprotected intercourse, 60–70 percent of couples will have become pregnant. Infertility, which is the inability to conceive after 1 year of unprotected intercourse, is common, however. An estimated 10–15 percent of couples who are trying to become pregnant will be infertile—perhaps 4.9 million Americans.

Infertility can cause emotional pain for many couples. Some feel as though they are failures if they cannot have children, and they spend much time and money on testing and treatment in their efforts to build a family. Sometimes infertility and the emotional response that often goes along with it strains relationships. Other couples find that infertility is not a big issue. They have happy, productive lives without having children.

Lately infertility has been in the news, and with good reason. Several factors have led to infertility being an increasing problem for couples today:

- The largest group of Americans ever, the baby boomers, are now in the middle of their reproductive years. This means that now more women of reproductive age may be trying to have babies.

- Sexually transmitted diseases (STDs), which can lead to pelvic inflammatory disease (PID) and infertility, are on the rise.

- More women are in the workplace, where they may be exposed to hazards that affect reproduction. Women and men are exposed to more hazards in the environment that can cause problems, too.

- Because so many couples have delayed having families until their thirties or even forties, there is more time for infections and other hazards to work against fertility. Even without such exposure, as couples age it takes longer for pregnancy to occur.

- Delaying childbearing leaves less time in which to have a family. Couples may feel more pressure to conceive in a shorter time.

- An increasing number of infertile couples now seek treatment.

To understand why there may be problems with having a baby, it helps to understand how a baby is conceived and what can go wrong at each stage. A woman and her partner can use this information to increase their chances of having a child and take advantage of medical care to diagnose and treat the problem. About 30–40 percent of all couples treated for infertility conceive at some point. For some causes, this proportion is much higher.

HOW CONCEPTION OCCURS

The conception of a baby depends on the coordination of many factors in both the man and woman (see "The Basic Steps of Fertilization"). The following sequence of events must occur:

1. *Ovulation.* The ovaries release a mature egg.
2. *Fertilization.* The egg is penetrated by a sperm. The cells of the fertilized egg begin multiplying.
3. *Implantation.* The fertilized egg implants in the wall of the uterus.

These three steps are shown in Figure 16.1.

Ovulation

A woman is born with a lifetime supply of immature eggs in her ovaries. Each month, one matures and is released in a process called ovulation. Ovulation is an important part of the menstrual cycle. In a typical 28-

day cycle, a woman's menstrual period begins on day 1. On day 14, ovulation occurs. On day 28, if the egg has not become fertilized, the menstrual cycle begins again with another period.

For ovulation to happen, different parts of the body must all work together. The brain and the ovaries both play roles in this coordination. The ovaries are the two almond-shaped glands sitting within reach of the fallopian tubes. Ovaries produce the eggs as well as the essential sexual hormones needed for menstruation and pregnancy.

Just before ovulation, the hypothalamus and pituitary glands in the brain signal the body to start producing hormones. Follicle-stimulating hormone (FSH) prompts fluid-filled chambers in the ovary called follicles to begin growing. In each follicle, a single ovum is growing as well. Luteinizing hormone (LH) triggers a follicle to rupture, releasing its egg (see Figure 16.1). Most months, only one egg is released.

Women ovulate about 14 days before their next menstrual period would be expected—day 14 on a 28-day cycle. Ovulation occurs within about a day

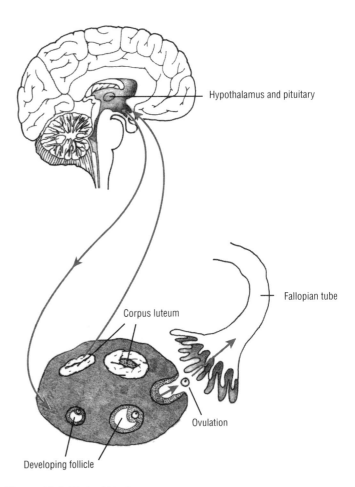

Figure labels: Hypothalamus and pituitary · Fallopian tube · Corpus luteum · Ovulation · Developing follicle

Figure 16.1 The Luteinizing Process
The menstrual cycle consists of a complex series of events that interact to stimulate ovulation, prepare the uterine lining for a pregnancy, and cause the uterine lining to be shed if pregnancy does not occur. Two glands in the brain, the *hypothalamus* and the *pituitary*, send *follicle-stimulating hormone* (FSH) and *luteinizing hormone* (LH) to the ovary just before ovulation to stimulate the development of a follicle and its release of an egg into a fallopian tube (ovulation). Follicles are the structures inside the ovary that produce the eggs to be fertilized and that release the hormone estrogen, which stimulates the lining of the uterus to thicken in preparation for pregnancy. After releasing the egg, the empty follicle, called the *corpus luteum*, begins producing progesterone. This hormone continues to stimulate the uterine lining to grow and thicken. If the egg is not fertilized, a sudden drop in estrogen and progesterone triggers the uterus to shed its lining as menstruation begins. This marks the start of the next cycle.

THE BASIC STEPS OF FERTILITY

Seven elements are essential to fertility:

1. A woman's ovaries must produce healthy eggs that are released regularly.

2. A man's testicles must be capable of producing healthy sperm that can reach the egg and then penetrate it.

3. During intercourse, the man's semen that contains his sperm has to be deposited at or at least close to the cervix. This puts the sperm in the best position to reach the egg.

4. There has to be a clear passage through the fallopian tube from the ovary to the uterus. This passage is used by both the egg moving down and the sperm moving up. Any obstruction in the fallopian tube interrupts the process of fertilization.

5. The man's sperm have to be able to move freely through the cervix. Any physical or chemical barrier can cause problems.

6. The ovum has 12 to 72 hours of life in which it can be fertilized. The sperm have up to 5 days in which they can fertilize an egg. Timing is critical.

7. Once the egg is fertilized, it has to find a suitable site for implantation in the lining of the uterus.

after the surge in LH. Drugstores carry home test kits that can help you track your ovulation hormones and time intercourse appropriately.

Both FSH and LH play additional roles in the menstrual cycle. They instruct the ovaries to produce estrogen and progesterone hormones that help ovulation to occur and the uterus to prepare for pregnancy. The uterus is a hollow organ, shaped like a pear and only about three inches long in a nonpregnant woman. Its lining, the endometrium, is richly supplied with blood vessels. The endometrium continually renews itself, building up in response to messages sent by estrogen and progesterone.

In the first half of a woman's menstrual cycle, estrogen makes the endometrial lining begin to thicken with a nutrient-rich bedding in case pregnancy should occur. Progesterone then takes over. It is produced mainly in the second half of the cycle by a temporary organ called the corpus luteum. The corpus luteum is formed in the ovary from the follicle that released its egg. Progesterone causes the lining of the uterus to thicken even more. Estrogen and progesterone both play roles in ovulation as well.

If the egg is not fertilized, it dissolves and is absorbed by the body. Then, hormone levels drop and the endometrium disintegrates without the hormonal nourishment. This shedding is the monthly menstrual period. The first day of a woman's period is the point at which her hormone levels are at their lowest.

Fertilization

For fertilization to occur, healthy sperm must be placed in a woman's vagina, near the cervix, around the time of ovulation (see Figure 16.2). Each sperm is about 1/1000 of an inch long; its whiplike tail moves it up through the cervix, into the uterus, and into the fallopian tubes. Only one sperm can fertilize an egg, but that one sperm must be strong enough to swim the equivalent of the English Channel at least three times without stopping. Though millions of sperm may start the race, only a few hundred survive the trip.

An egg recently released in ovulation is usually picked up by a nearby fallopian tube. Most women have two fallopian tubes, each about 4 inches long. They are positioned just above the ovaries and come equipped with featherlike fingers called fimbria (that's Latin for fringes) at the ends nearest the ovaries. The fimbria and the inside of the tubes are lined with cilia, millions of tiny hairs. These hairs move the egg from the ovary into the tubes. An egg can be fertilized for only about 12–72 hours after its release.

Mucus, fluids, and cilia move the egg down into the tube. The fallopian tubes have muscular ligaments throughout their lengths. In the middle, they actually

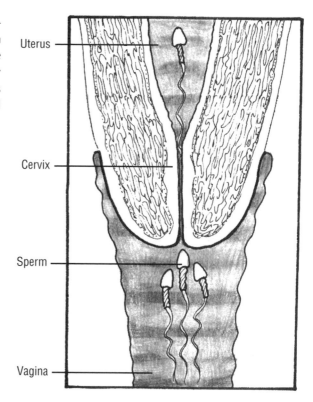

Figure 16.2 Sperm Entering Uterus
For pregnancy to occur, sperm cells (shown here many times their actual size in relation to the cervix) must find their way through the cervix and uterus and into a fallopian tube to the egg.

contract to help the sperm and egg move closer together and toward conception. At the end nearer the uterus, they tighten to close off and keep eggs from being released into the uterus too soon.

When sperm are present, they cluster around the egg. They release enzymes from their heads to help make a hole in the egg to allow penetration. Once one sperm enters the egg, a reaction occurs that prevents other sperm from entering.

Implantation

Inside the fertilized egg, cells begin to divide. If all goes well, the fertilized egg then journeys from the fallopian tube to the uterus where it implants itself in the spongy lining of the uterus. There it grows and develops into an embryo (weeks 2–8), then a fetus for the rest of the pregnancy, and 9 months later, a baby.

Numerous structural and hormonal factors play a part in fertility. What may look like the simplest of human activities—conceiving a baby—can become a miraculous chain of events, especially to a couple having problems getting pregnant.

THE CAUSES OF INFERTILITY

The causes of infertility are multiple, and some are hotly debated in medical circles. In some cases, the reasons are found in the woman (female-factor infertility); in other cases, the cause lies in the man (male-factor infertility). In still other couples, the infertility may be due to a combination of medical problems in both partners (see "Causes of Infertility"). For some couples with infertility, a cause is never found. This can be very upsetting.

One important cause of infertility in both men and women is sexually transmitted diseases (see Chapter 19). Even STDs with no symptoms can cause scarring in a man or woman's reproductive system; such scars block passageways for sperm or eggs. Having several sexual partners increases the chance of getting an STD. An STD can lead to a pelvic inflammatory disease (PID), a severe infection of the uterus and tubes; it can scar and block the tubes, causing infertility later on. To avoid getting STDs, limit sexual partners and use a condom during sex.

Even if a man produces healthy sperm, exposure to certain conditions or subtances may kill them. For example, heat is harmful to sperm. Fevers, long soaks in hot tubs, and tight underwear that keeps the testicles close to the body all can result in temporary drops in sperm counts. It takes 90 days for sperm to mature, so any man who has had a high fever within 3 months may have a low sperm count also (see also "Agents Harmful to Sperm"). Some substances have a permanent effect, while others are only temporary. A man trying to father a child may want to consult with his doctor if he has been exposed to any of these agents.

Other men have difficulty in getting the sperm to the right place. Some are impotent or cannot maintain an erection sufficient to allow intercourse. Others have blockages in the tubes that carry the sperm from the testicles through the penis. These blockages may be caused by infections, some sexually transmitted. In other men, a condition called retrograde ejaculation results in sperm going the wrong way once they reach the penis. Instead of going out the penis, they move backward up into the bladder.

Male-Factor Infertility

Male-factor infertility includes problems with the man's sperm. The difficulty may be with the sperm themselves or the delivery system that takes them from the testicles, where they are formed, through the penis and into the woman's vagina. (See the male reproductive system and a sperm in Chapter 15).

Normally, there are at least 20 million healthy sperm in each milliliter of semen ejaculated. Some men produce no sperm at all or very few. Others may have sperm that are oddly shaped or unable to move properly. Any of these problems can cause infertility.

Female-Factor Infertility

Ovulation Factors

As women age, their ovaries and the immature eggs contained therein age as well. Unlike men who produce new sperm on a regular basis, women are born with all the eggs they'll ever produce. Their eggs may become damaged from years of exposure to hazards such as chemicals or radiation.

Too little estrogen also can cause infertility. As a woman ages and nears menopause, the amount of estrogen produced drops gradually. With less estrogen, the ovaries may not produce an egg each month. The result is fewer babies as a woman ages. Another cause for low estrogen levels is too little body fat. Women who exercise too much or diet excessively—sometimes due to eating disorders—may not produce enough estrogen for ovulation to occur.

Other women with ovulatory problems have sufficient supplies of estrogen but lack other hormones, such as FSH, LH, and prolactin, that affect other aspects of the cycle.

CAUSES OF INFERTILITY

Male factors (30–40 percent)
Tubal and peritoneal factors (25–30 percent)
Ovulation factors (15–20 percent)
Cervical and uterine factors (10 percent)
Antibodies against sperm (5 percent)

AGENTS HARMFUL TO SPERM

Chemotherapy
Radiation treatment
Alcohol
Antibiotics (nitrofurantoin, sulfa drugs)
Ulcer treatments (cimetidine)
Marijuana
Nicotine
Diethylstilbestrol (DES)*
Anabolic steroids (used for body building)
Some lubricants used during sex

* A man's reproductive system can be affected if his mother took DES while pregnant with him.

Certain kinds of birth control continue to reduce ovulation even after they are no longer used. For example, some women who take birth control pills find that it takes them a few months to begin ovulating again once they've stopped taking the pill. After 2–3 years off the pill, however, their rates of ovulation are the same as for other women who use barrier contraception. Contraceptive implants that contain hormones offer a rapid return of fertility. On the other hand, contraceptive injections of hormones may substantially delay the return of fertility. It can take anywhere from 4 to more than 30 months for fertility to return.

Tubal and Peritoneal Factors

Conditions affecting the fallopian tubes or the peritoneum sometimes cause infertility. The peritoneum is a strong sac that lines the inside of the abdomen. It forms a sort of bag that contains the digestive organs and runs alongside the fallopian tubes.

Scarring or blockage in the tubes may cause infertility. One of the most common causes of damaged tubes is infections. When STDs are untreated, they can worsen and move up the uterus into the tubes. This is pelvic inflammatory disease, a major cause of blocked tubes. Use of an intrauterine device increases the risk of infection, especially in young women with several sexual partners. Some researchers say that smoking cigarettes changes the lining of the fallopian tubes, inflaming them and making them less hospitable to conception.

When tubes are damaged, an ectopic pregnancy is more likely if conception occurs. In an ectopic preg-

nancy, the egg is fertilized as in a normal pregnancy but it does not implant in the uterus. Instead, often because the fallopian tubes are damaged, it implants in the tube or somewhere in the peritoneum and begins to grow there. Because it can burst the tube, ectopic pregnancy can be life threatening. If you have a history of pelvic infections, your chances of ectopic pregnancy are four times greater than normal. (See Fig. 16.3.)

Other problems include adhesions, in which nearby organs or tissues bind themselves together. An adhesion that causes another organ to pull on a fallopian tube may move the tube away from the ovary. This prevents the tube from catching the egg when it is released. Adhesions may be caused by infection, previous surgery on the pelvic organs, or endometriosis.

The role of endometriosis in infertility is the subject of great debate among doctors. In endometriosis, tissue like that lining the uterus moves to other places in the abdomen where it begins growing in response to hormones, just as the endometrium does. Such growth can cause pain and inflammation. Up to one-third of infertile women are found to have endometriosis. We do not know if this is just a coincidence or if the endometriosis helps cause the infertility. Severe or extensive endometriosis can cause adhesions. Severe disease is definitely thought to be linked to infertility.

Cervical and Uterine Factors

The cervix is the narrow neck that forms the opening of the uterus to the vagina. It produces mucus that either helps or hinders the movement of sperm, depending on where a woman is in her menstrual cycle. As a woman nears ovulation, mucus thins and becomes slippery and stretchy to help move the sperm through the cervix. The mucus looks much like raw egg white. If the mucus is thick or scanty instead, it is much more difficult for the sperm to move. High levels of nicotine have been found in the cervical mucus of women who smoke. Nicotine can be poisonous to sperm.

Surgery on the cervix may also interfere with fertility. Some types of operations, such as conization (removing a wedge of tissue from the cervix), may result in scarring or little to no mucus production.

The uterus may be affected by infections or adhesions. An infection of the lining of the uterus, endometritis, can be caused by STDs such as gonorrhea. Tuberculosis also can cause endometritis. Overgrowth of the uterine lining, called endometrial hyperplasia, or endometrial cancer can cause infertility as well.

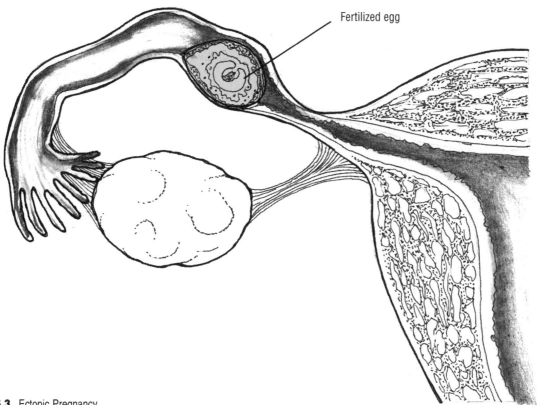

Figure 16.3. Ectopic Pregnancy
In an ectopic pregnancy the fertilized ovum becomes attached in a place other than inside the uterus. Most ectopic pregnancies occur in a fallopian tube. Infertility can result if the tube ruptures or if surgery is needed to repair or remove it.

If a woman has had the lining of her uterus scraped (a D&C or dilation and curettage) after a pregnancy or for abnormal bleeding, the lining may not grow back properly. Adhesions may form, or the lining may be thin; either condition can contribute to infertility.

Growths in the uterus, such as fibroids, have been studied as possible causes of infertility. Although they may play a small role, if any, in infertility, a doctor may remove them if no other cause for infertility is found.

An abnormally shaped uterus, such as one with a thin wall (septum) running down its middle, can affect a woman's ability to have a child. Affected women are born with these defects that cause miscarriage (loss of the baby before it is ready to be born) rather than inability to conceive.

Antibodies against Sperm

Some women and men produce antibodies against sperm. When the immune system malfunctions, it sees the sperm as a foreign threat and produces antibodies to fight them. The antibodies affect the ability of the sperm to move freely.

Unexplained Infertility

Sometimes a reason cannot be found for a couple's infertility. Even without knowing a cause, however, certain steps can be taken to increase the chance of conceiving. Some measures a couple can take themselves. Each month, approximately 3 percent of couples with unexplained infertility conceive on their own.

SELF-CARE FOR INFERTILITY

In some couples, infertility may be the result of a complex medical problem. In others, it may be due to something easily correctable. These suggestions can help you create the best possible conditions for conception:

- Both women and men should avoid getting sexually transmitted diseases, a cause of infertility. If either partner has symptoms of an STD (see Chapter 19), avoid having sex and see a doctor. Early treatment is important to prevent STDs from damaging the reproductive system.

- You are most likely to conceive around 14 days before your next menstrual period is due to begin. If you have a 28-day cycle, this would be days 13–15 of your menstrual cycle (with day 1 being the first day of the last menstrual period). Mark the dates when pregnancy is most likely on a calendar and make time for sex without stress. There is no need for your partner to save up sperm by delaying intercourse before these times. Just try to have intercourse during the middle of your cycle.

- Because sperm need to be kept cool, your partner should avoid tight clothing or underwear, long hot baths, and especially soaks in hot tubs, whirlpools, or saunas.

- During intercourse, all positions can produce pregnancy. After ejaculation, stay in bed for at least a half hour. Don't use any jellies, douches or creams because they can inhibit sperm. Some lubricants affect sperm as well.

- Both you and your partner should avoid the use of any illicit (street) drugs. Some affect fertility, and others harm the fetus if conception occurs.

- Stop smoking and limit your alcohol consumption, since they may interfere with ovulation and sperm production. Some experts even suggest limiting caffeinated beverages, but less is known about the effects of caffeine.

- Maintain a normal weight. Women who are either very overweight or underweight may have problems becoming pregnant.

- Avoid exercising excessively as too much exercise can interfere with ovulation.

Infertility may not be permanent. Many couples simply have reduced fertility and take longer to get pregnant.

FINDING HELP

If pregnancy has not occurred after a year of intercourse without birth control, you may wish to consult a doctor. Because fertility naturally declines with age, couples in their late thirties or forties may not want to wait this long to seek help.

Some couples are able to conceive almost immediately during the two to three months that it takes for the initial medical workup. Others need several months of diagnostic testing and treatment. About 30–40 percent of couples treated for infertility are able to conceive eventually.

Today, even the most difficult cases often can be treated successfully because of medical advances in the study and treatment of infertility during in the last 30 years. Your likelihood of getting pregnant depends on several factors: how long you've been trying to conceive, how old you are, and the exact cause of your infertility.

A variety of physicians may be able to help you find the cause of your infertility and treat it. Start with your obstetrician–gynecologist. She or he can perform the initial series of tests and refer you for further procedures if needed. Although men sometimes seek the assistance of urologists, some gynecologists can help them, too, as a part of treating the couple.

QUESTIONS FOR FERTILITY SPECIALISTS

- Are you board certified in obstetrics and gynecology, reproductive endocrinology, or urology?

- Are you a member of the American Fertility Society? Do you belong to any other special groups in your chosen area?

- How many infertile couples have you treated? What is your overall success rate for live births? (A pregnancy rate may not be as important to you because you are interested in a baby, not just the number of times this doctor has helped a couple get pregnant. Not all pregnancies end in success.)

- What is your hospital affiliation?

Some gynecologists have special interests or training in fertility issues and can coordinate most of the needed care themselves. Some have extra training in reproductive endocrinology, the study of how hor-

THE EMOTIONAL SIDE OF INFERTILITY

Although infertility is quite common, being one among millions may be small comfort. In addition to dealing with the concerns that come up with any medical problem, infertility can pose emotional concerns for some couples. Not every couple is devastated by infertility, however.

Couples that are affected emotionally may feel that their bodies are letting them down. Each menstrual period may remind them that another month has gone by without conceiving. You and your partner may blame each other, leading to strains in your relationship. Problems with fertility can embarrass you and put you on the spot when relatives and friends inquire about your family plans. Wanting to have a child and being unable to can harm a woman's self-esteem, or a man's. If you've been diagnosed with an infertility factor, or if your inability to become pregnant is unexplained, you experience predictable stages ranging from disbelief and denial, to frustration and anger and only after a considerable time, to acceptance.

Share your emotional concerns with your physician or other members of the health care team. Sharing your thoughts and your stress can be a helpful part of the healing process. A caring doctor can help heal the soul as well as the body.

You may want to seek counseling. Many couples contact support groups. The infertility group Resolve, Inc., can provide suggestions.

QUESTIONS TO ASK ABOUT TREATMENT

- What are my chances for getting pregnant? (Ask that the doctor provide information in a way that makes sense to you.)
- How long will the treatment take?
- How much will it cost?
- Is it covered by my insurance?
- What other options are available?
- What are the side effects—both physical and emotional? In the case of fertility drugs, this is a very important question to ask. The risk of multiple births rises dramatically when certain medications are used. If your doctor has suggested this treatment, ask how many women have given birth to twins, triplets, or even quadruplets while taking this particular drug.
- What are the possible complications?
- If surgery is recommended, where will it be performed? Will it require an overnight stay or can it be done on an outpatient basis? Who will perform the surgery?

mones affect fertility. This is a subspecialty of obstetrics and gynecology in which the doctor is required to complete 2 additional years of training in infertility after 4 years of obstetric and gynecological residency, passing both written and oral examinations.

If your own gynecologist does not specialize in infertility, she or he can refer you to a fertility specialist.

Your family physician, a local medical center, or your state or county medical society can suggest referrals as well. The American Fertility Society also can assist you in locating a professional. The infertility workup may take many months to complete. Before you select a doctor as your fertility specialist, consider asking him or her some key questions (see "Questions for Fertility Specialists").

Infertility can be an emotionally trying experience (see "The Emotional Side of Infertility"). The right physician with a competent staff can reduce the anxiety associated with infertility.

DIAGNOSING INFERTILITY

Before any therapy begins, a doctor conducts a complete investigation of both partners; therefore, both must be present at the first visit. It is essential that both be committed in any quest for conception and willing to support each other through the emotional ups and downs of therapy.

The basic workup for infertility involves four areas:

1. Semen analysis
2. Evaluation of ovulation
3. Postcoital test
4. Evaluation of tubes

A detailed medical and sexual history are taken, and various tests and procedures performed to check each area. Even if a difficulty is found in one area, the whole workup is completed in the event other problems need to be considered. If a man produces few sperm, for instance, it would not be helpful to try artificial insemination when his partner has blocked tubes.

Initial Visit

At the initial visit for infertility, the doctor takes a thorough family and personal medical history. Set aside at least 3 to 4 hours for your first visit and be prepared to provide information such as:

- Length and regularity of menstrual cycle
- Any unusual pain or cramping, vaginal discharge, or bleeding
- Previous marriages or pregnancies
- Contraception used
- Sexual habits (frequency, technique, use of lubricants during sex)
- General health (any operations, infections, injuries to reproductive organs)
- Any drug or medication usage (including alcohol and tobacco)
- Length of time you've been trying to get pregnant
- Birth defects in either partner or families

Don't hold back any information out of embarrassment. In fact, before you go, try to think back over your sexual, reproductive, and medical history. Even information that may seem unrelated may be helpful. For example, tuberculosis can affect the uterus as well as the lungs.

Though laboratory tests may be done at that first visit, testing often is scheduled for later. Often, tests must be precisely timed for certain days during the woman's menstrual cycle.

Basic Testing

Testing is a process of elimination in which the doctor rules out problems that may be causing infertility. Some tests are done on the man, and some on the woman.

Some are timed to the woman's menstrual cycle. Others follow sexual intercourse; some are even done at home.

Basic testing looks for problems in the four areas of the workup. Different methods can be used to examine these areas. When a problem is found in one of the four basic areas, additional specialized testing may be needed.

Basal Body Temperature

Developed in the 1930s, the basal body temperature (BBT) test is based on the fact that a woman's body temperature rises with ovulation. Most women have lower readings in the beginning of their menstrual cycles, before ovulation. Then, there is a small rise of 0.5–1°F just after ovulation. Because this test measures a change that occurs *after* ovulation, it cannot help predict when ovulation will occur in a given cycle. However, looking at the results for the past few cycles can show a pattern. Ovulation can be anticipated from this pattern.

For this test, a woman should measure her body temperature each morning while she is still in bed and before eating, drinking, smoking, or going to the bathroom. The temperature may be taken with an ordinary thermometer or with a special one designed for this purpose. If you aren't comfortable reading a mercury-based thermometer, buy one of the varieties that offers an instant digital readout. Whichever you choose, however, be prepared to use the same one each day.

Record the temperature carefully. You may find that it helps to keep track on a chart. Your doctor's office may be able to provide one for you. Because a lack of sleep, drinking alcohol, a fever, or any illness or emotional upset can affect your temperature, mark these changes on your chart, too.

Although keeping a BBT chart may prove to be boring or a nuisance, it can provide valuable information. Record your results each day and bring your chart with you for every visit. Not only can it help your doctor determine when or if you are ovulating but a BBT chart also can suggest hormonal problems interfering with conception.

Blood Tests

Blood tests may be done for both partners. Often the purpose is to measure the levels of hormones that play a role in fertility. These tests may be done at the beginning, middle, and end of the menstrual cycle. Some of the wide variety of hormones that may be tested include:

- FSH (follicle-stimulating hormone)
- LH (luteinizing hormone)
- Prolactin
- Progesterone
- Testosterone
- Thyroid-stimulating hormone

Blood tests also can detect the presence of antibodies to sperm.

Cervical Mucus Tests

Your doctor will examine the cervical mucus when you are most likely to be fertile, around ovulation. At that time, mucus is abundant, clear, glistening, and slippery. The doctor measures how far the mucus stretches. Mucus that stretches a lot is better for fertilization than mucus that is not stretchy. At other times during the menstrual cycle the cervical mucus is less hospitable to sperm. It is thick and cloudy and does not stretch so easily. (Infection, contraceptive creams, and douching cut down on the mucus.)

Endometrial Biopsy

In an endometrial biopsy, a small piece of tissue is taken from the lining of your uterus and studied for evidence of ovulation. This biopsy is performed during the last phase of your cycle, 10–12 days after the LH surge (around days 21–26). The result of an endometrial biopsy is usually compared with the BBT and a blood test for progesterone.

By testing the thickness of the uterine lining, the endometrial biopsy shows whether enough progesterone is present. If there isn't enough progesterone, this may be called a luteal phase defect. Even though it is linked to infertility and miscarriage, this defect is poorly understood. It can be treated with ovulation drugs or progesterone. Endometrial biopsy also can test for endometritis, endometrial hyperplasia, and endometrial cancer.

Hysterosalpingography

Hysterosalpingography (HSG) is a series of X-rays performed to see a woman's reproductive organs. It is sometimes referred to as the dye test. A technician injects a radio-opaque dye into the cervix. This dye fills up the uterus and travels up into the fallopian tubes. On an X-ray, it reveals any scarring or blocking. Done on an outpatient basis, a HSG helps the doctor find blockages in your tubes and any abnormalities in the uterus such as polyps (small growths in the uterus) or fibroids. Conditions detected by HSG are often confirmed by hysteroscopy, a procedure that allows the doctor to look directly inside the uterus.

Laparoscopy

In laparoscopy, a thin, lighted tube (like a telescope) is inserted into a small cut in the abdomen. By looking through the scope, the doctor can inspect the ovaries, tubes, and the outside of the uterus. Laparoscopy can check for endometriosis, blockages in the tubes at the end near the ovaries, and adhesions.

Postcoital Test

The postcoital test often is performed along with cervical mucus tests. It is done soon after intercourse, around the time of ovulation. The doctor examines the mucus and checks the number of active sperm cells in the vagina, cervix, and uterine cavity. If the cervical mucus is inhibiting healthy sperm, this will be clear from the test. Tests (2–8 hours after intercourse) can show how well the sperm get through the mucus. Later tests (12–18 hours after intercourse) can check how well the sperm survive.

Semen Analysis

Semen analysis determines the concentration, normal movement or motility, and percentage of normal sperm cells in semen. Usually, a sample of sperm is collected through masturbation at the lab. Men opposed to masturbation or who cannot perform on demand can use special collection pouches during sex. A sample not produced at the lab should be brought in within 1 hour.

The sperm count is conducted by examining the sample under a microscope. The shape of the sperm is another important factor. Most experts believe that abnormally shaped sperm can't fertilize an egg. How well the sperm move also is studied.

Ask to see a written comprehensive semen analysis report from your doctor. Keep in mind that sperm production is not always the same even in the same man. Probably the doctor will want to do the semen analysis at least three times over a 2- to 4-week period. The only exception to this might be if a man has a zero sperm count. When this happens, the doctor could halt the analysis after two tests, instead of prolonging the process.

Specialized Testing

Once the initial tests have been completed, the doctor usually has a good idea of what may be causing a couple to be infertile. She or he may suggest extra tests to confirm the diagnosis. Alternatively, all tests may be normal, and additional tests may be done to find a cause.

Cultures for Infection

Cultures can identify the type of organism causing an infection. Some of the organisms that may cause infection include *Chlamydia, Gonorrhea, Ureaplasma,* and *Mycoplasma,* as well as the organism that causes tuberculosis. Knowing the cause of infection is the first step toward proper treatment.

If there are signs of infection in the cervical mucus tests, cervicitis (inflammation of the cervix) may be interfering with the production of mucus. Cultures may be done to find out what type of infection, if any, is present. Cultures also may be done if an endometrial biopsy suggests endometritis. In men, cultures of the semen are sometimes done as well.

Hysteroscopy

With hysteroscopy, the doctor uses a thin, lighted telescopelike tube to examine the inside of the uterus. After the scope is passed through the cervical opening, the doctor inspects the uterus, its lining, and the opening of the tubes into the uterus. Because the procedure allows viewing the uterus itself, and not just an image of it, it can confirm other tests such as hysterosalpingography.

Imaging Techniques

When the doctor suspects a blockage in the man's reproductive system, imaging techniques such as ultrasound or special X-rays may be used. Ultrasound uses high-frequency sound waves to form clear images of the reproductive tract. In a woman, ultrasound also can monitor follicle development to see if ovaries are producing eggs ready for ripening and fertilization. Using a series of ultrasound scans a few days apart, experts have even found that up to 30 percent of women with previously undetermined infertility produce eggs that ripen but never release from the ovaries. Ultrasound can show how thick or receptive the uterine lining is at midcycle. Pelvic abnormalities or adhesions can be detected as well.

Sperm Antibody Testing

If the doctor suspects an immunological cause for the infertility—or if no cause has been found—sperm antibody testing may be done. In this test, the semen and sperm are mixed with special substances, such as beads coated with an antibody. The sperm are then checked to see if they bind to the beads.

Sperm Penetration Tests

If the ability of the sperm to fertilize an egg needs to be examined, sperm penetration tests may be done. In these tests, sperm are mixed with specially treated hamster eggs to measure how often penetration of the eggs occurs. (The difference between humans and hamsters is so great that nothing grows from the penetrated egg.) Similar tests can be done with human eggs.

TREATING INFERTILITY

Based on the findings of testing, the doctor will come up with a plan for therapy and will try to treat the problem causing the infertility. Drug treatment, hormone treatment, or surgery may be suggested. If that doesn't work, it may be possible to conceive with one of the new assisted reproductive technologies (ARTs).

Whatever the treatment plan, be prepared to ask questions about it (see "Questions to Ask About Treatment"). Listen carefully to the answers. Try to listen with your head and not your heart. Choose treatments carefully, for treatment failures can be demoralizing for

many couples. Some of the treatment options you may have are described here.

Medical Treatment

Some conditions, such as an under- or overactive thyroid, can be treated with medication. Other possible medical treatments include antibiotic therapy for any infections that may have become evident during the workup.

GENERAL PUBLICATIONS ON INFERTILITY

Allen, M., and S. Marks. *Miscarriage. Women Sharing from the Heart.* New York: John Wiley & Sons, 1993.

Berger, Gary S.; Marc Goldstein; and Mark Fuerst. *The Couple's Guide to Fertility.* New York: Doubleday, 1990.

Franklin, Robert R., and Dorothy K. Brockman. *In Pursuit of Fertility.* New York: Henry Holt, 1990.

Glazer, Ellen S. *The Long-Awaited Stork: A Guide to Parenting After Infertility.* Lexington, Mass.: Lexington Books, 1990.

Harkness, Carla. *The Infertility Book: A Comprehensive Medical and Emotional Guide.* 2nd ed. Berkeley, Calif: Celestial Arts Press, 1992.

Karow, William G.; William C. Gentry; Christopher Hsiung; and Andrienne Pope. *A Baby of Your Own. New Ways to Overcome Infertility.* Dallas: Taylor Publishing Company, 1992.

Levin, Paul. *Infertility—Exploring the Male Factor.* 7 Moore Road, Hopewell Junction, New York, NY 12533. 1993. VHS video, 47 minutes.

Liebmann-Smith, Joan. *In Pursuit of Pregnancy.* New York: Newmarket Press. 1989.

Novotny, Pamela Patrick. *What You Can Do About Infertility.* New York: Dell Publishing, 1991.

Office of Consumer/Business Education, Bureau of Consumer Protection, The Federal Trade Commission. *Facts for Consumers: Infertility Services.* Washington, DC 20580. 1990.

Robin, Peggy. *How to Be a Successful Fertility Patient.* New York: William Morrow, 1993.

Rosenberg, Helane S., and Yakov M. Epstein. *Getting Pregnant When You Thought You Couldn't.* New York: Warner Books, 1993.

Scher, Jonathan, and Carol Dix. *Preventing Miscarriage: The Good News.* New York: Harper Perennial, 1991.

Sha, Janet L. *Mothers of Thyme: Customs and Rituals of Infertility and Miscarriage.* Ann Arbor, Mich.: Lida Rose Press, 1990.

Ovulation Induction

If a woman does not ovulate, one thing that can be tried is using drugs or hormones to bring on, or induce, ovulation. This also is done with ART to prompt the body to produce more than one egg at a time. One of the most common medicines used for ovulation induction is clomiphene citrate. Others include:

- Gonadotropins
- Bromocriptine
- Gonadotropin-releasing hormone

These medicines are taken for certain days during the menstrual cycle. While using any of these treatments, a woman is tested to identify if and when ovulation occurs. BBT, progesterone tests, LH tests, and ultrasound can be used for this.

With most of these methods, about 80–90 percent of women begin ovulating. The pregnancy rate is lower—the exact rate depends on other factors that could be adding to the infertility. Several of the methods may result in more than one egg being released and thus increase the chance for multiple pregnancies.

Surgery

Several conditions can be treated by surgery, including blocked tubes, adhesions, and growths or defects in the uterus. The operation may involve a traditional opening in the abdomen, or it may be performed through a laparoscope or a hysteroscope.

Artificial Insemination

If the man produces few healthy sperm or none at all, artificial insemination by a donor may allow the couple to conceive a child. In this method, sperm from carefully selected donors is placed in the woman's uterus (see Figure 16.4). The American Fertility Society

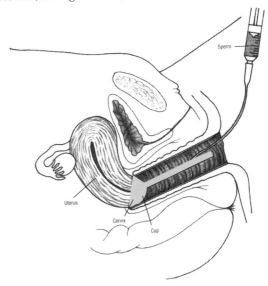

Figure 16.4 Artificial Insemination
Artificial insemination is one method by which a couple who have been unable to conceive may achieve pregnancy. A small cup attached to a hollow stem is inserted into the vagina. The cup is fitted over the cervix, and sperm are introduced into the uterus through a long tube attached to the stem. The stem is then withdrawn, leaving the cup in place over the cervix. It can be removed by the woman after 2-3 hours.

recommends using frozen sperm. This allows the sperm donors to be monitored for STDs before the sperm is used. In some cases, if the male partner has some healthy sperm, special washings and concentrating treatments can allow the use of his sperm in artificial insemination.

Assisted Reproductive Technologies

In the past two decades, the miracle of test-tube babies has revolutionized fertility treatment. Test-tube babies are created through one of the several types of ARTs. Centers all over the world, and perhaps in your own neighborhood, specialize in ART. These technologies can help get around situations like blocked fallopian tubes, cervical problems, low sperm counts, and unexplained infertility. They have provided a ray of hope for many infertile couples.

In ART, sperm and eggs taken from a man and woman are combined either in the woman's body or in a lab. Depending on the cause of the couple's infertility, the egg and sperm can come from the couple or from donors. For a woman, the process of obtaining the eggs can be complex. She must take medications that prompt her body to produce more than one egg. If an egg is used from a donor, the infertile woman's menstrual cycle needs to be altered to the same rhythm as the donor's. While all this is occurring, events may be monitored with blood tests of hormone levels and ultrasound.

Although ART is one of the fastest growing areas of infertility treatments, it has been largely unregulated. In a few cases, unscrupulous practitioners have preyed on the desperation of couples seeking to have a baby. Success rates vary widely, based on how they are reported. For instance, a center may describe its success rates in pregnancies, but not all of those pregnancies result in the birth of a baby. Some pregnancies do not continue to term or are lost so early that they are only recognized by a chemical test. Be sure to investigate before signing up for ART procedures at any clinic or program. Find out what the chance is of actually having a child—ask about the "take home baby" rate. If you are over 40, your chances of success with any ART are less than those of a younger woman. ART does not work for everyone.

While ART does not work for some women, for others it works too well. In many forms of ART, a fertilized egg is placed in the woman's body. To increase the chances of success, more than one may be placed. If all the eggs take, a woman can have twins, triplets, or

even more babies. Another problem with ART is its cost. Each attempt at pregnancy may cost thousands of dollars. Often, ART is not covered by health insurance.

Just as with other treatments, ART works best in certain situations. The different types of ART and when they work best are described next.

In vitro fertilization

In vitro fertilization, or IVF, comes from the Latin for "within a glass." It refers to combining the eggs and sperm in a small glass dish in a laboratory. The fertilized egg or eggs that result are placed in the woman's uterus (see Figure 16.5).

Once this technique was available only to women with defects in their fallopian tubes preventing the sperm and egg from meeting. Now, other couples may benefit from IVF, too:

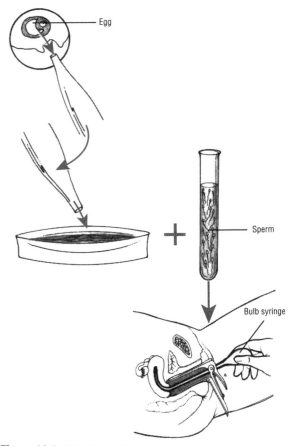

Figure 16.5 In Vitro Fertilization

In vitro fertilization (IVF) can be used to treat infertility in certain couples. The woman is given medication to help stimulate the production of multiple eggs. The eggs are then collected and placed in a laboratory dish, mixed with sperm, and incubated for 1 or 2 days. The fertilized eggs are then introduced into the woman's cervix with a bulb syringe.

- Men with inadequate sperm counts—With IVF, the sperm can be pooled together to increase the numbers.

- Women who do not ovulate—Donor eggs can be used and combined with the man's sperm.

- Women with cervical mucus that hinders sperm—IVF places the fertilized egg in the uterus, so the cervix is bypassed.

According to the American Fertility Society, the pregnancy rate for women who had undergone IVF in the United States is about 15 percent per treatment cycle. Higher rates are found in women younger than 40 years old whose partners had no problems. Some women require only one series of IVF treatments; others choose to have several IVFs. However, successful pregnancies vary from program to program. The price of IVF also differs depending on where you are treated; generally, costs can climb up to $8,000.

Gamete intrafallopian transfer

Gamete intrafallopian transfer, or GIFT, is an alternative to IVF for women with at least one functioning fallopian tube. Since the pregnancy rate is higher with GIFT than with IVF, some experts now recommend GIFT in other circumstances as well. When there is some question about the ability of the sperm to fertilize the egg, IVF is most likely be used.

Using much the same procedure as IVF, gametes (a male and female sex cell or a sperm and egg) are removed from each partner. Then, these gametes are injected together directly into the woman's fallopian tube without trying to bring them together in a laboratory dish for fertilization. The natural movement of the fallopian tube sends the fertilized egg to the uterus for implantation.

This technique may be more acceptable to people who do not want to interfere with nature by having conception take place in a laboratory. Pregnancy is more likely with GIFT than IVF. The pregnancy rate for women who have undergone GIFT is about 27 percent per treatment cycle.

Other variations

Other variations of IVF and GIFT exist. All involve removal of either a woman's own ripened eggs or a donor's, some type of artificial insemination using either her mate's or a donor's sperm, and then transfer of the egg and sperm back into her body.

WHEN TREATMENT FAILS

Even though today's medicine can help many couples have babies, some couples go through all the testing and all the treatment and are still infertile. They may invest years and thousands of dollars in fruitless efforts. For many of these couples, it is hard to give up the search for the one new test or treatment that may finally give them a baby. Although it can be very painful to finally admit that having a baby is not going to be possible, there comes a time for each infertile couple when this is the wisest and kindest step to take.

After taking some time to adjust and accept their situation, some infertile couples realize that they can have a full and happy life without children. Others seek to involve children in their lives in other ways. Some adopt, serve as foster parents, or use a surrogate to have a baby. Still others take a more active role with their nieces or nephews or volunteer with an organization that works with children.

Adoption can be a complex process; couples who are considering it should seek advice from their doctors or reputable adoption agencies. There is a waiting period while the adoption application is processed and reviewed, and fees must be paid. The demand is highest for healthy infants, so couples who wish to adopt one of these children may have to wait longer. Because of the smaller demand for children with disabilities and older children, couples wishing to adopt such children may have a shorter waiting period.

A fairly new option is using surrogate parents. The couple can contract with a woman to bear a child for them. The couple will be the child's genetic parents if they donate the sperm and egg placed in the surrogate's uterus. Or, if both donor eggs and sperm are used, neither partner will be related to the child. Surrogacy presents many complex legal and ethical issues for a couple to consider. It requires careful thought and planning, as well as legal advice.

FOR MORE INFORMATION

Several groups can provide you with information and support for infertility:

- The American Fertility Society can answer any concerns you might have about reproductive medicine or biology. Write to American Fertility Society, 1209 Montgomery Highway, Birmingham, AL 35216-2809; 205-978-5000. The society has compiled an extensive list of publications, a few of which are listed under "General Publications on Infertility"). Look for them at your local library or bookstore or contact the publishers noted.

- The American College of Obstetricians and Gynecologists offers a resource center that can provide you with pamphlets and answers to basic questions about infertility and women's health. Write to American College of Obstetricians and Gynecologists, 409 12th Street SW, Washington, DC 20024-2188; 202-638-5577.

- RESOLVE, Inc., is a group designed to bring infertile individuals together to share resources and stories. It can be a good source of support for couples struggling with infertility. For the group nearest you, write to Resolve National Headquarters, 5 Water Street, Arlington, MA 02174.

CHAPTER 17

Pregnancy and Childbirth

Susan Aucott Ballagh, M.D.,
& Barbara Bartlik, M.D.

Few words trigger a wider range of emotional reactions in women than, "You're pregnant!" Some women are simply ecstatic about their new pregnant state and almost ready to name the baby they won't meet for many months. Other women are frightened and uncertain about their condition and not quite ready for the upheaval a child can bring. Yet no matter how a woman reacts psychologically, ignorance is never bliss when it comes to pregnancy and childbirth. The more information a woman has about this special time, the better equipped she is to meet its challenges.

In almost no other stage of life are there so many changes and challenges in such a brief time. For most women, pregnancy lasts approximately 40 weeks or 280 days, counting from the first day of the last menstrual period (see "How to Calculate Your Due Date"). Compared to the number of years in a healthy woman's life, 280 days isn't a very long time.

During pregnancy, a woman is really two people at once; she's eating, breathing, and being responsible for her own health as well as that of her baby. It is an exciting time, but one that can be filled with conflicting emotions. Most pregnant women face uncertainties

HOW TO CALCULATE YOUR DUE DATE

To calculate your due date...

- Count 280 days from the first day of your last period.

or

- Count back three months from the first day of the last menstrual period and add seven days.

This is only a guide. Very few women actually deliver their babies on this expected day of arrival.

about pregnancy and some anxiety about what the future holds. You can be better prepared if you plan for your pregnancy and what it will entail, understand the changes that are taking place and learn ways to cope with them, and become actively involved in your prenatal care.

PRECONCEPTIONAL CARE

A woman who is planning to become pregnant may benefit from preconceptional care (see "Components of Preconceptional Care"). Such care is usually provided by an obstetrician-gynecologist. It is designed to identify risks or problems before pregnancy, provide information about any special needs a woman may have to prepare for pregnancy, and make sure a woman is as healthy as possible before she becomes pregnant.

Preconceptional care is important because the organs of the fetus (unborn baby) begin to form as early as day 17 of the pregnancy. The fetus may be exposed to health risks before a woman or her doctor even know she is pregnant. Preconceptional care is especially important for women who have certain medical conditions, such as hypertension and diabetes, which can affect the health of the fetus if they are not under control before pregnancy. Multivitamins containing at least 400 micrograms of folic acid reduce fetal malformations.

COMPONENTS OF PRECONCEPTIONAL CARE

The following items may be covered during a preconceptional visit:

- Assessment of medical, reproductive, and family history; nutritional status; drug exposures

- Possible effects of pregnancy on existing medical conditions

- Genetic concerns

- Immunization against infections

- Laboratory tests

- Nutritional counseling

- Discussion of social, financial, and psychological issues and concerns

IN THE BEGINNING

Every month, at about day 14 of a 28-day menstrual cycle, one of a woman's ovaries releases an egg; this is called ovulation. If a man's sperm penetrates the egg, fertilization takes place. The sperm fuses with the egg and forms a single cell. This cell begins to divide and travel down the fallopian tube. It reaches the uterus about the fourth day after fertilization. Now a cluster of about 100 fluid-filled cells, the egg floats until day five to eight when it becomes implanted in the lining of the uterus (endometrium).

The outer cells start to spread into the lining to form a blood supply right next to the mother's blood system, called the placenta. The placenta is actually a life-support system because it provides the fetus with food and oxygen and takes away waste products. The placenta also produces human chorionic gonadotropin (hCG), the hormone which signals the beginning of a new life. This hormone maintains the corpus luteum in the ovary which provides progesterone to the growing fetus.

The placenta connects the mother and the fetus. The umbilical cord links the fetus to the placenta. The fetus floats in a sac of amniotic fluid throughout pregnancy. This fluid regulates the unborn baby's temperature and acts as a shock absorber, protecting the fetus from injury.

CONFIRMING PREGNANCY

Even though every woman is different, in the first weeks after conception, some early signs of pregnancy occur. Some of these symptoms may disappear completely after the end of the first three months of pregnancy.

- Missing a period (it is possible to be pregnant and still bleed around the time a period would normally occur)
- Tender breasts
- Nausea and vomiting, often (but not always) in the mornings
- Fatigue
- Need to urinate frequently
- Aching or heaviness in the pelvic area

Kits for home pregnancy testing are available in most pharmacies. All rely on a chemical that, when combined with your urine in a little test tube, changes colors in the presence of hCG. Follow the directions of home kits carefully. Though up to 98 percent correct, if the test is performed too early, before hCG levels have risen, the results can be falsely negative. The test should be done at least 10–14 days after a period has been missed. It may be necessary to repeat the test.

About two weeks after a missed period, a doctor, nurse-midwife, or health care practitioner can confirm the pregnancy by testing a sample of blood or urine and examining the pelvic organs to detect changes that occur during pregnancy. Make plans then to begin a prenatal care program.

PROFESSIONAL SUPPORT

Care during pregnancy and birth can be provided by an obstetrician, a family practitioner, or a nurse-midwife. Ideally, a health professional should be selected before pregnancy. If you don't already have a doctor or nurse-midwife in whom you have confidence and trust, start searching for one right away. Recommendations can be made by family and friends, as well as the local medical society.

The American College of Obstetricians and Gynecologists can provide a list of specialists in the area. Write to their resource center at 409 Twelfth Street SW, Washington, DC 20024. To find a nurse-midwife, contact the American College of Nurse-Midwives, 1522 K Street NW, Washington, DC 20005, and send a self-addressed, stamped envelope.

To check the credentials of any physician in a specialty, phone the American Board of Medical Specialists' toll-free number, 800-776-2378. Specialists like obstetrician-gynecologists have 4 years of extra training beyond medical school and have passed certifying exams in their area of expertise. This information is available via the hotline.

Following are some points to consider when selecting a health care provider:

■ In what hospital does the doctor or midwife have privileges to practice? Is the location convenient?

■ How much will care cost and what does the fee include? What type of insurance is accepted? What does it cover?

■ What type of birthing rooms are available? Are there choices regarding the setting?

■ What are the health professionals' policies regarding episiotomies (a cut made between the vagina and the anus near the end of labor to help the baby's head pass through)? What options are available for pain relief?

■ Can special care be provided for any complications that you may have?

■ Is there a special neonatal unit or, if not, where will any baby who needs extra help be transferred?

The setting for giving birth should also be considered. Some hospitals have equipped labor rooms, called birthing rooms, with special beds and technical supports so labor and delivery can take place in one room, instead of moving the woman to a delivery room for birth. An alternative birthing center is a facility separate from the hospital where women give birth. Some have a relationship with a hospital so facilities can be shared and others do not. Most have comfortable settings for childbirth.

An interview with a provider being considered may be useful to answer these questions or any others that arise. Once a provider has been selected, prenatal care (a program of care for a pregnant woman before the birth of her baby) should begin.

PRENATAL CARE

With an uncomplicated pregnancy, visits to the doctor or nurse-midwife usually take place once a month during the initial six months and then every two or three weeks thereafter. The first visit is longer than the others and includes a health history, a thorough physical examination (including blood pressure, height and weight measurements), and tests. The internal reproductive organs are examined to check for changes in the cervix and the size of the uterus. Tests performed at the first visit include:

■ Blood tests to check for the blood type, Rh factor, anemia, immunity to rubella (German measles), hepatitis B virus, and some sexually transmitted diseases (STDs).

■ Urine tests to give information about sugar (which might be a sign of diabetes), protein (signaling possible kidney changes), and signs of infection.

■ A Pap test to detect changes in the cervix that could be an early sign of cancer.

Some tests may be repeated at subsequent visits. Other tests may be offered based on risk factors (see "Prenatal Care"). These tests include those to detect genetic disorders, some of which are offered routinely and some of which are recommended for special circumstances. (See Chapter 14).

After the first visit, most visits can be brief. Each one, however, is a good opportunity to ask questions and gather information on prenatal classes (see "Childbirth Preparation"). Each prenatal visit includes:

■ Sampling urine to check for sugar and protein

■ Measuring blood pressure to see if levels are normal

■ Assessing weight to be sure you are gaining enough

■ Listening to the heartbeat of the fetus (after 12 weeks)

■ Checking the size and position of the uterus and fetus

PRENATAL TESTS

The following prenatal tests may be offered to certain women based on their patient histories and the results of routine tests:

Maternal Serum Screening. Certain tests can be performed on the mother's blood to detect substances from the fetus that could signal a birth defect. These tests are usually offered to all women at about 15–18 weeks of pregnancy. One of the substances tested is alpha-fetoprotein (AFP). High levels could be a sign of a neural tube defect, which results when the brain or spinal cord do not develop properly. Low levels could be a sign of Down's syndrome. In some cases, the AFP test is combined with other tests to give more accurate results. Abnormal results require further testing, but most babies tested turn out to be normal.

Ultrasound. Ultrasound creates a picture of the fetus by beaming sound waves into the body and reflecting them on a screen. It is done if there is a question about the status or age of the fetus or to confirm the results of other tests. It can be done at various times during pregnancy, depending on the reason. A thin layer of jelly is rubbed on the mother's belly, and a handheld instrument, called a transducer, is passed over it. Ultrasound determines whether the baby is growing normally, positioning in the womb, abnormalities, or if there is more than one fetus.

Amniocentesis. For an amniocentesis test, the fetal cells in the amniotic fluid are analyzed for signs of birth defects. This test is performed between the 14th and 18th week of pregnancy. A small amount of fluid is removed with a needle from the sac surrounding the baby. The test is recommended for women 35 or older at the time of delivery because they have a higher risk of having a baby with Down's syndrome. In addition, it is given to women who have had a previous child with a birth defect, or who have a family or personal history that places them at risk for an inherited disease. Amniocentesis also may follow abnormal serum tests. There is a small risk of miscarriage with the test. (See Fig. 17.1)

Chorionic Villus Sampling (CVS). A sample of chorionic villi, the fetal blood vessels that form part of the placenta, is removed and analyzed for this test. It is done at 10–12 weeks of pregnancy. CVS is offered for chromosomal screening. This test may not be available in all areas, and there is a slight risk of miscarriage. Some women choose this test over amniocentesis because the results are available earlier.

Fetal Monitoring. Two forms of monitoring may be done during pregnancy, usually in the last 10 weeks, to check the well-being of the fetus. One is the nonstress test, which measures the fetal heartrate in response to its own movements. The other is the contraction stress test that measures how the fetal heart rate responds to the stress of a uterine contraction. For both tests, a device is strapped to the mother's abdomen and the results are recorded on a tracing. For the contraction stress test, mild uterine contractions are induced with a drug called oxytocin.

At each prenatal visit you should discuss with your doctor any changes that may have occurred since the last visit. Also, share any concerns you have and discuss how you should modify your lifestyle to promote a healthy pregnancy.

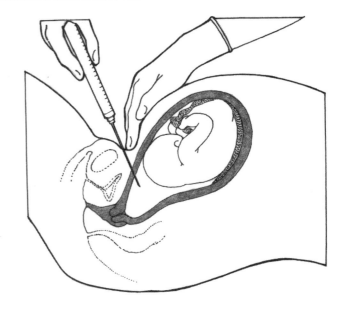

Figure 17.1 Amniocentesis
A needle is inserted into the uterus to obtain a sample of the amniotic fluid. This fluid contains cells of the fetus that can be studied to detect disorders.

CHILDBIRTH PREPARATION

Childbirth preparation can include lectures, exercise instructions, and tours of maternity/obstetrics departments. They may combine several theories of how to manage labor. There are various techniques. Most courses can be taken in a hospital or privately.

Lamaze. Named after a French doctor, Fernand Lamaze, these classes stress breathing exercises for each stage of labor, along with relaxation techniques. Also emphasized is the need to focus on something almost hypnotically to take your mind off your labor pains.

Dick-Read. Grantly Dick-Read is a British doctor whose theories and classes emphasize abdominal breathing and focusing on the feelings and signals the body sends during labor.

Bradley. The method developed by Denver obstetrician Robert Bradley is closer to Dick-Read than to Lamaze in theory. Couples learn how to relax and breathe deeply. Emphasis is on doing what comes naturally, the presence of fathers at labor and delivery, nutrition during pregnancy, and knowing all the options beforehand.

La Leche. The Spanish phrase, *the milk,* is the name of this organization founded in the 1950s to promote breast-feeding in the United States. Its local groups and books provide information as well as emotional support for breast-feeding mothers.

GROWTH AND DEVELOPMENT

When the fertilized egg becomes implanted in the uterus it begins to divide and grow. For the first 8 weeks of pregnancy, the egg is called an embryo. After that, it is called a fetus, which literally means "young one."

First Month (See Fig. 17.2)

- Inside a fluid-filled sac, the embryo has a simple brain, spine, and central nervous system.
- The circulatory system as well as the start of a digestive system have begun to form.

Second Month (See Fig. 17.3)

- The heart begins to beat in the tiny body, somewhere between the size of an apple seed and a green grape (½ inch).
- Spots appear where eyes will form and a face is almost recognizable.
- Arms and legs are present as little buds growing longer each day.
- An outline of the nervous system is present and major internal organs appear in a simple form.

Third Month (See Fig. 17.4)

- The fetus is the size of a tennis ball, about 2½ inches long and weighs about one-twentieth of a pound (14 grams).

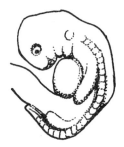
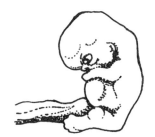

Figure 17.2 Five-Six Weeks   **Figure 17.3** Seven-Eight Weeks

- Fingers and toes are now in place.
- Ears, as well as earlobes, are developed.

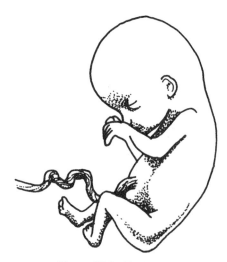

Figure 17.4 Twelve Weeks

- Eyelids close over the eyes and the muscles of the face are mature enough to allow movement of the face and lips.
- Vocal cords are complete.

Fourth Month (See Fig. 17.5)

- The fetus is fully formed and approximately 5 inches long, weighing about 4 ounces (110 grams). Using the placenta as a lifeline, the fetus now takes in lots of oxygen, food, and water.
- The fetus can suck a thumb.
- Eyebrows and eyelashes are growing.
- The fetal heart beats twice as fast as the mother's and can be heard with a special listening device (doppler unltrasound).

Fifth Month (See Fig. 17.6)

- An old-fashioned term referring to fetal movement is *quickening,* generally thought to mean "feeling life." It feels like a faint flutter, a slight tickling sensation, or perhaps even bubbles.

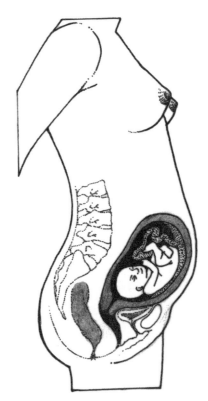

Figure 17.6 Five Months

- The unborn baby has hair on the head and is developing teeth. It is 6½ inches long and weighs ¾ of a pound (350 grams).
- A white, greasy substance called vernix covers the skin and protects it.
- Fine hair called lanugo covers the fetus.
- Facial features are wrinkled and shriveled.

Sixth Month (See Fig. 17.7)

- The fetus tries out leg and arm muscles often and can have periods of frenzied activity, kicking, punching, and even turning somersaults.
- Ten inches long and about 2 pounds (1000 grams), the fetus can cough, hiccup, and respond to sudden noises.

Seventh Month (See Fig. 17.8)

- The baby's eyes have opened and taste buds are forming. The part of the brain that controls intelligence and temperament is developing. Soon evidence of a personality appears.
- The baby's skin is wrinkled but an underlayering of fat is slowly building. Lungs are better

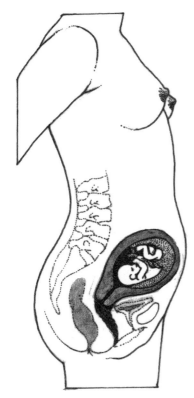

Figure 17.5 Four Months

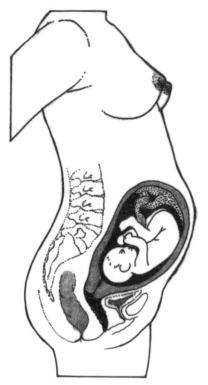

Figure 17.7 Six Months

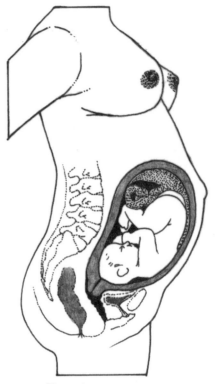

Figure 17.9 Eight Months

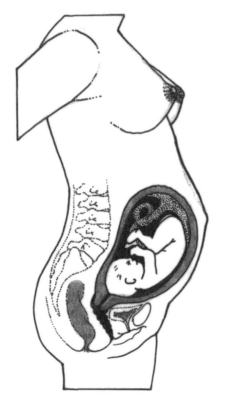

Figure 17.8 Seven Months

developed, but a substance called surfactant is still missing. Surfactant keeps newborn lungs from collapsing between each breath.

■ The baby is now 12 inches long and weighs about 3½ pounds (1700 grams).

Eighth Month (See Fig. 17.9)

■ The fetus is probably in the position in which most babies are born: head down, pushing on the pubic area, especially if this is a first birth. This is the cephalic position.

■ Bones harden, but the head bones remain soft and flexible for delivery.

■ The baby measures about 16 inches and weighs about 5½ pounds (2500 grams).

Ninth Month (See Fig. 17.10)

- The baby gains about an ounce a day now. If it's a boy, the testicles have descended.

- Nails have grown to cover fingers and toes.

- The lanugo hair and most of the vernix disappear.

Full Term

- A substance called meconium is now present in the baby's intestines. This becomes the first bowel movement after birth.

- At term (40 weeks) the average baby is about 20 inches long and weighs 7½ pounds (normal range is 6–9 pounds).

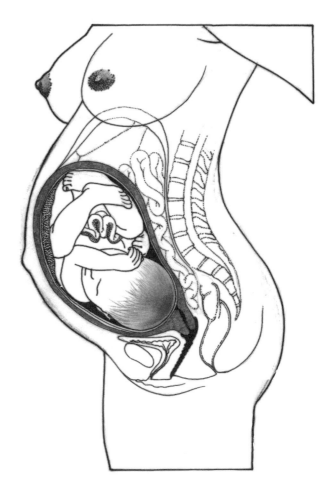

Figure 17.10 Nine Months
The fetus drops into the birth position as your due date nears.

GOOD HEALTH DURING PREGNANCY

There are ways a pregnant woman can help ensure the health of her baby. They include avoiding things that could be harmful to the fetus in crucial stages of development. During the first three months of pregnancy, often referred to as the first trimester, the unborn baby's organs are forming. Anything that the mother eats, drinks, and breathes is passed on to the fetus. For this reason, pregnant women should avoid things that can cause complications during pregnancy or be harmful to the fetus:

- Do not smoke tobacco, drink alcohol, or take any form of drug unless it is prescribed by a doctor. Tobacco deprives the fetus of oxygen. Alcohol can lead to fetal alcohol syndrome (mental retardation plus other effects). Drugs can prevent the baby from developing properly. Babies can also be born addicted to drugs.

WHERE DOES THE WEIGHT GO?

A woman of average weight should gain about 30 pounds during her pregnancy. Here is how it's distributed:

- 38% baby
- 22% blood and fluid
- 20% womb, breasts, buttocks, legs
- 11% amniotic fluid
- 9% placenta

- Avoid sources of infection. Certain infections can cause birth defects when passed to the fetus during pregnancy or birth. They include toxoplasmosis, an infection caused by a parasite in cat feces and raw meat, rubella (if a woman is not immune), syphilis, hepatitis B, and other sexually transmitted diseases.

- Avoid hazards in the workplace. They include chemicals, gas, dust, fumes, or radiation. Also, avoid lifting heavy loads or standing all day.
- Avoid household hazards such as cleaning products, fumes, or paints.
- Avoid high body temperature whether due to illness, baths, saunas, or hot tubs.

To maintain your health and that of your baby eat right to support the growth of the fetus, exercise to strengthen muscles and ease discomforts, and get enough sleep.

A woman of normal weight should gain approximately 30 pounds during pregnancy (see "Where Does the Weight Go?"). Women who are overweight should gain less. Teenagers and women who are underweight or carrying twins should gain more. Pregnancy is not a time to try to lose weight. You need about 2,400 calories per day during pregnancy (about 300 calories more than a nonpregnant woman). You also need extra iron, folic acid, and calcium to provide nutrients for the fetus.

Exercise can help a pregnant woman prepare for birth and make her more comfortable during pregnancy. Although this is not the time to take up a hard new sport, if you had been exercising before becoming pregnant, you could continue to do so. Your exercise program may need to be modified because of some of the changes that take place during pregnancy. Your center of gravity, and thus your balance, changes with the added weight, and the hormones of pregnancy cause joints to become more flexible and subject to injury. When exercising, avoid becoming overheated or very tired, drink lots of water, and move more slowly and without jarring motions. Moderate exercise, such as swimming and walking, are good choices; exercises to strengthen back muscles can relieve back pain. However, exercise while lying on the back reduces blood flow to the fetus and is best avoided.

CHANGES DURING PREGNANCY

A woman goes through many emotional and physical changes during her pregnancy. Each woman is different, however, and these changes don't occur in all women or at the same times. Many of these changes are related to the pressure exerted on various parts of the body as the fetus grows.

Emotions

Pregnancy is a turning point in a woman's life. As with other phases of transition, psychological issues may resurface during this time. Often the woman revisits her own childhood experience and recalls the way in which she was raised.

The first three months of pregnancy are a time of adjusting to, or coming to terms with, the pregnancy. The middle of pregnancy is a relatively quiet time, during which the woman begins the process of bonding with the baby. Knowing the sex of the child in advance, which is available through some prenatal tests, may promote bonding. The pregnant woman may withdraw from outside activities and focus on her relationship with the baby's father and her home life. These feelings continue to grow into the last part of pregnancy. There may be increased anxiety and fear of problems about the delivery at this time.

Sexuality

Sexuality changes during pregnancy. For some women, the increased levels of hormones enhance their desire for sex during pregnancy. For others, sexual functioning increases at certain phases and decreases at others. A number of factors may interfere with sexual functioning. They include nausea, physical discomfort, fear of harming the fetus, feeling less desirable with increased weight, and bodily changes. Changes in the partner's responsiveness are also a factor. Some men draw closer to their partner during pregnancy and the postpartum period, but others may go through psychological changes, causing them to withdraw from the relationship. The woman's new maternal role, and her new physical appearance, may bring out unresolved conflicts in her partner.

Some couples are concerned that having sex during pregnancy can harm the fetus. In most cases it will not because the fetus is cushioned by the sac of amniotic fluid. A couple may find it more comfortable to try different positions that don't place pressure on a woman's abdomen. If there is a complication or concern, the doctor or nurse-midwife may suggest that the couple abstain from sex.

Sleeping Problems

Early pregnancy is often associated with prolonged sleep and fatigue. Sleep disturbance is also noted during pregnancy. For some women it may be the first symptom of pregnancy. It is quite common for women to have difficulty falling asleep or staying asleep at any given time during the pregnancy. Sleep may be particularly disturbed as term approaches. Some women dream vividly. Sleeping medications are best avoided because they could harm the fetus, especially during early pregnancy. Warm baths, relaxation exercises, and lying on one side propped by a pillow may help. (See Fig. 17.11)

Backache

As they get ready for the strain of delivery, joints and ligaments in your body relax. The result could be a backache. Exercises can help promote good posture and relieve aching muscles. To avoid back injury, avoid lifting whenever possible. If you must lift, bend from the knees, keeping the back straight. Do not lie flat on your back because the supine position can make it hard to breathe, and reduce blood flow to the baby.

Breast Changes

One of the first signs of pregnancy is tender breasts. The breasts continue to grow and change throughout pregnancy to prepare for breast-feeding. The nipples and surrounding skin might become darker, and the nipples and veins become more prominent. A woman's bra size may increase to twice the original size during pregnancy. Wear a comfortable cotton bra with wide shoulder straps and deep bands under the cups. Late in pregnancy, a woman may notice a yellow, watery fluid leaking from her nipples. This is called colostrum, and it nourishes the baby in the first days of life. It is rich in protective substances, called antibodies, which fight infection.

Breathing Problems

The pressure of the uterus on the bottom of the rib cage can cause a feeling of shortness of breath. The lungs do not have room enough to expand and take in enough air. In late pregnancy just before birth, the fetus drops and this often relieves that feeling.

Gastrointestinal Problems

Most women have morning sickness—nausea and vomiting—during the first three months of pregnancy. It usually, but not always, goes away in the middle of pregnancy. The condition is worse when the stomach is empty. Eating a number of small meals a day may help.

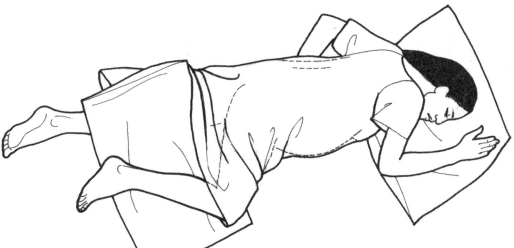

Figure 17.11 It may be more comfortable to sleep on one side with one leg propped up on a pillow.

Heartburn, or indigestion, has nothing to do with the heart. It is caused by acids from the stomach that cause a burning sensation in the throat and chest. Changes in the hormone levels during pregnancy slow digestion and relax the muscles that keep the stomach acids where they belong. Again, more frequent small meals instead of fewer large ones may bring some relief. Avoid large, spicy meals or fried foods. Also, avoid exercising or going to bed within two hours of eating. Your doctor or nurse-midwife may be able to suggest something to counteract the acidity in your stomach.

Many pregnant women are constipated during pregnancy. This is partly because of the pressure from the fetus on the bowel and the hormones of pregnancy that slow the passage of food. Exercise, eating foods high in fiber, and drinking fluids can help relieve constipation.

Hemorrhoids are enlarged or weakened veins near the anus. The baby's head creates pressure on these veins, causing them to swell during pregnancy. Straining during bowel movements makes the situation worse, causing itching, soreness, and perhaps even bleeding. Increasing fiber and fluid intake, using products for treating hemorrhoids and relieving constipation may help. You should of course consult your doctor before taking any medication.

Skin Changes

A dark line, called the linea nigra, may appear down the center of the stretched stomach, and the skin may itch. Skin on the abdomen and breasts must expand, often causing streaks called stretch marks. There is no way to prevent these marks; many lighten after birth. In some women, the hormones produced during pregnancy cause a brown mask on the face called chloasma that often fades after birth when hormones return to normal.

Varicose Veins

Swollen and painful veins, called varicose veins, often occur in the calves, thighs, and the vagina. They are made worse by poor circulation in the legs, especially during long periods of standing. Special support stockings can be worn to relieve aching, sore legs. Also helpful is lying on your side, with legs elevated, as is floating in water. While standing, move around as much as possible, lifting heels or toes to promote circulation.

Swelling

Most women have some degree of swelling in the legs or the hands during pregnancy. The face also may puff up because of the body's tendency to retain fluid. Although extreme swelling can be a sign that the kidneys are not working properly, some swelling is normal. Resting on your side with the feet elevated can help. In the third trimester, floating in water can help relieve swelling.

Other Changes

- Swollen gums that bleed more easily
- Muscle and leg cramps
- Numbness and tingling in the extremities
- Thicker hair growth
- Need to urinate more often (remember, sudden increases may signal infection)

SPECIAL CONSIDERATIONS

Some pregnancies require special care. In some cases this is known in advance. In others, warning signs occur during the course of pregnancy and are detected during prenatal care. Any warning signs should be reported to the clinician right away (see "Warning Signs").

Miscarriage

Miscarriage, also called spontaneous abortion, is the loss of a pregnancy before the fetus can live on its own. It occurs in about 15 percent of pregnancies, usually in early pregnancy. Most miscarriages occur in the first

WARNING SIGNS

Any of the following symptoms could be a sign of a problem and require immediate medical attention:

- Vaginal bleeding can be a sign of a miscarriage or a problem with the placenta.
- Vaginal discharge—either a change in the type or an increase in the amount—could be a sign of preterm labor or infection.
- Cramps and back pain could signal miscarriage or preterm birth.
- Swelling, headache, blurred vision occur with high blood pressure in pregnancy.
- Severe, sharp abdominal pain should be evaluated if it doesn't improve with position changes.
- Fever or chills may be symptoms of infection.
- Fluid discharge from your vagina may signal that the amniotic sac has ruptured and labor may begin soon.
- Decreased fetal movement for 12 hours after week 28 could mean the unborn baby is in trouble.

trimester, before 12 weeks. After week 16, the chance of having a miscarriage is low. The risk of miscarriage increases with age.

Miscarriage usually cannot be prevented and often occurs because the pregnancy is not normal. A miscarriage doesn't mean that a woman can't have children in the future. There is no proof that stress or physical or sexual activity causes miscarriage.

An early warning may be vaginal spotting. Other signs of a miscarriage are pain in the lower back, cramps in the lower abdomen, and heavy bleeding with clots. After a miscarriage, a procedure called dilation and curettage (D&C) may be necessary to open and clean the uterus. Loss of a pregnancy through miscarriage is traumatic, emotionally as well as physically. Discuss any concerns about current or future pregnancies with your health care professional. Special tests, procedures, or medicine may be needed if a woman experiences a loss after 12 weeks or if she loses several pregnancies in a row.

Preterm Labor

If labor begins before the 37th week of pregnancy, the baby may be born early. Often, labor can be stopped to allow the fetus more time in the uterus, where it has the best chance of growing and developing normally. Treatments to stop labor include bed rest, fluids given intravenously, and special agents to relax the uterus. The goal is to prolong the pregnancy until the fetus is fully developed. Today, even very early preterm infants can survive in neonatal intensive care units and drugs are available to help their lungs function better.

Problems with the Placenta

In late pregnancy, bleeding can be a sign of problems with the placenta. The placenta may pull away from the wall of the uterus (placental abruption), or it may cover the cervix (placenta previa). Both of these conditions can interfere with the oxygen supply of the fetus and require medical attention. These conditions may be best treated with a cesarean section.

Medical Conditions

High blood pressure and diabetes can develop during pregnancy in women who did not previously have these conditions. They often go away after delivery, although they can recur. These conditions can become worse in women who had them before they became pregnant. In either case, they require treatment.

High blood pressure, coupled with protein in the urine and swelling, is called preeclampsia. Symptoms include headaches, swelling of the hands and face, dizziness, blurred vision, sudden or uneven weight gain, and stomach pain. It can cause seizures and preterm birth and should be treated right away.

Diabetes that occurs during pregnancy is called gestational diabetes. Women with this condition have too much sugar in their blood because the hormones of pregnancy alter the way in which the body processes sugar. When blood sugar is high, the baby may become too large to pass through the mother's birth canal. Diabetes may be controlled through diet, exercise, or insulin (the hormone that processes sugar in the blood). Pills to control glucose are best avoided in pregnancy.

Rh Disease

Antigens are proteins found on the surfaces of blood cells that cause an immune response. One type of antigen is the Rh factor. If the mother's blood lacks the Rh antigen (Rh negative) and the father's blood contains it, the fetus can get the antigen from the father and be Rh positive.

The blood cells from an Rh positive baby can cause an Rh negative mother to produce anti-Rh antibodies as if she were allergic to the fetus. This is called sensitization. Her antibodies cross the placenta, causing anemia or Rh disease. This disease can be prevented by giving the mother a blood product called Rh immunoglobulin (RhIG). This product should be given at any time fetal blood might mix with mother's blood—for example, after an abortion, amniocentesis or chorionic villus testing—to keep antibodies from forming. Once antibodies are formed, they do not go away. RhIG is recommended at 28 weeks of pregnancy for women who are Rh-negative and not sensitized, unless the baby's father is also Rh negative. If her baby has Rh-positive blood, she should be given another dose shortly after she gives birth.

LABOR AND BIRTH

No two women experience exactly the same sensations during labor. Nor are all labors and the accompanying contractions the same length of time. Even expectant mothers who already have children can't be too sure about what might happen. Each baby is different, just as each birth experience holds surprises. What's important is that you understand the various stages of labor and delivery and, if possible, have someone available for support.

Once contractions begin, start timing how long each one lasts and how long it is from the start of one to the start of the next and note the times. If the contractions last 30–70 seconds, if they occur regularly, and if they don't go away with movement, it's probably the real thing. Contact your clinician. A first labor lasts on average 12–14 hours. Labor may be shorter for subsequent births.

There are three stages of labor. Changes take place in each stage, although they vary from one woman to another.

Stages of Labor

There are two main parts of the uterus: the upper part is muscular and can expand—its very top part is called the fundus—and at the bottom of the uterus the opening or cervix. In active childbirth, both parts of the uterus work together, contracting and pushing the baby down until the cervix dilates, or opens. The cervix is closed by a ring of muscles that gradually opens and thins (or effaces) during labor. (See Fig. 17.12)

A woman's body gradually prepares for labor and delivery during the last weeks of pregnancy. In those last weeks, the uterus may start to cramp. The cramps become stronger as the due date approaches. These are called Braxton-Hicks contractions or false labor. These contractions differ from true labor in a number of ways (see ''True versus False Labor'').

About 24 hours before active labor begins, the tiny mucus plug that has guarded the entrance to the cervix may break loose. This is called *bloody show* because blood could be present in the mucus.

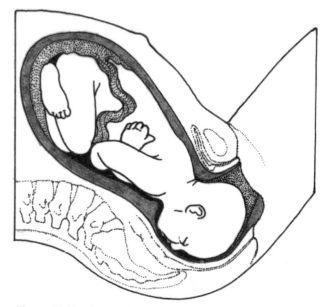

Figure 17.12 Second Stage of Labor
Contractions of the uterus push the baby through the fully opened cervix.

TRUE VERSUS FALSE LABOR

In true labor, contractions are

- Regular and get closer together
- Continuous in spite of movement
- Usually felt in the back and move to the front
- Increasing steadily in strength

In false labor, contractions are

- Irregular and do not get closer
- Stopped with movement or a change in position
- Often felt in the abdomen
- Weak and do not get stronger

First Stage

The first stage of labor begins when the cervix starts to open and ends when it is fully open. It occurs in three parts: early, active, and transition. In the hospital or clinic, an exam is done to see how labor is progressing.

- *Early Phase.* Contractions are usually mild, lasting 60–90 seconds and occurring every 15–20 minutes. They gradually become more regular and occur less than 5 minutes apart.
- *Active Phase.* Contractions are much stronger, lasting for about 45 seconds and occurring every 3 minutes. Tensing or pushing during this phase is discouraged.
- *Transition.* Transition is the most difficult stage of labor. The cervix is fully dilated, and contractions occur 2–3 minutes apart and last about 60 seconds. A wave of nausea is commonly noted, which passes rapidly.

Second Stage

The cervix is fully dilated and the baby is ready to be pushed out. Though it's tough physical work—especially in a long labor—it may be more rewarding and contractions may seem less intense. This stage includes the birth of the baby.

- The second stage may last 2 hours or longer
- Contractions slow to 2–5 minutes apart and last 60–90 seconds.

- Pushing should only be done during contractions, with resting and deep breathing between contractions.
- Maternal coordination and effort can speed delivery.

As the baby's head moves closer to the vaginal opening, it bulges and bumps against the pelvic floor with each contraction. In between contractions, the head may slip back inside. This back and forth motion is normal.

Pushing should stop as soon as the head crowns or becomes visible, to prevent tearing of your skin. At this point an episiotomy, or surgical cut, may be performed to widen the opening. (See Fig. 17.13) You may notice a stinging sensation or numbness as the baby is born because the skin has stretched so much.

In a normal birth, the baby's head slips out first, face down. The attendant checks to make sure the umbilical cord is not wrapped around the neck. The head turns so one side is lined up with the shoulders. Fluid or mucus may need to be sucked from the baby's mouth and nose. With the next contractions, the body slides out.

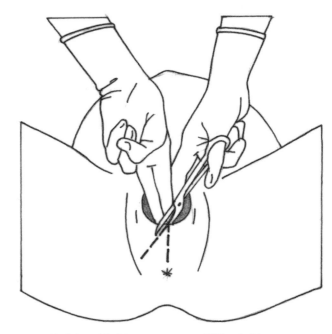

Mediolateral Incision   Midline Incision

Figure 17.13 Episiotomy
The skin in the perineum (area between the vulva and the rectum) may be cut just before birth to provide more room. Either a slanted (mediolateral) or straight (midline) incision may be used. The cut is closed with stitches after birth.

Third Stage

After the baby is born, the placenta is expelled. This stage may last up to 30 minutes.

- Contractions are closer together and may be less painful.
- The placenta is usually expelled as it separates from the wall of the uterus.
- A check will be made to ensure that the entire placenta is out and that no harmful tears are present in the vagina or cervix.

Pain Relief

Natural childbirth has come to mean an awake, aware, undrugged mother. It does *not* mean, as some people believe, a painless birth. (In childbirth, some women have a lot of pain and some have much less.) Many women wrongly feel they've failed if they can't stand the pain and need medication. There are various options available, and you need not hesitate to take advantage of them.

Epidural Block

Epidural anesthesia relieves pain during labor, by numbing the area from the waist down. It takes about 10 minutes for an anesthesiologist to administer the medication through a tube inserted between the vertebrae of the backbone. (See Fig. 17.14) An intravenous line is inserted so fluids and medication can be given to prevent blood pressure changes. Complications can include a drop in the mother's blood pressure, which may affect the baby's heartbeat, and a

headache, relieved by lying down for a few days after the birth.

Spinal Block

Similar to an epidural, a spinal block is injected into the spinal fluid sac and anesthesizes the body from the waist down. (See Fig. 17.14A) Pain relief lasts about 1–2 hours. The injection is given only once during labor, so it is best suited for pain relief during delivery. Complications are similar to those of epidural block.

Pudendal Block

An injection is given shortly before delivery to block pain in the vagina and rectum as the baby is born. It is one of the safest forms of anesthesia.

General Anesthetic

Medications that produce loss of consciousness can be used during cesarean delivery if there is an emergency. One complication is aspiration, when food from a woman's stomach enters the windpipe and lungs, causing injury. This is why a woman should not eat once active labor has begun.

Pain Medications

Drugs can be injected into a muscle or vein to relieve pain. These drugs can have side effects and slow the

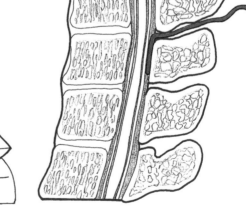

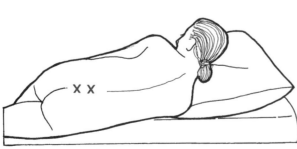

Figure 17.14 Spinal and Epidural Block Anesthesia
Both spinal and epidural anesthesia are given by an injection in the lower back (A). Spinal anesthesia is injected into the fluid surrounding the spinal cord. Epidural anesthesia is injected into the space outside the spinal cord covering (B).

baby's reflexes and breathing. They usually are given in small doses and avoided just before delivery.

Monitoring the Fetus

During labor, the status of the baby is monitored by listening to its heartbeat. This process, called auscultation, is done with a special stethoscope, or an electronic fetal monitor, a machine which records the heartbeat.

Auscultation

The heartbeat is monitored by a doctor or nurse, who listens to it at regular intervals. Usually the heartbeat is checked and recorded after a contraction. The frequency of monitoring depends on the stage of labor.

Electronic Fetal Monitoring (EFM)

The two kinds of EFM are external and internal. With external monitoring, an instrument using sound waves (doppler ultrasound) is attached to the mother's abdomen to record the heart rate of the fetus. With internal monitoring, a small device called an electrode is attached to the scalp of the fetus. Sometimes a tube called a catheter is inserted into the uterus to measure uterine contractions. External and internal monitoring techniques may be used together. Both techniques are done to assess whether the fetus is getting enough oxygen and prevent distress. With internal monitoring, the amniotic sac is broken for the device to be inserted in the uterus.

Assisted Delivery

Sometimes the mother needs a helping hand. If she is having trouble during labor, or if labor is delayed, the doctor may use certain tools designed to help speed delivery.

Forceps

Forceps are used to guide a baby through the birth canal; these metal instruments look a little like two big spoons hooked together. Often forceps are used if a baby seems to be in distress. During the pushing stage of labor, forceps can help an exhausted mother.

Vacuum Extraction

A plastic or metal suction cup is placed on the baby's head during delivery; vacuum extraction also helps speed up a delivery.

Oxytocin

Also called pitocin, it is a drug that causes contractions. It can be used to induce labor if a woman needs early delivery or has passed beyond 42 weeks of pregnancy and labor has not begun. Oxytocin also can be used to make the contractions stronger if the labor is not progressing well or the contractions are too weak. It is given intravenously to the mother a little bit at a time.

Cesarean Delivery

In a cesarean birth the baby is delivered through an incision in the mother's abdomen. Sometimes cesarean deliveries are arranged and scheduled in advance. On other occasions, the decision for a cesarean delivery will be done on an emergency basis because labor is not proceeding normally or the baby is having difficulty. Some of the reasons for cesarean delivery include:

- Cephalopelvic disproportion, in which the baby is too large to pass safely through the mother's pelvis.
- Fetal distress caused by the baby having difficulty withstanding labor or compression of the umbilical cord.
- Placental problems.
- Abnormal presentation, in which the baby lies bottom or feet first in the mother's birth canal (sometimes, the baby can be repositioned to allow a vaginal delivery).

Because cesarean deliveries are surgical procedures, recovery takes longer. Today, most clinicians encourage women who had a previous cesarean delivery to try a vaginal delivery, provided there are no reasons not to do so.

AFTER THE BABY IS BORN

Having a baby is hard work. New mothers need sleep, nourishment, quiet unpressured time to see and touch their new babies, and lots of support. The mother's body undergoes dramatic physical changes as it tries to shift gears and go back to its previous state. Many hospitals now send mothers home within the first 24 hours, which can be both a blessing and curse. While it can be comforting to be home, taking care of an infant is a 24-hour-a-day, seven-day-a-week proposition. Someone should be there to help with the beginning stages of motherhood. The body undergoes various physical changes over the next 6 weeks to return to a nonpregnant state.

Weight

Most women lose at least 13 pounds immediately after birth and an additional 3–4 pounds in the first days of the baby's life. Weight loss during the first six weeks after birth (postpartum) can be dramatic, especially for breast-feeding mothers.

Breast-feeding

Women who breast-feed need extra vitamins, minerals, and calories to support the baby. Breast milk is the best source of nutrition for a newborn baby because it has special nutrients that help the baby grow and combat diseases (see Chapter 18, Breast-feeding). If it is not possible to breast-feed at all times, consider storing your breast milk so it can be given to the baby with a bottle.

Cramps

As the uterus contracts to its prepregnant size, cramping sensations, called afterpains, may occur in the lower abdomen for a few days. This happens more often if a woman is breast-feeding. The cramps can be relieved with a mild painkiller. However, most painkillers are passed along into breast milk and may be hazardous to the newborn. Check with your pedatrician before taking medication.

Painful Urination

After childbirth, the bladder, bowel, and pelvic floor may be tender and sore, making every trip to the bathroom something to dread. What's more, eliminating all the built up extra fluid causes more frequent urination. A warm shower can relax the muscles and help ease urination, especially with an episiotomy.

Bleeding

Vaginal bleeding occurs for several weeks; anywhere from two to six is considered normal. If the mother is breast-feeding, bleeding might stop sooner. The flow is bright red and heavy at first, turning brownish as the days pass and healing begins. Nothing should be placed in the vagina, including tampons, until healing is complete. Intercourse should be avoided.

Bowel Movements

It may take a day or so for stool to pass after delivery. Drinking lots of water, walking, and eating high fiber foods can stimulate the system and get it back in working order. Straining should be avoided. A laxative or stool softener may help.

Episiotomy

Stitches take up to 2 weeks to heal and dissolve. Soreness can be relieved by applying ice to the area and lying down to keep pressure at a minimum. The area should be kept as clean as possible.

Sexuality

A woman can resume sexual activity as soon as she has healed. The physical effects of increased levels of hormones in breast-feeding women may reduce sexual desire and function. Many women need extra lubrication. A woman may not have menstrual periods if she is breast-feeding but she could become pregnant. Select a method of birth control and begin using it soon after birth.

Postpartum Depression

About 30–80 percent of women feel down or depressed following delivery (see Chapter 8). This is called postpartum blues. These symptoms usually go away spontaneously within 10 weeks of birth, without professional help. If symptoms persist beyond that point, or if a woman thinks about hurting herself or others, she should seek professional help and possibly antidepressant medication.

Postpartum depression occurs in approximately 10 percent of women after birth. If a woman has had a previous postpartum depression, the risk increases to approximately 30 percent. Panic disorder and obsessive-compulsive disorder also may arise during the postpartum period. Some of the symptoms of postpartum depression are feelings of worthlessness, anxiety, low self-esteem, insomnia, unusual weight loss, digestive problems, social isolation, feelings of inadequacy as a mother, obsessions about the baby's health or a dissatisfying relationship, mourning the loss of her former appearance or lifestyle, and, at times, suicidal thoughts. It is important to contact your clinician for help.

Postpartum psychosis is the most severe form of postpartum psychiatric illness. It affects a very small percentage of women who deliver. Postpartum psychosis is a medical emergency and requires prompt professional attention. There may be severe agitation, insomnia, and paranoia, as well as delusions and hallucinations that can lead to suicide or an impulse to kill the baby. Despite its severity, the prognosis for full recovery from postpartum psychosis is excellent.

Resources

Every new mother should pick up at least one good book on child care. Your doctor or midwife can give recommendations.

- *The Good Housekeeping Illustrated Book of Pregnancy and Baby Care* (Hearst Books), edited by Maryann Bucknum Brinley.
- *Dr. Spock's Baby and Child Care* (Dutton) A practical, easy-to-read guide, Benjamin Spock's book has been updated at various times during the last 50 years.
- *Your Baby and Child: From Birth to Age Five* (Knopf) by Penelope Leach, a British psychologist.
- *What To Expect When You Are Expecting* (Workman) by Arlene Eisenberg, Heidi Eisenberg Murkoff, and Sandee Eisenberg Hathaway. Now part of a series of three books by this mother-daughter team, these books are packed with pertinent advice and information.
- *Caring for Your Baby and Young Child, Birth to Age 5, The Complete and Authoritative Guide* from The American Academy of Pediatrics, edited by Steven P. Shelov, M.D., F.A.A.P.

CHAPTER 18

Breast-Feeding

Ruth A. Lawrence, M.D., F.A.A.P.

All mothers need to make an informed decision about how they want to feed their infant. You may have thought about it before becoming pregnant, but once the pregnancy is well established, it's important to discuss the question with your physician, your spouse, and other members of your family. If no one in your family has breast-fed before, you may find it helpful to contact one of the local groups such as International Childbirth Education Association (ICEA), La Leche League International (LLLI), or Nursing Mother's Counsel. Your obstetrician's office also can provide information about available childbirth classes in which the topic is thoroughly covered.

WHY BREAST-FEED?

The advantages of breast-feeding are numerous. Mother's milk is the ideal nutrition for a growing infant. The newborn human, one of the least mature of all the mammals, experiences the greatest brain growth in the first year of life. Human milk has the perfect ingredients to develop the brain. It has exactly the right elements to build strong bodies and to develop the brain and nervous system.

Mother's milk contains many active enzymes that help the infant to digest milk and help the infant's intestinal tract to mature and absorb the nutrients. Mother's milk, however, is more than just good nutrition. It contains antibodies to protect against infection. Breast-fed infants have fewer diarrhea and gastrointestinal infections, fewer otitis media (ear infections) and upper respiratory infections, and even have fewer urinary tract infections. They have fewer hospitalizations and fewer visits to a physician's office for illness. Infants are never allergic to their mother's milk, so breast-fed infants have fewer allergies.

Studies of chronic illness in childhood also indicate that infants who have been exclusively breast-fed for 4 or more months have less incidence of childhood onset diabetes, Crohn's disease, and childhood cancers (especially leukemia and lymphoma). In some studies, premature infants who receive their mother's milk early in life have been shown to score better on intelligence tests than those receiving only formula.

There are benefits for the mother as well. Women who breast-feed seem to have a lower incidence of breast cancer and ovarian cancer. Breast-feeders are less likely to become obese and less likely to develop calcium problems in later life than those who did not breast-feed or did not bear children.

Finally, breast-feeding can create a special relationship between mother and infant, which provides nurturing as well as nutrition and results in intimate contact many times a day.

An Informed Decision: Breast-Feeding Versus Formula

The alternative to breast-feeding is formula feeding. Today, commercially available formulas provide adequate nutrition as determined in laboratories. Most formulas (except the hypoallergenic ones) are made with cow's milk, which is altered to make it digestible for a human infant. While breast milk is always readily available at the correct concentration and temperature, formula requires preparation and the sterilization of bottles and nipples.

Some women prefer formula feeding, because their babies can be fed by other caregivers. In some ways, formula feeding is easier, because others can take over when the mother cannot be present. This may be important if the mother plans to return to school or work. Breast milk can be expressed, or pumped, from the breast and fed to the infant in a bottle or small cup.

The Role of the Father

When the infant is breast-fed, the role of the father is very important but different from the mother's. The father provides cuddling and comforting when the infant does not need to be fed. Most infants have a fussy period each day, usually in the evening (5:00 to 10:00 P.M.), when they need to be held, rocked, and stroked. The infant will nuzzle and root to be fed and may remain unsettled if she or he can smell milk. Babies settle down quickly if held by someone who is not lactating (making milk).

PRENATAL PREPARATION TO BREAST-FEEDING

As soon as pregnancy begins, the hormones produced to support the pregnancy, the placenta, and the uterus also have an effect on the breasts. The breasts begin to enlarge, the ducts that will carry the milk develop, and the cells that will produce the milk increase in number. By 16 weeks of pregnancy, the breast is ready to provide milk when the baby is born even if the infant arrives prematurely. The woman's nipples and areolas are also prepared for lactation. They become more pigmented and the Montgomery glands, which are invisible when not pregnant or lactating, enlarge and secrete a special sebaceous material that softens and lubricates the surface of the nipple and areola to protect them when the infant suckles. The nipple and areola also develop elastic tissue that will help the infant in drawing these tissues into the mouth during suckling.

If you're thinking of breast-feeding your unborn child, simply bathe and dry your breasts as you normally do. Do not use any ointments, oils, or medicines unless prescribed by your doctor. Normally, you do not need to do nipple exercises, nipple rolling, or buffing with rough cloth. These practices may cause irritation or, toward the end of pregnancy, may stimulate the uterus to contract. You should, however, have your breasts examined by an obstetrician.

Breast Examination

Breast examination is part of prenatal care. You may have questions about your breasts that you should discuss with your obstetrician early in pregnancy. Breasts, for example, come in many different different sizes and shapes. Usually one is slightly bigger than the other, but a major discrepancy in size and shape should be discussed with your physician.

Of more common concern is the size and shape of the nipples, which also vary among women. If your nipples do not protrude, a simple procedure will identify their ability to become erect so they can be easily grasped by the infant and drawn into her or his mouth. Support your breast with your fingers at the level of the areola, with the thumb above. Compress the areola. Does your nipple protrude? If your nipple becomes more inverted or indented, this suggests a true inverted nipple. Discuss this with your obstetrician, who may wish to suggest some treatment after evaluating your nipples. (Some doctors prefer to wait until after deliv-

ery and rely on the infant and an electric breast pump to draw the nipple out.)

If the uterus has been very irritable or there is concern about premature delivery, it is best to delay treatment with breast shells until delivery. A *breast shell* is a simple device that consists of a plastic disc about the size of the areola that has a hole in the center for the nipple. A dome of plastic with air holes in it fits over the disc. The shell, worn under your brassiere, gently encourages the nipple to protrude. (See Figure 18.1)

Flat nipples may also be of concern. They respond to simple treatment with breast shells or an electric pump used just before the infant begins to feed. After

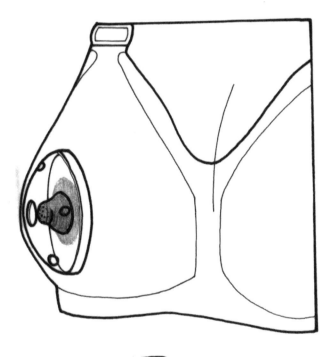

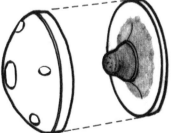

Figure 18.1 Breast Shells
Breast shells, worn under a bra, are used to encourage inverted nipples to protrude in preparation for breast-feeding. A disk with a hole in the center is placed over the nipple, and a small plastic dome with air holes fits over the disk.

the infant has been successfully nursing for a few days, these special procedures should no longer be necessary, as the nipple will become erect on stimulation.

Surgery

The question of previous surgery is always an important one. Simple procedures to remove a cyst or other benign mass usually present no problem to successful breast-feeding. If a small duct was cut during the procedure, a collection of milk could form behind it during lactation, forming a lump called a *galactocele*. Galactoceles can be drained by your physician with a needle and syringe if you become uncomfortable.

When contemplating surgery to reduce the size of your breasts, the matter of breast-feeding should be discussed with the surgeon. If you wish to breast-feed in the future, remind the surgeon so that the procedure will preserve the duct system to the areola and nipple. That is, these structures will not be removed but will be centered on the remaining breast tissue, allowing a normal flow of milk through the ducts.

Augmentation mammoplasty, or surgery to increase the size of the breasts, usually presents no problem when a woman wishes to breast-feed. The implant is placed between the glandular tissue and the chest wall; the duct system is not disturbed, and the nerve supply is not interrupted. Silicone implants, however, have been the subject of considerable concern and controversy because of reports of rupture and associated scarring of the breast tissue. Extensive scarring may interfere with milk production and release. Whether the silicone itself is the problem remains an open question. If the implant is intact, breast-feeding is safe. If there is any question, the milk can be examined in the laboratory for the presence of silicone.

Burns to the chest wall and other causes of breast scarring should be evaluated by your obstetrician. Breast-feeding is usually successful, and most women will find that with a little extra instruction, they can enjoy this special relationship with their infant. Your physician may refer you to another member of the staff experienced in breast-feeding or to an independent licensed lactation consultant.

Supporting the Breasts

Ordinarily, during pregnancy and lactation most women find that wearing a suitable brassiere relieves the "weighty" feeling in their breasts. Nursing bras, specially designed to allow you to feed the infant without getting completely undressed, can be purchased during the last trimester. They have adjustable shoulder straps and a long series of hooks in the back so they accommodate any changes in size that occur from the end of pregnancy into lactation. Many women wear their nursing bras day and night for weeks or even months. Avoid nursing brassieres that have narrow shoulder straps or built-in plastic-lined guards in the cup.

When lactating, it is wise to wear a disposable pad inside your bra so that milk does not leak through onto your clothing. It is also smart to avoid wearing pure silk or any other fabric that may show a ring of wetness. Many styles of blouses and dresses open in the front, have hidden zippers, or can be pulled up from the waist so that your infant can be nursed at any time or any place without undue exposure or disruption of your clothing. Flowered or print blouses have the obvious advantage of obscuring any signs of moisture.

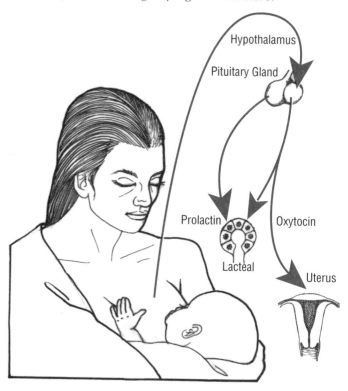

Figure 18.2 Breast-feeding
The breast-feeding cycle stimulates the production of milk in response to the infant's suckling, After delivery, a sudden drop in the hormones estrogen and progesterone begins to trigger milk production. The baby's suckling stimulates the hypothalamus and pituitary gland to release the hormones prolactin and oxytocin. These hormones in turn stimulate the production of milk and its transport through the alveoli and milk ducts. At the same time, the uterus is stimulated to contract and to begin to return to its normal size under the influence of oxytocin.

Preparatory Classes

Infants are born knowing how to breast-feed, but women must learn; it is not a reflex. In some mammalian species, females learn by observing other breast-feeding females that live with them. Today, women in the United States may have to learn how to breast-feed from a special organization. Furthermore, their own mothers may not have any advice, because they themselves did not breast-feed. La Leche League International, International Childbirth Education Association, and Breastfeeding Mother's Council have local branches that can be contacted about prenatal classes and assistance after delivery.

AFTER THE BIRTH: BREAST-FEEDING IN THE FIRST FEW DAYS

Breast-feeding begins shortly after birth. Infants are born with the right reflexes and instincts to breast-feed. In a normal delivery of a healthy child, the newly born infant will find his or her way to the breast and latch on, if left undisturbed on the mother's abdomen after the umbilical cord is clamped and cut. When in the uterus, infants suck and swallow amniotic fluid during the second and third trimesters. They are born with a rooting reflex, which means they will try to suck any object that stimulates the surface around their mouths. Their sucking motion, or undulating motion of the tongue, triggers the back of the throat to swallow.

Unless you have witnessed other women breast-feeding, you may need help in properly holding your baby for feeding. Hold your infant so that she or he is facing your breasts. Rest your infant's head in the crook of your elbow and support her or his buttocks. With your other hand, you may want to swaddle your child in a light blanket, because it has a calming effect. Draw the infant to your breast with the her or his face squarely facing it. (See Fig. 18.2) With your other hand, support your breast and compress the areola so that the infant can draw the nipple and areola into her or his mouth. (See Fig. 18.3) As the nipple and areola elongate to form a teat, the infant's tongue compresses it against the hard palate and suckles. The undulating motion of the tongue causes the milk to move along the ducts and be ejected from the nipple. (See Fig. 18.4)

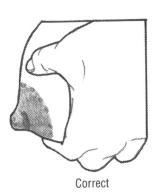

Correct

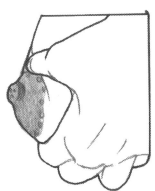

Incorrect

Figure 18.3 Positioning
To allow your baby to draw the nipple into her or his mouth, place your hand around one of your breasts with four fingers beneath the areola and your thumb on top. Gently press with fingers under the breast (top) to cause the nipple to protrude. Do not press in with your thumb (bottom), as this will tend to draw the nipple up and away from the baby's mouth.

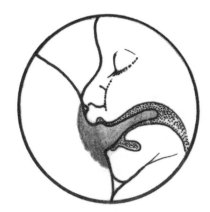

Figure 18.4 Suckling
When the baby latches onto the breast, the nipple is elongated and drawn back into her or his mouth. The baby's suckling motions stimulate the flow of milk through the milk ducts and out of the nipple toward the back of the baby's throat.

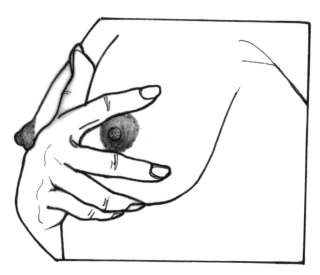

Figure 18.5 Scissors Grasp
One way to support the breast during breast-feeding is with the thumb and forefinger above the areola and the other three fingers beneath it. This is sometimes called the "scissors grasp."

You may feel comfortable supporting the breast with three fingers below the breast and the thumb and index finger above and well behind the areola. (See Fig. 18.5) An alternative position is to place all four fingers below the breast and the thumb above. (See Fig. 18.6) Choose the grasp most comfortable for you, en-

suring that your fingers do not block the infant from getting most of the areola in the mouth. Whether you lie down or sit up to nurse, the same principles apply: The infant's total body faces your breast, and your hand supports the breast and compresses the areola without obstructing the infant from getting a proper grasp.

To encourage the infant to latch on, stimulate the center of the infant's lower lip. (See Fig. 18.7) The rooting reflex will stimulate the infant to move forward, extend the tongue, and draw the nipple and areola into the mouth and begin suckling. If a good comfortable latch on is not achieved the first time, break the suction by slipping your finger into the corner of the infant's mouth and then repeat the process of positioning, stimulating the rooting reflex, and latching on.

The Let-Down Reflex

The infant will begin to suckle as soon as he or she is latched on. When the nipple is stimulated by the infant suckling or by a breast pump, this stimulation triggers what is known as the *let-down reflex*. The let-down reflex sends a message through the nerves in the nipple to the mother's brain. The mother's pituitary gland releases two hormones: prolactin and oxytocin. Prolactin stimulates the milk-producing cells in the breast to make milk, and oxytocin stimulates the duct system to move the milk to the nipple and eject, or let it down. (See Fig. 18.2) A little oxytocin is released when a woman hears or sees her baby, thus a little milk will

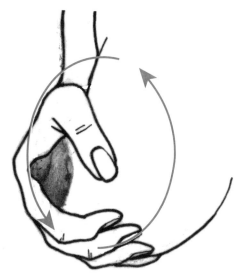

Figure 18.6 Alternate Grasp
Some women prefer to hold the breast with four fingers underneath the areola and the thumb on top. Choose the position that is most comfortable and effective for you.

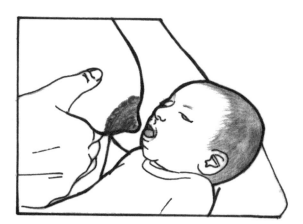

Figure 18.7 Latching On
Stimulating the baby's lower lip will help encourage her or him to latch on. When the baby is ready to feed, she or he will move forward, open her or his mouth and extend the tongue, and draw the nipple into the mouth.

drip. A new supply of milk, however, is not produced unless the nipple is stimulated by the infant or a pump.

It is important in the early days of breast-feeding to lie down or sit comfortably and to relax before feeding the infant. Feed your baby when he or she is ready, not when he or she has begun to cry frantically. Stress and discomfort can interfere with letting down.

You can prevent the development of sore nipples by proper positioning. If your nipples do get sore, evaluate and adjust your position. While there are several ways to hold an infant while feeding, find one or two that are best for you and your baby.

In the hospital, the nursing staff in the birthing center, postpartum floor, or newborn nursery can assist in getting you started. If you have problems such as flat or inverted nipples, a sleepy baby, or a baby with a cleft palate, talk to your physician. She or he can evaluate the situation and, if necessary, call for an appropriate consultant.

Because there are many things to learn about a new baby, it's difficult for a new mother to retain all the information that the health care staff provides. In addition, women are often discharged from the hospital with their new babies 24 to 48 hours after birth. There is simply not enough time for the doctors and nurses to assess the newborn and its needs completely. It is important, then, to make an appointment with the baby's doctor in the 1st week after birth. Ideally, try to schedule a home visit from an office nurse practitioner or a visiting nurse who is skilled at looking at mothers and babies in the first few days postpartum.

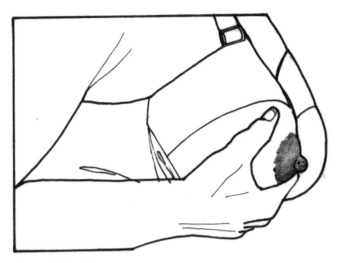

Figure 18.8 Colostrum
Colostrum is a thin, yellowish fluid that begins to be produced in the middle of pregnancy. Expressing milk can be done with the same grasp used to feed the infant.

and receives the colostrum, the breast makes more and more fluid. About the third or fourth day after birth, you will be aware of an increase in the size of your breasts and the increased flow and change in texture and color that indicate transitional milk. This means your milk has "come in." Mothers who have nursed other infants will find that their milk comes in earlier. While some swelling and engorgement of the breast is to be expected, excessive swelling can be uncomfortable. Your physician or nurse can suggest some means of relief.

When the Milk Comes In

At about 16 weeks of pregnancy, a small amount of milk can be expressed or may seep from the nipples. This early milk is called *colostrum*. Colostrum increases in volume so that at birth, after the placenta has been passed, the infant can suckle and obtain up to 0.5 ounce. Colostrum is yellowish, a little thicker than milk, and contains a lot of protective antibodies and cells that will protect the infant against infections and disease. It has more protein but a little less fat than later milk. Colostrum persists for 4 or 5 days and is gradually replaced by mature milk. (See Fig. 18.8) (The interim milk is called transitional milk.) Mature milk is available after about 10 days.

Right after delivery, the breasts feel soft, but over the next day, the body increases the blood supply to the breasts and they become full. As the infant nurses

Is Your Baby Getting Enough?

While it is not possible to measure the exact amount of milk that the infant gets at each breast-feeding, there are ways to tell if it is enough.

Feeding patterns vary, but a baby should be fed at least every 3 to 4 hours or a minimum of 6 times a day in the 1st month of life. Most breast-fed infants feed every 2 to 3 hours, resulting in 8 to 12 feedings a day. Often the infant will feed frequently for a few hours, especially between 5:00 and 10:00 P.M. and then stretch it out to 2 or 4 feedings overnight until 6:00 A.M. Feedings usually last 20 to 30 minutes, but others may be shorter. The actually vigorous suckling time usually adds up to about 90 minutes a day.

Breast-fed infants should wet at least six diapers a day, soaking at least one. (It is easier to keep track of wettings with cloth diapers than with disposable ones, especially the super-absorbent kind.) The urine should be pale in color. It should not be dark, concentrated, or leave a dusty deposit. A breast-fed infant also has a bowel movement every day in the first 4 to 6 weeks. Most breast-fed infants pass a stool with every feeding, because of the physiologic stimulus to the intestinal track. Right after birth, the infant passes a substance called *meconium*, which is a dark green, almost black material that is smooth and sticky. It should be totally passed by 3 days, and stools then become green brown (transitional stools) and then yellow and seedy. Yellow, loose, and seedy is the normal breast-fed stool, and it should begin by the third or fourth day. Failure to stool every day and to have loose yellow stools by the fourth day should be reported to your pediatrician. Failure to wet enough diapers and failure to feed long enough should also be discussed with the doctor.

Home scales are not very accurate, so take your infant to the physician's office for a weight check. Most infants lose weight after birth. A loss of 5 percent of birth weight is acceptable (5 ounces for a 7-pound baby). If the infant loses 7 to 8 percent of his or her birth weight, have the infant checked by the baby's physician. A loss of 10 percent is the maximum before aggressive interventions are introduced. Usually problems can be solved by adjusting the pattern of feeding, the frequency, or the positioning. The physician will want to check the infant every day or two until the milk supply is well established and weight gain persists. By 14 days, the infant should have returned to birth weight.

There are many community resources for nursing mothers to call for reassurance and guidance in the art of breast-feeding. La Leche League and Nursing Mother's Council have members who have nursed and who are willing to share their experiences. Management advice, however, should come from a certified licensed practitioner that your physician recommends and who will work with your physician to solve the problem.

DAY-TO-DAY BREAST-FEEDING: SPECIAL CARE AND TREATMENT

Ordinarily, no special treatment is necessary for the nipples, areola, or breasts. During normal showering or bathing, avoid putting soap directly on the nipples. Dry breasts gently but thoroughly. Between feedings, allow the milk to air dry on the skin. Bras should be kept dry and a dry nursing pad placed in the cup. As time goes on, there will be less leaking and less fullness. This does not mean the milk has dried up but that the breast is adapting to the process of producing and releasing milk on a continual basis.

If the nipples become sore, seek help before there are cracks and further trauma. Remember, it should not hurt to breast-feed. If it does, get advice from the nursing staff or from a lactation consultant referred by your doctor.

Occasionally, a lump may appear in the breast that does not go away. (The lactating breast feels lumpy but usually the lumps change.) The lump may be a milk-filled cyst caused by a plugged duct. Gentle but firm massage will usually drain it, especially after applying warm compresses. If you become feverish or feel sick or if the lump is painful, red, and warm, it may be mastitis. Mastitis must be treated. Call your physician promptly. You may have to take special antibiotics for 10 days to 2 weeks. Continue to breast-feed on both sides; start with the unaffected side and end up fully emptying the involved side. The most important part of the treatment is *rest*. Mastitis usually occurs when you have taken on too much activity or have become exhausted from caring for your baby. You'll need help with the baby and you will need to be relieved of other

WORKING AND BREAST-FEEDING

You may have to return to work, but it is still possible to continue to breast-feed. The baby's schedule can be adjusted to fit the requirements of the job. Breast-feeding can also be adjusted, depending on your work hours, breaks, and lunch hours. Some women continue to nurse or pump so the baby receives only mother's milk. Others may provide formula and breast-feed only while at home. There are no hard-and-fast rules. The feeding should be comfortable for you, the baby, and the child care provider. For best results, you need to find safe child care where breast-feeding is understood and supported. You should be able to nurse at day care when you drop off your infant, before you leave, and when you return to pick up the child. If your job permits, you should be able to breast-feed at other times during the day. Any amount of mother's milk continues to provide special nourishment, antibodies and protection against disease.

chores until you are rested and feel better. Hot or cold compresses will relieve local discomfort. Aspirin or ibuprofen can be taken for the fever, pain, and headache.

When the nipples become raw and painful, local treatment may be necessary. Treatment differs in different parts of the country. If the climate is very dry, as in desert areas, then treatment with bland ointments (Vitamins A and D or purified lanolin) will provide relief. In areas with high humidity, drying may help. Air drying or gentle blowing with a hair dryer on low heat and low air may be soothing. Your local health care provider will recommend the best skin treatment for the environment in which you live.

CHAPTER 19

Sexually Transmitted Diseases

Carol Widrow, M.D.

Sexually transmitted diseases (STDs) are spreading rapidly. Although they are more common now than ever before, many people fail to understand how to protect themselves from contracting an STD. Furthermore, many people do not recognize the early symptoms, or do not know how to get diagnosed and tested for such problems.

Parents often fail to discuss STDs with their children, because they are afraid of talking about sex. The information and education on STDs are limited in some school systems, although these diseases should be fully addressed in junior highs and high schools. The increased sexual promiscuity in the United States over the past 25 years has also helped the STD epidemic grow. Having more than one sexual partner greatly increases the risk of contracting an STD. Although women now have many options for birth control, only the use of condoms, a barrier precaution, greatly reduces the risk of contracting disease.

Some of the most dangerous STDs, including syphilis and gonorrhea, may occur without symptoms. Sexually active persons can carry an STD from one relationship to the next, infecting their new partners, while remaining completely unaware of the presence of disease.

Although most types of STD can be cured with antibiotics, there can be long-term, serious consequences. Many viruses are incurable, and a growing number of STDs can cause infertility in women. The best protection against STDs is to prevent them from occurring and, when they do occur, to obtain treatment immediately.

PREVENTION

The surest way to avoid an STD is to avoid sex. Some women may find abstinence an undesirable option, however. Sexually active women should practice safe sex:

- Limit your sexual partners.
- Know your partner's sexual history.
- Use condoms.

Practicing safe sex means being responsible for yourself as well as your partner. Safe sex can keep you from contracting one of the many types of STDs, including chlamydia, gonorrhea, herpes, syphilis, and genital warts. These types of STD are highly contagious and can be contracted easily. There is no vaccine that can prevent them. Practicing safe sex can also help protect against becoming infected with human immunodeficiency virus (HIV), which causes AIDS (see Chapter 20).

Other than abstinence, monogamy with an uninfected partner is the best way to avoid picking up an STD. Having several sexual partners greatly increases your risk for STDs. Ask your sexual partners if they have ever had an STD or if they are having sex with others.

Condoms, when used properly, are the most effective method to keep an STD from spreading. A woman should insist that a male sexual partner wear a condom, even if she is using another form of birth control. This is also true for women who do not need birth control, such as those who have gone through menopause or who have had their uteruses removed. If a male sexual partner does not want to use a condom, there is now a condom that women can use (see "The Female Condom," below). Women must learn to refuse to have sex with a man unless a condom is used.

Condoms are readily available over the counter in most drug stores, and there are many kinds. Condoms made of natural materials do not keep some viruses from passing between you and your partner, so latex condoms should always be used. A spermicide used with a condom may offer additional protection.

THE FEMALE CONDOM

There is now a condom that women can use themselves rather than relying on their male sex partners. Called the female condom, it consists of two rings with a latex sheath between them. The closed end of the sheath is inserted into the vagina, and the ring is placed high up around the cervix. The open end of the sheath remains outside the uterus. (See Fig. 19.1)

Like the condom for men, female condoms can be bought in drugstores without a prescription. It should be used once and then thrown away. Used as directed, it can be effective in preventing STDs and pregnancy.

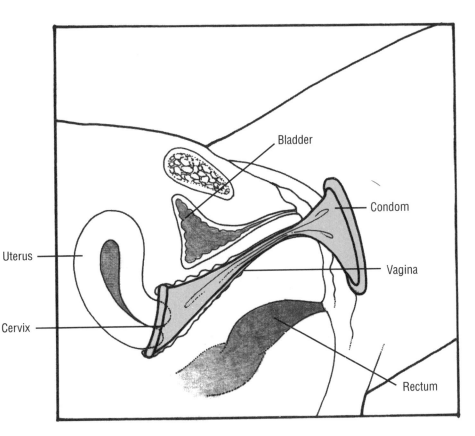

Figure 19.1 Female Condom
The *female condom* is a plastic sheath connected by rings on either end. One ring fits inside the vagina against the cervix (opening of the uterus), and the other ring anchors the sheath outside the body.

You cannot catch most types of STDs from nonsexual contact, such as hugging or holding hands. Most STD organisms cannot survive outside the body for long, so catching an STD from sitting on a toilet seat is very unlikely.

In addition to taking steps to prevent getting or passing on an STD, it is important to recognize the symptoms of these diseases. The better a woman understands her body, the better prepared she is to recognize such symptoms.

TYPES OF STDS

The following discussion covers the major types of STDs along with their symptoms, causes, diagnoses, and treatment. Some general guides apply to most STDs (see "General Management of STDs," below).

Chlamydia

Symptoms
Chlamydia often has no symptoms, and women are less likely to have symptoms than men. Signs of infection may only be noted during a doctor's phisical ex-

amination. The type of symptoms depends on the type of chlamydia infection and the area it attacks. One of the most common signs in women is a creamy white discharge from the vagina.

When symptoms do occur, they usually appear 1 to 3 weeks after infection. Women usually report a thin vaginal discharge, abdominal pain, and burning during urination. Men often report a burning sensation during urination and a urethral exudate. Men are more likely to display symptoms, women usually learn that they are infected only when their male sexual partner begins to show signs of infection.

Chlamydia commonly results in a genitourinary infection, such as nongonococcal urethritis (NGU), which is marked by a thin penile discharge in men and mild vaginal discharge in women. Chlamydia can in-

GENERAL MANAGEMENT OF STDS

Some guidelines about STDs apply regardless of the type of disease. For the best results, follow these recommendations:

- While taking antibiotics for an STD, complete the recommended treatment, even if symptoms go away before all the antibiotics have been taken. Stopping too soon can allow infection to return and prompt the bacterium or virus to develop resistance to the treatment.

- Sex partners of persons with STDs should be tested and treated. Both partners should be given antibiotics at the same time. This keeps the partners from passing the infection between themselves.

- To prevent reinfection, abstain from intercourse until all antibiotics have been taken and symptoms have diasppeared.

- Use condoms to prevent reinfection.

- Those who have one STD should probably be tested for others. Having one STD puts a person at a risk for others. In particular, gonorrhea and chlamydia commonly occur together. Diseases that cause open sores on the genitals increase the chance of getting AIDS from an infected partner.

fect the cervix (the opening of the uterus) a condition called cervicitis. If the cervicitis is not treated, the infection can move up into the uterus and the fallopian tubes. Infection of the tubes can cause a dangerous condition called pelvic inflammatory disease (PID) which may result in infertility.

Men and women who have anal sex, can have chlamydia infections of the rectum (proctitis). Swelling and soreness of the lymph nodes and rectal bleeding are signs of infection.

Newborns who get chlamydia from their mothers develop pneumonia and eye infections. Chlamydia is the leading cause of blindness in babies born in developing countries.

Cause

Chlamydia infections are caused by the bacterium *Chlamydia trachomatis*. This infection is the most common STD in the United States, and can be spread through vaginal or anal sex. It often is transmitted along with gonorrhea and contributes to a condition called pelvic inflammatory disease (see "Pelvic Inflammatory Disease"). A woman can pass chlamydia to her baby during its birth. In men chlamydia can cause such manifestations as epididymitis (infection around the testicle) and proctitis.

Diagnosis

Diagnosis of chlamydia is often difficult because it may have no symptoms. A woman may be tested if her partner has been found to be infected. Or she may be tested if she has symptoms, such as vaginitis, or PID.

A sample of discharge can be taken from the vagina or the cervix and tested. A culture is the most accurate way to diagnose chlamydia.

Treatment

The antibiotics recommended for treatment of chlamydia are doxycycline or azithromycin. Doxycycline must be taken for 7 days, but azithromycin—which is newer—can be taken in one dose.

Pregnant women with chlamydia infection are advised to use erythromycin, since tetracycline can adversely affect the fetus.

All sex partners should be informed of the infection. They should be tested if possible, but if testing is not available, they should be treated for chlamydia infection even if they have no symptoms.

Gonorrhea

Symptoms

Both men and women can contract gonorrhea. Women may have no symptoms; however, they usually occur and can include vaginal discharge and dysuria (painful urination). Women may delay treatment because they do not think the discharge is serious.

Men may have no symptoms for a 3- to 6-day period (called the incubation period). At the end of this time, they often develop a tingling sensation in the urethra followed by painful urination and a white discharge. With some strains of gonorrheal bacterium there may never be a discharge.

Symptoms vary, depending on the site infected. Men and women who have anal sex may have rectal discharge and discomfort; men and women who engage in oral sex may experience sore throat, pain on swallowing, cervical lymph nodes, and red tonsils with a discharge, often confused with strep throat. Women who have infection of the reproductive organs can have severe lower abdominal pain and fever. These signs may be the beginning of PID, a common cause of infertility in women. Infection of the fallopian tubes occurs in nearly 15 percent of the women who contract gonorrhea.

In its advanced stages, gonorrhea can enter the bloodstream and spread throughout the body, causing complications. It can attack the heart and joints, but these developments can be prevented through treatment.

Cause

Gonorrhea is caused by the bacterium *Neisseria gonorrhoeae*. It is second only to chlamydia in terms of number of cases in the United States. About 45 percent of people with gonorrhea also have chlamydia, and the risk factors of infection are similar. Even though the number of cases of gonorrhea seems to be dropping, about 1 million new cases are still reported each year. It is most common in people between the ages of 15 and 30. Babies born to mothers with the disease can contract an infection called gonococcal ophthalmia neonatorum at birth when they pass through the vagina. This condition can affect the baby's eyes, causing blindness, and requires a different antibiotic than that used to treat chlamydia infection in the newborn.

Diagnosis

Gonorrhea is diagnosed from a specimen taken from the infected area. A swab is used to take a sample of discharge from the urethra, cervix, rectum, or throat, depending on which areas were exposed. A sample(s) will be cultured so that every involved area can be definitively diagnosed.

Treatment

Women with gonorrhea as well as their sex partners should be treated. Anyone with gonorrhea should avoid all sexual activity while under treatment, because the disease is very easily spread.

Many types of drugs are used to fight gonorrhea. Although once antibiotics such as penicillin and tetracycline were the mainstays of treatment, today a large percentage of gonorrhea bacteria are resistant to these drugs. Therefore, newer drugs like ceftriaxone are used. Because gonorrhea and chlamydia often occur together, doctors usually recommend that patients also take doxycycline to eliminate any undiagnosed chlamydia.

Pregnant women can be safely treated with ceftriaxone. In case they also have a chlamydial infection, they are usually treated with erythromycin as well.

In women with simple infections whose symptoms are cleared by treatment, further testing is not needed. However, women who continue to have symptoms should be tested to see if the bacteria persists, and if so, what types of antibiotics are likely to eliminate it.

Genital Warts

Symptoms

Genital warts begin as tiny red or pink bumps. After about 2 months (the incubation period can range from 1 to 6 months), they become moist on the surface. The warts will spread if left untreated. In males they are usually located on the scrotum or on the shaft or tip of the penis. In women they grow on the vulva, on the cervical and vaginal walls, and around the anus. The virus can also cause growths on the cervix.

Cause

Also called venereal warts or condyloma, genital warts are caused by the human papillomavirus (HPV). This virus causes warts on the skin of men and women and is easily transmitted by sexual contact. There are many different types of HPV that can cause warts. Some types have been linked to a risk of cervical cancer. (See Chapter 15).

Diagnosis

Genital warts look similar to typical skin warts. A trained eye often can diagnose genital warts without any tests. Painting the area with a weak acid solution causes the warts to turn white, which can help in diagnosis. Warts on the cervix can be detected by a Pap test, in which a sample of cells is removed from the cervix for study under a microscope. A sample of the wart can be taken and studied to reveal what type of HPV is causing the infection.

PELVIC INFLAMMATORY DISEASE

When an STD moves from the vulva and vagina up to the uterus and fallopian tubes, it causes pelvic inflammatory disease (PID). PID can cause infertility in a woman even without symptoms.

Most cases of PID occur when *Chlamydia trachomatis* or *Neisseria gonorrhoeae* spreads up the fallopian tubes, but they can be caused by other STDs as well.

The use of an intrauterine device (IUD) for birth control can increase the risk of PID, with the greatest risk coming a few months after the IUD is inserted. Women who develop PID after using an IUD are usually advised to have it removed.

A woman may have no symptoms of PID until its advanced stages. Then, it can cause abdominal and low back pain and fever. White blood cells, working to eliminate the infection, may cause a discharge.

PID is one of the major preventable causes of infertility in women. The infection in the fallopian tubes can cause abscesses and scar tissue to form in the tubes that may block sperm from passing through them, leaving the woman infertile. Approximately 13 percent of women who have one attack of PID are left infertile. Those who suffer three attacks of PID have a 75 percent chance of becoming infertile.

PID is diagnosed during a gynecological exam and lab testing for STDs. Although chlamydia and gonorrhea are commonly diagnosed as the causes of PID, these two types of organisms can die quickly. They may not be easily cultured at the time testing is done. The common bacterium *Escherichia coli*, found in the digestive and genital tracts of healthy women, is often the only type of bacteria noted at the time of the diagnosis.

PID is treated with antibiotics that may be administered orally or intravenously, depending on the severity of the infection. In some cases, surgery is required to remove abscesses that remain after antibiotic treatment.

Treatment

Genital warts are treated by removing the warts from both partners. Medications that are placed on the wart include a natural resin called podofilox (which inhibits wart growth) and acids such as trichloroacetic or bichloroacetic acid (which dry up the warts). Podofilox should not be used by pregnant women.

Other options include laser surgery and freezing the warts, called cryotherapy. Electrodesiccation (sending an electrical current through the tissue, which then dries up) is also used to remove the warts.

Although the visible warts can be removed, this does not cure the virus. As yet there is no cure or vaccine for HPV. Since the virus may remain in the body, warts may come back and require further treatment. Because of the risk of cancer, women who contract the virus should have frequent and regular Pap tests.

Genital Herpes

Symptoms

The symptoms of genital herpes first appear after a 3- to 7-day incubation period. Genital herpes is characterized by pain and itching in the genital area along with blisters or open sores. When these are present, a person is said to be having an outbreak. The first outbreak of genital herpes is usualy marked by additional flulike symptoms, including fever, headache, and swollen lymph nodes in the groin area. Recurrent outbreaks tend to have more localized symptoms.

The symptoms are usually preceded by a tingly or burning sensation in the area, that will later develop into tiny red blisters in both men and women. These blisters then grow into larger pimplelike bumps that have a watery yellow center. The blisters rupture, and within 3 or 4 days a crust forms.

In both sexes, the blisters can appear in the genital area and on the thighs, abdomen, buttocks, and anus. In women blisters usually appear on the labia and around the clitoris. In men, they may appear on the penis and scrotum. Sometimes blisters near the opening of the urethra and on the tip of the penis will swell up, making urination difficult and painful.

Blisters may also develop internally on the female cervix and vaginal walls or inside the male urethra. These internal lesions may make it difficult for men to urinate and difficult to detect the virus in women.

The entire process of a herpes outbreak, from initial tingle to dried-up crust, can last about 3 weeks, but the virus may still be active—and the infected person contagious—for 2 weeks after the symptoms disappear. Although the virus is most contagious during the blistering stage, it can be transmitted during the early phase of burning and tingling as well.

Even though the symptoms subside, the virus moves to the nerve cells in the base of the spinal cord, where it is dormant. During a recurrent outbreak, the virus travels down the nerves to the genital area and causes a new set of blisters and more distress. Between 50 and 75 percent of those who have an initial outbreak will suffer a recurrent infection within 3 months. The cause of the recurrent attacks is unknown, but there does seem to be a correlation between outbreaks and stress or a weakened immune system.

There is no cure for genital herpes, but each successive outbreak has fewer and weaker symptoms. After a number of years, the outbreaks may disappear.

If a pregnant woman has open herpes lesions, she runs the risk of infecting her baby as it passes through the vagina at birth. If infected, the baby may suffer brain damage, blindness, or death if not treated. A pregnant woman with herpes will be examined when she is in labor. If she has active sores, she should have her baby by cesarean section.

Cause

About 150 million people in the United States are thought to have been exposed to herpes simplex virus, the virus that causes genital herpes. Each year, about 300,000 new cases are diagnosed. Herpes simplex virus type 2 causes about 80 percent of cases of genital herpes. The other 20 percent is caused by herpes simplex type 1 virus, better known as the cause of sores on the mouth and lips.

The virus is transmitted through sexual contact—vaginal, anal, or oral—and can also enter the body through mucous membranes or cuts in the skin. Genital herpes can also infect the eyes if fingers carrying the virus touch the eyes. Active genital herpes is highly contagious. Transmission is known to occur during inapparent activation of the infection, even when blisters or open sores are not visible.

Diagnosis

A diagnosis of genital herpes is made by taking a sample culture from a liquid-filled blister or a sore in its early phase.

Treatment

Genital herpes has no cure but a vaccine for prevention is being developed. Keeping the infected area clean and dry can help improve a person's comfort when having an outbreak. Use of the oral drug acyclovir can reduce the length of time the virus can be transmitted, shorten the healing time, and decrease the severity of symptoms. Pregnant women are best served by using the topical form. Persons who have frequent recurrences can take acyclovir daily to prevent attacks. Because the infection is usually contracted while sores are present, abstaining from sex until sores are completely healed can help stop the spread of herpes. Transmission, however, can occur during active disease without blisters or symptoms; therefore the safest approach is to use a condom.

Syphilis

Symptoms

Syphilis occurs in three stages: primary, secondary, and tertiary. The signs of primary syphilis are painless sores called chancres on the genitals, tongue, lips, breast, or rectum, along with swollen lymph nodes in the adjacent area. If the sore is located in a woman's vagina, it can easily go undetected. The incubation period for primary syphilis is 2 to 3 weeks and sometimes as long as 8 weeks.

Secondary syphilis begins in 2 to 6 weeks after the chancre heals, usually without treatment. The signs of secondary syphilis may include fever, headache, aching joints, and a skin rash. The skin rash appears diffusely as well as on the bottoms of feet and the palms of hands.

An infected person then can go through a period when syphilis is latent, that is without signs or symptoms. They may be followed by tertiary syphilis if the person is not treated. Latent syphillis can be life threatening because the bacteria by this time has spread throughout the body and into the blood system, and brain. Tertiary syphilis, which appears years later, can cause a number of problems, including nerve and brain damage and heart disease. These severe symptoms are not very common in the United States, since syphilis rarely progresses to this late stage.

Women infected with syphilis can pass the infection to their unborn fetus during pregnancy. About 50 percent of those fetuses infected will be born prematurely or stillborn. Those infants that do survive may appear healthy at birth but develop problems later.

Cause

Until the recent arrival of acquired immunodeficiency syndrome (AIDS), syphilis was the most serious of the STDs. It is caused by the bacterium *Treponema pallidum*. Although it was once a very common infection, today syphilis is rarer than chlamydia and gonorrhea. In the past few years, however, the incidence of syphilis has increased, especially within the homosexual community.

Syphilis is contracted during sexual contact, through cuts or sores in the skin or mucous membranes. The disease is very contagious. It can also pass through the blood and to an unborn fetus from an infected mother.

Diagnosis

Infection is suspected based on the presence of sores (for primary syphilis) or rash and flulike symptoms (for secondary syphilis). A positive blood test is necessary to diagnose syphilis. Even if a person has no symptoms, a blood test can usually detect syphilis.

Some states require syphilis tests before issuing marriage licenses, so some people learn only then that they have syphilis at that time. Others are tested for syphilis when they enter a hospital. Because of the danger of syphilis for the fetus, all pregnant women are tested for syphilis.

Treatment

Penicillin given intramuscularly is effective for primary and for secondary syphilis. Latent syphilis can also be treated with penicillin to prevent complications, but must be given longer and at higher doses to achieve success during this phase. Penicillin can be used safely to treat pregnant women and prevent transmission to their fetus. It can also be used to treat infected infants. Penicillin is the most commonly used antibiotic for syphilis, but doxycycline or tetracycline can be used for those who are allergic to penicillin.

Because syphilis can be spread when open lesions are present, sexual contact of any kind should be avoided during this time. Routine blood tests are required for one year following the initial syphilis infection to determine whether treatment has been successful.

Trichomonas

Symptoms

Common symptoms in women include an abundant yellow frothy musty smelling discharge. Sores may form on the cervix. The vulva may itch, and urinating may be painful. Most men with trichomonas infection do not have symptoms.

Trichomonas infection is caused by a small organism called *Trichomonas vaginalis.* It affects about 15 percent of sexually active women and 10 percent of sexually active men. It causes symptoms like those of vaginitis (see Chapter 15). Because the organism can live outside the vagina, nonsexual transmission may also occur.

Diagnosis

To diagnose trichomonas infection, a sample of the discharge is taken and examined under a microscope.

Treatment

Trichomonas infection is not usually serious and can be treated easily with metronidazole. Usually just one dose is needed, but some doctors choose to give a lower dose for 7 days. A woman and her sex partner(s) must be treated. They should avoid having sex until they have completed their treatment and no longer have symptoms. Anyone who is taking metronidazole should avoid drinking alcohol, which can cause severe nausea and vomiting when mixed with metronidazole.

Cytomegalovirus

Symptoms

CMV often has no symptoms. Women who do have symptoms may have a mild illness similar to the flu. Although CMV is not harmful for most women, it causes special concerns for a pregnant woman, who can pass CMV to her fetus through the umbilical cord. CMV is most risky if a woman first becomes infected while she is pregnant. If this happens, the fetus can be harmed. CMV can also be passed to the infant during birth and later through breast milk. Approximately 50 percent of mothers who have CMV pass it on to their infants, and of those infants 5 to 15 percent will have abnormal central nervous systems at birth.

Cause

Cytomegalovirus (CMV) is caused by a virus with the same name. Up to 70 percent of people have evidence in their blood that they have been infected with CMV. Children can contract the disease from an infected mother. One of the most common ways a woman gets CMV is by being exposed to children, for example, in day care. CMV also may be passed on through blood transfusions or through sexual activity with an infected partner.

Diagnosis

Cytomegalovirus is diagnosed through a blood test for CMV antibodies. Infection in the fetus can be diagnosed by testing blood or the amniotic fluid.

Treatment

There is no cure for CMV. Because a fetus can develop severe abnormalities if infected with the virus early in development, tests are performed early in pregnancy. Infection of the fetus late in pregnancy may lead to childhood hearing and learning problems.

Chancroid

Symptoms

The initial symptoms are one or more painful swellings (boils) that appear in the genital area. If ignored, these lesions will rupture and release pus.

Cause

Rare in the United States but common in the tropics, chancroid is caused by the organism *Haemophilus ducreyi*, which is passed during sex across genital mucus membranes. It moves through the lymphatic system into the groin area to infect the glands.

Diagnosis

A microscopic examination of the pus is necessary to determine the cause of any lesions. Syphilis has similar symptoms, so this examination will rule out syphilis.

Treatment

Azithromycin, ceftriaxone, or erythromycin is most comonly given to treat the patient and prevent spread of the disease. Gentle pressure on lesions can also help accelerate their healing. Even if they don't have symptoms, sex partners of women with chancroid should also be examined and treated.

CHAPTER 20

AIDS and Women

Carol Widrow, M.D.

nfection with human immunodeficiency virus (HIV) leads to a condition called acquired immune deficiency syndrome (AIDS). The infection causes the body's immune system, which fights disease, to weaken, leaving it open to a range of other diseases. It can take 8 to 10 years from the initial infection with HIV to the development of symptoms of full-blown AIDS. During that time, a person with HIV can pass the virus to others. The infection is transmitted through sex, exposure to blood or blood products of individuals who are infected, and from a mother who is HIV positive to her infant. Although treatment is available to help limit the progression of the conditions that occur with AIDS, there is no cure.

Since its discovery in 1984, AIDS has reached epidemic proportions throughout the world. The World Health Organization, which is devoted to promoting better health internationally, estimates that 13 million men, women, and children worldwide are infected with HIV. In the United States, 1 million individuals are estimated to be infected with HIV. More than 400,000 individuals have AIDS, and over 245,000 have died from it according to the Centers for Disease Control and Prevention (CDC), a federal agency that monitors the disease and issues guidelines for its management.

In the U.S., infection with HIV affects all groups, although it occurs in minority populations more than it does in white populations. Through 1992, 47 percent of all reported AIDS cases were among African-Americans and Hispanics, although these two groups represent only 21 percent of the total population. Although the disease was originally prevalent mostly in homosexual men, heterosexual sex is now the most common mode of infection worldwide and is the fastest growing mode of transmission in the United States. The increase in heterosexual transmission has led to a dramatic increase in HIV infection in women, who comprised almost 13 percent of the AIDS cases diagnosed in 1992. In the U.S., AIDS is the fourth leading cause of death in women of reproductive age and the leading cause of death in black women of reproductive age in New York and New Jersey. (See Table 20.1)

AIDS is also among the top 10 causes of death for children aged 1 to 4 years. Infants of mothers who are HIV infected have a 15 to 30 percent risk of acquiring the virus and will also become motherless as a result of AIDS.

As can be seen, HIV infection and AIDS are enormous public health issues. In the absence of an effective vaccine, the best way to bring the spread of HIV under control is through prevention. This can be done by avoiding practices that pose a risk for transmitting the virus.

HOW HIV IS TRANSMITTED

HIV can be found in the body fluids of an infected individual. These fluids include blood as well as semen, saliva, vaginal secretions, amniotic fluid (which surrounds the fetus in the mother's abdomen during pregnancy), breast milk, and urine. It is transmitted three ways:

1. Exposure to body secretions of individuals who are infected during sexual activity.
2. Exposure to blood or blood products, such as through a transfusion or when sharing needles with other intravenous drug using individuals.
3. During pregnancy, when a mother who is infected can pass the virus to her fetus, or during delivery or breast-feeding.

The virus is not spread through casual contact. It is not transmitted through sharing food and drink; touching everyday objects such as linens, telephones, doorknobs, and toilet seats; using swimming pools or hot tubs; hugging or casual kissing; coughing or sneezing; being exposed to another person's tears or sweat; by getting bitten by an insect. (See Table 20.2)

Sexual Activity

Women are at greater risk than men during heterosexual sex, because the virus seems to be much more easily transmitted from men to women than from women to men. Any interruption or break in the skin or mucous membranes of the genital tract (the vagina, penis, and anus) increases access of the virus via infected semen, blood, or vaginal secretions. These interruptions can occur through traumatic sex, which causes tearing of the skin or lining of the genital tract,

TABLE 20.1   AIDS AMONG WOMEN

Age at diagnosis (years)	White, not Hispanic No.	(%)	Black, not Hispanic No.	(%)	Hispanic No.	(%)	Asian/Pacific Islander No.	(%)	American Indian/ Alaska Native No.	(%)	Total No.	(%)
Under 5	360	(3)	1,362	(5)	535	(5)	6	(2)	7	(5)	2,277	(4)
5-12	101	(1)	230	(1)	127	(1)	6	(2)	–	–	466	(1)
13-19	113	(1)	358	(1)	91	(1)	1	(0)	1	(1)	565	(1)
20-24	802	(6)	1,737	(6)	751	(7)	15	(5)	16	(11)	3,325	(6)
25-29	2,316	(18)	4,786	(16)	2,053	(18)	27	(10)	29	(20)	9,222	(17)
30-34	2,970	(23)	6,975	(24)	2,746	(25)	56	(20)	38	(26)	12,806	(24)
35-39	2,381	(18)	6,377	(22)	2,150	(19)	45	(16)	21	(14)	10,995	(20)
40-44	1,403	(11)	3,804	(13)	1,289	(12)	42	(15)	14	(10)	6,561	(12)
45-49	765	(6)	1,614	(6)	627	(6)	25	(9)	8	(6)	3,044	(6)
50-54	444	(3)	878	(3)	362	(3)	15	(5)	3	(2)	1,705	(3)
55-59	380	(3)	504	(2)	219	(2)	10	(4)	4	(3)	1,119	(2)
60-64	295	(2)	320	(1)	112	(1)	13	(5)	3	(2)	743	(1)
65 or older	685	(5)	328	(1)	118	(1)	16	(6)	1	(1)	1,149	(2)
	13,015	(100)	29,273	(100)	11,181	(100)	277	(100)	145	(100)	53,978	(100)
Total	198,130		130,384		68,903		2,706		944		401,749	

Source: U.S. Dept of Health and Human Services, Public Health Service, CDC, Atlanta, GA 30333.

TABLE 20.2   WAYS WOMEN GET AIDS

Exposure category	White, not Latino No.	(%)	Africa American, not Latino No.	(5)	Latino No.	(%)	Asian/Pacific Islander No.	(%)	American Indian/ Alaska Native No.	(%)	Totals No.	(%)
Injecting drug use	5,426	(43)	14,160	(51)	4,923	(47)	43	(16)	65	(47)	24,660	(48)
Hemophilia/coagulation disorder	56	(0)	20	(0)	6	(0)	1	(0)	–	–	83	(0)
Heterosexual contact:	4,536	(36)	9,014	(33)	4,479	(43)	118	(45)	46	(33)	18,217	(36)
Sex with injecting drug user	2,131		4,968		2,798		35		30		9,976	
Sex with bisexual male	766		576		220		34		3		1,601	
Sex with person with hemophilia	168		26		14		2		2		212	
Sex with transfusion recipient with HIV infection	203		79		67		12		–		363	
Sex with HIV-infected person, risk not specified	1,268		3,365		1,380		35		11		6,065	
Receipt of blood transfusion, blood components, or tissue	1,489	(12)	725	(3)	389	(4)	62	(23)	10	(7)	2,676	(5)
Risk not reported or identified	1,047	(8)	3,762	(14)	722	(7)	41	(15)	17	(12)	5,599	(11)
Total	12,544	(100)	27,681	(100)	10,519	(100)	265	(100)	138	(100)	51,235	(100)

Source: U.S. HIV and AIDS Cases Reported through June 1994, U.S. Department of Health and Human Services, Public Health Service, CDC, Atlanta, Ga 30333.

or through sores that occur with sexually transmitted diseases such as herpes or syphilis. Types of intercourse that have a high risk of trauma, such as anal intercourse, also have a high risk of infection with HIV. Bisexual men who engage in this activity also have sexual contact with women, who can then acquire the infection.

Lesbians appear to be at much less of a risk of contracting the virus from sexual contact, provided they know the risk factors of their partners. Most women with HIV who have had sexual contact only with other women have a history of intravenous drug use or have received blood products. There is a slight risk of transmitting the virus through sexual intercourse during menstruation when one partner is HIV positive and through practices such as digital manipulation or sharing of mechanical devices. In general, when one partner of a lesbian couple is infected, there is a real but low risk that the virus can be transmitted to the uninfected partner.

Exposure to Blood and Blood Products

Intravenous drug use is a major cause of HIV infection. If needles are shared, small amounts of contaminated blood can transmit the virus from one person to another. An intravenous drug user also can transmit the virus to sex partners. More than 50 percent of the women who have contracted AIDS from heterosexual transmission had a sex partner who was an intravenous drug user. In addition, many of these women are themselves intravenous drug users. Women who are HIV positive can transmit the virus to their children. Over 70 percent of children with AIDS have mothers who are intravenous drug users or mothers who are sexual partners of intravenous drug users.

Before 1985, blood donated to blood banks was not tested for HIV, so people who received blood transfusions were at risk for infection. Since then, all donated blood has been tested for HIV, and the blood donors are screened for their risk of transmitting the virus. The blood supply is now considered to be quite safe (99 percent).

Individuals with blood disorders, especially those with hemophilia, depend on donated blood to obtain clotting factors, which control bleeding. Clotting factors are produced in blood products derived from blood donations. Since 1985, clotting factors have been heated, inactivating HIV and making the blood products generally safe.

Health care workers are also at risk of being exposed to the blood of an infected individual during emergency and routine medical procedures. Surgery and dental work can result in accidental exposure to HIV. All health care workers are advised to follow what are called "universal precautions," a set of guidelines established by the CDC to protect them from exposure to HIV and other viruses.

Pregnancy

A woman who is HIV positive has about a one in three chance of infecting her child with the virus. During pregnancy, viruses may cross the placenta (which passes nourishment to the fetus from the mother) and infect the fetus. The newborn may become infected by exposure to the mother's blood and vaginal secretions during birth. Breast-feeding can cause infection, especially in mothers who contracted HIV shortly after the baby's birth. Therefore, it is recommended that women who are infected do not breast-feed their infants.

It is difficult to tell at the time of birth if a child is infected, because the mother's antibodies (part of the immune system) are present in the newborn's blood. Thus all infants born to women who are HIV positive have HIV antibodies in their blood. If the child is *not* infected, he or she will test HIV negative by the age of 15 to 18 months, when the mother's antibodies have been replaced by the infant's own. An 18-month-old child who tests positive, however, is almost certainly infected. Children who are infected usually have symptoms within the first 3 years of life, although some do not develop signs of AIDS for 7 or more years. In general, the course of disease and survival rates are worse for children who show signs of the disease within the first year of life.

Because HIV can be spread through semen, women who undergo artificial insemination, in which semen from a donor is placed into the cervical area, can be infected with HIV in this way. Not all sperm banks screen donors for HIV, so there is a risk of infection. It is imperative for a recipient to ascertain if donors are screened at month 0 and a later time before they accept semen.

TESTING FOR HIV

A person can be tested to determine whether HIV infection has occurred. The test detects antibodies in the blood. Antibodies are proteins produced in response to a foreign protein of the virus. Once a person is infected, the body begins to produce antibodies, which can be detected in the blood 6 to 12 weeks after infection. These early weeks are called the "window period," which is the time when a person is infected but an antibody test is negative.

Two tests are used to detect HIV. The first test is an enzyme-linked immunosorbent assay, usually referred to as ELISA. It is used as a screening test, which may be repeated if the test is positive. The second test is called a Western blot, which is used to confirm the positive results of the ELISA test. Both tests detect antibodies to HIV in the blood, but the Western blot is more specific than the ELISA test.

Although these tests are over 99 percent accurate, false-positive results (showing the infection is present when it isn't) and false-negative results (showing the infection is not present when it is) can occur. One of the reasons for false results is the period between the time when a person becomes infected and when antibodies appear. If a person is tested soon after infection, antibodies may not yet have been produced to show up on the test.

Some doctors suggest that everyone be tested for HIV, regardless of individual risk. Anyone who is exposed to risk factors should be tested for HIV. Testing is also recommended if a person shows signs of HIV infection. Because the virus can be passed from mother to baby, a woman who is pregnant or considering pregnancy may wish to be tested, since new information shows treatment can significantly reduce the baby's risk. If there is a question about a sex partner's history the testing is worth considering. Many women who test positive for HIV do not have a history of any risk factors except having had sex with a man, which confirms the importance of the heterosexual route of transmission.

If you choose to have an HIV test, be sure to receive counseling before the test and after the results are provided. Counseling should include information about risk behaviors and how to change them. It also should explain how to get special health care and how to avoid passing the virus to others, if the tests are positive. If test results are positive, you should take steps to ensure your health as well as the health of others with whom you may come in contact. Because of potential discrimination against individuals who are HIV positive, conveying results of tests is strictly confidential, except as provided by law in certain states.

PREVENTION OF HIV INFECTION

As the number of people infected with HIV increases, individual risk of contracting the virus also increases. This is a fatal disease and has no cure, so the best protection is through prevention: Practicing safe sex, avoiding intravenous drug use, ensuring the safety of blood products, and having a healthy pregnancy.

Practicing Safe Sex

Safe sex practices can lower your risk of HIV infection. These practices involve limiting the number of your sex partners, knowing the history of your sex partners, always using a condom, and avoiding certain practices that could cause trauma.

The history of a sex partner can also pose a risk. If you have sex with someone who has had sex with someone who has risk factors, there is a possibility that you could be infected with HIV. It is best to question sexual partners about their history: Ask whether they have ever used intravenous drugs or had sex with someone who did and ask about other sex partners or bisexual practices. Always ask your partners to use a condom, and if they refuse, limit your sexual activities to touching, kissing, or other forms of sexual expression that do not involve intercourse.

Condoms should always be used during sexual intercourse. It is important that condoms be used consistently and properly—most condom failure is the result of incorrect use. Condoms not only prevent pregnancy but also offer protection against sexually transmitted diseases such as herpes, syphilis, and chlamydia as well as AIDS. Although condoms cannot totally eliminate the risk of transmission of HIV, if used correctly, they decrease the risk of infection by eliminating your contact with semen and any penile lesions your partner may have.

Latex condoms provide better protection than natural membrane condoms, which although they appear intact can have pores through which the virus can pass. If lubricant is required with condom use, use only water-based lubricants, because oil- or petroleum-based lubricants can weaken the latex and allow the virus to pass through. Condoms should be used with the spermicide nonoxynol-9. Spermicide use increases the contraceptive effectiveness rate of the condom as well as helps kill HIV. Oral contraceptives, diaphragms, and intrauterine devices are all good methods of birth control, but they do not offer any protection against HIV or sexually transmitted diseases. Always supplement these methods with the use of condoms.

When you become involved in a mutually faithful relationship, you will want to know when you can stop using condoms. Before condom use is discontinued, it is advisable that both you and your partner be tested for HIV 3 to 6 months after either of you has had sexual contact with a different partner.

Specific sexual practices can also increase your risk of HIV infection. There is a great likelihood of trauma

RISK FACTORS

The following factors, whether they apply to an individual or to an individual's sex partner, increase the risk of infection with HIV:

- Injecting drugs, especially with shared needles
- Current or past sexual contact with
    More than one partner
    Someone who has tested positive for HIV or who has AIDS
    A man who has had sex with another man, whether he is mainly heterosexual, bisexual, or homosexual
- Receiving blood or blood products before 1985
- Current or past sexually transmitted diseases such as gonorrhea, chlamydia, syphilis, or hepatitis B

A DIALOGUE ABOUT AIDS

Talking with partners about the risk of AIDS is key to a healthy relationship. AIDS can be a difficult thing to talk about, but it can be deadly not to discuss it. Here are some points for women to raise:

- Have you ever had sex with a man?
- Have you ever used drugs? Do you use drugs now?
- Have you ever had a sex partner who was a drug user?
- How many sex partners have you had in the past year?

If the answers aren't reassuring or if your partner will not consent to the use of a condom, set limits and tell your partner about your decisions. Your partner should accept your choices; if not, it may be better to stop having sex for a time than to risk your health. If your partner becomes abusive because of your choice to have safe sex, this is a sign that the relationship is not a healthy one between adults who care about each other. Exercise good judgment: People are not always exactly truthful when they want to have sex with someone.

with anal sex, and the virus is easily absorbed into the bloodstream through the rectum. Condoms are also likely to break during anal sex. HIV can also spread through oral sex, especially if there are cuts, tears, or sores in the mouth. For oral sex with a man, condoms should be used. For oral sex with a woman, a condom cut open, plastic wrap, or a dental dam (a square of latex used for oral surgery) should be used. If a sexual device (dildo or vibrator) is shared, it should be disinfected with bleach or rubbing alcohol every time it is used. Some type of protection should be used if there is a risk that sex acts may draw blood or tear skin.

Avoiding Drug Use

About 50 percent of the women who test positive for HIV are infected through intravenous drug use. If needles are shared, HIV-infected blood left in needles after injecting drugs can infect the next person who uses the needle.

If you do use drugs, never share needles or any of the equipment used to inject drugs. All equipment should be sterilized. Needles can be sterilized by flushing twice with pure laundry bleach. Bleach should be removed by flushing twice with tap water. Because of the risk of HIV infection with intravenous drug use, many municipalities are distributing clean needles to drug-addicted individuals as a means of controlling the spread of AIDS.

Ensuring the Safety of Blood Products

Since 1985, the risk of HIV infection through blood transfusion has been low. A slight risk does exist, however. One of the ways to avoid infection by blood transfusion is to donate your own blood before any planned surgery so that, if blood is needed, your own blood can be used. Health care workers should follow the universal precautions, which include wearing masks, gloves, and protective clothing during certain medical procedures as protection against exposure to infected blood.

Having a Healthy Pregnancy

Sperm can transmit HIV. Thus a woman who is trying to become pregnant may become infected. The best way to protect yourself against infection is for both you and your partner to be tested for HIV before having unprotected sex.

If you choose to become pregnant by artificial insemination, that is, by having semen inserted into your cervix, the donor should be tested before it is used.

If you are pregnant and HIV positive, you have a risk of passing the virus to your fetus during pregnancy. Preliminary studies show that this risk can be reduced by 66 percent by giving treatment during pregnancy. Treatment is most effective when it is given to women who do not have advanced disease. HIV infection or AIDS does not seem to have an effect on the pregnancy itself. Because of the risk to the fetus, however, if you are infected with HIV or at risk of being infected, you should seek special prenatal care.

THE AIDS PROCESS

HIV infection means that the virus has entered the bloodstream and has begun to break down the immune system. The immune system helps protect your body from viruses, bacteria, parasites, and fungi. If any infection occurs, special white blood cells, called T cells, are activated to defend your body against the infection.

HIV infects T cells that have a specific surface protein called CD4. HIV binds to the CD4 protein on the white blood cell, thus beginning the course of infection. Once attached, the virus enters the cell and multiplies, eventually killing the T cell. As more and more of the T cells die, the body's ability to fight certain types of infections weakens. This leaves a person who is HIV positive open to so-called opportunistic infections. Such infections are able to take hold, because of the person's weakened immune system.

A person with HIV infection may remain healthy for many years. It can take 8–10 years or even longer after the initial infection with HIV until serious illness and infections appear. These illnesses tend to occur after HIV has left few T cells alive. Until then, a person with HIV may show signs of certain types of infection that come and go, as their immune system starts to weaken.

The Initial Infection

Once HIV infects the cells, 40 to 60 percent of individuals will develop antibodies to the virus within about 1 to 8 weeks after exposure. Symptoms similar to flu or mononucleosis occur, including fever (with or without swollen glands), rash, sore throat, fatigue, muscle aches, nausea, vomiting, and/or diarrhea. These symptoms last between 3 and 14 days. After recovery from the primary infection, the individual who is HIV positive usually has no symptoms for some time. The virus is being shed or passed into body fluids, however, and can be passed to others. Antibodies to HIV develop in almost all individuals who are infected within 2 to 3 months.

Early Markers of HIV Infection

As the immune system decreases in efficiency, individuals who are HIV-infected begin to show signs of HIV disease. Early signs of immune system deficiency include generalized lymphadenopathy—a persistent swelling of the lymph glands—as well as fever, night sweats, diarrhea, weight loss, and fatigue. These signs occur in both men and women. Effects specific to women have not been fully studied, but those that have been observed often appear as routine gynecologic problems. Their presence should alert both women and their physicians to the possibility of HIV infection in those who otherwise may not have risk factors. Some early markers of HIV infection in women include the following conditions.

Recurrent Vaginal Candidiasis

Candidiasis is commonly known as a yeast infection, which women often get when they take antibiotics, are pregnant, or have diabetes. The symptoms are a thick white or yellow discharge, vaginal itch or burning, and pain when urinating. Such infections may be HIV related when they occur more than three times in a 6-month period or are difficult to treat. HIV infection may be suspected if no other cause for yeast infection can be identified.

Cervical Disease

It is unclear if cervical intraepithelial neoplasia (CIN), a precancerous lesion on the opening of the uterus, occurs more often in women with HIV. It is clear, however, that when CIN occurs in women infected with HIV it is more advanced, persistent, and difficult to treat, and it recurs more often than in women who are not infected with HIV. There are a number of risk factors besides HIV infection that are related to CIN. Women with more advanced CIN, however, may wish to be tested for HIV. CIN can lead to invasive cancer, which can be prevented if cervical disease is detected in its early stages. All women should have a Pap test yearly to screen for cervical disease. Women with HIV should consider having a pelvic exam every 6 months.

Herpes and Human Papillomavirus

Certain viral diseases, such as herpes and human papillomavirus (HPV), may be more serious in women who are infected with HIV. The herpes virus enters bodily fluids (sheds) more frequently and may be a chronic problem requiring long-term therapy. Human papillomavirus, which causes genital warts, has been linked to cervical cancer and thus can become a serious problem for women whose immune system is not fully functional.

The Final Stage

The final stage of HIV infection is full-blown AIDS. People who are HIV positive are said to have AIDS when they are sick with serious illnesses and infections caused by the effects of the virus. Since it is the CD4 cells that are destroyed by the virus, these cells are counted and the result is a rough estimate of the state of a person's immune system. The number of CD4 T cells in a healthy person who is not infected by HIV is 800 to 1,200. Individuals who are HIV positive and have CD4 counts of less than 200 are considered to have AIDS.

Certain disorders have been identified by the CDC as representing a diagnosis of AIDS when they appear in individuals who are HIV infected (see "AIDS-defining Diseases"). These disorders appear in both men and women but not always in the same frequency. They have mostly been studied in men and only recently have disorders specific to women been included. It seems that AIDS is the same in men and women, but there are few studies to show that there are any specific gender differences in response to HIV infection or treatment. Because many women with HIV have no stated risk factors, the diagnosis is often delayed and a disorder may be severe by the time they seek treatment.

Pneumocystis carinii Pneumonia

Pneumocystis carinii pneumonia is the most common AIDS-defining disorder in both men or women. It is an infection of the lungs, and symptoms include fever, cough, and shortness of breath. Treatment may be given both to treat as well as to help prevent this disorder.

AIDS-DEFINING DISEASES

The CDC has identified the following conditions as diagnostic of AIDS when they occur in people who are infected with HIV. These conditions are also used to determine who is eligible for disability benefits.

- Cancer, invasive, cervical
- Candidiasis
    Bronchi, trachea, or lungs
    Esophageal
- Coccidioidomycosis, disseminated or extrapulmonary
- Cryptococcosis
    Extrapulmonary
    Chronic intestinal (greater than 1 month's duration)
- Cytomegalovirus
    Disease (other than liver, spleen, or lymph nodes)
    Retinitis (with loss of vision)
- Encephalopathy, HIV related
- Herpes simplex, chronic ulcers (greater than 1 month's duration) or bronchitis, pneumonitis, or esophagitis
- Histoplasmosis, disseminated or extrapulmonary
- Isosporiasis, chronic intestinal (greater than 1 month's duration)
- Kaposi's sarcoma
- Leukoencephalopathy, progressive multifocal
- Lymphoma
    Burkitt's
    Immunoblastic
    Primary, brain
- *Mycobacterium* species
    M. avium complex or *M. kansasii;* disseminated or extrapulmonary
    M. tuberculosis, any site
    Other or unidentified species
- Pneumonia
    Pneumocystis carinii
    Recurrent
- *Salmonella,* recurrent septicemia
- Toxoplasmosis, brain
- Wasting syndrome

SOURCE: Centers for Disease Control and Prevention, "1993 Revised Classification System for HIV Infection and Expanded Surveillance Case Definition for AIDS among Adolescents and Adults," *MMWR. Morbitity and Mortality Weekly Report* 41, no. RR-17 (1992): 1–9.

Esophageal Candidiasis

Esophageal candidiasis is a yeast infection in the esophagus, the passageway from the throat to the stomach. The symptoms can be difficulty swallowing, pain in the chest, and weight loss.

Tuberculosis

Tuberculosis (TB) is a bacterial infection seen in all stages of HIV infection. Populations at risk for HIV infection are also at risk for TB; the current rise in the number of reported TB cases is related in part to AIDS. In early stages, the symptoms are cough, fever, and weight loss, and the disease is limited mostly to the lungs. In later stages of HIV infection, when the immune system is weakened, TB can spread outside the lungs to the lymph nodes, bone marrow, liver, spleen, and gastrointestinal tract.

Mycobacterial Infections

Infection from *Mycobacterium* species occurs in up to 50 percent of AIDS patients, usually after there has been severe damage to the immune system. The mycobacteria are acquired either by ingestion or by inhalation. They then move from the lungs to other parts of the body, causing fever, weight loss, diarrhea, anemia, and enlargement of the liver and spleen.

Cytomegalovirus

Cytomegalovirus is often found in people with poor immune function. It can infect many organ systems, including the lungs, brain, adrenal glands, and gastrointestinal system. Most often, it infects the eyes, causing blurring and loss of vision. It begins in one eye and tends to cause disease in the other.

Toxoplasmosis

Toxoplasmosis infection is caused by a parasite that is acquired by eating undercooked food. It can also be transmitted from cat feces. Initially, symptoms of infection are fever, night sweats, sore throat, and swollen lymph glands. The symptoms can then disappear, but the parasite remains and is reactivated whenever the immune system becomes less able to function. The parasite grows in the brain, causing headaches, seizures, and weakness in various parts of the body.

TREATMENT FOR AIDS

Although there is no cure for AIDS, early medical consultation and medication can prolong the time that a person who is HIV positive can be free of symptoms. In addition, treatment focuses on preventing certain conditions from occurring, slowing the damage to the immune system, and treating conditions as they occur.

Immunizations, such as flu shots, can be given to help keep people with HIV from getting other infections that could do damage in the presence of a weakened immune system. There is also treatment to help prevent *pneumocystic carinii* pneumonia, which is given to people with a CD4 count below 200. In general, individuals who are HIV infected should avoid being around people who are sick, because any infection could be life-threatening, even chicken pox or measles.

Drug therapy is intended to stop HIV from reproducing and destroying the immune system and includes AZT (zidovudine), didanosine (ddl), and dideoxycytidine (ddC). These drugs have side effects and are often changed or used in combination, depending on the person's reaction to them.

Infections and other conditions associated with AIDS are treated as they arise, just as they would be in any other individual. Because the infections can be severe and often recur in people with HIV, however, such patients may need to take the medicine for the rest of their lives.

THE FUTURE

New information continues to evolve about HIV and AIDS and new treatments are emerging. There is no cure, however, and the key to combating the disease is through prevention. Education is the most important preventive measure available. It has proved to be effective in the homosexual population, which through public awareness and educational campaigns has reduced the incidence of HIV infection. The same approach can benefit the general population, where there are an increasing number of women who become infected with HIV today by contracting the virus through heterosexual transmission.

AIDS INFORMATION

For updated information about AIDS call one of the following hot lines.

- National AIDS Hotline: 800-342-AIDS
- Spanish-language hot line: 800-344-AIDS
- Deaf access hot line: 800-AIDS-TTY

Or write to the CDC National AIDS Clearinghouse at P.O. Box 6003, Rockville, MD 20849-6003.

PART IV

THE HEALTHY BODY: SYMPTOMS, DIAGNOSES, AND TREATMENTS

CHAPTER 21

Accidents and Emergencies

Diane Sixsmith, M.D., M.P.H., F.A.C.E.P. and Christina Gertrud Rehm, M.D., F.A.C.S

One of the leading causes of death in the United States, accidents are the main cause of death in children and young men. More teenage women die in motor vehicle accidents than from any other cause. Although injuries occur to women of all ages, elderly women are more prone to accidental injuries and suffer serious consequences from them.

When accidents or emergencies occur, a prompt response can be life saving. In some cases, a matter of minutes can make a difference. In an emergency, assessing a situation and reacting quickly and calmly re-quires knowledge, experience, and training (see "Emergency Procedures" and "What to Do").

You can learn first aid and life-saving techniques such as cardiopulmonary resuscitation (CPR) in regularly scheduled classes with qualified instructors. Classes are available through schools, community organizations, and hospitals. Other sources include the American Red Cross and the American Heart Association. Experts estimate, however, that nearly one-half of all accidents could be prevented by removing hazards and by practicing some basic safety techniques.

HOW TO PREVENT ACCIDENTS

You can prevent many accidents by recognizing and eliminating the sources of possible danger in the home and workplace. Basic safety practices can make hobbies, such as swimming, boating, and camping, safer for your entire family.

Safety in the Home

The home can be a major source of accidents, especially for children and the elderly. Some basic precautions can make your home safe and secure.

Fire

Install a smoke detector near the kitchen and in a two-story building at the top of the stairs. Check the detectors periodically to be sure they are working. Place a working fire extinguisher in your house, preferably in or near the kitchen. Have an escape plan that protects family members in the event of fire. Make sure that adults and children know the escape routes; rehearse the plan every so often. To prevent a sudden combustion, do not use heating devices with exposed coils and do not allow oil rags or debris to accumulate. Never smoke in bed or permit anyone else to do so.

Electrical Hazards

Replace any frayed electrical cords or loose plugs. Use extension cords sparingly and avoid overloading electrical sockets. When replacing fuses, always use a fuse of the same amperes. Appliances such as hair dryers should not be used near water. Any outlets near water should be equipped with circuit breakers that disconnect the electrical supply when exposed to water. Make sure all major appliances are grounded.

Kitchen Hazards

Never leave a stove in operation unattended. Check to make sure no pot holders, paper goods, or other inflammable items are on or near the stove. Turn the handles of pots toward the stove, not facing out where they could be hit and dislodged in passing. When trying to reach high places, use a sturdy stool or ladder designed for that purpose. Do not stand on a chair.

Hazardous Substances

Store pesticides, weed killers, and petroleum products in well-ventilated areas away from the heat. Keep poisonous substances in a locked cupboard away from small children (see "Poisons"). Containers of unused products should be disposed of properly, in accordance with the instructions on the label. Never place these products in other containers, especially cans that formerly held food. Do not flush these substances down the toilet.

Falls

All stairways should have secure stair rails. Make sure the stairways are adequately illuminated, both at the top and the bottom. Stairs and landings should never be waxed. Inspect carpeted stairs periodically for worn, frayed, or loose areas. Secure all rugs throughout the

EMERGENCY PROCEDURES

When breathing or circulation stops for 6 minutes, brain damage and death can result. Therefore, most life-or-death accident situations center on your ability to maintain the working of the lungs (respiration) and the heart (circulation). If the victim is not breathing, her heart has stopped beating or she is bleeding badly, immediate action is required to maintain these vital functions.

If a person has stopped breathing, it may be the result of choking, drowning, or heart attack. Taking action to restore respiratory and circulatory functions requires these ABCs:

- **A**irway—Remove any obstruction so a person can breathe.
- **B**reathing—Perform artificial respiration to restore breathing.
- **C**irculation—Compress the chest to restore the heartbeat and blood circulation.

Artificial respiration, also called rescue breathing or mouth-to-mouth resuscitation, can restore breathing. Chest compressions can initiate a heartbeat when there is none. Artificial respiration combined with chest compression is called *cardiopulmonary resuscitation* (CPR) (see Figure 21.1). Used to manually restore the victim's breathing and circulation, CPR should be learned in a certified training program.

house to the floors to prevent slippage and use rubber matting under scatter rugs and small carpets.

Safety in the Workplace

Certain jobs involve handling hazardous substances or working with dangerous equipment. If you work under possibly hazardous conditions, wear protective clothing and equipment at all times, including goggles, ear plugs, masks, and gloves. Never operate machinery when you feel drowsy or ill, or if you are taking medications that can cause drowsiness. Certain substances in the workplace are especially hazardous to pregnant women or to women planning to get pregnant. These substances include methyl mercury, lead, polychlorinated biphenyls, polybrominated biphenyls, and organic solvents. Various forms of radiation also can harm the fetus. If you think you are pregnant, or may soon be pregnant, and are exposed to hazardous substances, ask for a transfer to a less hazardous working environment.

Safety on the Road

Automobile accidents are a major cause of deaths. About one-half of all auto crashes are related to driving under the influence of alcohol and other drugs. *Never* drink and drive, or allow someone to drive who is impaired by alcohol or drugs. In addition, many deaths and major injuries could be prevented by using safety belts. They should be worn at all times by all passengers including children and pregnant women.

WHAT TO DO

When an accident occurs, determine whether the person is conscious and in need of assistance. If the victim is conscious and breathing, no further action is needed unless bleeding needs to be controlled. The victim's ABC's—airway, breathing and heartbeat—should be monitored to decide if CPR must be done. When the victim is unconscious and not breathing but has a pulse, perform rescue breathing. If the victim has no pulse and is not breathing, begin CPR.

Also consider the possibility of a spinal cord injury. If you suspect a neck or back injury, do not move the victim unless it is absolutely necessary, for example, if you must perform CPR or if the area is unsafe. When you must move the victim, place the patient on a blanket or board and drag the blanket or board. Keep the head, neck, and back immobile and the body straight and in line with the head. If CPR is necessary, open the airway by lifting the chin, not by tilting the head. If the person is unconscious and does not appear to have a neck or back injury, place the body in the recovery position, on the stomach, supported by an arm and a leg at right angles to the body. Tilt the head back to keep the airway open.

Artificial respiration, cardiopulmonary resuscitation, and clearing obstructed airways to relieve choking are important emergency medical procedures. Every adult should be trained in how to use them through programs endorsed by the American Heart Association or the American Red Cross.

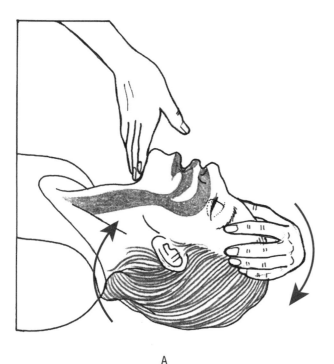

A

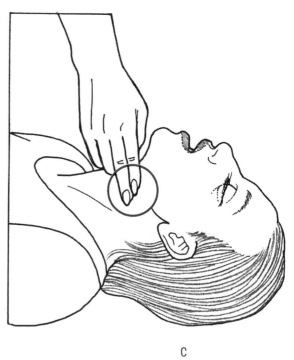

C

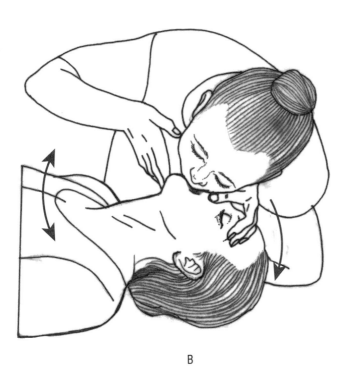

B

Figure 21.1 Cardiopulmonary Resuscitaton (CPR)
Start cardiopulmonary resuscitation immediately when a person has stopped breathing and does not have a heartbeat. Continue until the person has resumed breathing.
• Place the person on her back and clear the airway by removing the tongue and any foreign matter from the back of the throat.

• Place one hand on the victim's forehead. Place two fingers of the other hand under the bony part of the victim's chin. Push on the forehead, and lift the chin to tilt the head back (A).
• Keeping the hands in place on the forehead and chin, squeeze the victim's nostrils closed between your thumb and forefinger (B).
• Take a deep breath and cover the victim's entire mouth with your mouth and give 2 quick breaths that last 1 to 1½ seconds. Watch the victim's chest rise with each breath, and let it fall before you give another breath.
• When the chest doesn't rise, retilt the victim's head and try again. If it still doesn't rise, the airway is blocked, and you must clear the obstruction (see "Choking").
• Check the carotid artery in the neck for a pulse (C). If there is a pulse, but the victim isn't breathing, continue rescue breathing about once every 5 seconds (12 breaths per minute). When the person's chest has expanded, stop blowing, remove your mouth, and turn your head over the victim's mouth so you can detect any breathing.
• Put your middle finger on the notch where the ribs meet the breastbone, and place your index finger next to your middle finger.
• Place the heel of your other hand next to the index finger, with one hand on top of the other. Only the heel of your hand should be touching, but not resting, on the chest (D).
• Lean over the victim with elbows locked, and bear down and up, down and up, in a ½ second cycle of holding and releasing compressions. Each compression should depress the chest 1½ to 2 inches to squeeze blood through the heart (E).
• After 15 compressions, perform two breaths as described for rescue breathing.
• Repeat the cycle of 15 compressions and 2 breaths for 1 minute (about 4 times), and then recheck the pulse. Continue this cycle until the victim recovers or help arrives.

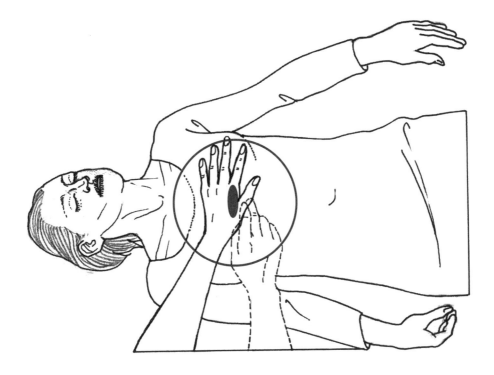

D

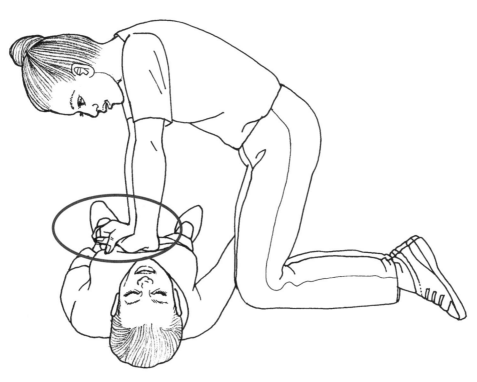

E

Because motorcycle and bicycle accidents cause severe injuries—especially head injuries—wear protective head gear while riding a motorcycle or bicycle. When riding a motorcycle, wear clothing that offers padding on the arms and legs. While riding a bike, obey all traffic signs and regulations and make sure you clearly signal your intentions to passing motorists.

Water Safety

Drowning and boating accidents often occur because people ignore basic U.S. Coast Guard regulations and safety guidelines. Even expert swimmers should follow these basic water safety rules:

- Never swim alone.
- Never leave young children unattended in the bathtub, around pools, or anywhere near deep water. In the water, they. should always wear flotation devices.
- Know your limits and don't exceed them.
- Don't dive into a pool or pond until you've tested its depth.

- Don't drink alcohol while swimming or boating.
- Don't go out in a boat unless there is someone on board who knows how to handle it.
- Always wear a life jacket on a boat.
- Follow all boating regulations.

The Great Outdoors

When camping or hiking you can be exposed to the elements for long periods, so you should be equipped for all possibilities in the event an accident occurs and you are not near help. Before leaving on a hiking or overnight camping trip, tell someone where you are going and when you plan to return. Obtain a good map and chart your course on it. In extreme temperatures, be alert to signs of overexposure—heat stroke, hypothermia, or frostbite—and take appropriate action (see "First Aid"). Take along a simple snake bite kit and salves for insect bites.

ADMINISTERING FIRST AID

Some emergencies may require life support measures, but the majority of minor accidents can be managed using simple first aid techniques. Again, the ability to accurately assess the severity of the situation and to respond appropriately and quickly can help avoid complications later.

The goals of first aid are

- Help the victim recover and restore and maintain vital functions (breathing, heartbeat)
- Prevent further injury or deterioration of the victim's condition
- Provide reassurance and make the person as comfortable as possible
- Get help

Begin by assessing the person's condition before summoning help (see "Steps to Take in an Emergency"). Or, preferably, one person can seek help while another administers first aid. The best source of help is an emergency medical service, which usually can be

reached by calling 911. Give the name, location, and telephone number to emergency personnel. If necessary, the victim can be transported to a hospital by the emergency crew.

In the event of poisoning, contact a poison control center. The number of the nearest center, as well as other emergency numbers, should be prominently displayed near the telephone. These numbers are usually listed in the front of a local telephone book.

Bites and Stings

Even though bites and stings from animals and insects are rarely life threatening, they can lead to complications from allergic reactions or infection. Some snakes and spiders are particularly poisonous, and their venom can cause serious reactions. You should be able to identify the insect or animal to medical personnel. In some cases, the victim may show signs of shock and should be treated accordingly. Other first aid recommendations:

HOME FIRST AID KIT

Keep the following items in an easily accessible place to treat minor emergencies:

- thermometer
- sterile gauze rolls and squares
- adhesive tape
- Ace elastic bandages
- band-aids in a variety of sizes
- iodine or an antiseptic with iodine in it
- antibacterial ointments or creams
- hydrogen peroxide
- safety pins
- clean towels
- clean cloth (old sheets) for slings
- tweezers
- ice packs
- hot water bottle
- basic drugs:
  —aspirin, acetominaphen, and ibuprofen
  —steroid cream for rashes or itching
  —antihistamine for allergies
  —antidiarrheal pills or liquid
  —antacid pills or liquid
  —a mild laxative
  —fluid replacement drink (electrolyte replacement)

- Treat stings from bees, hornets, or wasps by removing the stinger from the skin. It can be scraped off using a blunt, firm instrument. Do not use tweezers because they may force more venom into the skin. When the victim shows signs of a severe allergic reaction (dizziness, weakness, or difficulty breathing or swallowing), you may have to apply mouth-to-mouth resuscitation or CPR until help arrives.

- Animal bites, especially deep puncture wounds, are dangerous and may result in tetanus or rabies. Report any animal to police or animal control authorities so the animal can be tested for rabies. Also, get a tetanus shot.

- Spider bites are not serious unless they come from a black widow spider (black with a red hourglass mark), a brown recluse spider (tan with a dark violin mark), or a tarantula (large and hairy). Scorpions are also poisonous. Keep the victim quiet and make sure the site of the bite is kept below the level of the heart. Place a cold compress on the site of the bite and administer CPR as needed.

- If improperly treated, poisonous snake bites can be fatal. Two poisonous snakes in the United States are pit vipers (rattlesnakes, copperheads, and cottonmouths) and coral snakes. Pit vipers have distinctive slanted eyes, fangs, and pits between their nostrils and eyes. Coral snakes are bright red, black, and yellow with white rings and black noses. They do not have fangs. Contrary to some Western movies snake bites should not be cut. Neither should cold compresses or tourniquets be applied. Instead, keep the victim quiet and keep the site of the bite lower than the level of the heart. Monitor the person's vital functions and administer CPR as needed until help arrives.

Bleeding

Severe and uncontrolled bleeding can lead to unconsciousness, shock, and eventually death. Arterial blood is bright red and escapes in spurts; venous blood is darker, and flows more slowly. If the blood is coming from an artery, it may spurt and flow too quickly for the blood to clot. The first step is to control bleeding either through direct pressure or through nearby pressure points (see Figure 21.2). Maintain pressure for 10 minutes.

The use of a tourniquet is not recommended unless bleeding cannot be controlled otherwise or an amputation is involved. If a part of the body is accidentally severed, control bleeding from the wound as much as possible. Immediately place the amputated part in a bag and place it in another bag filled with ice. Take the victim and the severed part to an emergency room as soon as possible, so the part can be rejoined.

Bleeding from a wound may be controlled by applying direct pressure in the following steps:

- Place the victim on her back, feet up, if possible, elevate the wounded area so gravity can help slow the bleeding.

- Press hard on the wound with a clean pad, holding edges of the wound together if they are gaping. If there is anything in the wound, exert pressure around, not on, the wound.

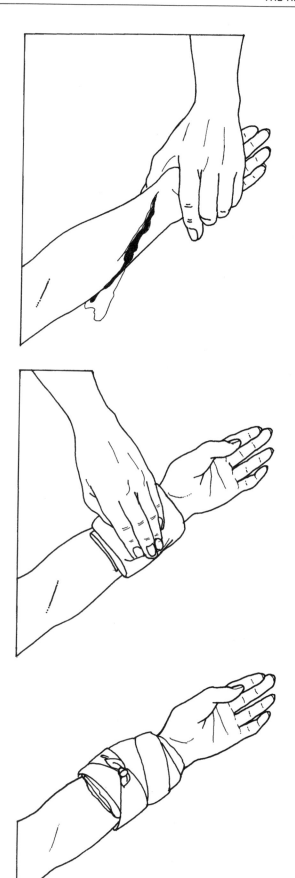

- Bind a pad firmly over the wound to maintain pressure.
- Placing pressure on an artery or pulse point directly above a wound if bleeding does not stop with direct pressure.

Burns

Burns can be caused by fire, steam, hot liquids, radiation, friction, electricity, or chemicals. The size of the burned area and its depth determine its seriousness. *First degree* burns involve only the outer layer of the skin, the epidermis. *Second degree* burns affect both the epidermis and the underlying dermis. *Third degree* burns involve the destruction of an entire area of skin and even the tissue underneath. Third-degree burns are always serious. Giving first aid right away may lessen the severity of the burn (see Figure 21.3). Minor burns can be very painful, whereas major burns often are painless because the nerves may be destroyed. First aid treatment involves removing constricting rings, bracelets, or shoes because swelling may make them difficult to remove later. Never apply any ointment, cream, oil, spray, or home remedy because it can interfere with healing. Flush minor burns with cool water, or apply cool, wet compresses. Dress the burned area with clean dry bandages that should be changed as needed. Should signs of infection develop, seek medical attention.

Place the burned part in cold water (not ice water) or wrap it in a clean, wet towel to cool the burn. Pat the area dry with a clean, preferably sterile, cloth and cover the burn with a dry, sterile, nonadhesive dressing.

Figure 21.2 Bleeding
Bleeding from a wound may be controlled by applying direct pressure in the following steps:
• Place the victim on her back, feet up; if possible, elevate the wounded area so gravity can help slow the bleeding.
• Press hard on the wound with a clean pad, holding the edges of the wound together if they are gaping. If there is anything in the wound, exert pressure around, not on, the wound.
• Bind a pad firmly over the wound to maintain pressure.
• Place pressure on an artery or pulse point directly above a wound if bleeding does not stop with direct pressure.

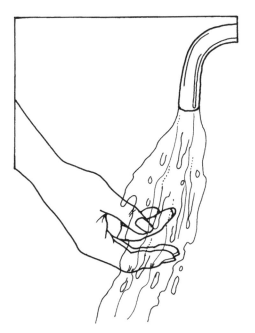 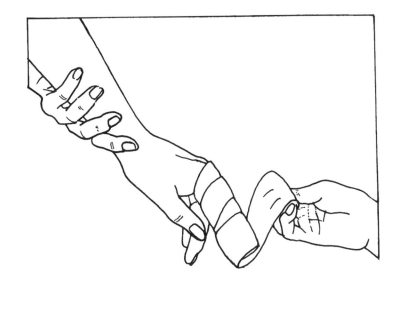

Figure 21.3 Burns
Place the burned part in cold water (not ice water), or wrap it in a clean, wet towel to cool the burn. Pat the area dry with a clean, preferably sterile, cloth and cover the burn with a dry, sterile, nonadhesive dressing.

Choking

A person whose airway is obstructed has difficulty breathing and may turn blue. If the airway is only partially blocked and the person is coughing, do not try to administer first aid. Some air is being inhaled and the obstruction may be coughed up. When the airway is totally blocked, the victim cannot cough or talk, may clutch at the throat, and eventually loses consciousness. This is a true emergency, and you must help immediately to save the person's life. Do not try to remove the obstruction with your finger. Instead, perform abdominal thrusts, also known as the Heimlich maneuver (see Figure 21.4). If this is not effective immediately, call for emergency assistance and continue trying the Heimlich maneuver.

When the victim is obese or pregnant, a chest thrust is safer. Place your hand in the center of the victim's breastbone, not on the ribs or abdomen.

Drowning

Only good swimmers should ever attempt to rescue a drowning person. Too often, the would-be rescuer drowns along with the swimmer. In most cases, you should follow these techniques recommended by the Coast Guard:

- Throw a flotation device—a life jacket, preserver, or anything that floats—tied to a rope to the floundering person so she can be pulled ashore.
- Row a boat to the swimmer as quickly as possible.
- Tow the person by giving her an oar, rope, or life preserver to hold onto.

When none of these techniques is possible and you can safely swim to the victim's aid, then do so. Or summon help immediately. If the victim has stopped breathing, begin rescue breathing immediately even though the person is still in the water. Do this by giving four quick breaths and then a breath every five seconds as you pull the person to shore. Once ashore, do CPR as needed until breathing and pulse resume. Once she is revived, keep the victim warm and have her hospitalized for observation.

A person who can't breathe, talk, or cough, could be choking. Take the following steps immediately:

- Stand behind the victim with your hands around her waist. Place your fist, thumb in, on the victim's abdomen midway between the waist and rib cage. (A)
- Place your other hand over your fist and thrust hard, inward and upward. (B)

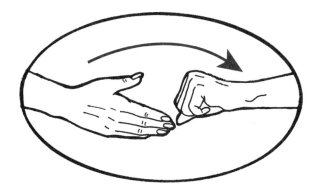

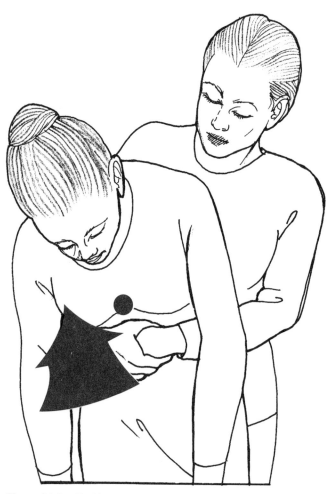

Figure 21.4 Choking

A person who can't breathe, talk, or cough could be choking. Victims who are choking often place their thumb and forefinger at the base of the throat. Take the following steps immediately:
• Stand behind the victim with your hands around her waist. Place your fist, thumb in, on the victim's abdomen midway between the waist and rib cage (A).

• Place your other hand over your fist, and thrust hard, inward and upward (B).
• Repeat abdominal thrusts as needed until the obstruction is cleared or the victim loses consciousness.
• Place an unconscious person on her back, clear the victim's mouth if necessary, and check for breathing.
• Tilt the head of a victim who is not breathing back, and lift the chin to prepare for rescue breathing.
• Breathe two full breaths into the victim's mouth. If the airway is still obstructed, your breaths cannot expand the victim's chest.
• Begin abdominal thrusts by straddling the victim's thighs and placing the heel of one hand against the middle of the victim's abdomen, just above the navel and below the tip of the breastbone.
• Place one hand over the other, fingers pointed toward the victim's head, and give 6-10 quick inward and upward thrusts.
• Sweep your finger inside the victim's mouth to remove any object. If breathing has not been restored, open the airway and give two more breaths. If the breaths do not go in, give another series of 6-10 thrusts, check the victim's mouth, and give two full breaths.
• Continue the sequence of thrusts, checking the mouth, and breaths until the object is dislodged.

■ Repeat abdominal thrusts as needed until the obstruction is cleared or the victim loses consciousness.

■ Place an unconscious person on her back, clear the victim's mouth if necessary, and check for breathing

■ Tilt the head of a victim who is not breathing back and lift the chin to prepare for rescue breathing.

■ Breathe two full breaths into the victim's mouth. If the airway is still obstructed, your breaths cannot expand the victim's chest.

■ Begin abdominal thrusts by straddling the victim's thighs and placing the heel of one hand

against the middle of the victim's abdomen, just above the navel and below the tip of the breastbone.

■ Place one hand over the other, fingers pointed toward the victim's head, and give 6–10 quick inward and upward thrusts.

■ Sweep your finger inside the victim's mouth to remove any object. If breathing has not been restored, open the airway and give two more breaths. If the breaths do not go in, give another series of 6–10 thrusts, check the victim's mouth, and give two full breaths.

■ Continue the sequence of thrusts, checking the mouth, and breaths until the object is dislodged.

Electric Shock

The human body is a conductor of electricity, just like water and metal; current traveling through the body damages to internal organs and skin. The victim can lose consciousness, stop breathing, sustain serious internal and external burns, and possibly die. Because wood and rubber do not conduct electricity, you can use a wooden pole or board to separate the victim from the source of current. Until you do this, never touch the victim because she is an electrical conductor and could cause you to be electrocuted. Instead, do the following:

- Shut off the electrical current, or use something wood or rubber to move the victim away from the source of the current.

- Check the victim's breathing and heartbeats. If needed, administer rescue breathing or CPR.

- Give first aid for any burns.

- Monitor the victim for shock and treat as needed. Summon help.

Overexposure to Heat or Cold

Extreme temperatures are often encountered by hikers, mountain climbers, and campers. Sometimes, though, the elderly, the very young, and the chronically ill are also affected. Heat exhaustion can lead to heatstroke, which can cause shock, brain damage, and death. Hypothermia occurs when a person is exposed to very cold temperatures and loses body heat faster than it can be replaced. Frostbite literally can freeze a limb, damaging tissues.

Heat exhaustion is caused by dehydration. The first signs are muscle cramps, heavy perspiration, lightheadedness, and weakness. If body temperature continues to increase, the victim becomes extremely thirsty and may suffer nausea, vomiting, and headache. Behavior becomes irrational and the victim lapses into unconsciousness. If the body temperature goes above 106°F, *heatstroke* can occur, causing the body's system for regulating temperature to become overwhelmed. The victim's skin is hot, dry, and red, and pulse and breathing may be rapid but weak. (See Fig. 21.5) Seizures and unconsciousness may follow. Heatstroke requires immediate medical attention:

- Move the person to a cool, shaded place.
- Wrap the person in cool wet towels or sheets

and place cold compresses on the neck, groin, and armpits.

- Fan the victim, either by hand or using an electric fan.

- Monitor the body temperature; if it rises, repeat the cooling process.

- Do not give the victim anything by mouth.

Hypothermia, the opposite of heatstroke, occurs when someone is exposed to subzero temperatures. Body temperature drops below normal, causing a gradual slowing down of physical and mental processes. Symptoms include clumsiness, confusion, drowsiness, and slurred speech. Eventually slow, weak breathing and heartbeat, and coma can occur. Once the victim is removed from the cold, apply first aid:

- Check the victim's breathing and heartbeat and give mouth-to-mouth resuscitation if her breathing rate is less than 6 breaths per minute. Otherwise, do not interfere. Do not perform chest compressions because they can trigger cardiac arrest.

- Wrap the victim in warm blankets or clothes and, in mild hypothermia, offer her warm, sweet, nonalcoholic drinks.

- Rewarming someone with severe hypothermia can be tricky. Do not use direct heat. Hot water bottles and body-to-body transfer of heat may work, but seek medical attention as soon as possible.

A victim of hypothermia also may have frostbite. Warm the frostbitten area in warm (not hot) water or with warm compresses. Do not warm with direct heat or rub frostbitten areas with anything, particularly snow.

Foreign Body in the Eye

A foreign object in the eye, even if invisible, can cause pain and injury until it is removed. Never rub the eye, and never attempt to remove an object embedded in the eyeball. The safest way to remove an object in the eye is to flush it out with sterile saline solution or, if that is not available, warm tap water. If the foreign body is not obvious, look inside the lower eyelid and either flush it out or remove it with a clean cloth (do not use

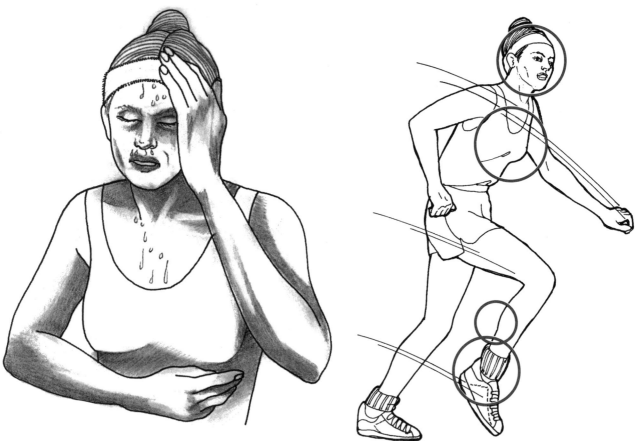

Figure 21.5 Heat Exhaustion
Heat exhaustion can be brought on by excessive sweating that causes a loss of salt and results in muscle cramps. Other symptoms of heat exhaustion include dizziness, headache, and rapid pulse rate and breathing.

a cotton swab or tissue). If you still cannot see it, inspect the inside of the upper eyelid (see Figure 21.6). If tearing or pain persists, see a doctor. (Chapter 23 has more information on eye emergencies.)

Inspect the inside of the upper eyelid to find a foreign body in the eye (A). While the victim is looking down, place a cotton swab on the upper eyelid and grasp the upper eyelashes (B). Gently pull on the eyelashes to fold the eyelid back over the swab. Remove the object by flushing or with a clean cloth.

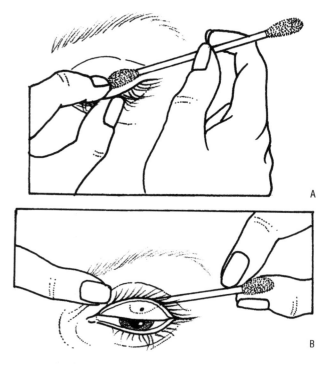

Figure 21.6 Removing Foreign Objects from the Eye
Inspect the inside of the upper eyelid to find a foreign body in the eye (A). While the victim is looking down, place a cotton swab on the upper eyelid and grasp the upper eyelashes (B). Gently pull on the eyelashes to fold the eyelid back over the swab. Remove the object by flushing or with a clean cloth.

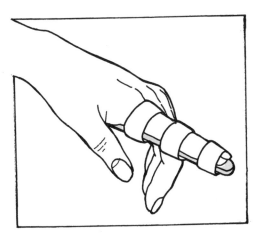

A

Figure 21.7 Splinting a Broken Bone
Immobilize a broken bone with a splint made with wood, magazines, or whatever rigid material is available. Tie the splint to the injured part with bandages or ties. A splint of the index finger (A) should keep the finger extended. A splint of the forearm (B) should extend from the elbow to beyond the wrist.

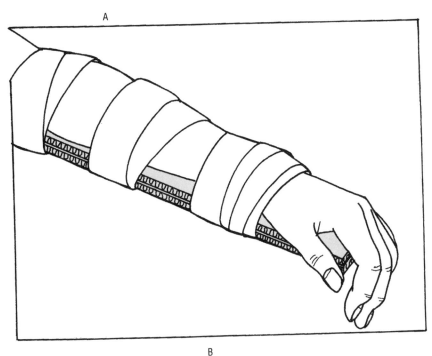

B

Fractures

When a bone is broken or fractured, if it cannot be used, the area affected becomes swollen, discolored, painful and tender. In compound fractures, the broken bone protrudes or is exposed through the skin. The goal of first aid with broken bones is to keep the bone protected and avoid further damage. You can do this by applying a splint (see Figures 21.7, 21.8). Do not attempt to move the bones back into place. For a hip, pelvic, or back injury, do not move the victim if possible. Call an ambulance as soon as possible. Monitor the person for shock and do not give anything by mouth.

Sprains

A sprain occurs when the fibers in a ligament become torn and cause pain, swelling, and bruising. The joint can still function, but it should be immobilized so that the torn fibers can heal. If the area is misshapen, the pain is extreme, or circulation is impaired, seek medical help. Otherwise, administer the following first aid:

- Apply cold compresses at once and reapply as often as possible for the first 24 hours to stop swelling. After 24 hours, apply warm compresses to further reduce swelling.

- Elevate the joint.

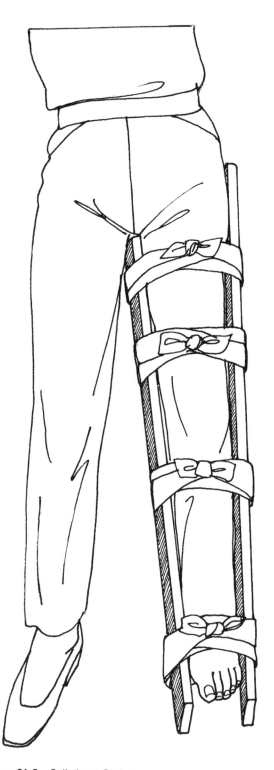

Figure 21.8 Splinting a Broken Leg

Make a splint of the knee or lower leg of two padded boards. Place one board on the outside of the injured leg and extending from the hip to below the heel. Place the other board on the inside of the leg. Secure the splint in at least four places.

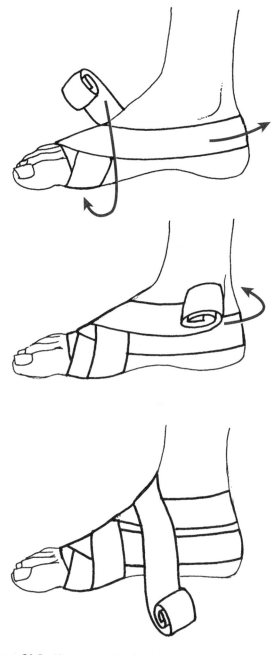

Figure 21.9 Wrapping a Sprained Ankle

Wrap a sprained ankle by applying a figure-eight bandage.

• Begin with one or two circular turns around the foot, then bring the bandage diagonally across the top of the foot and around the ankle.

• Continue wrapping the bandage around the ankle over the top of the foot and under the arch.

• Continue figure-eight turns with each one overlapping the last, and fasten with clips.

■ Wrap the joint with a bandage to provide support (see Figure 21.9).

Wrap a sprained ankle by applying a figure-eight bandage.

■ Begin with one or two circular turns around the foot, then bring the bandage diagonally across the top of the foot and around the ankle.

■ Continue wrapping the bandage around the ankle over the top of the foot and under the arch.

■ Continue figure-eight turns with each one overlapping the last and fasten with clips.

Nosebleeds

Most nosebleeds are usually caused by minor trauma or by certain medical conditions, such as high blood pressure, allergies, or colds. Nosebleeds do not require medical attention unless the bleeding persists or is caused by a more extensive injury. Otherwise, first aid should be adequate. Put the head back, pack the nostril with gauze or a clean cloth, and avoid blowing the nose for some time afterwards. Persistent nosebleeds merit medical attention. (See Fig. 21.10)

Head Injuries

Head injuries can be internal or external or both, they involve bleeding and damage to the brain. Any injury to the head may also involve a neck or spinal injury. Always consider this possibility in an accident and do not move the victim unless it is absolutely necessary.

In addition to signs of trauma, symptoms of head injury include severe headache, vomiting, confusion, personality changes, drowsiness, slurred speech, stiff neck, convulsions, double vision, and weakness in an arm or leg. In some cases, fluid may drain from the ears, nose, or mouth. These symptoms may occur at the time of the accident or be delayed, so you should closely observed the victim for 24 hours after an accident. If symptoms occur, seek medical attention. Otherwise, give first aid based on the victim's condition:

■ Check the person's breathing and heartbeat and begin rescue breathing, CPR, or control of bleeding as needed.

■ If the victim is unconscious, stabilize her head by placing your hands on both sides of the victim's head; keep the head in line with the spine and prevent movement.

■ The skull may be fractured, so do not press on it to stop external bleeding. Instead, gently wrap the head in a bandage. If there are superficial scalp wounds, apply light pressure with a cloth to stop bleeding.

■ If the victim is vomiting, make sure the airway is clear.

■ Apply ice to any swelling.

Heart Attack

A heart attack is a life-threatening emergency. A quick response can make the difference in the amount of damage done to the body by the ensuing lack of oxygen to vital organs. Symptoms of a heart attack include a crushing, constant pain in the chest (versus a sharp pain that comes and goes), shortness of breath, nausea and vomiting, and sweating. Even though a person with these symptoms may not be having a heart attack, summon emergency care immediately. Tell emergency medical personnel the victim may be having a heart attack so they can bring life-support equipment with them.

When a possible heart attack victim is unconscious and not breathing, start artificial respiration immediately. If there is no pulse, apply CPR. If the victim is conscious, place him or her in a sitting position and be reassuring, as you wait for help. Do not give her anything to eat or drink.

Poison

Poisoning can be caused by swallowing poisonous substances, inhaling gases, exposing the skin to chemicals and toxic substances, and from injecting drugs. Acids, alkalis, and petroleum products are all poisons commonly found in the home. Acids and alkalis include cleaning products such as oven and toilet bowl cleaners and detergents. Petroleum products include solvents, gasoline, and kerosene. Over-the-counter medications also are poisonous if taken in large doses, as inquisitive small children sometimes do. Pesticides

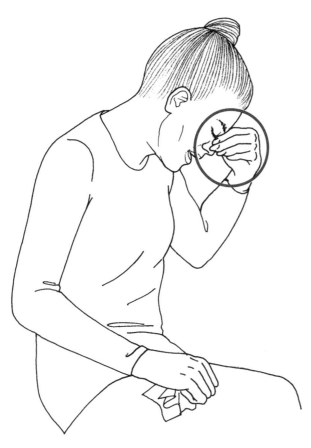

Figure 21.10   Stopping a Nosebleed
To stop a nosebleed, have the victim sit down and lean forward. If there are blood clots in the nostrils, ask the victim to blow them out. Hold the soft part of the bridge of the victim's nose firmly for 15 minutes. Place cold compresses on the bridge of the nose. If the bleeding persists for more than 15 minutes, repeat the procedure. If this fails to stop the bleeding, seek medical help.

and weed killers contain strong poisons and can be toxic if swallowed, inhaled, or exposed to the skin.

If you suspect someone has been poisoned, contact your local poison control center or emergency medical service and follow their directions carefully. Tell them the name of the poison, how much was taken, and when. Do not induce vomiting or give the victim anything to eat or drink unless you are specifically told to do so.

If the victim has been overcome from inhaling smoke or chemical gas fumes, move the person into the fresh air and perform rescue breathing. Call emergency medical services and inform them that the victim needs oxygen.

Shock

The normal flow of blood through one's body can be reduced by a heart attack, trauma, infection, or allergy. When this happens, shock results. Because the amount of oxygen circulating to the organs is sharply reduced, shock is a life-threatening aftermath to many accidents. Shock can follow any severe injury, especially when there has been blood loss. Shock also occurs when the body suffers severe stress, caused by poisonous bites or exposure to extreme heat or cold. Consider the possibility of shock when any injury occurs and take measures to prevent it.

Symptoms of shock include decreasing alertness, restlessness, anxiety, confusion, cold and clammy skin, paleness, blue lips and fingernails, chest pain, rapid and shallow breathing, numbness, paralysis, nausea and vomiting, and thirst. The victim can eventually become unconscious. Emergency attention includes:

- Administer rescue breathing, CPR, and bleeding control as needed. Call for help.
- Lay the victim flat, face up, and elevate her feet 8 to 12 inches unless she has a head, neck, or back injury.
- Loosen clothing and cover the victim in a blanket to prevent heat loss. Do not apply direct heat.
- Keep the person calm. Avoid asking unnecessary questions.
- Do not give the victim anything by mouth.

Unconsciousness

A person may lose consciousness because of an injury, blood loss, or a lack of oxygen caused by drowning or an airway obstruction. Certain medical conditions, such as diabetes or a neurologic illness can cause someone to slip into a coma and become unconscious. Fainting is a temporary form of unconsciousness that can be caused by a number of triggers.

When people lose consciousness they lose control of their muscles and reflexes, thus blocking their airways. When an unconscious person is not breathing, give immediate artificial respiration. If the victim is breathing, loosen her clothing and place her on her stomach with both arms and one leg at right angles to the body and the head back so that her chin is lower than her body. Monitor the victim to ensure she is breathing until help arrives.

SPECIAL CONCERNS FOR WOMEN

Generally, women are as susceptible to accidents and injuries as anyone else, and the same guidelines for first aid apply to them as to men. Some special circumstances, however, require special attention in women. For example, older women are more likely to have brittle bones because of a condition called osteoporosis. The bones break under little pressure or even on their own from the mere weight of the body on the joints. Elderly women should take special precautions to remove any hazards from their homes that could cause falls and to avoid injuries.

Pregnancy also poses special concerns for women. A pregnant woman's sense of balance changes because of the alteration in weight distribution in her body, so she is more at risk of falling. If you are pregnant, wear flat or low-heeled shoes, be careful climbing stairs, lifting heavy objects, and washing windows; and avoid walking on wet floors when housecleaning. Always wear a safety belt while driving to protect yourself and your unborn baby.

If an accident does occur, you may need to modify first aid procedures for a pregnant woman. For instance, if she is choking, the abdominal thrust should not be used. Instead, use a chest thrust to dislodge a blockage. When a pregnant woman has an injury that results in blood loss or emergency care, this calls for special precautions.

Pregnancy results in certain changes in the function of a woman's body. The overall amount of blood in her body and her heart rate increase, which means that it may take longer for blood losses to become obvious. Blood flow through the uterus and placenta to the fetus also can decrease sharply before changes in heart rate and blood pressure occur in the mother. Internal blood loss can occur silently while the woman still feels well and shows no signs of problems. For this reason, certain injuries to pregnant women should always receive medical attention:

- Motor vehicle accidents
- Falls
- Assaults, especially if the woman is knocked unconscious or has been beaten in the abdomen
- Head injuries, especially if the woman loses consciousness, does not remember the accident, or acts abnormally
- Chest pain or trouble breathing
- Any blow to the abdomen
- Spinal pain that does not go away or also involves loss of sensation, tingling, or weakness in arms or legs
- Burns from a fire in a closed space or burns that involve blisters over an area greater than the palm of the hand

STEPS TO TAKE IN AN EMERGENCY

- Determine if a person is conscious and in need of assistance by asking, "Are you OK?"
- Control any severe bleeding (see "Bleeding").
- Clear the airway if breathing has stopped and begin resuscitation.
- Perform CPR if the heart has stopped beating (if trained to do so).
- Take steps to guard against shock (see "Shock").

Place an injured woman in the later states of pregnancy on her left side so the uterus does not compress the vein that returns blood to the heart. If she has vaginal bleeding or the amniotic sac of fluid that holds the baby ruptures due to trauma, fetal monitoring is needed to check the uterus and the baby's heartbeat. Some hospitals have special units for monitoring pregnant women at risk of problems, or the monitoring may be done in the emergency room.

When used during pregnancy, some medications can cause problems with the baby. These include drugs that affect blood circulation, blood thinners, and narcotics. Carefully consider the risks and benefits of these drugs to reach an informed decision about their use.

In an emergency, the pregnant woman's condition is the top priority because if she is not well the baby won't be either. Informed decisions should be made in consultation with the doctor after considering all the options. A baby born after 24 weeks has a chance of life on its own. If the pregnant woman's condition is serious, it may be best to deliver the baby. When the mother's heart and breathing have stopped, the baby can survive only about 15 minutes and should be delivered immediately. These situations require careful consultation with the trauma team, the obstetrician, and a neonatologist, who specializes in the care of newborns.

CHAPTER 22

The Brain and Nervous System

Carolyn Barley Britton, M.D., M.S.

Among the most complex of the body mechanisms, the nervous system is responsible for thought, intellect, language, movement, sensation, and certain workings of other organ systems. Because the brain and nerves together act as a kind of control center for the body and its functions, any disorders of the systems may have far-reaching effects in different parts of the body.

Nervous system disorders can be *primary,* that is due to intrinsic dysfunction of the components of the nervous system. Or they can be *secondary,* that is, due to systemic illness, nutritional deficiency, exposure to toxic substances, or injury, among other causes. Neurological symptoms or disorders are present in 10 percent of outpatients, 12 percent of emergency room patients, and 15 percent of hospitalized patients.

STRUCTURE AND FUNCTION OF THE NERVOUS SYSTEM

The nervous system is comprised of several subsystems:

- The *central nervous system,* which consists of the brain and spinal cord (see Fig. 22.1).

- The *peripheral or neuromuscular system* comprising the cranial and peripheral nerves, emanating from the brain and spinal cord respectively; the neuromuscular junction (the synapse or connection of peripheral nerves to muscles); and muscle (see Fig. 22.2).

- The *autonomic nervous system,* which consists of sympathetic and parasympathetic fibers that arise from the spinal cord and terminate on internal organs such as the heart, gastrointestinal tract, bladder, and sex organs. This system affects heart rate, temperature regulation, blood pressure, and bowel, bladder, and sexual functions.

The brain itself is a complex organ that consists of cerebral hemispheres controlling thought, language, memory, spatial orientation, sensation, and movement. Its basal ganglia and the cerebellum are responsible for motor tone, postural control, and coordination; the brain stem controls consciousness, respiration, heart rate, temperature regulation, and cranial nerve function (see Fig. 22.3). Motor and sensory fibers also pass through the brain stem, ascending from the spinal cord or descending from the cerebral hemispheres.

The brain and spinal cord are bathed in cerebrospinal fluid (CSF), which extracts nutrients such as glucose from the blood to supply the cells of the nervous system and removes cellular wastes. For protection, both are covered by three membranes and encased in bony structures, the skull and vertebral column, respectively. Nerves issuing from the brain stem supply the special sense organs (eyes, ears, nose), the facial muscles, and muscles of chewing, speech, and swal-

THE DECADE OF THE BRAIN

The U.S. Congress has designated the years 1990 to 2000 as the *Decade of the Brain.* The intent is both to focus public attention on neurological disorders and to recognize the tremendous advances in the understanding and treatment made possible by modern molecular biological techniques and improved management, including preventive therapy. For example, the incidence of stroke can be reduced by improved medical management of hypertension, the most common risk factor. Genetic research has led to the discovery of genes responsible for or strongly associated with several chronic degenerative diseases: muscular dystrophy, Huntington's chorea, and Alzheimer's dementia. This information is valuable for genetic counseling and will be useful for the development of therapeutic intervention, including gene therapy.

Although some neurological diseases are incurable, improved medical management and rehabilitative measures can be effective in prevention or improved survival, with a better quality of life for many patients.

lowing (cranial nerves). From the spinal cord, nerves emanate to supply muscles of the limbs and trunk (peripheral nerves) and internal organs (autonomic nerves). The vertebral column surrounding the spinal cord is a segmented structure resembling interlocking blocks separated by a gelatinous material, the intervertebral disc, which is held in place by strong, fibrous bands (see Fig. 22.4). Ligaments help to maintain the stability of the column and allow for movement.

The basic functional unit of the nervous system is the *neuron,* or nerve cell. Because neurons do not di-

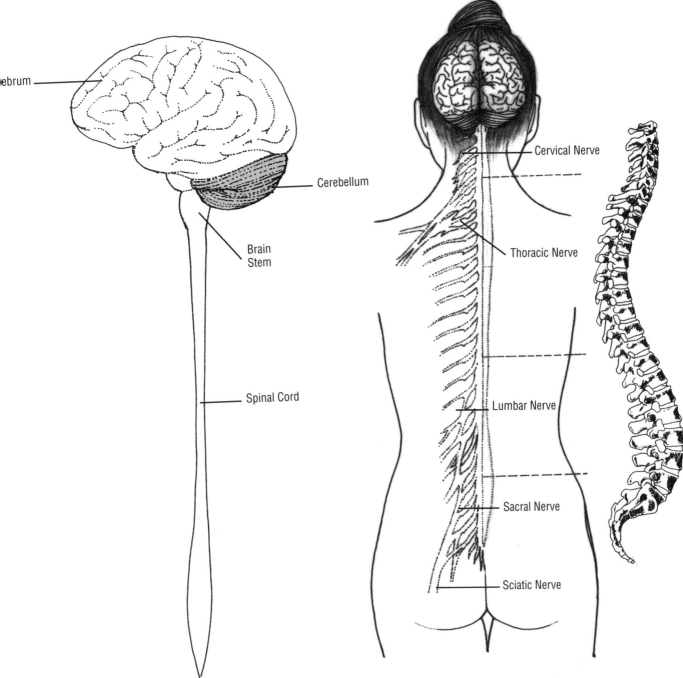

Cerebrum

Cerebellum

Brain
Stem

Spinal Cord

Cervical Nerve

Thoracic Nerve

Lumbar Nerve

Sacral Nerve

Sciatic Nerve

Figure 22.1 Functions of the Nervous System
The spinal cord conducts nerve signals between the body and the brain. The brain stem, at the juncture of the spinal cord and the brain, is responsible for breathing, heart function, and sleep cycles. Just above the brain stem, the cerebellum manages coordination, balance, and posture. Above the cerebellum is the limbic system, which controls primitive urges (such as self-preservation, emotions, moods, some senses, and certain bodily functions such as reproduction). The cerebrum is the largest and most highly developed part of the human brain. It allows impulses, thoughts, and ideas. The cerebrum is divided into two parts or lobes, each of which is responsible for different functions. (See Fig. 22.3)

Figure 22.2 The Peripheral Nervous System
Nerves extend from the spinal cord between each vertebra in the spinal column and bring sensation to various parts of the body. The nerves are identified by the region of the spine from which they arise.

vide and have limited regenerative capacity, their loss may result in permanent neurological disability. Billions of neurons in the brain and spinal cord communicate with each other—by contacts or *synapses*—and with the muscles and internal organs. The spinal cord and sense organs also send impulses to the brain, generating neural activity responsible for all aspects of human behavior. Impulses from neurons in the cerebral hemispheres of the brain are sent through branching nerve fibers called *axons* that terminate on other neurons in the basal ganglia, brain stem, or spinal cord. Messages are relayed via their axons to the cranial or spinal nerves (see Fig. 22.5). Some axons are several feet long, stretching from the brain to the lower spinal cord, and many are covered by a sheath called *myelin* that enhances the speed of conduction of nerve impulses. Other supporting cells in the nervous system, called *glia*, modulate neural activity and provide nutritional support. When a nerve impulse reaches the end of an axon, it causes the release of specific chemicals, the "messengers" of nerve activity.

The nervous system is dependent on a continuous supply of oxygen and glucose delivered by the blood. Because the brain has no capacity to store oxygen or glucose, interruption of blood flow for a few minutes may result in permanent neurological damage. The brain alone receives approximately 20 percent of the cardiac output of blood. The major blood vessels to the brain are the two internal carotid arteries and the two vertebral arteries. The carotid arteries supply the hemispheres of the brain, and the vertebral arteries supply the brain stem and cerebellum. The two circulations meet in a structure at the base of the brain called the *circle of Willis.*

Disorders of the brain and nervous system can cause various conditions.

1. Cell death or dysfunction (stroke, Alzheimer's disease, Parkinson's disease) due to loss of blood supply, oxygen, degenerative disease, trauma, infection, tumor, or toxins
2. Loss of critical support structures such as myelin, resulting in slowing of nerve impulse transmission (multiple sclerosis) and, if massive, cell death
3. Loss of appropriate cell-to-cell regulation, resulting in spontaneous or inappropriate neural activity (e.g., epileptic seizures)
4. Loss of critical nutrients such as vitamins, leading to cell malfunction or death.

KEEPING YOUR NERVOUS SYSTEM HEALTHY

Some degenerative or genetic neurological disorders are intrinsic to the nervous system, but others can be prevented by regular health maintenance, early treatment of systemic illness, good nutritional habits and avoidance of injury.

Lead a Healthy Lifestyle

Good health habits are important for the prevention of many neurological diseases. For example, your stroke risk is reduced by not smoking, avoiding excessive alcohol consumption, and seeking effective medical management of hypertension, heart disease, diabetes, and elevated cholesterol.

A good diet is essential. Deficiency of certain vitamins may cause neurological injury. Vitamin deficiency may occur because of malnutrition, restricted food intake, or malabsorption. Strict vegetarian diets, for example, may be deficient in B-12, which is found

WHERE VITAMINS AFFECT THE NERVOUS SYSTEM

Vitamin	Site Affected
B-1 (thiamine)	Brain, possibly peripheral nerves
B-6 (pyridoxine)	Brain (seizures, mental retardation, stroke), peripheral nerves
B-12	Optic nerve, brain, spinal cord, peripheral nerves
Folic Acid	Possibly peripheral nerves
Vitamin E	Eye, brain (cerebellum), peripheral nerves
B-3 (niacin)	Brain (cerebellum)
Biotin	Brain

primarily in animal protein; supplements may be necessary (see Chapter 3). Excessive vitamin intake also poses a risk, especially with fat-soluble vitamins, which are stored in the body. For example, excess vitamin A may cause brain swelling. Excess pyridoxine (Vitamin B-6) may damage peripheral nerves.

Sexually transmitted diseases can involve the nervous system. Safer sex practices using barrier methods (condoms) are necessary to prevent damaging infections. Both syphilis and the human immunodeficiency virus (HIV), which causes AIDS, may damage the brain, spinal cord, and peripheral nerves and may be transmitted to an unborn child. For this reason, if you are sexually active and/or pregnant, and are not in a long-term, monogamous relationship, you should seek counseling and testing for sexually transmitted diseases, including AIDS.

Minimize Your Exposure to Toxic Substances

Most people require prescribed medications from time to time, and many commonly use over-the-counter drugs. The potential occurrence of side effects should not cause you to avoid necessary medications. Rather, you should have a good understanding of why you require a particular drug, as well as its potential risks and potential interactions if you are taking several drugs at one time. It is also important that you have regular medical follow-ups when taking prescription drugs. All persistent new symptoms that occur when taking a new medication should be discussed with your physician. Examples of neurological symptoms or disorders related to commonly prescribed medications include the following:

- Dizziness due to antihypertensives (may indicate excess dosage)
- Headache precipitated or exacerbated by high-estrogen birth control pills
- Involuntary movements caused by haloperidol (Haldol), an antipsychotic drug
- Peripheral neuropathy (nerve degeneration) caused by phenytoin (Dilantin), a drug commonly used to treat epilepsy.

Exposure to neurotoxins may occur in the workplace or at home. In the workplace, occupational safety regulations require explicit labeling of toxic components. Workplace rules that ensure safety should be followed at all times. In the home, read labels carefully and follow instructions regarding protective clothing, ventilation, and disposal when using cleaning agents, paints, varnishes, artist's supplies, pesticides, or any potentially toxic substance. Known neurotoxins include carbon monoxide, methyl alcohol, benzene, carbon tetrachloride, lead, and certain pesticides.

Recreational drugs and alcohol are especially toxic to the nervous system. Regular and excessive use of alcohol can cause seizures, dementia, degeneration of the brain, and peripheral neuropathy. It may also predispose a person to certain infections. Cocaine use can result in stroke, brain hemorrhage, brain infection, and psychiatric disorders. Intravenous drug use may lead to bacterial infection of the brain and spinal cord, and is an important risk for transmission of HIV. Addiction to any of these substances is a serious medical problem with many secondary medical and social consequences. If you suspect that you have an addictive or substance abuse problem, seek medical assistance from appropriately trained personnel as soon as possible. (See Chapter 7).

Think Safety

Traumatic injury to the nervous system may occur in the home, at work, or during leisure activities. To avoid potential severe damage, pay attention to safety measures and make sure that they are a part of your daily routine. Everyday safety precautions should include use of the following:

- Safety belts in automobiles
- Helmets when recommended for a sport, such as cycling or skating
- Other protective clothing when recommended, such as goggles, protective padding, and gloves.

If you have a neurological condition that impairs vision, balance, or coordination, discuss any planned physical activity with your physician.

Back pain is a common ailment, often related to lifestyle factors such as lack of exercise, obesity, poor posture, and engaging in activities or work that results in back strain. Attention to diet, maintaining proper weight, and an exercise regimen that strengthens abdominal and back muscles may reduce the risk of injury and any resulting involvement of the nervous system.

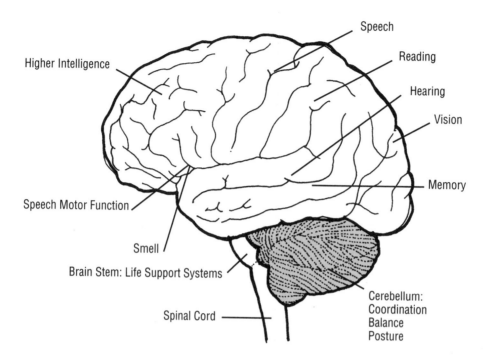

Figure 22.3 The Brain
Different parts of the brain control various functions in the body.

NEUROLOGICAL EVALUATION AND DIAGNOSIS

Since many apparent neurological disorders may be due to a systemic illness, consult a primary care physician first for a general evaluation and for referral to a neurologist, if appropriate.

Confirming a specific neurologic disease is sometimes an arduous process, requiring the expertise of several specialists. Those who may be necessary include the following:

- Ophthalmologists (eye)
- Otolaryngologists (ear, nose, and throat)
- Neurosurgeons
- Neuroradiologists
- Psychiatrists
- Orthopedic surgeons
- Vascular surgeons
- Speech and swallowing pathologists
- Rehabilitative medicine specialists

- Medical subspecialists: rheumatology, infectious disease, cardiology, and others
- Geneticists

The growth of neurological knowledge since the 1970s is due in part to neurological subspecialists who are experts in the management of particular diseases, such as epilepsy, Parkinson's disease, muscle diseases, and multiple sclerosis. A general neurologist may be able to diagnose and treat most nervous system disorders, but difficult or atypical cases may be referred to a neurological subspecialist for management advice or continued care.

When consulting a specialist such as a neurologist, it is useful to make notes before the visit of the symptoms you wish to discuss. The sequence and timing of these symptoms or other events is important neurological information to include. The physician will ask you specific questions relating to a detailed clinical history. If mental or language impairment is present, a family member or friend should provide medical information.

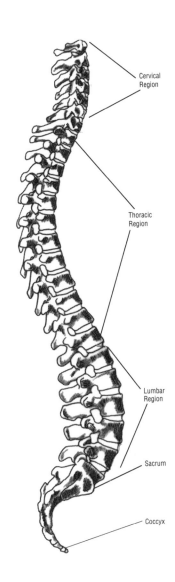

Figure 22.4 The Spinal Column
The spinal cord is enclosed with the 33 vertebrae, bones that make up the spinal column: seven cervical, twelve thoracic, five lumbar, five sacral, and four which form the coccyx at the base of the spine.

Medications, drug and alcohol use, and potential exposures to toxic or infectious substances are important to report. Family history is important for diagnosis of genetic disorders, and even travel history may be relevant.

The preliminary physical exam will test how well the various parts of your nervous system are functioning. Tests may include your tendon reflexes, muscle strength and tone, sensory functions, and your mental state.

SPECIALISTS IN NEUROLOGICAL DISORDERS

Your primary care physician may refer you to a number of specialists who treat various aspects of diseases of the nervous system and their symptoms. Depending on the nature of the problem, they may work as a team. The team may include any or all of the following health care professionals:

- Neurologist—a doctor who specializes in the nervous system and its disorders
- Neuroradiologist—a doctor who specializes in imaging tests of the nervous system
- Neurosurgeon—a doctor who specializes in surgery of the nervous system, including the brain and the spinal cord
- Psychiatrist—a doctor who specializes in mental disorders
- Physical therapist—a trained professional who helps patients with movement disorders through manipulative exercises
- Speech therapist—a trained professional who provides guidance and therapy to overcome speech problems and to relearn speech patterns.

COMMON NEUROLOGICAL SIGNS AND SYMPTOMS

The goal of the diagnostic evaluation is to determine the cause of a specific symptom. *Symptoms* are the subjective feelings that you may experience as a patient. *Signs* are objective abnormalities detected by the physician. Symptoms such as dizziness, headache, or other pain may be disabling but not result in abnormal signs or be due to neurological injury. Other symptoms, such as loss of sensation, paralysis, or language disturbance are suggestive of neurological injury. Treatment may be directed to the underlying cause, or to amelioration of the symptom if a specific cause is not identified or cannot be treated. Sometimes, despite aggressive efforts, a cause cannot be determined.

Headache

Most people experience headaches at one time or another. In most cases, headaches are benign, temporary, and spontaneously resolve or respond to over-the-counter pain medications. In some cases, however, the symptom is incapacitating, chronic, or recurrent. Headache can also be a symptom of a serious medical condition. Age of onset and the character of the headache (quality, location, duration, and time course) are important for a specific diagnosis. Associated or precipitating factors are also useful information:

- Head trauma
- Relationship to menses
- Ingestion of hormonal active medications such as birth control pills
- Diet
- Alcohol
- Medications
- Use of illegal drugs
- Exposure to toxic substances.

The characteristics of headaches due to serious medical problems, such as a brain tumor, tend to overlap those of benign origin, such as tension or migraine. Brain tumor headaches may be mild; conversely, migraine or tension headaches may be severe. Medical evaluation is indicated for chronic headache especially if the pain is present when lying down or on arising, if the headache is of sudden onset, or if it is associated with symptoms such as fever, vomiting, behavioral change, visual disturbance, or loss of motor strength, sensation, or balance.

Your primary care physician or internist can refer you to a specialist, such as an ophthalmologist or neurologist, when necessary. A clinical history, physical examination, and baseline laboratory data such as a blood count and blood chemistry profile (including serum glucose) may be sufficient for diagnosis. Specialized diagnostic procedures may be ordered on the basis of the physician's assessment of your history and examination. These procedures may include brain imaging with computerized tomography (CT), magnetic

resonance imaging (MRI), lumbar puncture, cerebral angiography, and biopsy of cerebral vessels or brain tissue. In most cases, however, these specialized tests are not required for diagnosis.

The management of primary headache disorders (migraine and tension headaches) is discussed later in this chapter. Secondary headaches due to an underlying disorder, such as hemorrhage, infection, tumor, or sinus disease, is managed by treatment of the underlying cause.

Dizziness, Vertigo, Hearing Loss

Dizziness is a nonspecific complaint that is differentiated from the more specific problem of true vertigo, although some may use these terms interchangeably. The differentiation of the nonspecific symptom of dizziness from true vertigo is based on careful history and physical examination.

Dizziness is a term used to describe diverse sensory experiences, among them giddiness, light-headedness, unsteadiness, faintness, and true vertigo. Certain types of seizures may be referred to as "dizzy spells" or may have a vertiginous component.

Vertigo is a sensation of movement of either the environment or the body. The room may seem to spin, for example, or to rotate, to and fro or up and down. Or you may experience a forcible pull toward the ground (impulsion). Associated symptoms usually include nausea, vomiting, imbalance, and an inability to walk. Tinnitus (a ringing or roaring sound in the ear) and hearing loss may occur. During attacks of vertigo, abnormal jerky horizontal or vertical eye movements, termed *nystagmus*, may be observed.

Normally, we maintain postural control and an awareness of the position of the body in space through a complex coordination of vision and sensory input from the eyes, ears, and specialized sensory organs (propioceptors) in the neck, muscles, and joints. These incoming sensory data are coordinated in the brain. Disturbance in any of these pathways may cause dizziness or true vertigo.

True vertigo is usually due to disturbances of the vestibular system, which includes the organs of the inner ear, the auditory nerve, and various vestibular nuclei in the brain stem. The goal of the initial evaluation of vertigo is to localize the site causing the symptom, whether it is in the labyrinth of the ear or in the central brain stem.

The labyrinth of the inner ear consists of three semicircular canals that are connected to saclike swellings, the utricle and saccule, that connect in turn to a spiral structure, the cochlea (see Fig. 22.6). These hollow canals are filled with fluid whose movement across specialized cells triggers impulses to the brain to maintain balance. Abnormalities in movement of the fluid, degeneration of the sensory receptor, and debris in the system are all potential triggers of vertigo. Often a viral inflammation is suspected.

Problems in the labyrinth may also involve mixed signals being sent from the nerve cells in the inner ear to the brain. They include a condition called Ménière's disease (see the section "Common Neurological Disorders"); positional vertigo, in which symptoms occur only when the body is in certain positions; vestibular neuronitis, acute, usually self-limiting attacks of vertigo that can follow a viral infection; and problems that are responses to certain antibiotics. Problems in the brain or its connecting nerves result when there is damage to the nerves or the brain stem and the messages are not reaching the brain. This can occur with a tumor, which can press on a nerve, or with a stroke. Other neurological diseases, such as multiple sclerosis and Parkinson's disease, can involve damage to the sensory nerves, which can result in dizziness as well as a number of other symptoms.

Certain drugs—among them salicylates (aspirin-containing compounds), quinine, and aminoglycoside antibiotics—may cause tinnitus, hearing loss, and vertigo. Nonvertiginous dizziness has many causes and requires a detailed history and examination to determine the cause. Most often, the cause is nonneurological—for example, severe anemia, low blood sugar, drug side effects, low blood pressure, or high blood pressure. Your primary care physician will seek to exclude these causes during the medical evaluation.

Diagnostic tests to investigate true vertigo include an audiogram, to test hearing; calorics, which involve irrigation of the ears with hot and cold water, to assess labyrinthine and brain stem function; electronystagmography, a test to detect abnormal eye movements (nystagmus); and tests to assess nerve and brain stem function. If imaging is necessary, an MRI with contrast is the procedure of choice.

Fainting, or Syncope

Syncope is a medical term referring to loss of consciousness and postural control, commonly called a *faint*. Prodromal (warning) symptoms usually occur, including light-headedness or giddiness, dim vision, and stomach discomfort or queasiness. Lying down may abort the attack. Although there is usually complete loss of contact with the environment during syncope, in some cases the person is vaguely aware of what is going on around her or him. With prolonged syncope (20 seconds or longer), brief muscle twitches may occur, simulating a seizure. Unlike seizures, however, there is no loss of bowel and bladder control, and the mind is clear as soon as the person awakens.

Diagnosis

Frequent fainting episodes require a thorough initial evaluation by an internist or primary care physician, with referral to a cardiologist or neurologist when a cause is not apparent. Nonneurological disorders are the usual causes, most of them affecting the circulatory system. Vasodepressor syncope, often seen in the young, is due to dilation of peripheral blood vessels accompanied by a decrease in cardiac output in response to a number of stimuli, including strong emotion, heat, and pain. Other nonneurological causes of syncope include postural hypotension (a drop in blood pressure when standing) due to medication, blood loss, or anemia; metabolic disorders such as Addison's disease; and prolonged bed rest. Cardiac arrhythmia, myocardial infarction, obstruction of normal cardiac output caused by a narrow outflow tract (aortic or pulmonic stenosis), low blood oxygen, severe anxiety, and hyperventilation are other causes. Unusual occurrences of syncope are following urination (micturition syncope), after a paroxysm of coughing (tussive syncope), and after eating (postprandial syncope). Abnormal slowing of the heart rate by excessive discharge of the vagus nerve (one of the nerves to the heart) is the suspected cause.

A neurologist is involved in the evaluation of syncope because neurological conditions may cause a fainting fit and seizure disorder must be excluded.

Syncope may occur in the context of stroke but is rarely the sole symptom. Distinguishing syncope from seizure is often difficult and requires taking a careful history. An electroencephalogram (EEG) is sometimes helpful, although a normal study will not entirely exclude seizures.

Sometimes, despite extensive investigations, a cause for syncope is not determined. In this case, regular follow-up is advisable, with repeat diagnostic testing as events warrant. In some cases psychiatric referral is necessary because panic attacks, anxiety, and other psychiatric problems may cause syncope or apparent syncope.

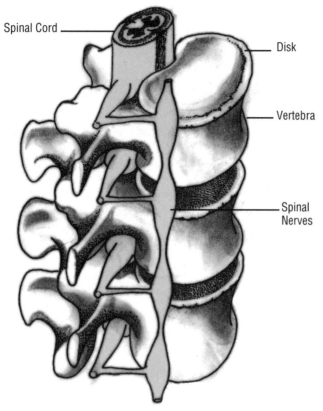

Spinal Cord

Disk

Vertebra

Spinal Nerves

Figure 22.5 The Spinal Cord
The spinal cord is protected by the vertebral column, which is made up of interlocking bones called vertebrae. Intervertebral discs provide cushioning between the vertebrae, which are connected by ligaments that allow movement of the spinal column.

Treatment

The prevention and treatment of syncope depends on the cause. Interventions include a change in medication, fluid or blood replacement, and glucose control. In hyperventilation, breathing into a paper bag prevents the extreme loss of carbon dioxide that causes dizziness and syncope. Measures useful for treatment of neurogenic low blood pressure are elevation of the head of the bed when sleeping; elastic stockings and abdominal binders to increase blood return to the heart; increased salt intake; and medications such as fludrocortisone acetate (Florinef), tyramine, monoamine oxidase inhibitors, beta-blockers, and indomethacin.

Pain

Neurological evaluation is often necessary for persons suffering from acute or chronic pain syndromes. Phy-

sicians who may be involved in pain assessment and care include internists or primary care physicians, orthopedic surgeons, neurosurgeons, physiatrists (rehabilitation medicine specialists), psychiatrists, and anesthesiologists. The neurologist is specifically concerned with pain in the head, neck, back, and limbs. In some cases of chronic pain, a multidisciplinary team of several specialists provides care.

Acute, Persistent Pain

Severe pain in the structures of the nervous system requires prompt evaluation. Consult your primary care physician to determine the appropriate referral. For some acute pain syndromes, however, immediate help may be needed. You may require an emergency room evaluation, especially if you have no primary physician or if the associated symptoms or signs suggest an emergency condition. Emergency conditions include brain or spine hemorrhage or infection, and pressure on the brain or spine due to tumor or other causes. In these conditions, pain is of sudden onset or builds in intensity over a few days. Associated signs or symptoms that may indicate an emergency situation are fever and change in mental function, strength, sensation, or gait. In spine compression, difficulty urinating may occur.

Assessment of acute pain always begins with a detailed history and examination. In emergency conditions, treatment may be initiated before diagnostic tests are ordered. The doctor will ensure that all the vital organs are functioning properly. In some cases, a tube will be inserted into the trachea and a respirator used to support ventilation. This technique is especially useful if there is brain swelling or mental function is depressed. A catheter may be inserted to drain the bladder and monitor urine output. Intravenous fluids may be given. Pain medications are sometimes withheld until the diagnosis is secure because mental function may need to be followed. If there is pressure on the brain or spine, steroids or mannitol may be given to reduce swelling. Studies that may be necessary include MRI, CT, angiography, and myelography. Whenever infection is suspected, lumbar puncture must be done without delay for diagnosis unless there is suspicion of a mass lesion, such as an abscess. Lumbar puncture is also useful for diagnosis of brain hemorrhage.

Emergency conditions may require the patient or the family to make decisions about procedures or surgery in the space of a few hours. It is important to recognize that when a neurological emergency exists, delays in treatment may cause irreversible injury or death.

Chronic Pain Syndromes

Intermittent, chronic pain requires multidisciplinary management. Important information for a correct diagnosis includes the location of pain and its radiation, character, and duration. Also important is your response to medications or different postures, and any association of the pain with neurological abnormalities such as change in mental function, sensation, strength, or gait. A prior history of trauma or medical conditions such as diabetes, cancer, or infections (Lyme disease, HIV, *Herpes zoster*) is also relevant. In some cases, history and examination are sufficient for diagnosis; in others, diagnostic tests are necessary, including imaging studies, lumbar puncture, and electromyography (EMG), a test of nerve function.

As stated previously, headache is the commonest cause of head pain. There are other pain syndromes called neuralgias, pains in a specific nerve pattern in the head. Sometimes the pain is caused by inflammation of the brain or blood vessels in the head, as in cranial arteritis. Temporomandibular joint (TMJ) problems may cause head pain and are diagnosed by examination and x-ray.

Trigeminal Neuralgia

Also known as tic doloreaux, *trigeminal neuralgia* occurs in middle age and later life, and is characterized by repetitive bursts of severe pain in the face, most often in the cheek. The pain is in the distribution of the fifth cranial nerve (trigeminal nerve), which has three branches: the first to the eye area (ophthalmic), the second to the cheek and nose area (mandibular), and the third to the lower face and chin (maxillary). Facial weakness and sensory loss do not usually occur. The pain is often triggered by stimulation to the face, mouth, and gums, as occurs in shaving, brushing the teeth, yawning, or chewing. Exposure to air may also precipitate episodes of pain. Attacks often occur in clusters that last for days, weeks, or months, followed by spontaneous remission.

A symptomatic tic may be due to a tumor, dental problems, multiple sclerosis, or an aneurysm; the cause is determined by examination and imaging studies, usually MRI. Sometimes the tic is caused by a blood vessel pressing on the nerve.

Several medications are useful for pain control, including antiepileptic drugs such as phenytoin (Dilantin) and carbamazepine (Tegretol); the tricyclic antidepressant amitriptyline (Elavil); clonazepam (Klonopin); and baclofen (Lioresal). Sometimes drugs are combined when a single drug is insufficient for pain control. Surgery is available for those with intractable pain. The traditional method of treatment involved injection of alcohol or phenol into the nerve root, resulting in loss of facial sensation. Two surgical methods currently used are the Janetta procedure, a technique of nerve decompression when pain is due to pressure by a blood vessel, and stereotactic radiofrequency thermocoagulation, a technique that heats the nerve. The Janetta procedure does not cause sensory loss.

Temporal Arteritis

This condition is a cause of headache in the older population, age of onset usually in the mid-50s, and is less common in women. Pain is caused by inflammation of the blood vessels. Diagnosis is by biopsy of the temporal artery, an uncomplicated office procedure. If it is not diagnosed, blindness may occur because of involvement of ophthalmic blood vessels. Involvement of large vessels in the brain can cause a stroke. Steroids are an effective treatment.

Herpes Zoster Infection (Shingles)

Shingles may involve the face and other parts of the body. This viral infection responds to treatment with acyclovir (Zovirax) or is self-limited. Some people, particularly women, develop a severe pain syndrome in the affected area that is called postherpetic neuralgia. In most cases the pain resolves after two to three months. In others, however, the pain may become chronic and intractable. Medical management is similar to that for tic doloreaux, with amitriptyline (Elavil) the preferred drug. Phenothiazine medications are also useful but may have unacceptable side effects. Topical treatment with capsaicin (a counter-irritant) or the use of local anesthetic sprays and a technique called transcutaneous electrical stimulation (TENS) may benefit some shingles sufferers. (See Chapter 35)

Back Pain

One of the most common ailments, back pain affects up to 20 percent of the U.S. population. It is the commonest cause of disability in people under age 45, with 6 to 8 million persons claiming disability for this problem.

Many women are at special risk because of sedentary lifestyles, pregnancy, household and child care activities, and postmenopausal thinning of bone (osteoporosis). Maintaining proper weight, regular exercise, and good nutrition with adequate intake of vitamin D and calcium reduce the risk of back problems. Because household chores and child care involve repetitive lifting, bending, and stooping, it pays to learn proper lifting techniques. In postmenopausal women, estrogen replacement therapy may lessen the severity of osteoporosis. (See Chapter 34)

In the evaluation of a patient with neck or lower back pain, the neurologist first determines if there is injury to the spinal cord or nerves. This may be obvious if there is weakness or loss of muscle tissue. Conversely, the damage may be detectable only by examination, which consists of inspection and palpation of the spine and joints; observation of gait; tests of spine mobility; attempts to elicit pain by palpation, punch, and spine or limb movement; tests of sensory perception by light touch, pinprick, application of heat and cold, and vibration; and tests of individual muscle strength and reflexes.

Severe back pain may also result from spasm of neck or back muscles. Strains or sprains can be caused by whiplash injury, heavy lifting, or twisting injury to the spine, even without structural injury to the spinal cord or nerves. Such pain results from the stretching or tearing of support structures such as ligaments and tendons. Pain that radiates down a limb in a localized distribution, called radiculopathy, suggests pressure on a nerve or root. Sciatica, pain radiating from the hip down the back of the leg, is an example. Pressure on the spinal cord causes pain over the affected area and may result in leg weakness, walking problems, or urinary incontinence.

Diagnosis

Diagnostic tests include X-rays, imaging studies (CT, MRI, myelography), and EMG. The extent and promptness of the testing depend on the history and examination, not just the severity of pain.

The purpose of the diagnostic tests is to identify a structural cause for the pain, such as disk bulge, tumor, infection, or arthritis. It is important to recognize, however, that structural abnormalities such as disk bulges and arthritis are common in adults and may not be responsible for the pain in question.

Treatment

Pain due to structural spine problems may be managed conservatively with rest, pain medication, and a supervised therapy program, or may require surgery. Both orthopedic surgeons and neurosurgeons evaluate and operate on spine problems. If surgery is recom-

mended, make sure you obtain more than one opinion, especially if the problem identified is arthritis or disc disease. If the spinal cord is compressed by a tumor, disk, or abscess, emergency surgery may be necessary to prevent irreversible paralysis and incontinence.

Most lower back pain is not due to structural spine disease. Lax ligaments, poor muscle tone, poor posture, and obesity are contributing factors. Psychological problems can also contribute to the severity and chronicity of the pain. Weight reduction and regular exercise are appropriate nonsurgical treatment of pain. Stress management, biofeedback, and acupuncture are also sometimes recommended. Nonnarcotic analgesics may be used for pain relief; amitriptyline benefits some. Narcotic drugs should be reserved for those with cancer and with severe pain.

Myofascial Pain Syndrome

This refers to localized areas of muscle pain and tenderness called "trigger points." It may exist with other pain syndromes, and the cause is uncertain. Prior trauma, such as whiplash injury, plays a role in some cases. The diagnosis is by clinical examination. Treatment consists of massage; acupressure; acupuncture; local application of heat, cold, or topical sprays; and an exercise regimen. Trigger point injections of local anesthetics and steroids are also helpful. Stress reduction and regular exercise prevent relapse.

Stupor and Coma

Stupor is an altered state of consciousness in which a person appears sleepy or lethargic but can be roused. *Coma* is a state of unconsciousness from which a person cannot be roused. Any abrupt change in mental state or level of consciousness requires prompt evaluation in an emergency room. Emergency transport personnel will assess the vital signs and administer appropriate treatment en route to the hospital. If breathing is compromised, a tube will be inserted into the trachea for delivery of oxygen. Narcan (a drug to reverse drug overdose), glucose, thiamine, and intravenous fluids are usually given. In trauma cases, the spine is immobilized in case there is unrecognized injury.

Once the patient is in the hospital, medical specialists and neurologists will determine if the coma is due to a systemic problem (drug overdose, diabetes, low blood sugar, exposure to a toxic substance) or a primary neurological event (meningitis, encephalitis, brain hemorrhage, or stroke). Recovery from coma is dependent on cause and duration. In prolonged coma, care includes nutritional support and prevention of pneumonia, skin breakdown and blood clots in the legs and lungs. Some causes of coma result in brain death. This diagnosis is determined by both clinical and electrical (EEG) criteria. (Most medical institutions have a protocol for determination of brain death.) Clinical criteria include no evidence of speech or comprehension; no volitional movement or response to pain; no spontaneous respiration; no eye movements or pupil reflexes; no limb reflexes. The examination is re-peated after several hours to determine irreversibility. The EEG is flat, indicating no cerebral activity.

Brain death cannot be diagnosed immediately after cardiac arrest or in the presence of severe hypothermia or high levels of sedative/hypnotic drugs. A person may meet all criteria for brain death and still show reflex leg or toe movements due to spinal reflexes.

In cases of coma with partial recovery, a persistent vegetative state may ensue. The person may exhibit spontaneous blinking, roving eye movements, and reflex limb movements in response to touch or pain, but no pattern can be established.

COMMON NEUROLOGICAL DISORDERS

Neurological disorders can be self-limiting (disappear on their own) or have symptoms that come and go over a long period. Sometimes the symptoms become progressively worse. In many cases, treatment is available to control symptoms and prevent progression of the disease.

Migraine Headache

Migraine headaches are common in the U.S. population, affecting 7.4 percent of women and 3.5 percent of men. The first attack is most often in the late teens or in young adulthood but may occur at any age. Childhood onset is not uncommon. In some women, the headaches occur in the premenstrual period. Fifty to 70 percent of cases are familial, indicating an inherited disorder.

Migraine is a recurrent, throbbing headache accompanied by complex symptoms suggesting a systemic disorder. In most sufferers, there are at least three distinct phases: the prodrome (symptoms that precede the headache), the headache phase, and the posthead-ache period. The symptom complex may last several days. The prodrome consists of an altered psychic state that may be reflected in sudden, increased energy a few days preceding the headache. Headache may then begin suddenly or build slowly after an *aura* or brief warning.

The aura may be visual, sensory, psychic, or motor, and usually lasts 10 to 20 minutes before onset of the headache. Visual auras, the most common, consist of zigzag lines, flashes of white or colored light, or other distortions that move across the visual field, leaving a blind spot or an inability to see to one side. Sensory symptoms consist of numbness and tingling of lips or limbs. Disturbances of mood, mental confusion, and language problems may also occur.

A migraine headache is classified as common, classic, or complicated. *Common migraine* is a headache without aura. It occurs in almost 90 percent of migraine sufferers. *Classic migraine* is migraine with an aura. There are other specific migraine patterns with associated neurological symptoms or signs, such as unilateral dilated pupil, droopy lid, and paralysis of eye movement (ophthalmoplegic migraine), vertigo and imbalance (basilar migraine), and unilateral limb paralysis (hemiplegic migraine). These types of migraine headaches are usually hereditary and often begin in childhood.

The migraine headache is usually very severe, often beginning in a localized area, such as above or behind the eye, then spreading to half the head before becoming generalized. Nausea and vomiting occur with both common and classic migraine. Sensitivity to light and sound is usual, and skin color and temperature changes sometimes occur. Most sufferers seek rest in a quiet, darkened environment. Once the headache has abated, fatigue and drowsiness are common complaints.

Diagnosis

The diagnosis of migraine is based on history and examination. If the neurological examination is normal, the diagnostic evaluation may be limited to examination and baseline blood studies. Diagnostic tests such

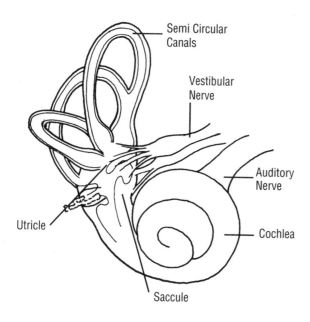

Semi Circular Canals

Vestibular Nerve

Auditory Nerve

Cochlea

Utricle

Saccule

Figure 22.6 The Labyrinth of the Inner Ear
The labyrinth is part of the vestibular system of the inner ear. It is made up of three semicircular canals that arise from the base of a rounded chamber called the vestibule. Within the vestibule are two fluid-filled sacs called the utricle and the saccule, which are connected to the cochlea.

as brain imaging with MRI or CT and angiography are indicated in older persons and those with complicated migraine. Lumbar puncture may be indicated because the migraine headache may mimic the headache of brain hemorrhage or infection.

Treatment

The management of migraine has three objectives: aborting the attack, pain relief, and prevention of further episodes. Migraine aura and other neurological symptoms are due to constriction of blood vessels in the brain; the pain is caused by excessive blood vessel dilation. Medications that abort headache prevent excess vasodilation.

Two drugs specifically abort headache: ergotamine tartrate derivatives and sumatriptin (Imitrex). One derivative, Cafergot, is a combination of ergotamine and caffeine. Ergotamine derivatives are available in tablets for oral or sublingual use, rectal suppositories and in-

jectable solutions. Imitrex is available for injection only and comes in a preloaded kit for self-administration. Your physician can provide training in self-injection techniques. A medication given by injection or a rectal suppository is preferred because tablets may not be well absorbed. The dosage of Ergot derivative and Imitrex is limited because of serious side effects from overuse. Pregnant women and those with complicated migraine should not use these vasoconstrictive medications.

A number of other medications are available for pain relief, and some of them are also effective in aborting attacks. Your physician will outline the types you may try, ranging from over-the-counter medications such as aspirin, acetaminophen (Tylenol), and nonsteroidal drugs like ibuprofen (Advil, Motrin) to prescription drugs. Avoid those with addictive potential, especially narcotics, unless they are absolutely necessary for pain control. Finding the appropriate medication is a trial-and-error process. Medication overdosage can worsen the headache. If you suffer from migraine and take several analgesic tablets daily, yet experience daily morning headache, you are likely suffering from medication overdosage.

Preventive therapy is necessary in cases of frequent migraine. Stress management, regular exercise, dietary changes, and biofeedback are beneficial. Possible food triggers for migraine include chocolate, nuts, aged cheese, citrus fruits, bananas, monosodium glutamate (present in some Chinese food and used as a flavor enhancer), dairy products, pickles, cured meats, and alcohol. Birth control pills and the antihypertensive drug reserpine may trigger or cause migraine.

Prophylactic drugs are usually given until a pain-free state is achieved for several months. Medication may then be tapered off and discontinued. Abrupt discontinuation of medication may provoke severe rebound migraine or *status migrainosus,* a syndrome of almost continuous headache that requires hospital management. Prophylactic medications for migraine include beta-blockers such as propranolol (Inderal); calcium channel blockers (verapamil, nifedipine); methysergide (Sansert), a long-acting ergot derivative; and amitriptyline (Elavil). Indomethacin (Indocin) is often useful in premenstrual migraine.

Cluster headache is a variant of migraine that usually affects adult men. This type of headache is among the worst, typically awakening the sufferer from sleep. Unlike migraine sufferers, those with cluster headaches are unable to rest and are agitated and restless, sometimes in such great pain that suicide is contemplated. *Tension headache* is regarded as a musculoskeletal contraction headache, with pain usually described as squeezing or viselike. Its characteristics may overlap those of migraine, and it may be as severe as, or coexist with, typical migraine.

Spine and Disc Disorders

Degenerative changes in the spine are an inevitable part of aging. Bone, ligaments, tendons, and the intervertebral discs are affected. The lower part of the neck and lower back are at greatest risk for degenerative change. Osteoporosis or multiple pregnancies in women are aggravating factors.

Osteoporosis causes thinning of bone that may result in painful vertebral collapse. Immobilization is the usual treatment, with gradual return to movement in a supervised therapy program. A cervical collar or a lower back support brace is prescribed.

Arthritic spine changes result in bony overgrowth that narrows the spinal canal, causing spinal stenosis. Pain in the legs when walking is a symptom of spinal stenosis. Pain is treated with bed rest, analgesics, cervical collar or back brace, and physical therapy. Prolonged use of a back brace is usually not recommended because it weakens abdominal muscles. Surgery is indicated for intractable, severe pain and for those with signs of nerve or spinal cord injury.

Disc disease may be due to degeneration of the disc itself or to degeneration of the ligaments that hold the disc in place. Disc herniation is extrusion of the disc into the spinal canal, where it may compress a nerve or the spinal cord. Disc disease and arthritis can exist together.

The nature and extent of surgical intervention depend on the spine problem. For spinal stenosis or disc degeneration and spinal stenosis, more extensive surgical procedures may be necessary to relieve pressure on the spine and nerve roots.

Sometimes surgery fails to relieve pain. This may not be due to a failure in surgical technique but to factors beyond the surgeon's control, such as postoperative scarring or a persistent, inflammatory reaction at the operated site (arachnoiditis). Persistent or recurrent postoperative pain requires reevaluation with imaging studies. If no new surgical problem is identified, long-term physical therapy is indicated.

Head and Brain Injury

Traumatic head injury requires prompt medical evaluation because of the potential for serious brain damage. Head injury may result from blunt trauma due to a blow or fall, indirect trauma such as blast injury or whiplash, or penetrating trauma, as with a bullet wound.

Head injury with skull fracture and penetrating head wounds have the highest potential for significant brain injury. There may be hemorrhage into brain tissue or between the membranes overlying the brain (subdural or epidural hematoma). Loss of consciousness usually occurs with significant brain injury, but in some cases is brief. This brief unconsciousness in an apparently lucid person may mask serious injury, however, and is characteristic of epidural hematomas that then suddenly enlarge, causing severe brain compression and death if untreated.

Concussion refers to the loss of consciousness after a head injury. *Contusion* refers to a brain injury similar to a bruise. After concussion, a person may show no symptoms or may experience symptoms of amnesia in regard to the injury and the immediate surrounding time period, dizziness, tinnitus, and headache. In some cases, mood changes, irritability, loss of interest in usual activities, slowed thinking, poor concentration, and depression may occur. The symptoms may last several weeks or months. This postconcussion syndrome is sometimes seen with even minor head injuries. Antidepressants may be beneficial for control of headache and depression. Neurological signs may occur with severe cerebral contusion, resulting in slow or incomplete recovery.

Complications of head injury include meningitis and brain abscess. Impact seizures occur at the time of injury and do not predict a future seizure disorder. Permanent seizure disorders are more likely with penetrating wounds. Seizures that occur more than a month after injury are called posttraumatic epilepsy.

Victims of significant head trauma are assessed and stabilized medically to ensure that other vital structures are not injured. Medications to prevent seizures and treat brain swelling are given. The neck should be immobilized until X-rays are taken because neck injury can escape detection in the unconscious head-injured person. Imaging studies, usually CT, are obtained. If a large hematoma is visualized, emergency drainage is performed. Small hematomas may be followed by means of periodic examination and scans. In some penetrating injuries, such as bullet wounds, surgery may be limited to removing dead tissue and cleansing the area because removal of the bullet or its fragments is too risky.

Recovery after head injury may be gradual and prolonged if neurologic deficits are severe. Cognitive remedial therapy is important for those with memory and language deficits.

Epilepsy

A seizure is a behavioral or neurological event caused by abnormal electrical discharge in the brain. Recurrent seizures are called epilepsy. The behaviors observed before and during a seizure include staring spells with inattention, repetitive automatic movements or gestures, repetitive jerks of a limb, and loss of consciousness with generalized jerking of the limbs and back arching. Tongue biting and urinary incontinence can occur. Confusion, amnesia, and agitation can follow a generalized seizure.

Diagnosis

Persons with possible seizures should be evaluated by an experienced primary care clinician, internist, or neurologist. The primary care physician or internist will look for toxic or metabolic causes of seizures. The neurologist will look for neurological abnormalities that could indicate a brain lesion. The history is the most important part of the diagnostic evaluation. Family history, birth injury, head trauma, and infection, among others, are important in determining if a single seizure will lead to epilepsy. Some seizure disorders are inherited.

Diagnostic tests include baseline blood tests (blood count, serum glucose, and chemistry profile), EEG, and brain imaging. Lumbar puncture is sometimes recommended. You may be asked to remain awake the night before an EEG and be given a mild sedative during the test. This is done to "activate" abnormal electrical discharges. During the test other activators, such as flashing lights and rapid breathing, are used. Without activation, an EEG is likely to be normal between seizures. Sometimes it is normal despite their use. Repeat studies are sometimes done, and in some cases video-EEG is performed. Video-EEG is done in a hospital setting with continuous EEG and camera monitoring for 24–48 hours. This is useful for determining if an event is a seizure and for localizing the seizure discharge.

The results of the history, examination, and diagnostic tests are used to classify epilepsy as partial, primary, or symptomatic. *Partial* seizures originate in a localized area of the brain but may spread to the whole brain, becoming secondarily generalized. Temporal lobe and complex partial seizures are examples of partial seizures. Seizures may also be diagnosed as *primary,* not associated with a brain lesion, or *symptomatic,* due to a brain lesion such as tumor, stroke, vascular malformation, trauma, or birth injury.

Treatment

The classification of the seizures determines the selection of the most effective drug therapy. There are several medications for treatment of epilepsy, but single-drug therapy is preferred. If the initial drug selected does not work, the neurologist will substitute another, rather than prescribe a combination of two. In difficult cases, multiple drugs may be necessary. Blood levels are monitored to ensure adequate dosage. Anticonvulsant medication may have side effects, so medical follow-up is necessary.

Symptomatic seizures may require treatment of the precipitating cause as well as medication for the seizures. Chronic alcoholism, for example, may lead to a seizure disorder that occurs only during periods of abstinence. Drug use and dependence may also cause seizures. These seizures usually remit with abstinence. Medication is not necessary unless there is a coexistent brain injury.

Surgery is performed for severe epilepsy that does not respond to medical management. Such surgery is available in specialized centers and requires careful evaluation, including brain mapping, to isolate the focus of the seizure discharge. Success rates may approach 50 percent with a cure or improved response to medication.

Persons with epilepsy who are neurologically normal and whose seizures are well controlled may live a normal life and participate in all activities. Some jobs and activities may pose a risk if there are occasional breakthrough seizures. Appropriate activities should be discussed with the doctor. Driving is not restricted if seizures are controlled. State laws should be checked for requirements of reporting and medical clearance.

If seizures are controlled for several years, your physicians may recommend gradual discontinuation of medication. The physician will consider several factors, including the seizure type and EEG findings. Never make this decision on your own without medical supervision. Abrupt discontinuation of seizure medication may cause *status epilepticus,* frequently recurring seizures with unconsciousness, a neurological emergency.

Strokes

Stroke is one of the most common disorders of the nervous system. The term is often used interchangeably with *cerebrovascular accident* (CVA), implying a vascular cause. Because not all neurological impairments that resemble a stroke are of vascular origin, the term *stroke syndrome* is preferred. Diagnostic tests are necessary to determine if a vascular event is the cause.

A stroke is a focal neurological abnormality that occurs suddenly or over a period of a few hours. Stroke-like symptoms that are transient and fully resolvable, lasting from minutes up to 24 hours, are called *transient ischemic attacks* (TIAS).

Vascular stroke is caused by hemorrhage in the brain or blockage of a blood vessel by a clot (embolus or thrombus). The neurological deficit occurs because a portion of the brain is deprived of oxygen or compressed by the bleeding. Bleeding into the brain may be caused by trauma, bleeding disorders like hemophilia, tumor, a ruptured aneurysm, vascular malformation, cocaine use, hypertension, a degenerative blood vessel disease, or amyloid. Inflammation of blood vessels (vasculitis) may also lead to hemorrhage or infarct. Stroke due to blockage of a vessel by clot is called cerebral infarction. A thrombus may form in a blood vessel narrowed by atherosclerosis or damaged by hypertension. The heart may be a source of an embolus, a clot that travels to a blood vessel from a distant site. Embolic infarctions may be associated with bleeding. Abnormal heart valves, irregular heart rhythms, and myocardial infarction may all lead to stroke. Conversely, those who have stroke are at significant risk for coronary artery disease.

The symptoms and signs of stroke depend on the area of the brain affected. There may be visual problems such as blindness in one eye, double vision, or inability to see to one side; difficulty understanding or speaking; weakness of an arm and leg; or unsteadiness when walking.

Diagnosis

Imaging studies such as CT or MRI determine the area of the brain that is affected and detect hemorrhage or other conditions, such as a tumor. Lumbar puncture is sometimes necessary. Angiography is used to identify the site of blockage as well as potential surgical problems such as aneurysm, vascular malformation, or narrowed carotid arteries. Other diagnostic tests will depend on the nature of the stroke and may include an echocardiogram to reveal abnormal heart valves or thrombus, an EKG or a 24-hour heart monitor to detect abnormal heart rhythms, an ultrasound of the large neck vessels (Doppler study), and an EEG. In some cases, special blood tests are done to detect in-

flammatory problems, such as lupus or blood abnormalities that are associated with a clotting tendency.

Treatment

Treatment of stroke begins with prevention, which includes control of blood pressure, reduction of serum cholesterol, management of diabetes mellitus, and cessation of smoking or illicit drug use. Aspirin therapy and anticoagulants (blood thinners) are prescribed preventively to those at risk for stroke, and therapeutically to those who have suffered stroke. Surgery on the carotid artery is performed for severe blockage in those who have TIAs or minor stroke due to the blockage, or for bleeding aneurysms. Surgery is not done if the vessel is completely closed.

Following stroke, rehabilitation should begin as soon as possible. For major deficits, inpatient treatment is necessary. For those with minor disability, home-based or outpatient treatment is sufficient.

Ménière's Disease

The classic labyrinthine form of vertigo, Ménière's disease, usually occurs in the 50s; women and men are equally affected. The attacks of vertigo are abrupt and usually associated with tinnitus, diminished hearing, or a sense of fullness in the ear. Nausea, vomiting, imbalance, or an inability to walk may also occur. Rarely, the attacks are so violent that they result in sudden falls. The medical examination may disclose hearing loss, usually in one ear and generally before the first attack of vertigo, and nystagmus. The clinical course is recurrent attacks and progressive hearing loss, although the severity of the attacks lessens as hearing loss increases. In 10 percent of cases, the hearing loss is in both ears. Rarely, the disease is inherited.

Diagnosis

Although the cause of Ménière's disease is uncertain, pathologic studies often show an abnormal collection of fluid in the affected ear. It is reasonable to suggest that vertigo is precipitated by membrane rupture and the release of the fluid into the space around the nerves, resulting in damages to the vestibular nerve and cochlear cells.

Treatment

This condition is treated by bed rest and antihistamine-type medications such as dimenhydrinate (Dramamine), cyclizine (Marezine), and meclizine (Antivert). Medication for nausea and anxiety may also be prescribed. Dietary salt restriction and diuretics are sometimes recommended but are of unproven benefit. Continuous disabling vertigo may be corrected by surgical labyrinthine destruction, a treatment of last resort for those with unilateral disease. This type of surgery causes deafness.

There are other types of labyrinthine vertigo.

- *Benign positional vertigo.* A rapid change in position can cause a vertigo that can be reproduced by similar maneuvers during examination. Hearing is normal. This disorder is attributed to the dislocation of small stonelike structures (otoliths) into one of the semicircular canals. Some specialists recommend trying to displace the otoliths by lying first on the side that causes vertigo for 30 seconds, then changing to the other side. Repeat this maneuver 5 times, several times a day.

- *Vestibular neuronitis.* This benign form of vertigo often follows an infection and is usually self-limited. Vertigo may, however, be severe and sometimes recurrent.

- *Labyrinthine apoplexy.* This term applies to a syndrome of sudden vertigo with resulting destruction of the labyrinth of the inner ear. The cause is unknown.

Vertigo of vestibular nerve origin may be due to a tumor, inflammation, infection, or compression of the nerve by an adjacent artery. The most common cause is a tumor known as an acoustic neuroma. Deafness usually precedes the vertigo, and other signs may be present. Vertigo of brain stem origin is usually accompanied by other signs and symptoms. Causes include stroke, multiple sclerosis, infection, and migraine.

Parkinson's Disease

Parkinson's disease is a degenerative disease of the elderly, with peak age at onset in the 60s, although some cases are identified in persons as young as 30. The prevalence increases with advancing age. Approximately 500,000 persons in the United States have Parkinson's. The disease is rarely familial.

Parkinson's is a disorder of movement. The main features are rigidity, tremor while resting, motor slowness, postural instability, and abnormal gait. Tremor may affect hands and legs; it is worse at rest and decreases with motion. Depression and dementia may coexist, their frequency increasing with disease duration in up to half of patients.

Diagnosis

Parkinson's disease is diagnosed by a medical history and examination. The onset of the disease is sometimes so gradual that symptoms are attributed to depression or "normal" aging. Diagnostic tests are used to exclude other disorders that cause Parkinsonian symptoms (symptomatic Parkinson's). These include hydrocephalus (enlargement of the water-filled brain spaces), stroke, and other brain lesions. CT or MRI imaging is usually done to exclude these causes. Some drugs also cause a Parkinsonian state, especially the phenothiazines.

Treatment

Because Parkinson's is due to a loss of the brain chemical dopamine, drugs used to treat Parkinson's replace this chemical or act to balance the ratio between dopamine and another brain chemical, acetylcholine. There are several useful drugs: a combination of levodopa and carbidopa (Sinemet), which lessens the risk of nausea caused by levodopa alone; bromocriptine (Parlodel); a drug that acts like dopamine; seligiline (Eldepryl), a drug that may slow the progression of Parkinson's; trihexiphenidyl (Artane), a drug that lowers the level of acetylcholine; and amantidine (Symmetrel), a drug that releases dopamine from cells. Vitamin E also has been recommended to slow disease progression but is of uncertain benefit.

The management of Parkinson's disease is complex and should be done by a physician experienced in use of the available drugs. Drug combinations may be required, and sometimes a "drug holiday," when all drugs are stopped, may be necessary. Overuse of drugs can accelerate the progression of the disease or lead to unacceptable side effects, such as low blood pressure, confusion, hallucinations, and abnormal movements. Depression improves with antidepressive medication and sometimes with electroconvulsive therapy (ECT). Physical therapy is also an important part of treatment. Dietary restriction of foods containing the chemical phenylalanine may be necessary.

Multiple Sclerosis

This is the most common neurological disorder of young adults, affecting 250,000 to 350,000 people in the United States. Two-thirds of those affected have a first attack between the ages of 20 and 40. The disease occurs rarely in childhood or as late as the 50s and 60s. Women are affected two to three times more often than men, and 15 percent of cases have an affected relative.

The cause of multiple sclerosis (MS) is unknown. Factors thought to play a role are viral infectious agents, genetics, and geographic location. The incidence of the disease is much lower in equatorial regions of the world and increases at more northern latitudes. An abnormal immune response that destroys the central nervous system substance myelin (the covering of nerve fibers) is thought to trigger attacks. Although many have suggested that a virus induces the autoimmunity, no consistent relationship between a particular virus and MS has been established. Some have suggested that initial attacks or relapses are triggered by infection, trauma, or pregnancy, but others question the association of these otherwise common events with MS.

The symptoms of MS depend on the area of brain affected. Visual loss due to optic neuritis (inflammation of the optic nerve) is a common initial complaint. Up to half of persons with this problem will develop MS within 5 years. Other symptoms include double vision, slurred speech, leg stiffness, incoordination, and limb numbness, tingling, or weakness. Bladder, bowel, and sexual functions may be affected. Paroxysmal pain syndromes such as tic doloreaux sometimes occur.

MS is an episodic disorder, meaning that symptoms begin abruptly and remit over several weeks. Chronic progressive MS, a less common presentation, is characterized by progressive disability without remissions. Some patients enjoy a benign course with few or nondisabling attacks, and some are asymptomatic for life, diagnosed with MS only incidentally at autopsy.

Diagnosis

Diagnosis is by clinical criteria based on neurological examination or by a combination of clinical and laboratory tests. Diagnostic tests include lumbar puncture, MRI scans of brain and/or spinal cord, and evoked potential studies. Lumbar puncture is done to test for olioclonal bands, an abnormal protein pattern found in MS but not limited to this disease. MRI identifies the white matter plaques of MS. Other tests show delay in nerve transmission caused by the loss of myelin.

Treatment

Intravenous or oral steroids can shorten acute attacks and speed recovery. Intravenous steroids are preferred for optic neuritis. Other immunosuppressive drugs sometimes given are azathioprine (Imuran) and cyclophosphamide (Cytoxan). The new drug Beta-Seron, a type of interferon, decreases the number of attacks in those who relapse. Baclofen (Lioresal) is used for spasticity. It may be given orally or intrathecally into the spinal space. Paroxysmal pain of MS may be treated with amitriptyline or other drugs.

Physical therapy and supportive services are important aspects of MS management. Bladder symptoms should be evaluated by a urologist. Drugs are available that may alleviate incontinence or retention. Diet, adequate rest, and avoidance of temperature extremes, especially heat, are also important.

Polyneuropathy

Polyneuropathy affects the peripheral or autonomic nerves. Peripheral neuropathy may affect sensation, motor strength, or both in the hands and feet. Symptoms include numbness, tingling, and weakness. Symptoms of autonomic neuropathy include sweating, diarrhea or constipation, difficulty urinating, and impotence.

There are many causes of peripheral neuropathy, including genetic disorders, alcoholism or the abuse of other drugs, exposure to toxic substances, nutritional deficiency, metabolic disorders, inflammation, infection, chronic illness, and cancer. Peripheral neuropathy also may be a remote effect of cancer or a complication of chemotherapy. *Guillain-Barré disease* is a form of peripheral neuropathy. It is a viral infection characterized by progressive numbness and weakness. When it is severe, complete paralysis and loss of respiration may occur.

Diagnosis

Neuropathy is determined by a medical history and examination. Electromyography (EMG), a test of nerve and muscle function, is used to classify the neuropathy and pinpoint the part of a nerve affected. A nerve biopsy and special blood tests may be necessary.

DEGENERATIVE DISEASES

Dementia

Dementia, a gradual decline and loss of intellectual and social functioning, affects millions of Americans in their later years. One of the most common causes of dementia is Alzheimer's disease, which accounts for about 50 percent of all cases of dementia. The disease begins with a gradual loss of memory, increasing confusion and anxiety, and a growing irritability. The disease progresses to the point where the person is unable to work, socialize, or communicate. The disease is due to a degeneration of brain cells, but the exact process is unknown. To date, there is no effective treatment or cure. Other causes of dementia are stroke, brain tumor, head injuries, and some infectious diseases of the brain.

Amyotrophic Lateral Sclerosis (ALS)

Commonly called Lou Gehrig's disease, amyotrophic lateral sclerosis is a progressive degeneration of the nerve cells controlling voluntary motor functions. The symptoms include difficulty in walking; swallowing, speaking, or breathing problems; and a gradual wasting away of the muscles of the arms and legs. Death usually occurs within 2 to 10 years after diagnosis. The cause is unknown, and there is currently no effective treatment.

Huntington's Disease

Huntington's disease, or chorea, is a progressive hereditary disorder characterized by abnormal involuntary movements, personality changes, and mental deterioration. It is an autosomal dominant disease, which means the child of an affected parent has a 50 percent chance of inheriting the disease. The onset of symptoms is usually between 35 and 40 years of age, and death occurs within 10 to 15 years.

Treatment

Treatment depends on cause. Some polyneuropathies, such as Guillain-Barré, are treated with plasmapheresis, intravenous gamma-globulin, or steroids. Recovery from Guillain-Barré may be complete, even in a severe case. Some genetic disorders are progressive. Physical therapy, adaptive equipment, and special shoes are sometimes necessary.

Tumor

Primary tumors of the nervous system originate there; secondary or metastatic tumors have spread from distant sites in the body. Primary brain or spinal cord tumors can be either benign or malignant; metastatic tumors are always malignant. Breast and lung cancers are especially likely to spread to the brain and spinal cord. Even a benign brain tumor may cause serious problems because of its size or inaccessibility to surgery.

Symptoms depend on the site affected. Headache, mental confusion, language impairment, visual change, weakness, or strokelike symptoms may indicate a brain tumor. Seizures may also be a presenting symptom. Spinal cord tumors cause back pain, difficulty walking, and bowel or bladder problems.

Diagnosis

Brain or spinal tumors are diagnosed by CT imaging or MRS. A pathologic diagnosis requires tissue confirmation, which may be done by a craniotomy, where the skull is opened, or by a stereotactic biopsy. A low-risk procedure when done by an expert, a stereotactic biopsy is done with the patient awake. A small hole is drilled into the skull and a probe is passed to the site to be biopsied, using the CT scan as a guide. Because the brain has no pain fibers, the procedure is not painful.

Treatment

Benign tumors are surgically removed unless their location precludes it. Malignant tumors may be treated with surgery, radiation, and chemotherapy, individually or in combination. Surgery is selectively used in cases of metastatic cancer.

Motor Neuron Disease

Motor neurons in the brain and spinal cord control movement. They are subject to a degenerative disease whose cause is unknown. Some cases are familial (inherited), and others may be the remote effects of a disease like cancer. Symptoms include a gradual wasting and weakness of muscles. All limbs are eventually affected. A bulbar form of the disease affects speech and swallowing. Mentation is always normal. There is no known treatment except in cases of remote effect where the cause is amenable to therapy. Progression is sometimes rapid, with death in 3 years due to respiratory failure. Others progress more slowly and are successfully managed with therapy, adaptive equipment, and portable ventilators for many years.

Myasthenia Gravis

A disease of the neuromuscular junction (the region between nerve and muscle) myasthenia gravis results in what is called fatigable muscle weakness. The term *fatigable* refers to weakness that occurs after repetitive use of a muscle, not to the generalized state of fatigue. Typically, the muscle weakness fluctuates during the

day. Symptoms may be confined to the eye muscles, with complaints of droopy lids and double vision. Or the disease may involve facial, speech, and swallowing muscles, causing facial weakness and difficulty in chewing, swallowing and speaking. Involvement of limb muscles occurs in generalized myasthenia.

Peak age at onset in women is 20 to 30 and in men, ages 60 to 70. The disease rarely occurs in childhood.

Diagnosis

Myasthenia gravis is an autoimmune disease. It is due to a defect in neuromuscular transmision—antibodies form against receptors in the muscle membrane, decreasing the response to the neurotransmitter acetyl-

NEUROLOGICAL TESTS

Tests used to assess neurological disorders include imaging studies such as CT scans and MRI, plus tests that study the electrical impulses of the brain, tests of nerve and muscle function, and procedures to assess nerve responses to stimuli. Other procedures include an examination of cerebrospinal fluid and a biopsy of brain, nerve, and muscle tissue. The tests performed depend on the symptoms and the findings of an examination. Their purpose is to identify the area of the nervous system affected and to determine the cause of the problem.

Biopsy
A biopsy is a surgical procedure used to confirm a diagnosis. A piece of tissue is removed and studied under a microscope. In some cases, cultures are done to look for infectious organisms. A brain biopsy is done to determine the nature of a suspected tumor or to look for disease in brain tissue, such as infection or a degenerative process. A biopsy is often necessary because scans of different brain processes may look similar. A brain biopsy may be open (craniotomy) or stereotactic (done with a probe). The open surgical approach depends on the site and nature of the lesion. The risk is less for stereotactic biopsy, but the procedure may not work as well because of the small amount of tissue obtained. A nerve biopsy can provide information on nerve defects that may relate to inherited, inflammatory, or metabolic conditions. A muscle biopsy is part of the workup of patients with muscle weakness.

Electroencephalography
Electrical activity of the brain can be recorded on an electroencephalogram, which provides a picture of the functioning of the brain. Abnormal patterns can show up when the brain is not functioning properly. The test is especially helpful in seizure disorders and can be used to assess stuporous or comatose patients. It is also used to monitor the state of the brain under anesthesia during surgery, and in cases of injury or drug intoxication. A flat pattern, showing no brain activity, is accepted as brain death.

For the procedure, electrodes are placed on the patient's scalp and attached to a machine that produces a tracing. A sedative may be given before the test. There is no risk, and the test may be done on an outpatient basis.

Evoked Potentials
The stimulation of certain areas in the body can produce a response that can be traced by electrodes placed along nerve pathways. Electrodes are usually attached to the scalp, the responses are recorded on a graph, and the results are analyzed by a computer to show the pattern and strength of brain waves. Each peak or wave corresponds to a particular sensory relay, and alterations in the waves can show a problem at a specific site in the body.

Visual evoked potentials involve stimulation of the eye to detect problems in the optic nerve. The test can also be used to assess sight and blindness, particularly

NEUROLOGICAL TESTS (Continued)

in the very young and the very old. Brain stem audio evoked potentials test hearing. A sound is made into an earphone, and the response is traced along the auditory nerve, inner ear, and parts of the brain that process sound. Somatosensory evoked potentials, used to monitor the spinal cord and brain stem, can help detect disorders or injuries, and may be used during surgery to ensure that these areas remain intact while being manipulated. The evoked potentials are also useful in patients with multiple sclerosis to detect delays in nerve transmission caused by loss of myelin.

Lumbar Puncture
The fluid that surrounds the spinal cord can show signs of infection, disease, bleeding, and pressure in the skull. A sample of fluid is obtained by placing a needle into the lumbar region of the spine through the membrane covering the spine (the dura). A local anesthetic is given before the procedure.

About 10 percent of patients have a headache following this procedure, and sometimes nausea and vomiting occur. Bed rest and a liberal intake of fluids are recommended to prevent post-lumbar puncture problems. In most patients, the symptoms resolve in a few days. In some, severe headache persists, called a post-lumbar puncture headache. This is due to persistent leaking at the puncture site, and can be treated with a blood patch, a minor procedure. Rarely, patients develop double vision, which is usually resolved in a few days or weeks.

Severe complications of lumbar puncture are uncommon. The procedure is safe and is usually performed in a doctor's office. There is no risk of injury to the spinal cord because the needle is inserted several segments below the termination of the cord. This test is contraindicated for patients with bleeding problems, large brain masses, and abscesses over the spine.

Imaging Studies
Several techniques are used for viewing the brain, spinal cord, and other areas of the body that relate to the nervous system. The test selected depends on the condition. Multiple tests are sometimes necessary.

Angiography
For this procedure, a catheter (tube) is placed into an artery and dye is injected through it. X-rays are then taken from different angles. This test can show a disruption or obstruction in the blood vessels, or the site of bleeding or an aneurysm. There is a small risk of neurological signs and symptoms of stroke, especially

for patients with atherosclerotic disease, but these are usually transient. Other complications include an embolism, cutting or tearing of an artery, and an allergic reaction to the dye. The procedure is usually done in a hospital under the direction of a neuroradiologist.

Computed Tomography (CT Scan)
This rapid and safe test provides images of the skull, cerebrospinal fluid, and brain. It can show structural defects, bleeding, fluid buildup, or tumors. Images of blood vessels can be enhanced and made clearer by intravenous injection of dye before the procedure. The technician takes pictures in small sequential slices, so that when they are reassembled by a computer, the image can show multiple planes. Risks are usually confined to dye reactions. A radiologist is present to treat such complications. The test can be done on an outpatient basis.

Magnetic Resonance Imaging (MRI)
For this test the patient is surrounded by a magnetic field through which pulses of radio frequency radiation are projected. Coils are placed on or near the patient's body to serve as antennae in detecting changes caused by the radio-frequency waves. The information obtained from the coils is reconstructed by computer into an image. The test can show differences in tissue and bone structure and help identify masses. A contrasting dye is injected to show certain vascular details. (There is less risk of reaction to this dye than to the contrast used for a CT scan.) The test carries little risk and can be used during pregnancy without the dye. It cannot be used if a person has any metal in his or her body, such as metal clips or plates, or a pacemaker. It also may pose a risk with prosthetic devices, such as cardiac valves and orthopedic devices. The test can be done on an outpatient basis. The tubelike enclosure of the machine may cause a problem for those with claustrophobia. A mild sedative may help. "Open" machines are available, but picture quality may be compromised.

Myelography
In this procedure, dye is injected into the lumbar or cervical (neck) area of the spinal column to assess the spinal cord, blood vessels, ligaments, and disks. An X-ray and/or CT scan of the area is then done to obtain the image. The test is useful for showing compression of the spinal cord (as with a protruding disc), osteoarthritic bones, tumors, or abscess. Headache, nausea, and

vomiting can occur but usually disappear within 24 hours. Seizures may occur but are rare. The procedure is thought to be relatively safe and is sometimes done on an outpatient basis or with an overnight hospital stay.

Nerve Conduction and Electromyography

This test is used to evaluate nerve and muscle function. For nerve conduction, a mild shocklike stimulus is applied to different nerves and an electrode records how fast the impulse travels along the nerve. Slowing, delay, and blockage of conduction can be identified.

This test is useful in diagnosing carpal tunnel syndrome, Guillain-Barré, and other disorders that slow conduction.

For the electromyograph, fine needles are inserted into different muscles and are attached to leads. A pattern is generated on an oscilloscope that shows if there is a nerve problem, a muscle disorder, or both. Interpretation of the pattern is critical and requires an experienced physician, knowledgeable in muscle and nerve problems.

The test is mildly uncomfortable but not severely painful. It is done on an outpatient basis.

---

choline. Antibodies to the acetylcholine receptor are found in almost 90 percent of patients with generalized myasthenia, 70 percent of ocular myasthenia. The edrophonium (Tensilon) test and EMG are used for diagnosis. The edrophonium test, done in the doctor's office, consists of an injection of a drug that partially reverses the weakness. Patients with myasthenia are evaluated for thyroid disorders and for thymoma, a chest tumor. Pulmonary function tests are done to assess respiratory status.

Treatment

Treatment may include anticholinesterase drugs such as Mestinon, plasmapheresis, steroids, and immunosuppressive drugs. The thymus is removed (thymectomy) when a thymoma is present, unless medically contraindicated. In those cases without tumor, a thymectomy is usually recommended because there is good chance of remission following the procedure. Sometimes the disease spontaneously remits, but generally only for short periods. Myasthenia requires expert management and should be handled in centers where physicians have special expertise with the disease.

CHAPTER 23

The Eyes

Penny A. Asbell, M.D., F.A.C.S. and
Ana Bartolomei Aguilera, M.D.

The eyes may be windows of the soul, as the poet says, but these vital sense organs are also our most important connections to the world around us. More than 80 percent of what we learn is conveyed to us through our eyes.

Often compared to a camera, yet far more complex, our eyes are able to receive and transmit millions of pieces of visual information in just an instant. These unique structures work by capturing light and transforming it into impulses that the brain then interprets as images. Our eyes work for us thousands of times a day, moving and focusing and capturing detailed, three-dimensional pictures that we use to establish our knowledge of the world and our place in it.

STRUCTURE AND FUNCTION OF THE EYE

The human eye is approximately spherical in shape, about 1 inch in diameter. It is composed of three major layers: the outer layer, consisting of the sclera and cornea; the middle uvea, consisting of the choroid and iris; and the inner retina (Figure 23.1).

One of the important functions of the outer layer of the eye is to protect the delicate inner structures. The *sclera*—or the white of the eye—covers most of the eyeball and is composed of extremely tough opaque tissue. The *cornea* is a curved transparent membrane that forms the outer coat of the front of the eye. The curvature of the cornea acts as a lens and provides much of the focusing power of the eye and governs how accurately we see. Another protective tissue, the *conjunctiva* covers the exposed front portion of the sclera.

The *choroid* is part of the middle layer of the eye. Richly supplied with blood vessels, its role is mainly to provide nutrition to the retina. The choroid is continuous with the *iris*, a flat, pigmented area with a round opening in the center called the *pupil*. It is the iris that

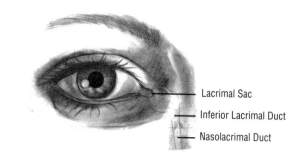

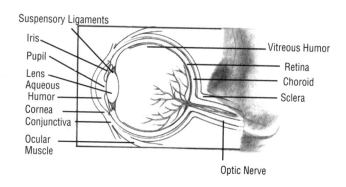

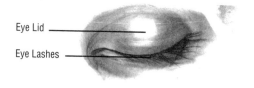

Figure 23.1 The eye and its parts. *Top:* External appearance of the parts of the eye. *Middle:* The parts of the eye are surrounded by a protective sphere, the *sclera*, the front of which (the *cornea*) is transparent. A protective film, the *conjunctiva*, extends from the inside of the eyelid over the front of the sclera. The inner lining of the sclera, the *choroid*, absorbs light and prevents scattering. Light enters the eye through the *pupil* and passes through the *lens*, is focused on the *retina*, and is transmitted through the *optic nerve* to the brain. Muscles in the *iris*, which forms a rim around the lens, control the diameter of the pupil. (The color of the iris, which may be various shades of blue, green, hazel, brown, or nearly black, depends on the amount of pigment inside it.) *Suspensory ligaments* control the shape of the lens as light passes through it. Two chambers of fluid—one inside the choroid (*vitreous humor*) and one in the chamber in front of the lens (*aqueous humor*)—aid in refracting light. *Bottom:* Eyelids serve primarily to protect the eye. They are lined with a thin layer of tissue, the conjunctiva, that distributes tear fluid over the cornea with each blink. Eyelashes help keep dust and debris away from the surface of the eye.

determines the color of the eye; the pupil appears as the black area in the center of the iris.

Behind the pupil and iris is the *lens*, a transparent structure that refracts, or bends, the incoming light and focuses it onto the retina. The elasticity of the lens naturally decreases with age, causing farsightedness, or presbyopia. Many middle-aged and older adults have trouble reading without their glasses.

Lying in front of the iris is the *anterior chamber*. This space is filled with *aqueous humor*, a watery fluid similar to blood serum. This fluid nourishes and lubricates the lens and the cornea. Behind the lens—and making up the bulk of the interior of the eyeball—is the *vitreous humor*, a transparent, colorless, gelatinous fluid. Occasionally, broken lines and squiggles or dots—called floaters—may swim into your vision. Floaters are usually harmless bits of debris left over in the vitreous humor from the development of the eye before birth or from changes in vitreous composition due to aging. (If floaters are accompanied with flashes of light, however, it's advisable to check with your doctor to make sure there is nothing seriously wrong; floaters may be associated with retinal detachments.)

The *retina* is the innermost layer of the eye. Composed of visual cells, nerve endings, connecting fibers, and a rich network of blood vessels, the retina serves as the receptor of visual stimuli, which it then transmits to the brain via the *optic nerve*.

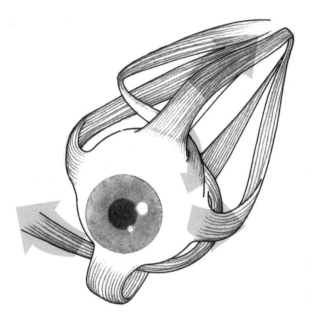

Figure 23.2 Muscles of the eye. Six *intraocular muscles* control the movement of the eye and allow it to move in any direction. Four *rectus* muscles (superior, inferior, lateral, and medial) move the eye up, down, and to either side. The two *oblique* muscles (superior and inferior) are responsible for diagonal or rotary movement. These muscles work as a group, rather than independently, and any one eye movement involves all six muscles to some degree.

We move our eyes by means of the six *extraocular muscles* (Figure 23.2). These muscles are responsible for every possible eye movement. The function of the

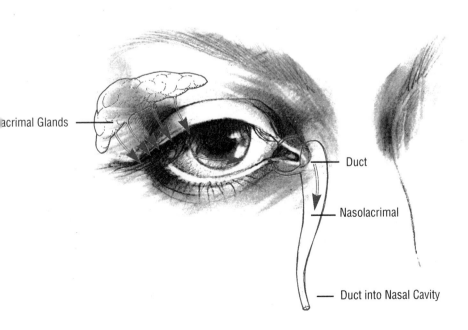

Lacrimal Glands

Duct

Nasolacrimal

Duct into Nasal Cavity

Figure 23.3 The lacrimal system. Fluid that lubricates the surface of the eye is produced by a system of structures surrounding the eye itself. Lacrimal fluid originates from the *lacrimal gland* above the eye, washes over the surface of the cornea, and pools in the corners of the conjunctiva. It then drains into the *lacrimal sac* and through the *inferior* and *nasolacrimal ducts* into the nasal cavity. During emotional stress or tension, stimulation of the lacrimal gland often produced excess lacrimal fluid, shed as tears during the act of crying.

eyelids is mainly protective. The *tear glands*—located in the outer upper eyelids—secrete the liquid that lubricates, cleans, and nourishes the eyes (Figure 23.3). The *eyelashes* act as a screen to filter particles and help keep the eye free of debris.

Each eyeball is suspended inside the *bony orbit*, a cone-shaped skeletal socket. This orbit is specifically designed to protect and shield the eye from a direct injury.

HOW WE SEE

As newborns, we can perceive light, shadow, and even shapes. But we have not yet acquired the ability to interpret or "read" the information that is supplied to our brains via the optic nerve. As we mature, our brains develop the ability to make sense out of the messages transmitted by our eyes, and we begin to understand the world around us.

First, there is light. Vision is the process by which light is perceived. We do not actually see objects, but see only the light that is reflected off objects. The less light, the less clearly we see a flower, a tree, a person. In total darkness, we see nothing at all.

Light enters the eye by passing through the cornea, the aqueous humor, and the pupil to be focused finally by the lens. It then travels through the vitreous humor and onto the retina. When the light strikes the retina, it stimulates chemical changes in the light-sensitive nerve endings, known as the photo receptors, or the *rods* and *cones*. The rods and cones interconnect and converge to form a network of about a million nerve fibers that make up the optic nerve.

It is the optic nerve that transmits visual data to the brain. Once the vision centers of the brain have interpreted the information, these centers relay signals to other parts of the brain. For example, you see that an object is moving toward you. Your eyes convey this information to your brain, which signals the motor cortex—the area of the brain that controls movement—to allow you to step quickly out of the way.

HOW TO PROTECT AND CARE FOR YOUR EYES

Too often, we take our eyes for granted. It is only when something happens to interfere with our clear vision of the world that we feel compelled to consult a physician. But everyone should have her eyes examined on a regular basis, whether there is a problem or not.

If you are under 40 and do not have any eye problems or relatives with eye diseases, have your eyes examined every two to three years. Between ages 40 and 60, have an eye exam every 2 years. After the age of 60, visit your eye specialist every year for signs of glaucoma or cataracts and other diseases that tend to show up with advancing age.

Besides regular eye examinations, you'll want to take various precautions to protect your eyes from infection and injury.

How to Avoid Accidental Injuries to Your Eyes

According to the National Society to Prevent Blindness, nearly 90 percent of all impact injuries to the eye could have been prevented by using proper eye protection. Many of these injuries occur during sports and recreational activities, particularly baseball, squash, tennis, and racquetball. If you are involved in any potentially hazardous sports, use the best possible eye protection. The material for the lenses should be polycarbonate plastic, and the frames should be made of a special safety material and designed specifically for the sport in question. You can obtain such glasses through opticians, eye specialists, and sporting goods stores.

Swimming, too, can lead to eye irritations and infections. For example, chlorine in pools can make your eyes feel uncomfortable. Infections can be contracted when swimming in freshwater. If you are a swimmer, use watertight swimming goggles. Prescription goggles are also available, and are a better alternative than using contact lenses when swimming. You can, of course, use an ordinary pair of watertight goggles over your contact lenses, if you prefer.

Some of the most common injuries to the eye occur in the home, while you are cleaning, gardening, cooking, or working in the yard. Grease can spatter, hazardous chemicals can splash or drift, wood chips can fly straight into your eyes. Household cleaning products, especially those that contain ammonia and chlorine, are particularly dangerous in this regard.

If a chemical has splashed into your eyes, rinse them with copious amounts of water and go to the nearest emergency room or see your ophthalmologist as soon as possible. Bring the bottle or write down the name of the chemical involved because, although acids and alkalis are initially treated similarly, injuries caused by these substances have a different prognosis. The damage caused by an acid occurs at the time it touches the eye, while an alkali continues to do harm long after it first makes contact with the eye, and the prognosis is much worse. To prevent potentially serious accidents, always use safety goggles when engaged in any activity that involves tools or dangerous chemicals.

The Sun and Your Eyes

Today, all of us know enough to stay out of the sun during peak hours and to use sunscreen when we do venture into the sun, whether in the backyard or on the beach. Such safety precautions are especially important when it comes to your eyes. You can sustain permanent eye damage from routinely staring at the sun on reflected water, such as when sailing or surfing.

High-quality sunglasses can prevent these problems. Make sure your sunglasses have ultraviolet protection and are dark enough to hide your eyes behind them. If you use a sunlamp or visit commercial tanning booths, always use special safety goggles. These artificial tanning devices are especially hazardous, because the ultraviolet light they emit is much more intense than natural sunlight. UV light has also been associated with the development of pterygium and cataracts. Wind and sun may also worsen cases of dry eyes.

FINDING THE CORRECT EYE SPECIALIST

For total eye care, seek out the advice of an *ophthalmologist.* An ophthalmologist is a medical doctor with at least four years of specialized training in the diagnosis and treatment of eye diseases and conditions. Ophthalmologists can prescribe corrective lenses, conduct eye examinations, treat diseases, and perform surgery on the eyes. Some ophthalmologists further specialize within the field of ophthalmology, becoming experts in problems of the retina or cornea or concentrating on children's eye problems or specific areas of surgery, such as surgery for cataracts.

Optometrists are not medical doctors, but are graduates of a school of optometry and earn a doctor of optometry (O.D.) degree. They are trained to test the eyes for nonmedical defects of vision and prescribe and dispense corrective lenses. Optometrists can also diagnose diseases of the eye, but an ophthalmologist will be able to evaluate more thoroughly ophthalmic signs of systemic disease.

An *optician* is a specialist who is trained to fill prescriptions for lenses, as written by ophthalmologists and optometrists. They grind and fit the lenses, but do not examine eyes. In some states, opticians are allowed to fit patients with contact lenses.

All of these professionals play an important role in the care of your eyes. If you do not have a regular ophthalmologist, ask your family doctor or primary physician for a recommendation. Or call a nearby teaching hospital and get several referrals. Most local libraries also have directories of medical specialists in your area. When you call an ophthalmologist to make an appointment, be sure to ask about fee schedules. Fees vary according to locality, but shop around if you think you have been quoted a fee that seems too high. Also, don't hesitate to get a second opinion, especially if surgery is a possibility. Make sure the specialist you consult for the second opinion has no personal or professional connection with the one who originally recommended surgery.

Cosmetics and Your Eyes

Our eyes are our most expressive feature, so it is only natural to want to emphasize them. There is no harm in using eye makeup, as long as you observe some commonsense rules about the use of eye cosmetics.

COPING WITH A BLACK EYE

A "black eye" is simply a bruise around the eye socket, which usually appears on the rim of the eye socket, below the eye. It may start out being bluish purple; it gradually fades in two weeks or so. Contrary to popular belief, a steak applied to the eye won't help the bruise to vanish any faster, although ice and cold compresses can help control the initial swelling.

If you sustain a hard blow to the eye, suffer more extensive cuts and lacerations around the eye, or notice changes in vision, pain on eye movement or double vision, see your ophthalmologist for a complete evaluation. Sometimes a black eye will indicate a more serious injury to the eye or even a skull fracture.

- *Never use anyone else's cosmetics.* The mascara may belong to your best friend, but don't use it. First, infections are transmitted in this way, and second, you may find that you are allergic to her particular brand of eye makeup.

- *Avoid using old eye cosmetics.* If you wear eye makeup regularly, you will probably use it up before it can cause problems. But if you wear eye makeup only for holidays and special occasions, you should be aware that old eye makeup can become contaminated. So throw it away to avoid any chance of infection.

- *Try to test new cosmetics before using them.* If you tend to have allergic reactions to cosmetics, look for products that are advertised as being hypoallergenic. Although none of these products can claim to be 100 percent free of allergy-causing substances, you may be able to avoid the particular ingredients that bother you. Purchase only a small amount or, if possible, get a free sample and try it. If you do experience an allergic reaction, discontinue using the product immediately.

- *Apply eye makeup carefully and properly.* When applying mascara or eyeliner, always keep the cosmetics out of the eye itself. You can do this by applying mascara only on the outer two-thirds of the lashes; do not start at the roots of the lashes. Similarly, never apply eyeliner—whether liquid or pencil—to the inner eyelid margins: use it only above the eyelashes of the upper lid and below the eyelashes of the lower lid. Take care not to apply eye makeup hastily, or you may run the risk of accidentally poking yourself in the eye, causing an infection or even damage to the cornea. If you use contact lenses, insert them before applying cosmetics and remove them before you remove the makeup. Contact lens wearers should also avoid using frosted eyeshadow. The iridescent particles can flake, get in the eyes, and attach themselves to the contact lens, causing enough friction to scratch the cornea. To remove eye makeup, you may use ordinary soap and water or one of the commercial products specially formulated for this purpose.

- *Other cosmetic hazards.* Try to avoid getting shampoos and other products for the hair into the eyes. Be especially careful to shield your eyes when using hair spray.

Lighting and Your Eyes

One of the myths of eye care is that improper lighting—the glare of an overhead light or the absence of adequate light—will damage your vision. Not so. Reading or doing close work in poor light cannot harm your eyes, although you may suffer discomfort and eyestrain from doing so.

IF YOUR EYES ARE RED

Exhaustion, lack of sleep, and the use of alcohol can all contribute to making your eyes red. If the redness is only occasional and clears up quickly, there is nothing to worry about. However, persistent redness, especially if accompanied by irritation or pain in the eye, may indicate problems that need immediate medical intervention.

For these reasons, it is not recommended that you use over-the-counter eyedrops to clear up redness in the eye. The drops may mask a condition that could develop into a serious problem later. For example, you might use the drops, not realizing that the redness is the result of a corneal ulcer. Ulcers need immediate medical attention to avoid permanent damage to your vision, or even loss of the eye. Similarly, the use of topical eye anesthetics is never recommended, because they affect healing and mask the symptoms of serious eye problems.

For comfort, position a light source behind you when you are reading. The light should be directed onto the page, and it should be reasonably bright, not glaring. If you are reading at a desk, use a shielded light that is positioned in front of you. The shield keeps the light on the page without allowing it to shine in your eyes.

When watching television, do not totally darken the entire room. Always keep the room softly illuminated, to avoid the eyestrain resulting from too great a contrast between the television screen and the surrounding area.

COMMON PROBLEMS OF THE EYE

The most common eye disorders involve refractive errors, such as nearsightedness, or myopia. Other types of vision impairment usually come with aging and include glaucoma and cataracts. Inflammation or infection of the eye or the surrounding tissues, trauma to the eye, and problems resulting from a systemic disease such as diabetes are other common eye disorders.

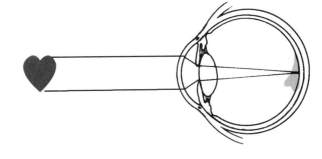

Refractive Errors

When light strikes the eye, it is refracted, or bent, by the cornea and lens so that the rays converge and are in focus when they reach the retina. The retina in turn sends a message of the visual image to the brain. Unfortunately, for a large number of people, the visual image may be blurred or unfocused, conditions called nearsightedness and farsightedess (Figure 23.4).

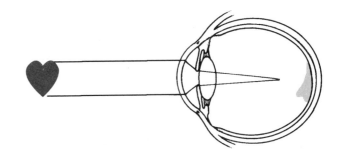

Nearsightedness

Also known as myopia, nearsightedness affects about 20 percent of the population and tends to run in families. It often first appears in early childhood, progresses through the late teens, then stabilizes through the 20s and 30s. After the age of 40, however, the effects of aging may cause the condition to worsen.

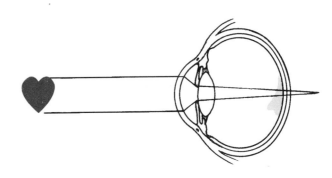

Symptoms
If you are nearsighted, objects in the distance appear blurry and indistinct. A severely nearsighted individual will clearly see only objects that are a few inches from her eyes.

Cause
Nearsightedness occurs because the eyes are too long in shape from front to back. This malformation

Figure 23.4 Near- and farsightedness. In a person with perfect vision, light is focused exactly on the retina (*top*). Nearsightedness, or *myopia*, occurs when the shape of the eye is elongated from front to back, causing light to focus on a point in front of the retina (*middle*). Objects that are far away appear blurry and indistinct. In farsightedness, or *hyperopia*, the eye is shortened from front to back, and light is focused on a point behind the retina (*bottom*). This causes near objects to be out of focus.

causes the light rays that are refracted by the cornea and lens to become focused before they get to the retina. From that point, they start to diverge and go out of focus.

Diagnosis

Your ophthalmologist or optometrist will conduct a complete eye exam to establish the degree of your nearsightedness (see "Diagnostic Eye Tests and Procedures").

Treatment

Nearsightedness can be alleviated by the use of corrective lenses, either eyeglasses or contact lenses. Another possible although more radical approach is a radial keratotomy, a new microsurgical technique that can correct myopia. You and your doctor should thoroughly and carefully discuss the procedure and its benefits and side effects before such surgery is undertaken. Be sure to get a second opinion as well.

Radial keratotomy

Radial keratotomy was devised in 1974 by a Soviet eye surgeon and later introduced to the United States. It involves making a series of delicate incisions partway through the outer sections of the cornea, the clear tissue that covers the external part of the eye. After the incisions heal, the cornea should be flatter than before, allowing the focal point of the light rays to fall on the retina. The operation is not without its risks, however, including infection, perforation of the cornea, and the undercorrection or overcorrection of the myopia. Myopic people may decide to wait a few years until the U.S. Food and Drug Administration has approved a computer-laser surgical intervention that promises greater accuracy with fewer side effects.

Radial keratotomy can be done in a doctor's office under local anesthesia. The operation takes about a half-hour. The procedure costs about $3,000 and is not covered by most private insurance carriers or by Medicare.

Farsightedness

Farsightedness, also known as hyperopia, occurs when the eyeball is too short from the front to the back, making the angle between the iris and the surface of the cornea too narrow. The rays of light are focused behind the retina instead of on it, so that objects at close range appear blurry. Hyperopia is generally congenital.

Symptoms

Farsighted people have difficulty focusing on objects that are close to them. They may experience symptoms of eyestrain, including headaches and aching eyes, after reading or doing close work.

Cause

In addition to a hereditary shape of the eyeball, farsightedness may also be caused by the inability of the lens to focus. As we age, our lenses lose their elasticity, which leads to presbyopia.

Diagnosis

Your ophthalmologist or optometrist will conduct a complete eye examination to determine the extent of your hyperopia (see "Diagnostic Eye Tests and Procedures").

Treatment

Farsightedness can be corrected by the use of eyeglasses or contact lenses made specifically to accomodate the problem.

Astigmatism

A highly common disorder, astigmatism is a refractive abnormality caused by the uneven curvature of the cornea. Frequently, it is an additional complication to hyperopia or myopia.

Symptoms

With astigmatism, your visual field may be blurred. Mild astigmatism causes little distortion, but you may suffer from headaches or eye fatigue when focusing at short distances.

Cause

Astigmatism occurs when different areas of the cornea need different optical corrections. Astigmatism may be congenital or may be developed due to trauma, scarring, or surgery.

Diagnosis

Your ophthalmologist or optometrist will conduct a complete eye examination to determine the extent of your astigmatism (see "Diagnostic Eye Tests and Procedures").

Treatment

Astigmatism can be corrected by the use of eyeglasses or contact lenses.

Presbyopia

Presbyopia, or "old sight," is not really a refractive error. It results from the hardening, or loss of elasticity, of the crystalline lens of the eye. Presbyopia is part of the natural process of aging, and it happens to everyone to some degree.

Symptoms

Increasing difficulty in focusing on objects at close range and eyestrain are among the telltale signs of the aging eye. You may notice the first signs of presbyopia when you can no longer read the small print of newspapers or find it difficult to thread a needle or read directions on a jar or package. If you are already farsighted, you may notice the changes earlier; if you are nearsighted, you may find that your eyes are increasingly tired after reading.

Cause

Presbyopia is the loss of our ability to bend the lens so it can focus on near or far objects. The result is that after the age of 40 it becomes increasingly more difficult to see nearby objects clearly and to read small print.

Diagnosis

Your ophthalmologist will conduct a complete eye examination to determine the extent of your presbyopia (see "Diagnostic Eye Tests and Procedures").

Treatment

Presbyopia is corrected with reading glasses. If you already wear glasses to correct nearsightedness or farsightedness, you may need to get bifocals or use two separate pairs of glasses—one for distance and one for close reading or viewing. Because presbyopia progresses gradually, you may need several changes in prescriptions as your ability to focus lessens. By the time you are 65, you will have lost most of your ability to accommodate, and your presbyopia will have stabilized.

Problems of the Aging Eye

Older adults suffer from the onset of presbyopia, a hardening of the lens that makes it difficult to focus on nearby objects (see previous discussion). But there are other more serious visual disorders that can occur in the later years, including ptosis (drooping eyelid), glaucoma, cataracts, macular degeneration, retinal detachment, optic neuritis, and retinitis pigmentosa (Figure 23.5).

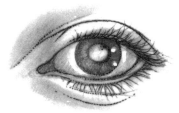

Cataract

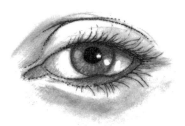

Stye

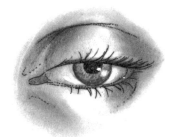

Ptosis

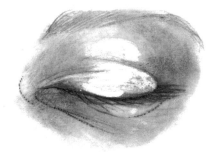

Orbital Cellulitis

Figure 23.5 Diseases affecting the appearance of the eye. From the outside, a cataract (*top*) appears as a cloudy area over the pupil. A sty (*second from top*) is an infection of the eyelid resulting in a painful reddish bump on the inside of the eye. Ptosis (*second from bottom*), or drooping eyelid, is a common effect of aging and is caused by a loss of elasticity in the muscles of the eyelid. Orbital cellulitis (*bottom*) is an infection of the eye socket; in its more severe forms, it can cause the eye lids to swell shut.

Drooping Eyelid

The abnormal drooping of the eyelid in either one or both eyes is called ptosis. Ptosis is a common effect of aging.

Symptoms

There are no significant problems with ptosis, unless the drooping eyelid interferes with vision because it blocks the pupil.

Causes

As you age, the muscles that support the eye gradually lose their tone, which causes mild ptosis. Eye surgery can also cause the condition, as can diabetes, stroke, and a brain tumor. Sometimes ptosis is an inherited condition.

Diagnosis

If you suddenly notice that one or both of your eyes are drooping, see your ophthalmologist. A complete medical may be required to rule out other causes, such as stroke, tumor, diabetes, or myasthenia gravis (a serious disease).

Treatment

A gradual drooping of the eyelids is a normal part of aging, and usually isn't serious enough to warrant correction. However, if you think the condition is unsightly or if your vision has been affected, cosmetic surgery (blepharoplasty) is available to tighten up the muscles that control the lid position.

Blepharoplasty

Blepharoplasty is a surgical procedure that removes the excess skin and fat from the upper and lower eyelids and corrects drooping eyelids. Although blepharoplasty has fewer complications than other forms of cosmetic surgery, there is always a risk of infection. In some instances, there may be overcorrection, resulting in ectropion (a turning out of the eyelid) or lagophthalmia (incomplete eyelid closure, which may lead to dry eyes and infection). For these reasons, it is essential that you choose a surgeon with extensive experience in this type of surgery. (See Chapter 36 for further information on cosmetic eye surgery.)

Glaucoma

Glaucoma is a group of diseases characterized by increased intraocular pressure in the eye (Figure 23.6). This pressure can lead to damage to the nerve of the eye and a corresponding decrease in vision. In the

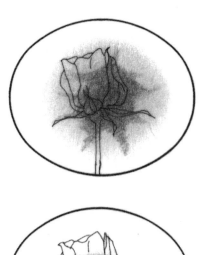
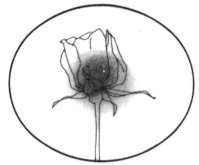
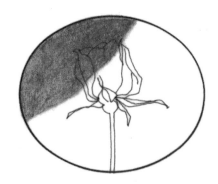
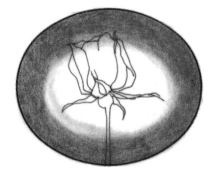

Figure 23.6 Effects of eye diseases on vision. Some eye disorders cause abnormalities in the field of vision. A cataract (*top*) causes opacity or clouding of the lens. Macular degeneration (*second from top*) affects the central field of vision and usually occurs in both eyes. A detached retina (*second from bottom*) may be marked by a shadow over a portion of the field of vision and also often causes flashing lights, floaters, and blurriness. Open-angle glaucoma (*bottom*) in its earlier stages causes a loss of peripheral vision.

ALL ABOUT EYEGLASSES

Spectacles were probably first made in Venice, the medieval center of the glass industry. As with many inventions of the day, they were first viewed with suspicion. However, as their usefulness became more apparent, the new lenses were rapidly adopted by the learned and the wealthy. Today, we all have access to standardized, machine-ground lenses that correct common visual impairments.

Eyeglasses are specially ground lenses that are tailored to the needs of the individual eye. These lenses are necessary to compensate for the defect in the eye and to deliver a focused image to the retina.

Most glasses use a single-vision lens, which means there is only one set of optical corrections in the lens. Bifocals, on the other hand, contain two sets of optical corrections—a prescription for reading (the bottom part of the lens) and one for distance (the top part). Bifocals with no obvious demarcation in the two lenses are available. Some people may prefer trifocals, which carry prescriptive lenses for near, middle, and far distances, although many people have difficulty adjusting to them. For those who need help only for reading, half-glasses may suffice.

Frames

When shopping around for new glasses, you should be aware of the shape of your face. Is it oval, round, heart-shaped, rectangular, or square? To find out, pull your hair away from your face, look in the mirror, and outline your face with a washable crayon or lipstick right on the mirror. Try to select a frame that is a different shape from your face, for example, a rectangular or squared-off frame will look better on a round face, whereas rounder frames may suit a square or rectangularly shaped face. You're lucky if your face is oval shaped, because most frames will look good on you. If you have a heart-shaped face, don't buy aviator glasses or very large frames; they will look overwhelming. You may also want to avoid large frames if your prescription is strong enough to distort the appearance of your eyes. Image distortion is also more of a problem with strong eyeglass prescriptions; smaller frames are recommended when the objects seen through the periphery of the lenses are distorted.

When choosing a frame color, look for less emphasis rather than more. Dark-haired people usually look better in darker frames, while lighter-haired individuals should stick to lighter-colored frames.

Types of lenses

Eyeglass lenses come in plastic and glass; each has advantages and disadvantages. Plastic lenses are lighter, more comfortable, and more protective than glass. They can also be tinted different colors. The main disadvantage of plastic is that it scratches easily.

Glass lenses are fairly resistant to scratching. Glass also comes in photochromatic lenses, which automatically darken and become clear in response to light. For example, when you go outside into bright sunlight, the lenses become dark. The chief problems with glass lenses is that they are heavier than plastic and are liable to break and splinter when broken. Often your choice of lens material depends on your lifestyle. Discuss your needs with your ophthalmologist, optometrist, or optician before choosing one or the other.

Sunglasses

Well-made, reliable sunglasses are a must for outdoor activities and for hours spent in the sun. It's especially important to protect your vision against sun damage by using sunglasses with ultraviolet (uv) protection. Be careful, though—buying sunglasses off the rack does not necessarily guarantee that they are coated for uv rays. Your best bet is to buy from a reliable ophthalmologist, optometrist, or optician. If you would rather not spend the money for prescription sunglasses, consider tinted clip-ons. These devices are readily available in drugstores and variety shops at reasonable prices and will protect you against the sun's glare while allowing you the benefit of your own prescription glasses.

Eyewear care

Prescription glasses are a sizable investment and deserve regular care and maintenance. Keep them clean using a soft cloth or special lens-cleaning papers available in drugstores and optical shops. Always keep your glasses protected in a case, especially if you carry them in a purse or pocket. See an ophthalmologist, optometrist, or optician if you notice that your glasses keep slipping or the frame seems loose or wobbly. Most professionals will adjust the fit of your glasses for free or at a nominal cost. If you travel extensively, it's a good idea to carry a prescription for your glasses in case you lose or damage them.

ALL ABOUT CONTACT LENSES

More than 25 million Americans now wear contact lenses, those little curved plastic discs that fit over the cornea and provide correction for such refraction errors as nearsightedness, farsightedness, and astigmatism. Contact lenses have some distinct advantages over regular eyewear—they provide a fuller, more unobstructed view and are convenient to use. Most important to many users though, is that they don't have to wear glasses. But there is much confusion about which type of lens is best to use, and there are lingering concerns about their safety.

The first step in buying contact lenses is the initial consultation with a trained, skilled professional. Contact lenses should be prescribed by an ophthalmologist or an optometrist who specializes in this kind of work. You should receive a thorough eye examination before being fitted for the lenses and have regular checkups afterward. It may take some time to feel comfortable wearing contacts; however, if you experience any pain or persistent discomfort, call the specialist who initially fitted you.

Types of contact lenses

There are two basic types of contact lenses: hard and soft. Hard lenses were the first contact lenses to be introduced. They are sturdy, last a long time, are easy to care for, and usually provide excellent visual correction. They may correct astigmatism better than soft lenses and may be the only type of contact lens that improves vision for patients with irregular astigmatism. They are also the least expensive type of contact lenses. But hard lenses require a longer period of adjustment than soft contacts and can be uncomfortable if a foreign body lodges under the lens.

Soft contact lenses were introduced about 20 years ago. They are usually much more comfortable to wear initially than the hard lenses but require far more cleaning and maintenance and are more costly. They also are not as sturdy as hard lenses and wear out more rapidly. Soft lenses may become uncomfortably dry in hot, windy weather conditions or while using a hair dryer.

Soft lenses are available as both daily- and extended-wear lenses. Extended-wear lenses can be kept in the eye a longer time, because they contain enough water in them to allow oxygen to pass into the cornea, even when you are sleeping. They provide good sight at all times, require less frequent handling, and are beneficial to people who are "on call" at all

hours. However, there is a distinctly greater risk of eye infection when using them, they require more monitoring by a doctor, they are more fragile, and they cost more than other types of lenses. The latest thing in contact lenses are the disposables, or frequent-replacement contact lenses, which are similar to the extended-wear type but are discarded after being worn for about 2 weeks. As for any type of contact lenses, follow your doctor's instructions on the proper handling of this product.

A more recent development is gas-permeable hard lenses. This type of contact lens contains openings to allow oxygen and carbon dioxide to reach the cornea. As a result, these lenses are more comfortable than the original hard lenses, but they are also more expensive. Gas-permeable lenses are easier to clean than soft lenses and tend to last longer. Most people who wear hard lenses wear the gas-permeable type.

Which type of contact lens is best for you? That depends on your particular optical problem, the condition of your eyes (for example, other diseases), your needs and lifestyle, your personality, and your pocketbook. Your doctor will recommend the best lens to fit your needs.

Maintenance and use

It is absolutely essential to follow carefully the doctor's instructions on the hygenic insertion and removal of contact lenses. It is also important to adhere to all directions concerning their proper cleaning and storage. If you do not, you run the risk of infection and possible permanent damage to your eyes. *Always* wash your hands before inserting and removing your lenses.

Clean hard lenses with a commercial cleaning solution, then place the lenses into a storage solution that will kill bacteria and keep the lenses moist. *Never* use saliva to moisten or clean the lenses. Soft lenses require more attention. Clean them each day with a disinfecting solution; a weekly soaking in an enzyme cleaner is also beneficial. Extended-wear lenses should be cleaned and sterilized periodically. Eyes sometimes become dry during sleep, so you may be advised to use lubricating drops at night and in the morning. Always follow your doctor's and the manufacturer's recommendations for the use of each type of contact lens solution.

Here are some other helpful suggestions about using and caring for your contact lenses.

ALL ABOUT CONTACT LENSES (Continued)

- If your eyes are red and irritated, remove your contacts immediately and wear your glasses instead. If the discomfort persists or if you have pain, discharge, or loss of vision, see your eye care specialist.

- Don't rub your eyes while wearing contact lenses, and try to avoid smoky rooms and dusty and windy environments.

- Do not wear the lenses while swimming unless you also wear watertight goggles.

- Do not switch solutions without your doctor's approval. Not all solutions are compatible with all contact lens materials.

- Always keep a backup pair of glasses around, in case you lose a contact or cannot wear your lenses for some reason.

- Be alert to any problems that may develop from wearing contact lenses, especially pain,

blurry vision, tearing, redness, and sensitivity to light. See your eye care specialist if you experience these symptoms.

Using eye makeup

You can use eye cosmetics when using contact lenses as long as you follow some simple rules. First, always put the lenses on before applying makeup and remove them before removing the makeup. Check to make sure there is no makeup on your fingers when you are handling the contacts, and use a clear soap to wash your hands before inserting or removing the contacts. Use water-soluble cosmetic products. Be extremely careful when applying mascara to the lashes—particles of the material may drop into the eye, causing irritation and contamination of the lens. Do not use aerosol sprays when you are wearing contact lenses. Be careful when you use nail polish and nail polish removers—they can give off fumes that are damaging to contact lenses.

United States, glaucoma is a leading cause of blindness, but the disease is preventable and treatable—if caught in time. Unfortunately, in its most common form, glaucoma has no symptoms until extensive damage has already occurred. For this reason, everyone over the age of 40 should have their eye pressure checked on a regular basis.

Glaucoma can be inherited; about 20 percent of people with glaucoma have close relatives with the disease. There are other risk factors: If you have diabetes, you are three times as likely to get glaucoma, and African-Americans have a significantly higher chance of developing glaucoma than people of other races. A form of secondary glaucoma can also occur after any trauma to the eye, including cataracts, retinal detachment, ocular surgery, inflammation, and injuries to the eye.

Open Angle Glaucoma

The most common form of glaucoma is open angle glaucoma, sometimes called simple or chronic glaucoma. This type of glaucoma affects more than 90 percent of all glaucoma sufferers.

Symptoms

Open angle glaucoma is painless and insidious in onset. You gradually lose your peripheral vision, but your central vision is unaffected until the disease is far advanced. Usually, the initial clue to a physician is increased pressure in the eye. (Examination of the optic nerve may indicate glaucomatous damage even in the presence of normal eye pressure.)

Cause

Glaucoma occurs when the aqueous humor is blocked from draining normally and pressure builds up within the eye. When this happens, it affects the optic nerve, destroying fibers that cannot be regenerated or replaced.

Diagnosis

If you have a family history of glaucoma, see an eye specialist for regular examinations. Anyone over the age of 40 should also have routine eye checkups. The ophthamologist (or, in some cases, optometrist) will conduct several tests to detect any abnormalities in the eye, including determining if an increase in intraocular pressure has occurred and checking the status of the optic nerve and visual fields, if necessary (see "Diagnostic Eye Tests and Procedures").

Treatment

If your eye specialist has found that you have only slightly increased intraocular pressure, he or she may choose to wait and carefully monitor your progress over the next year or so. Some ophthalmologists prefer to begin treatment when the first signs of definite damage appear, but others prefer to avoid any damage by beginning treatment soon after diagnosis, if they believe the condition warrants it.

The principal treatment is the use of eyedrops. These eyedrops—in differing strengths depending on the progression of the glaucoma—must be taken for the rest of your life. If the eyedrops do not stabilize the glaucoma, oral medication may be recommended or added to the drops. Finally, surgery is available in more advanced cases that do not respond to the medications.

Narrow Angle Glaucoma

Also known as acute glaucoma, narrow angle glaucoma is far less common than the chronic or open angle type. The onset of acute glaucoma can be sudden and painful, and its occurrence is clearly a medical emergency.

Symptoms

The eye suddenly becomes red and cloudy, with the vision obscured. Halos appear around lights and sometimes the cornea becomes rock-hard and painful. Nausea and vomiting may develop.

Cause

The pressure in the eye increases suddenly because the passage of the aqueous humor is blocked. This can occur when the anterior chamber is very narrow.

Diagnosis

Loss of vision and sudden onset of pain in the eye, with possible vomiting, signal a serious eye condition. See your doctor immediately or go to a hospital emergency room as soon as possible.

Treatment

Acute glaucoma is usually treated with immediate surgery. The procedure, known as an iridectomy, creates a small opening in the eye. An iridectomy can be done in the doctor's office under a local anesthetic using a laser or it may be done surgically in an operating room.

Cataracts

Cataracts are a major source of blindness throughout the world. But fortunately, most cataracts can be easily and successfully treated.

A cataract is any opacity or clouding of the lens of the eye that prevents the formation of a clear image and causes a decrease in vision. Normally, the human lens converges the light rays that come through the eye. An opacity of the lens will scatter or block these rays. If the opacity or clouding is small and at the lens periphery, there will be little or no interference with vision. If the cloudiness is larger and denser, vision will be noticeably blurry. Cataracts are a common disease of aging. As the lens becomes less and less resilient, it loses its transparency and clarity.

Symptoms

People with cataracts develop blurry vision and have difficulty seeing at night or in a very bright light. They also may experience halos around lights, which is caused by the changes taking place in the lens. Another symptom, often referred to as "second sight," involves the growth of a cataract in the center of the lens, which temporarily serves to increase the focusing power of the lens. Over time, however, this renewed ability to focus tends to lessen. You may not be aware that you have cataracts until your physician tells you; you will know only that you are not seeing as clearly as you used to. Symptoms usually develop gradually, with a painless progressive decrease in vision.

Causes

Most cataracts occur with age. In fact, everyone over 60 probably has some degree of cataract formation. Recent research indicates that exposure to ultraviolet light—usually sunlight—can play a part in the development of cataracts. Other lifestyle habits have also been implicated in cataract formation, including smoking and exposure to radiation. Obviously, wearing sunglasses with protection against UV rays is warranted, as is eating a nutritious diet (including vitamin A), limiting your exposure to infrared light and other sources of radiation, and not smoking. The so-called senile cataracts of the later years are probably caused by a combination of the aging process and an individual's lifelong habits and environment.

There are other causes of cataracts besides aging,

although they tend to be rare. A congenital cataract, one which is present at birth, is the result of some event during fetal development. If a pregnant woman contracts a rubella infection (German measles), her fetus may develop congenital cataracts. Secondary cataracts can occur after an injury to the eye or as the result of an intraocular infection in the anterior chamber or in the vitreous fluid of the eye. Chronic use of medications can also cause cataracts, specifically those of the corticosteroid group of drugs used to treat chronic illnesses like rheumatoid arthritis and lupus. Because women have a higher incidence of autoimmune diseases than men, they use more oral steroids to control their symptoms and thus also have a higher incidence of steroid-induced cataracts. Hyperparathyroidism can also cause cataracts.

Diagnosis

Your doctor will conduct a complete eye examination, including a slit-lamp evaluation and an ultrasound test if needed (see "Diagnostic Eye Tests and Procedures"). A slit-lamp exam enables the physician to see the condition of the lens. If it appears opaque or clouded, another test, ultrasound, can be done to make sure the back of the eye appears normal.

Treatment

Once vision is impaired by the cataract, surgical removal is the most effective treatment (see "Cataract Surgery" below). However, until loss of vision is severe enough to disrupt daily activities, other less radical treatment may suffice, such as a change in eyeglass prescription or in some cases the use of medicated eye drops to widen the pupil. The drops allow more light to enter the lens, and mitigate the glare of bright lights on the clouded lens.

Cataract surgery

Cataract surgery is generally recommended when an individual cannot perform daily activities because of deteriorating vision. The operation doesn't depend on a specific level of vision or on the "ripeness" of the cataract, but on individual needs and circumstances. More than 1 million cataract operations are performed every year in the United States, making it the most frequent surgery performed on people over 65 years of age. The procedure is generally quite safe, nearly painless, and very successful—about 95 percent of individuals who undergo cataract surgery experience a marked improvement in their vision.

A small incision is made at the outer edge of the cornea and the lens is removed. At the same time, an artificial, plastic lens, called an intraocular lens, is implanted in the eye. The intraocular lens helps provide vision after the surgery. Once the lens is implanted, the incision is sutured closed. (Some newer techniques use no sutures at all.) The surgeon uses medications to keep the pupil dilated, to prevent infection, and to reduce inflammation.

Cataract surgery generally is performed under local anesthesia in a hospital setting on an outpatient basis. The operation takes about 1 hour. If you are particularly nervous or apprehensive about the procedure, you may require general anesthesia.

There are alternatives to lens implantation, namely special eyeglasses and contact lenses. These devices have significant drawbacks, however. The glasses do not fully correct your vision and can cause distortion. Your vision remains very poor without the glasses, which are not particularly attractive. The contact lenses may work well, but they require frequent handling for insertion and removal and have a greater risk of infection and other complications. Both of these options are considered when surgery cannot be performed because of a complication or another eye condition. Intraocular lenses offer the best correction for vision at this time.

Macular Degeneration

Macular degeneration is a common cause of visual loss in people over 60; it is usually bilateral, but asymmetric. The macula is the area of the retina that is used for direct, central vision, which is the area of visual loss. Damage to this area won't make you totally blind, since you will still be able to use your peripheral vision to function.

Symptoms

Macular degeneration first shows up as difficulty in reading small print and seeing distant objects. Objects tend to be distorted.

Cause

The macula gets its nutrition from blood vessels in the choroid. Any condition that restricts blood flow, therefore, will damage the macula. This condition—called the "dry form"—often occurs because of aging and associated arteriosclerosis. In another form of macular degeneration—called the "wet form"—abnormal blood vessels grow under the retina, causing retinal bleeding and a gradual loss of vision.

Diagnosis

Ophthalmologists test for macular degeneration by examining the retina with an ophthalmascope and with a fundus contact lens. If changes are noted, a fluorscein test is done to reveal the blood vessel pattern in the eye so any abnormalities may be detected.

Treatment

There is no effective treatment for the dry form of macular degeneration. In the wet type, laser therapy is used to coagulate the abnormal blood vessels and prevent further bleeding. However, new blood vessels often grow after the surgery. Regular eye examinations aid in early detection of macular changes so that treatment may be instituted soon enough to prevent significant damage.

Disorders of the Retina and Optic Nerve

Retinal Detachment

Retinal detachment is a serious medical emergency (Figure 23.7). It occurs when the retina—the thin, transparent membrane in the back portion of the eye—peels away from the wall of the eye. The retina detaches when a hole or tear in it allows fluid to collect between the retina and the layer of wall behind it. Retinal detachments are more common in men than women.

Symptoms

If a retinal detachment occurs, you experience a sensation of flashing lights, many floaters, and blurry vision. You also may notice the appearance of a shadow over a portion of your field of vision. If you ever suffer from these symptoms, see your ophthalmologist immediately or go to the nearest hospital emergency room. There is no pain associated with detached retina, as the retina does not contain pain receptors.

Causes

Most cases of retinal detachment are caused by trauma to the eye due to accidents. People who are nearsighted (myopic) are more at risk than those with normal vision or other refractive errors, probably because their retinas are more tautly stretched. Diabetics with retinal disease may also develop detachments. Recent cataract surgery is another risk factor.

Diagnosis

Your eye care specialist will use eyedrops to dilate your eyes. This allows the doctor to make a complete evaluation of your retina, using an indirect ophthalmoscope.

Treatment

Once the retina is detached, you will need prompt surgery to repair the damage. If the tear is small and the detachment minimal (which sometimes occurs when

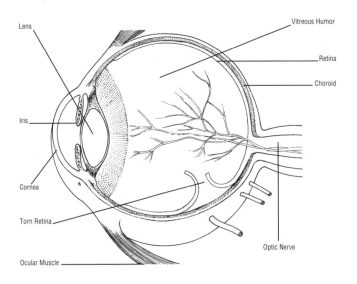

Figure 23.7 Retinal detachment. A torn or detached retina results from the collection of fluid between the retina and the layer of tissue behind it (the choroid). This fluid buildup results from a hole or tear in the retina, most often from an injury. A detached retina is painless but causes visual disturbances such as sparks of light, floaters, and blurry vision. Any of these symptoms requires prompt medical attention.

the condition is detected early), a laser is applied around the hole in the retina and forms a scar. The scar prevents the retina from continuing to detach or separate. If the detachment or tear is too large, laser surgery is not an option. In that case, conventional surgery is needed to repair the retina. A local or general anesthesia is used, depending on the extent of the detachment and the surgery needed. The most common type of operation uses a technique called scleral buckling, in which the wall (sclera) of the eye is indented (buckled) over the defect. In some complicated cases, there may be an injection of special gases into the eye to keep the retina attached while it heals. Depending upon the location of the tear or the detached area, the patient may be instructed to lie face down continuously for several weeks, so that the gas floats upward and keeps the retina in place. In most cases, however, patients can leave the hospital a few days after the procedure, although they must avoid strenuous activities for 3 or 4 weeks.

Retinal Vessel Occlusion

The cells of the retina are nourished by tiny blood vessels. Occasionally these vessels become blocked by a blood clot or fatty deposits. When this occurs, the retina stops functioning, causing blindness in part or all of one eye. The blocking of a retinal artery is a medical emergency, because without a blood supply, the cells of the retina die. The blocking of a retinal vein is less immediately serious, but there is a danger that the blocked vein may rupture, spilling its contents into the vitreous humor and causing a clouding or loss of vision.

Symptoms

If you experience a retinal occlusion, your vision will suddenly become clouded or blurred in a portion of the visual field of one eye. You may also lose your vision entirely in that eye.

Causes

Retinal vessel occlusion occurs most often in the elderly, who are more likely to suffer vascular complications from chronic diseases such as diabetes and hypertension.

Diagnosis

If you notice a sudden blurring of your vision, see your ophthalmologist immediately. Your doctor will give you a complete eye examination to determine the source of the problem and the appropriate mode of action. You may also have to undergo a complete medical exam to identify any systemic problems that may be causing the problem.

Treatment

An occlusion of the retinal arteries needs to be attended to within 1 to 2 hours after its occurrence so that blood flow can be restored. After that amount of time, the cells of the retina may be irreparably damaged, and no other treatment is possible to restore vision.

Retinitis Pigmentosa

A disorder of the photoreceptors of the eye, retinitis pigmentosa is an inherited condition. This rare disorder involves the gradual degeneration of the retinas in both eyes, beginning with defective night vision. In many cases, the disease will eventually lead to legal blindness.

Symptoms

Difficulty seeing at night and loss of peripheral vision over a period of several months are the most typical symptoms of retinitis pigmentosa. As the disease progresses, peripheral vision may be lost as well, leading to tunnel vision.

Causes

Most cases of this condition are inherited. There are several genetic types of retinitis pigmentosa, including X-linked, autosomal dominant, and autosomal recessive. Each affects the individual differently. Others have no known cause.

Diagnosis

Some cases of retinitis pigmentosa show up early in childhood, usually starting with a loss of night vision. If this disorder runs in your family, have your child tested regularly by an ophthalmologist. The doctor will perform a complete eye examination, using an electroretinogram (ERG), which records the actions of the retina in response to light stimuli.

Treatment

At present, there is no effective treatment for this disease. Newly developed glasses are available, however, that widen the field of vision and allow retinitis pigmentosa sufferers to function on a daily basis. Physicians also recommend the use of sunglasses to prevent further deterioration of the retina.

Optic Neuritis

Optic neuritis occurs when the optic nerve—the nerve in the eye that carries visual impulses to the brain—becomes inflamed. The vessels that provide blood and oxygen to the eye may also be affected.

Symptoms

The most common symptoms of optic neuritis are an acute loss of vision in one eye and/or pain on movement of the eye.

Causes

There are many different causes of optic neuritis. Some cases are caused by a virus; other cases may be the result of a chronic disease such as multiple sclerosis. Many cases occur in elderly people who are suffering from a condition known as temporal or cranial arteritis. Arteritis occurs when an artery in the head, often near the temple, becomes inflamed and blocks the blood flow to the eyes. High blood pressure, high cholesterol levels, and diabetes are often contributing factors to arteritis.

Diagnosis

Your physician will conduct a series of tests to determine the source and extent of the problem. Optic neuritis is often associated with multiple sclerosis, so your doctor may recommend a complete medical exam as well. Older people, especially those over 60, should be tested for temporal arteritis.

Treatment

If the optic neuritis results from temporal arteritis, your doctor may prescribe corticosteroid medications to prevent involvement of the other eye. If the condition is not caused by arteritis, there is no known treatment. Sometimes the condition clears up on its own, and vision is restored. If the source of the problem is multiple sclerosis, the inflammation may recur, causing further damage to the eye.

Disorders of the Cornea

The cornea, the curved, transparent cover of the front of the eyeball, is subject to injuries from a number of causes. These injuries can range from less serious conditions such as an inflammation or small abrasion to more critical conditions such as an ulcer or infection.

Keratitis

Keratitis is an inflammation of the cornea. This condition is fairly common among people who use contact lenses and who suffer from chronic dry eyes.

Symptoms

The signs of keratitis are decrease in the field of vision, sensitivity to light (called photophobia), a general discomfort in the eye, and the sensation of a foreign body in the eye.

Causes

Keratitis can be the product of dry eyes, infection, an injury to the eye, a nutritional deficiency, or an exposure to toxic materials.

Diagnosis

Your ophthalmologist will conduct a series of examinations to determine the source and cause of the condition.

Treatment

Depending on the cause of the inflammation, there are several treatments available for keratitis. These include antibiotic eyedrops, antiviral medications to control (but not cure) the problem, and various lubricants to soothe the discomfort.

Corneal Abrasions

A corneal abrasion is usually a scraping of the cornea by a foreign object. You'll feel that "something" is under your upper eyelid, but you can't see it or remove it by blinking or flushing it out. Do not try to flush out the foreign body unless you use a sterile solution.

Symptoms

If you suffer a corneal abrasion, you'll experience some pain, tearing or watering of the eye, and a sensitivity to light. Any motion of the eyeball or blinking may increase the discomfort as the upper eyelid passes over the damaged area of the cornea.

Causes

Foreign bodies—a grain of sand, a particle of wind-blown dirt—can cause the initial injury. Contact lenses may also produce abrasions if they do not fit properly, are worn too long, or if the user does not insert or remove them according to instructions.

Diagnosis

If you can't seem to dislodge the foreign object by blinking or flushing, you probably have an abrasion or scratch on the cornea. See your doctor as soon as possible to avoid any possibility of further damage to the eye. Your physician will examine the eye under magnification to determine the extent of the injury. Sometimes the doctor will use special eyedrops containing a dye to make the abrasion more visible.

Treatment

An abrasion or scratch on the cornea is usually treated with antibiotic drops or an ointment to prevent infection. If the injury is large and painful, the doctor will apply an eye patch or a "bandage" contact lens to keep the eyelid from rubbing against the injured part of the cornea. A bandage contact lens is a special lens that is used to protect the surface of the cornea. The lens may dissolve on its own (called a collagen shield) or it may need to be removed by the ophthalmologist. Corneal abrasions usually heal without scarring after several days. A more serious injury, one that causes scarring of the cornea, may require surgery.

Corneal scarring

Corneal scars may be congenital or, more commonly, develop as the result of trauma to the eye. A deep scratch on the cornea, for example, may involve other layers of the cornea and leave a scar—an opaque area—that obscures vision.

Depending on the location and severity of the scarring, treatment may consist of a new prescription for eyeglass lenses or the use of hard contact lenses. Hard lenses provide a "new" smooth surface to the eye and help correct any astigmatism caused by the corneal scar. Soft lenses, on the other hand, conform to the eye and do not correct any refractive changes caused by the scar. If the scar is too deep, however, you may require a corneal transplant.

Corneal Transplant

This surgical procedure is recommended if your eyesight has been greatly impaired by scarring of the cornea (Figure 23.8). In this operation, a healthy cornea from a deceased donor is transplanted into your eye. The surgery is performed at the hospital, under a general anesthetic, and takes about 2 hours from start to finish. (Elderly patients with multiple medical problems may need a local anesthetic.)

In the procedure, the surgeon removes the central part of the injured cornea, using a circular cutting instrument called a trephine. A graft of a corresponding size is then fashioned from the donor cornea, and the graft is placed in the hole in the recipient's cornea and sutured into place. The eye is patched for about a day;

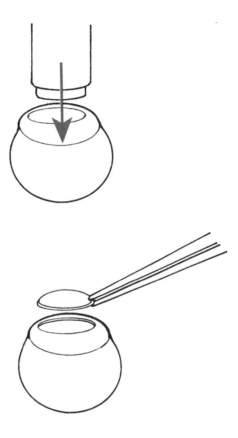

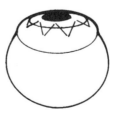

Figure 23.8 Corneal transplant surgery. Scarring of the cornea sometimes requires corneal transplant. In this procedure, the damaged part of the cornea is removed with a special cutting instrument (*top*), and a graft obtained from a donor cornea (*middle*) is then sutured into place (*bottom*).

when the patch is removed, drops are started to prevent infection and rejection of the transplanted cornea. Vision may improve in several weeks, but it may take up to six months before a complete improvement is achieved.

Corneal Ulcers and Infections

A corneal ulcer is an open sore on the cornea. This is a serious matter and should be treated as soon as possible by an ophthalmologist. If left untreated, the ulcer may damage the cornea permanently. A deep ulcer can even erode through the cornea, infecting the entire eyeball and leading to the loss of the eye.

FOREIGN PARTICLES IN THE EYE

Occasionally, specks of dust or sand will blow into your eyes, causing discomfort and irritation. Normally, these small particles will wash out on their own. Sometimes, however, the particle is more difficult to dislodge. In that case, try to find a well-lighted mirror. Do not rub the eye or try to remove the debris with your fingers. If the particle is easily visible, you can try to remove it using the corner of a clean handkerchief. This may be difficult for you to do on your own, as your eyes will blink and tear involuntarily. If you have no one to help you, try using an eye cup to flush out the foreign body. *Never attempt to remove a foreign body that is embedded on the white of the eye or on the cornea.* You could cause an abrasion or other injury.

If the particle is difficult to remove, go to the emergency room of a hospital for help or to your ophthalmologist. If you do remove the object, but pain, redness, and irritation persist, see your doctor.

Symptoms

Corneal ulcers may cause redness in the eye, a decrease in vision, sensitivity to light, and severe pain. Some ulcers can be seen with the naked eye; they appear as a round depression or white spot on the cornea.

Causes

Most ulcers are caused by a corneal abrasion that becomes infected. The improper insertion/removal of contact lenses is one common cause of abrasions. Infectious ulcers are usually caused by bacteria or viruses, most commonly the herpes simplex virus. Noninfectious ulcers are the result of diseases such as rheumatoid arthritis and lupus. Blepharitis—an infection of the eyelid—can also increase the likelihood of developing a corneal ulcer.

Diagnosis

Any inflammation of the eye or opacity on the cornea is a serious matter. If you experience any discomfort while wearing contact lenses, remove the contacts immediately and consult your ophthalmologist. If an ulcer is suspected, your doctor will perform a series of tests to reveal the ulcer and establish its cause; a bacterial ulcer is usually more severe than one caused by a virus. A fluorescein stain may be necessary to detect an ulcer caused by the herpes simplex virus.

Treatment

Bacterial ulcers are usually treated with antibiotic eyedrops. If the infection is viral, your physician will prescribe antiviral drops or ointment. This treatment helps control the immediate condition, but like other herpes infections, the ulcer may recur. *Never* use steroid drops on a corneal ulcer. *Never* use eyedrops that were previously prescribed for an inflamed eye for a second inflammation without your doctor's approval. Using the wrong drops can exacerbate your condition. If the cornea becomes irreparably damaged, it may be necessary to undergo a corneal transplant to replace the injured cornea (see "Corneal Transplant").

Other Eye Inflammations and Infections

The terms *inflammation* and *infection* do not mean the same thing. Inflammation occurs when the body attempts to defend itself against an invading organism or other foreign substance. Infection, on the other hand, occurs when the body, or a part of it, is invaded by a bacteria, virus, or fungus that multiplies and spreads to other areas. There are numerous types of eye inflammations and infections, from the common problem of conjunctivitis to the rarer conditions of iritis and orbital cellulitis (Figure 23.9).

Conjunctivitis

Also known as "pink eye," conjunctivitis is a superficial inflammation of the conjunctiva, the tissue that

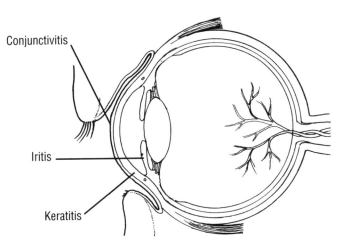

Conjunctivitis

Iritis

Keratitis

Figure 23.9 Common eye disorders. Conditions resulting from inflammation of the eye include conjunctivitis (*top*), an inflammation of the transparent layer of tissue covering the cornea; iritis (*middle*), caused by an inflamed iris or uveal tract (the layer just below the sclera); and keratitis (*bottom*), caused by infection with herpes simplex virus.

covers the eyeball. The conjunctiva lines the eye up to the margin of the cornea and covers the inner eyelids as well. Conjunctivitis can be highly contagious, especially among children.

Symptoms

The most typical signs of conjunctivitis are redness in the eye, a burning sensation, itching, and a discharge that may cause the eyelids to stick together, especially upon awakening. Viral conjunctivitis is sometimes associated with a cold or upper respiratory infection and usually produces a watery discharge. Bacterial conjunctivitis causes much thicker and more viscous matter. Conjunctivitis that is the result of an allergy produces more intense itching, and some swelling and tearing of the eyes.

Cause

Conjunctivitis can be caused by viruses or bacteria. It can also be caused by allergies or toxic substances.

Diagnosis

If you experience the symptoms of conjunctivitis, see your eye doctor as soon as possible. To determine which type of infection you have, your physician may have to take a sample from the conjunctiva for analysis.

Treatment

You can soothe the immediate discomfort of conjunctivitis by applying cool, clean compresses to the eyes. Depending on the cause of your infection, your doctor will probably prescribe medication in the form of eyedrops. For the allergic form of the disease, eyedrops containing antihistamines and an agent that constricts blood vessels may shorten the course of the attack. Bacterial conjunctivitis usually responds to antibiotic drops. The viral type of conjunctivitis is typically self-limited; there are no medications that would make much difference in its course.

Conjunctivitis is an annoying condition, but is usually harmless to your sight. It is very contagious, however, so if you suspect you have contracted conjunctivitis, see your physician for an immediate diagnosis and early treatment. To avoid spreading the disease among family members and friends, make sure you wash your hands often and try not to touch or rub your eyes with your hands. Change your towels, facecloths, and pillowcases once a day. Don't use other people's cosmetics and make sure you discard all eye makeup, particularly mascara, if you used it while you had conjunctivitis.

Uveitis and Iritis

Uveitis is an inflammation of the uveal tract, the layer of the eye immediately below the sclera. The uvea is composed of the iris (the colored part of the eye), the ciliary body, and the choroid. When only the iris is inflamed, the condition is known as iritis.

Symptoms

Redness of the eye, blurry vision, and sensitivity to light are the most common symptoms of iritis.

Cause

The herpes simplex or herpes zoster virus can cause an inflammation in this part of the eye. In addition, uveitis may occur in conjunction with a systemic disease such as rheumatoid arthritis and Crohn's disease.

Diagnosis

Your ophthalmologist will examine your eye, perhaps using a slit-lamp test, to see the extent of the inflammation. You may need a complete physical examination to determine if there is an underlying disorder that has caused the condition.

Treatment

Topical and systemic steroids and antibiotics are used in the treatment of uveitis or iritis. Prompt treatment can lessen any complications, such as glaucoma or cataracts, that can develop from the inflammation.

THE HERPES VIRUS AND YOUR EYES

The herpes simplex virus commonly causes fever blisters—known as "cold sores"—around the mouth. But this virus can also produce a serious inflammation of the cornea, keratitis, which can result in loss of vision if it remains neglected or untreated. If you notice a redness or burning in your eyes, accompanied by an increased sensitivity to light and a decrease in vision, see your ophthalmologist without delay. You may need antiviral, anti-inflammatory, and/or antibiotic drops to avoid superinfection.

The herpes zoster virus can cause a painful skin inflammation, popularly known as "shingles." This condition may affect the forehead, nose, upper face, eyelids, and eye, as well as other parts of the body. To avoid eye involvement and complications, see your ophthalmologist immediately for antiviral medications. The sooner the treatment is started, the less the chance of damage to your vision.

Orbital Cellulitis

Cellulitis is an acute infection of the eye socket that often affects children, although it can occur in people of any age. This is a serious condition that usually requires hospitalization.

Symptoms

The first signs of an orbital infection are swelling, redness of the eyelids and eye socket, pain, and decreased vision. Sometimes the eye actually protrudes from the socket as a result of the swelling.

Cause

Cellulitis is caused by bacteria that enter the eye through an infection of the sinuses, of the eye or eyelid, or from a foreign object that contaminates the eye.

Diagnosis

After a series of tests, your ophthalmologist can determine the nature and extent of the infection.

Treatment

Orbital cellulitis is an eye emergency. Consult your ophthalmologist immediately or go to the nearest hospital emergency room if you or any member of your family suffers from swelling and redness of the eye and eye socket. Antibiotic medications are used to treat the condition, and sometimes surgery is needed to drain the abcess, if any.

Endophthalmitis

Endophthalmitis is a rare but serious condition involving the inflammation and infection of the tissues inside the eye.

Symptoms

The most common signs of endophthalmitis are redness of the eye, severe swelling of the eyelid, pain, and a decrease in vision.

Cause

This widespread infection most commonly occurs after surgery on the eye or from some other trauma to the eye.

Diagnosis

The ophthalmologist will take a culture of the vitreous humor inside the eye. The sample of fluid is sent to the laboratory to determine the organism causing the infection and its sensitivity to different antibiotics. This procedure may be done at the office or in the operating room depending on the severity of the infection and the facilities available.

Treatment

Topical, intraocular, and intravenous antibiotics and steroids are used to treat the infection. If the infection is extensive, surgery may be necessary to remove the infected contents of the eye. Called a vitrectomy, this procedure is usually done at the hospital with local or general anesthesia.

Dacryocystitis

Inflammation and infection of the tear sac, dacryocystitis, is found most commonly in babies and in elderly women. In both cases, the condition results from prolonged obstruction of the tear drainage system, whether because of the narrowness of the sac (babies) or the results of aging on the tear ducts (elderly women). If the duct is obstructed or closed, tears accumulate in the sac or eye, and the retained secretions may become infected.

Symptoms

The eye waters profusely and there is a milky white discharge usually accompanied by a redness and swelling of the tear duct, which may extend to the eyelids and the conjunctiva.

Cause

The condition is caused by the plugging of the tear drainage system because of infection, injury, tumor, or just because it is too narrow.

Diagnosis

Under a topical anesthetic, the ophthalmologist will irrigate the tear ducts to test their functioning.

Treatment

Warm compresses and topical or oral antibiotics will both soothe and eventually help to clear up the inflammation. Older women may require surgery to relieve the obstruction of the tear duct and to allow tears to drain from the eye.

Toxoplasmosis

Toxoplasmosis is an infection, transmitted by a parasite, that can affect the central nervous system and the eye. The infection may be congenital—transmitted to the fetus during pregnancy—or acquired.

DRY EYES

Whenever you blink, tears clean and lubricate your eyes. Tears, in fact, are essential for the proper functioning of the eyes, because the cornea must stay wet to stay healthy. If there aren't enough tears—or the blink reflex is somehow decreased—you suffer from a condition known as "dry eyes." Your eyes feel gritty, irritable, and uncomfortable; your vision also may be affected.

Dry eyes are most common in women after menopause, when their tear production decreases. This condition also affects people after cosmetic eye surgery, when the blinking reflex has been affected. Contact lens wearers, too, may experience dry eyes.

If you are bothered by excessively dry, swollen, or irritated eyes, consult your ophthalmologist. She will probably prescribe lubricating eye drops that can give you relief. Some eye medications for this condition are also available without prescription, but they should be used only under a doctor's supervision.

Symptoms

Acquired toxoplasmosis usually has few noticeable symptoms. It's detected only when there's intense eye inflammation resulting in redness of the eyes, pain, sensitivity to light, and a decrease in vision. The active lesion appears white on the retina.

Cause

Toxoplasmosis can be transmitted by inadequately cooked meat, by cat feces, or by an infected mother to her infant. Prevention, then, includes avoidance of uncooked meat. Pregnant women should avoid any contact with cat feces; if you have a cat, have someone else empty the litter box.

Diagnosis

The ophthalmologist will conduct an examination of the eyes, including a dilated exam, to identify the characteristic retinal lesions.

Treatment

This serious condition is treated with oral antibiotics including sulfas and clindamycin. Oral and topical steroids also may be necessary, depending on the degree of inflammation and location of the lesions. Treatment is more aggressive if the lesions are near the macula or optic nerve. Toxoplasmosis usually leaves a scar on the damaged retinal tissue.

Disorders of the Eyelid

The eyelids are vital to the proper functioning of your eyes. First, they protect your vision by the quick reflex of blinking. When the nerves in the cornea sense even the slightest disturbance, the signal goes to your eyelids to close. Second, the eyelids clean and lubricate your eyes by distributing tears. Last, but not least, the eyelids shut out the light and allow your eyes to rest, even for the space of a blink. Occasionally, however, the eyelids develop problems of their own.

Sties

Sties, the most common of all eyelid infections, feel and look like pimples. In some ways, the sty is similar to an acne lesion; it first appears as a painful red lump on the edge of the eyelid and gradually develops into a whitehead.

Symptoms

You will first notice a discomfort or pain around the eyelid area, followed by a reddening lump that gradually develops a head of whitish pus.

Cause

Sties are usually caused by a bacterial infection of an eyelash follicle. If sties are frequent, the cause may be an underlying chronic infection of the eyelid.

Diagnosis

Sties are almost always harmless to your sight and usually can be treated at home. If the sty does not go away or your sight is affected, see your ophthalmologist promptly for an eye examination. Also check with your doctor if you suffer from recurrent sties.

Treatment

You can treat a sty at home by applying a warm compress to the sore area for about 10 minutes four times a day. Do not squeeze the sty, but allow the pus to drain out on its own. If the sty is stubborn or recurs often, your ophthalmologist may prescribe an antibiotic cream and/or eyedrops. In some cases, the doctor may lance and drain the sty.

Chalazion

A type of internal sty, a chalazion appears as a red lump on the upper eyelid. Chalazia are larger than sties and usually are not painful, just unsightly.

Symptoms

A red, painless lump appears on the upper eyelid. It feels like a tiny pea and may be tender to the touch.

Cause

A chalazion occurs when a gland in the upper eyelid becomes plugged. The blockage may occur after other eyelid infections, such as blepharitis (see below). Recurrent nonhealing lumps on the eyelid may indicate the presence of a tumor, so see your ophthalmologist if the red lump does not disappear on its own within a month or two.

Diagnosis

Sometimes it is hard to know if you are suffering from a sty or a chalazion. Your ophthalmologist can determine this from a clinical examination.

Treatment

Most chalazia disappear on their own in a few months without medical intervention. If the nodule is small and causing no symptoms, treatment may not be required. Home treatment consists of pressing warm to hot compresses on the lump until it dissolves or disappears. Sometimes, however, a chalazion continues to enlarge and becomes unsightly, or fails to disappear on its own. In that case, your doctor can remove it in a simple surgical procedure with local anesthesia.

Blepharitis

Blepharitis is an inflammation and infection of the edges of the eyelids. It is not contagious, is rarely threatening to sight, and is usually easy to treat.

Symptoms

The eyelids become sticky, crusty, and reddened. The eyelids emit the sticky secretions at night, so many people with this condition literally have to pry their eyes open in the morning. Often conjunctivitis, sties, and chalazia accompany this condition. In severe cases, a corneal ulcer may develop.

Cause

Blepharitis is usually caused by a bacterial infection that affects the tiny glands and hair follicles that open onto the surface of the eyelids. It is similar to dandruff, and it often afflicts people who have dandruff of the scalp, eyebrows, and external ears. Blepharitis can also be the result of a localized allergic reaction (usually from eye cosmetics) and exposure to dust, smoke, and irritating chemicals.

Diagnosis

Blepharitis should not be neglected, because abscesses and secondary infections of the eye may develop from the initial condition. If you are suffering from crusty, sticky eyes, especially upon awakening in the morning, see your ophthalmologist. Your doctor will examine your eyes and eyelids and prescribe an appropriate course of action.

Treatment

If the condition is caused by bacteria, topical antibiotics can clear up the basic infection. You can also treat the problem at home by scrubbing the eyelids frequently with a special over-the-counter solution made for that purpose. Blepharitis is a chronic condition and can recur, so you probably should continue to bathe your eyelids on a regular basis, using a clean washcloth and warm to hot water, even after the immediate infection has disappeared.

Blepharospasm

A blepharospasm is an involuntary closure of the eyelids, either intermittently or continuously.

Symptoms
This progressive condition usually affects both eyes at once. In severe cases, the blinking of the eyes and the squeezing of the lids may become so severe as to interfere with a person's daily activities and functioning.

Cause
In most instances, the cause of the spasm is unknown. The symptoms, however, seem to be made worse by stress, fatigue, prolonged driving, and bright lights. In some cases, blepharospasm may be linked to a neurological disorder, such as Parkinson's disease.

Diagnosis
Your ophthalmologist will do a series of tests to determine the cause of the disorder. You may have to consult a neurologist to rule out other causes, such as Parkinson's disease.

Treatment
The treatment of this condition depends on any associated eye problems, such as dry eyes or blepharitis (see above). Surgery is available for those people who do not respond to medication. Severe cases may require injection of botulinum toxin, a drug that partly paralyzes the muscles and relieves the intense spasms caused by the disease. The effects of the toxin last about three months, depending on the patient.

Entropion and Ectropion

Sometimes the upper or lower eyelids turn in, causing the eyelashes to scratch the cornea. This condition is called entropion. The reverse situation is ectropion, when the lower lid turns out, causing tears to flow out of the eye instead of lubricating the eye.

Symptoms
In entropion, the turned-in eyelashes may irritate the eyes and cause scratching of the cornea. You may first experience red and crusty eyes, especially in the morning. In severe cases, the irritation may lead to keratitis or the formation of corneal ulcers. In ectropion, there is excessive tearing and eye irritation. The lower lid may also become loose, pulling away from the eye.

Causes
Entropion and ectropion are usually problems of the elderly, and their occurrence depends on how an individual's skin ages over the years. In a small number of cases, scarring of the eyelid after injury can cause the skin to contract and pull the lashes in, causing entropion. While most cases of ectropion are also related to aging, underlying medical conditions such as atopic dermatitis or lupus erythematosus can also cause the problem to develop.

Diagnosis
An ophthalmologist will conduct a series of tests to discover the source of your discomfort.

Treatment
Both entropion and extropion can be corrected surgically. The procedure is relatively simple, and can be performed under a local anesthetic in a hospital or out-patient setting.

HOW SYSTEMIC DISEASES AFFECT THE EYE

Any disease that affects the body as a whole is likely to have some effect on the eyes and vision. The most important of these diseases are diabetes, multiple sclerosis, AIDS, hypertension, and dysfunction of the thyroid gland.

The Eye and Diabetes

One of the leading causes of blindness in the United States is diabetic retinopathy. This condition is not a symptom of diabetes, but rather a long-term complication stemming from the disease itself. Diabetic retinopathy involves damage to the blood vessels of the retina and may lead to hemorrhages. Unfortunately, the symptoms may be subtle until the disease is fairly well advanced. In fact, all stages of the retinal deterioration may be asymptomatic (that is, without symptoms) if they do not involve the macula, which is the area of central vision of the retina. When the macula is affected, the vision decreases regardless of the stage of the eye disorder. In addition, retinal detachment may also occur as a result of diabetic retinopathy. That is why, if you are diabetic, you should see your ophthalmologist for a checkup on a regular basis, at least once a year.

Management of the underlying disease—diabetes—is the first goal for you and your physician (see Chapter 30). Treatment, depending on the type of diabetes you have, may involve insulin, oral medication, nutrition, and exercise therapy. Specific treatment for diabetic retinopathy may include laser therapy to close off areas of leaking blood vessels and to arrest the growth of the abnormal blood vessels around the retina.

The Eye and Multiple Sclerosis

Multiple sclerosis, a progressive disease, affects the central nervous system, destroying the myelin sheath around the nerves (see Chapter 22). More commonly found in women, multiple sclerosis affects young adults between the ages of 20 and 40. The disease can affect the optic nerve itself, causing poor vision and blind spots, or the muscles that coordinate eye movements,

causing double vision. Fortunately, many people with multiple sclerosis have periods of remission, when their symtoms improve or disappear entirely. Defects in vision originating with the disease can be controlled by the use of steroids.

The Eye and AIDS

The main eye problem for people suffering from acquired immune deficiency syndrome (AIDS) is their susceptibility to infections of all kinds. The complications can include corneal diseases, hemorrhages of the retina, and lesions on the conjunctiva. Antibiotics can usually control the opportunistic infections that occur over the course of the disease. For this reason, people suffering from AIDS who experience eye pain, inflammation, or difficulty in seeing should see an ophthalmologist immediately.

The Eye and Melanoma

Melanomas are usually thought of as skin cancers, but they can also occur within the eye. The eye can be the

TWITCHES, RED SPOTS, AND FLOATERS

Our eyes (and eyelids) are occasionally affected by sensations and symptoms that are annoying but are usually harmless. Chief among them are twitches, or tics, of the eyelid; subconjunctival hemorrhage, or red spots in the eye; and floaters, or spots before the eyes.

Twitches

Every so often you may notice that your eyelid quivers involuntarily for a short period several times in a day. No one knows exactly what causes this fibrillation, or quivering, of the muscles around the eye, but it is generally assumed that tension or anxiety plays a role. Eyelid twitches and tics are harmless and usually nothing to worry about, although they can be distracting when they occur. Some people find that gently massaging the affected eyelid can significantly decrease the problem.

Red spots

The sudden appearance of blood in the white of the eye is a common, if sometimes alarming, occurrence. Called a subconjunctival hemorrhage, this problem

develops when a tiny blood vessel in the eye bursts and the blood seeps into the white of the eye. While unsightly, the hemorrhage is almost always harmless, once systemic hypertension and blood clotting diseases are ruled out. The blood is usually reabsorbed within 10 to 14 days, and there is no effective treatment to make it disappear any faster. If you experience pain or change of vision in the eye, however, see your physician promptly.

Floaters

Almost everyone at some time or another will experience floaters, those tiny dots, squiggles, and strands that float across the vision and then vanish. These "spots before your eyes" are usually bits of debris floating in the vitreous humor and are harmless in themselves. However, if you suddenly experience many of these floaters, perhaps accompanied by flashes of light, check with your ophthalmologist as soon as possible. These signs may indicate the beginning of a retinal detachment, which, if not treated immediately, could lead to permanent damage to your eyesight.

primary site of the cancer, or it can spread to the eye from another location in the body. Melanoma is an extremely fast-growing and lethal form of cancer, so early detection and treatment is essential.

Unfortunately, the signs of melanoma are not always obvious. If you notice a brown or black spot on your iris, or experience a red, painful eye, or have problems with your vision in one eye, see your ophthalmologist without delay.

Small tumors can be treated with radiation and chemotherapy. In some cases, the entire eyeball will have to be removed to prevent the spread of the cancer.

The Eye and Hypertension

Hypertension, or high blood pressure, affects the whole body and can affect the eyes as well. In severe hypertension, the tiny arteries in the retina become narrow and constricted. In some cases, retinal hemorrhages occur, leading to the formation of scar tissue, which may eventually cause a retinal detachment. The only way to prevent these problems is to treat the hypertension from the very beginning, and to have frequent checkups with an ophthalmologist to prevent, if possible, further eye complications.

The Eye and the Thyroid

The thyroid gland secretes thyroid hormones that regulate the body's metabolic system. When the gland becomes overactive and secretes too much of the hormones, Graves' disease is the result. This disease produces a wide range of symptoms, including nervousness, an intolerance to heat, weight loss, and eye problems. In Graves' disease, the eyes tend to protrude abnormally. There may also be double vision and a dry, gritty feeling in the eyes. Primary treatment consists in controlling the overactivity of the thyroid gland. If the eye symptoms are mild, ointments and sometimes steroids can help soothe and correct the condition. In more severe cases, surgery may be necessary.

DIAGNOSTIC EYE TESTS AND PROCEDURES

Regular eye examinations should be a routine part of your general health care. Periodic checkups are especially important as you grow older and are more susceptible to certain disorders of the eye, such as glaucoma and cataracts. In both these conditions, early detection and appropriate treatment is vital to preserving your sight.

The Routine Eye Examination

When you first visit an ophthalmologist's or optometrist's office, you will be asked to fill out a lengthy questionnaire about your general health and medical history. The doctor will then question you about the condition of your eyes. Do you wear glasses or contact lenses? How often? Do you use any medications for your eyes? Have you had any recent eye problems, or do you have any symptoms that worry you? If you wear glasses, you will be asked to produce them so that the prescription can be noted and compared with the results of the examination.

In the examining room, your eye care specialist will have you read aloud from the Snellen chart—that well-known row of letters and numbers that diminish in size from top to bottom—to check on your ability to see from a certain distance, both with and without glasses. The doctor will then physically examine your eyes, noting any evidence of disease or any structural abnormality. This examination is done using a penlight, special lenses, and finally, the slit lamp or biomicroscope. This instrument allows the doctor to take a magnified look at your eyelids, eyes, pupils, corneas, and conjunctivas.

At this point, some eye doctors will put drops into your eyes to dilate them. This helps these doctors see inner tissues of the eyes more clearly. The doctor examines the inner eye to detect lesions or changes due to myopia, diabetes, hypertension, inflammation, or trauma. While the pupils remain dilated, your vision will be blurred and you will be sensitive to light. The effect can last several hours to several days, depending on the medication used.

If you are over 40, you should have your eye pressure checked. The pressure test, called tonometry, measures your eyes for intraocular pressure, a sign of glaucoma. There are several different types of tonometry. The most common instrument used is a tonometer attached to the biomicroscope. Your eyes are anesthetized with drops and the tonometer is placed directly on the eye. Other methods include the Schiotz tonometer and the air-puff tonometer. None of these tests is painful, but some people find the air-puff tonometer uncomfortable.

Other tests may be performed, depending on specific findings from the examination of the inner eye pupil dilation and from the slit-lamp exam.

Specialized Tests

Fluorescein Angiography

Fluorescein angiography evaluates the conditions in the back of the eye. It's particularly useful for detecting diabetic retinopathy and vascular occlusions. The physician injects a fluorescent dye intravenously—usually in the arm—and then takes serial photographs of the inner eye. There may be some nausea and discomfort after the dye injection, but this passes quickly. The procedure takes about 20 minutes, but blurred vision caused by the drops used to dilate the eyes may take about 8 hours to disappear.

Ultrasonography

Ultrasound is used to evaluate the inner eye when the presence of a corneal scar, dense cataract, or vitreous hemorrhage does not allow direct visualization. It can also help in the diagnosis of a retinal detachment or the detection of intraocular masses (tumors). It may be used to measure the thickness of the cornea and the length of the eye before intraocular lens implantation in cataract extraction.

Fundoscopy

Fundoscopy, which uses a device with a special lens and a bright light, aids in the evaluation of the retina. Eye drops are placed in the eyes to dilate the pupil. The bright light may be uncomfortable, but the test takes 5 minutes or less. There are no side effects, other than the usual effects of the dilating drops, which generally wear off in a few hours.

THE BENEFITS OF LASER SURGERY

The prevention and treatment of various eye ailments and conditions have benefited greatly from the advances made over the last decade in laser technology. Laser surgery uses high-powered beams of light to seal or repair torn tissue or to create tiny holes in tissue to relieve pressure. Lasers are used for the treatment of acute glaucoma, for example. In this procedure, a small opening is made in the iris to relieve and control eye pressure. Laser surgery is also used to relieve intraocular pressure in chronic glaucoma.

There are other applications for laser therapy. Laser surgery is frequently used to control the leakage of blood and overgrowth of blood vessels in the retina caused by diabetic retinopathy and is also used to help seal tears in the retina that precede a detachment. After cataract surgery, a laser capsulotomy removes the opaque membrane instantly without the need of another intraocular surgery.

Most laser procedures are done in the doctor's office. The exception is some retinal laser therapy that is combined with conventional surgery. Laser therapy can be performed using a local anesthetic, thus avoiding the risk that accompanies the use of a general anesthetic. Laser surgery has some complications, including possible increase in eye pressure, the possibility of retinal detachment, and hemorrhage. These complications are rare, however, and the benefits of the surgery in most cases far outweigh the risks.

CHAPTER 24

Ears, Nose, and Throat

Melissa Susan Pashcow, M.D., F.A.C.S,
Gwen Korovin, M.D. and
Lynn C. Kase, M.A., C.C.C.-A.

The ear, the nose, and the throat work together to perform a variety of functions. They are treated as a single system within the specialty of otolaryngology because they are interrelated. A disorder in one organ often affects another and should be treated accordingly.

STRUCTURE AND FUNCTION

The ear, nose, and throat are connected through various channels in the head and neck. They overlap in terms of function, structure, and nerve supply. Collectively, the ear, nose, and throat are responsible for hearing and balance, smell, taste, speaking, and swallowing.

Ear

The ear consists of three parts: the external, middle, and inner ear. Each part begins where the other ends. They work together in a complex process that permits a person to hear sounds. (See Fig. 24.1)

The external ear acts as a sound–gathering funnel. The visible part of the ear, called the pinna, is composed of skin and cartilage. It delivers sound into the external ear canal. This canal carries sound from the pinna to the middle ear. It contains glands that produce wax and hairs that protect the middle ear. It also modifies the air that enters the inner ear so that it maintains a constant temperature and level of humidity.

The middle ear is made up of the eardrum, or tympanic membrane, and tiny bones called ossicles: the malleus, the incus, and the stapes. These bones amplify and conduct sound signals to the inner ear. The eustachian tube is the connection between the middle ear chamber and the back of the nose. When a person swallows, the eustachian tube opens so that air pressure in the middle ear and nose is equalized. This mechanism protects the middle ear from harmful pressure differences, such as those that occur with takeoff and landing in an airplane.

In the inner ear, the vestibular labyrinth, also called the semicircular canals, contains sensory cells that are largely responsible for balance. The cochlea, a spiral, snail-shaped structure, contains the sensory cells that are responsible for hearing. It transforms sound vibrations into nerve impulses, which are then conveyed to the brain via the auditory nerve.

The auditory nerve is a bundle of nerve fibers that connects the inner ear with the brain. Auditory signals are sent to the cortex of the brain, which is responsible for interpreting speech, music, and other higher mental faculties.

Sound energy is transmitted through air when air molecules are disturbed. Sound waves are received by the external ear, pass through the external canal, and strike the tympanic membrane (eardrum), causing it to vibrate. The human ear can pick up sounds that move the tympanic membrane by very slight vibrations, such as those made by dropping a pin. These vibrations are transmitted to the bones of the middle ear, where they are amplified so sound waves can reach the inner ear and be transformed into electrical impulses to the brain.

Nose

The nose is formed by a triangular framework of bone and cartilage, covered with skin, and lined with mucous membrane. The olfactory nerve works with the nose to allow odors to be detected. (See Fig. 24.2)

Air enters the body through the nostrils, two identical openings that are separated by a partition known as the septum. This wall between the nostrils is composed of cartilage and bone, and is coverd by a layer of mucous membrane. Three thin, scroll-like structures, called turbinates, curve from the outer wall of the nose toward the septum. They act to warm and humidify air moving through the nasal passages. In the nasal passages, air is directed from the nostrils, past the sinus openings, and back toward the upper airways. Behind the nasal cavity, on the back wall of the nasal passage, are the adenoids, two spongy masses of lymph tissue that involute by adolescence.

The sinuses are hollow spaces in the bones of the face and the skull. They have the same type of lining as the nose and are connected to the nose by tiny openings. There are four sinus cavities: frontal, ethmoid, maxillary, and sphenoid.

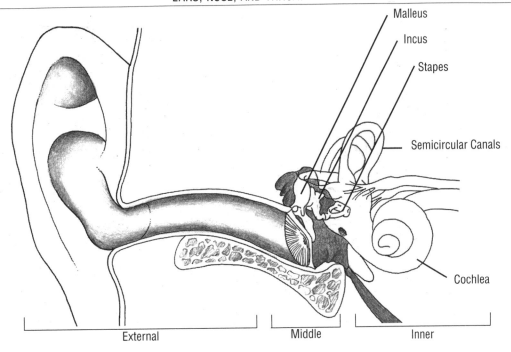

Figure 24.1. The External, Middle, and Inner Ear
The bones of the middle ear include the malleus, incus, and stapes. The inner ear is responsible for balance and hearing, which are controlled by the seimcircular canals and the cochlea, respectively.

DEALING WITH EAR WAX

''Never put anything smaller than your elbow in your ear.''

This old saying is still true. Placing sharp or pointed objects in the ear may burst the eardrum. There are other ways to deal with ear wax.

The skin of the outer ear canal has special glands that manufacture ear wax. The wax traps dirt that may enter the ear canal and prevents debris from reaching the eardrum. If left alone, ear wax will build up, then dry out and leave the ear.

In some people, the wax accumulates and blocks the ear canal, interfering with hearing. Such blockages are best treated by a physician. Ear drops may be prescribed prior to the cleaning to soften the wax.

A commonly used home remedy for softening wax is hydrogen peroxide. After softening, the wax can be washed or suctioned out by a doctor or removed by special instruments. Perforations (holes) in the eardrum can be caused by self-treatment with drops and ear washing. It is better to get the wax completely removed and then start a program to prevent future buildups by instilling softening drops regularly to keep the wax moving.

In the upper portion of the nose is the olfactory nerve. It transmits smells to the olfactory bulb, a structure located at the front of the brain, just behind the nose, which processes the sense of smell. (See Fig. 24.3)

The nose is the major organ of smell. In addition to being a source of pleasure, the sense of smell can warn of impending danger, such as fire or hazardous fumes. It also contributes to the sense of taste. When the ability to smell is obstructed, as with a cold, 80 percent of the ability to taste is gone as well.

Special nerve cells in the nose, mouth, and throat transmit messages to the brain, where specific smells or tastes are identified. Cells that detect smells are in the nose and connected directly to the brain. Cells that detect tastes are in the taste buds concentrated on the tongue. Nerve cells on the moist surfaces of the nose, mouth, and throat also contribute to taste and smell by helping to identify sensations of certain foods, such as the heat of spicy food. Together, these cells help to identify four basic taste sensations—sweet, sour, bitter, and salty—along with other characteristics that produce flavors.

The nose brings air into the respiratory tract and filters, warms, and moistens the incoming air. Sneezing is a reflex by which irritating matter is ejected from the

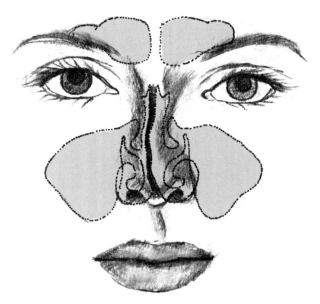

Figure 24.2. The Nose
The nose is a framework of bones and cartilage connected through tiny openings to the sinuses.

body, at a rate of up to 200 miles per hour. The nose's resonating chambers, above the roof of the mouth, contribute to speech.

The sinus cavities within the bones of the face also give resonance to speech. Connected to the nose and the throat, they produce mucus that helps cleanse the airways of dust, bacteria, and other impurities. The mucus runs from the sinuses, through the nose, down the throat, and into the stomach, where it is processed by the digestive system.

Throat

The throat, or pharynx, is part of the system that delivers air to the lungs, food and drink to the stomach, and sounds from the vocal cords to the mouth. This 3- to 5-inch muscular tube is an important junction for the passageways leading into the body. The nasal passages and the mouth cavity lead to the pharynx. The throat is also linked with the middle ear by the eustachian tubes. The throat is a direct link to the esophagus, a muscular tube that extends to the stomach, and the trachea or windpipe, the air passage leading to and from the lungs. (See Fig. 24.4)

Air and food enter through the mouth and are first sensed by the tongue, a mobile organ made up of muscle and supplied by nerves that control movement, sensation, and taste. It is important for swallowing as well as for taste. The uppermost part of the throat is the nasopharynx. It contains the adenoids and the openings of the eustachian tubes of the middle ear. Tonsils are almond-shaped lymph structures on either side of the palate (roof of the mouth). There are also small masses of lymph nodes near the root of the tongue.

The throat regulates the passage of air through the trachea (windpipe) and the passage of food through the esophagus. A small flap of cartilage, called the epiglottis, serves as a safety valve for this function. When a person swallows, it closes off the vocal cords and windpipe. Food is then propelled down the esophagus to the stomach. When the swallow is completed, the epiglottis opens so breathing can continue.

The larynx, known as the voice box, is mainly comprised of vocal cords. The Adam's apple sits in front of the vocal cords. The larynx is responsible for the basic sounds of speech. It also acts to protect the airways by allowing only air to enter the lungs.

STAYING HEALTHY

The ears, nose, and throat are responsible for important functions in a woman's life. You can improve the health of these organs and the senses they supply by protecting them from harm.

■ Avoid getting and spreading colds by practicing good hygiene. Wash your hands frequently if you are around a person with a cold or if you have a cold yourself. Colds are spread more readily by hand contact than through the

air. Don't share utensils or towels with a person who has a cold.

■ Control symptoms of allergies if you have them. They are usually seasonal, such as allergies to pollens. Avoid contact with allergens, and stay in an air-conditioned environment. Using antihistamines and sleeping with your head elevated to promote drainage may be helpful. For severe, recurrent allergy symptoms,

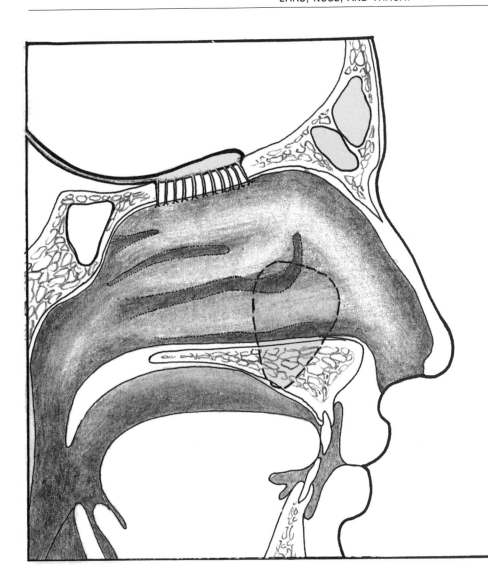

Figure 24.3. Olfactory Bulb
The olfactory bulb, located behind the nose, controls the sense of smell.

a series of shots to help prevent the reaction may be considered.

- Avoid irritants to the nose, especially tobacco smoke. Chronic irritation of the nose, throat, and larynx increases the risk of infection and complications from colds, such as sinusitis, laryngitis, and bronchitis. Smoking also depresses the senses of smell and taste. It may cause cancer, especially in those who are heavy alcohol drinkers as well.

- Don't drink alcohol, or drink moderately. Alcohol causes chronic irritation and is linked with cancer of the throat and mouth.

- Protect your ears. Prolonged exposure to loud noise can cause deafness and should be avoided. Wear earplugs, even if exposed to loud noise for short periods.

- Do not fly if you have ear pain or an ear infection. See your doctor and get treatment before you travel. During airplane travel it is important to equalize the pressure on both sides of the eardrum. The highest risk is when the airplane is descending. If you are experiencing nasal or ear problems, you may want to carry nasal spray and spray each nostril at the beginning of the descent. Chew gum, yawn, and drink liquids to open the eustachian tubes, which will equalize the pressure in the ears.

- Keep wax from plugging ears. If you have a problem with wax buildup, take measures to keep the wax soft and loose, and visit your ear doctor (see box).

SIGNS AND SYMPTOMS

Problems in the ears, nose, and throat can cause symptoms in any or all of them. In some cases, such as a cold, the problems affect the entire system. Although a cold is not serious, it can lead to complications that may require medical attention (see "Upper Respiratory Infections"). Any symptoms that affect hearing, smelling, or talking may require medical attention if they are not related to a simple cold or allergy.

Ears

Problems in the ears can be related to infection, to pressure inside the ear, or to the many disorders that can cause loss of hearing. In some cases, a disturbance in the nerve that connects the ears to the brain may be involved and disrupt balance.

Earache
Both the outer ear and the middle ear can be infected by bacteria, a virus, or a fungus. A condition referred to as "swimmer's ear" may result when water gets trapped inside the ear canal, causing pressure and pain, and creating conditions for a fungal infection. Ear discomfort can also result from a buildup of wax.

Pain in the ear can arise while flying. This pain is often related to a problem in the eustachian tube. An upper respiratory infection causes congestion around the eustachian tube opening and may lead to a feeling of fullness in the middle ear and sometimes severe pain, particularly when the plane is descending. "Barotrauma" is the term for bleeding into the eardrum caused by pressure changes. Preventive measures include chewing, swallowing, or yawning during descent to open the canal and equalize the pressure. Use of some nasal decongestant sprays can shrink the mucous membranes.

Any sudden injury, or trauma, to the ear can lead to perforation of the eardrum. This can result in sudden pain, bleeding, and hearing loss, and should receive immediate medical attention.

Hearing Loss
Hearing loss affects millions of people. Although it can occur at any age, hearing loss is an undeniable factor of the aging process. Over 90 percent of the population over 80 years of age has some degree of hearing loss. In older people, hearing loss usually is secondary to loss of function of the nerve that conducts sound impulses to the brain. In children, the cause of hearing loss is usually middle ear disease. Hearing loss, both temporary and permanent, can result from trauma to the head, tumors that involve the auditory nerve, and ear infections. Short-term exposure to high-intensity sound can cause temporary hearing loss. Those who have long-term exposure, such as construction workers and rock musicians, can have permanent damage. Some common drugs, such as aspirin and antibiotics, can damage hearing. Others affected by hearing loss include individuals with heart disease, diabetes, and thyroid problems.

The signs of hearing loss include difficulty understanding conversation, resulting in missing words or giving inappropriate answers to questions. Frequently not hearing the phone or doorbell may be a further sign of hearing loss. A hearing-impaired person may become withdrawn and avoid socializing because of fear of not hearing well.

Any dizziness, ringing in the ears, or change in hearing should be evaluated. Any individual who suspects a hearing loss should first consult a physician, preferably an otologist or an otolaryngologist, so that any underlying medical problems can be ruled out as the cause. Most states require that a signed medical clearance be obtained before an audiologist or hearing aid dispenser can dispense any hearing instrument. Hearing aids can help those with some amounts of permanent hearing loss.

Tinnitus
Noise in the ears, often described as a ringing sound, is a common problem. It may come and go, and can vary from a low roar to a high squeal or whine that is heard in one or both ears. Tinnitus is usually more bothersome in quiet surroundings, especially at night in bed.

There are many possible causes of tinnitus. A small plug of wax may be a temporary cause. In most cases, there is accompanying damage to the microscopic endings of the auditory nerve in the inner ear. Tinnitus is most often associated with a hearing loss. Exposure to loud noises is a common cause of tinnitus. It can also be associated with a middle ear problem such as infection, a hole in the eardrum, a buildup of fluid, or stiffening of the middle ear bones. Ménière's disease affects the labyrinth and produces tinnitus, vertigo, and hearing loss. Ringing in the ears can be a symptom of

SOUND

Sound has three properties:

Pitch is a function of the frequency of sound waves that strike the eardrum. The human ear detects frequencies from about 20 to about 20,000 cycles. The human voice is about 100 (for men) to 150 (for women) cycles per second. The higher the frequency, the higher the pitch of the sound.

Intensity, or loudness, is measured in decibels. Here are some examples:

- Ticking watch
    20 decibels
- Conversation
    70 decibels
- Car horn
    100 decibels
- Rock music
    140 decibels
- Jet takeoff
    160 decibels

Timbre depends on secondary vibrations. A piano, flute, or trumpet sounds different even when each plays the same note. Timbre helps a person to recognize voices.

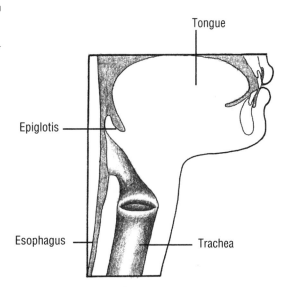

Figure 24.4. The Throat
The throat connects with the trachea and the esophagus, bringing air to the lungs and food to the stomach, respectively.

(Tongue, Epiglotis, Esophagus, Trachea)

roid disease, and autoimmune disease), infections, and trauma. A thorough medical exam is required for anyone suffering from vertigo. Factors that are important to the diagnosis include the onset of the symptoms, which often are associated with nausea, vomiting, sweating, and collapse but not loss of consciousness. Treatment is based on the underlying cause and relief of symptoms.

an aneurysm (a weakening or bulging in the wall of a blood vessel) or a rare noncancerous tumor that grows on the auditory nerve (acoustic neuroma) (see Chapter 22, "The Nervous System"). Certain medications and medical conditions also may cause tinnitus, which can go away when the condition is treated or the medication discontinued.

If the cause is not identified, treatment is aimed at the symptom. Many physicians will suggest listening to music at low volume or finding some kind of "white noise" to compete with the head noises.

Vertigo

A feeling of motion while standing still, as well as dizziness, can be caused by inner ear problems such as infections and tumors of the acoustic nerve. A sense of balance depends on complex interactions between the labyrinth of the inner ear and other parts of the nervous system. Any conflict in the messages from any of the components may cause a disturbance in balance.

Vertigo can also be caused by certain medical disorders (such as cardiovascular disease, diabetes, thy-

Nose

Symptoms related to the nose may be most obvious when they cause the discomfort associated with colds and allergies: sneezing, congestion, runny nose. These symptoms can lead to more serious complications, such as sinusitis and bronchitis, and should receive medical care if they persist. Other problems relating to the nose include bleeding, loss of smell, and nasal obstruction.

Anosmia

Almost everyone has experienced a loss of smell when suffering a common cold, allergies, or an infection of the nasal passages. Any nasal condition that interferes with the passage of air to the roof of the nose, where the olfactory nerve is located, will cause a loss of smell. Nasal congestion is the most common temporary cause, and cigarette smoking is a common chronic cause. When the sense of smell is affected, there is also a loss of the sense of taste. Persistent anosmia requires a medical examination.

Nasal obstruction

One of the many reasons for breathing through the mouth, rather than the nose, is an obstruction in the nose. A physical blockage of the air passageways of the nose may be secondary to factors including structural problems (deviated septum), nasal tumors, infection, or allergies. If the septum is obstructing a nostril, the problem can be corrected by surgery. Many women have prolonged bouts with a stuffy nose when they are pregnant. This is related to high levels of the hormone progesterone during pregnancy. Several weeks after the birth of the baby, the nasal congestion with obstruction disappears. Postmenopausal women may experience excessive dryness of the nose.

Nosebleeds

A common cause of bleeding from one nostril is local trauma secondary to excessive blowing or picking. Other causes, which can lead to bleeding from both nostrils, are congestion and irritation of the very delicate blood vessels in the nose. A common cause is hypertension. Bleeding disorders, vitamin deficiency, and drug abuse can also cause nosebleeds. Pinching the soft part of the nose above the nostrils is most effective in stopping the bleeding. Occasionally, packing in the nose, which is usually done in the emergency room, may be required. A condition called *vicarious menstruation* manifests itself by nosebleeds. It is caused by congestion of nasal blood vessels secondary to circulating estrogen.

Throat

Problems in the throat can occur with upper respiratory infections, or the throat itself can become infected. A sore throat, difficulty swallowing, hoarseness, and swelling in the neck can be signs of more serious problems.

Dysphagia

Difficulty swallowing is usually caused by severe sore throat. In older women, disorders of muscles and nerves, and tumors must be considered. The diagnosis is based on difficulty in swallowing liquids or solids and other symptoms such as pain, loss of weight, or decrease in energy. The exam may include direct inspection and X-rays of the swallowing mechanism.

Hoarseness

A deepening or harsh quality of the voice may be related to a short-term illness, such as an upper respiratory infection and the laryngitis (inflammation of the larynx) that often accompanies it. Hoarseness that lasts over time may indicate a more serious condition. It may occur because of overuse and abuse of the voice, as may happen with singers and teachers. Such benign vocal cord growths are called polyps or nodules. Most significantly, although more rarely, cancer of the larynx may be seen.

Neck Mass

A swelling or lump in the neck is usually due to glands responding to inflammation in the throat. Other causes of swelling in this area are conditions of the thyroid or cysts in the throat. Swollen glands usually go away soon after the soreness does. Any persistent lump should be evaluated by a physician.

Sore Throat

The throat can become directly infected with viruses and bacteria (strep throat, tonsillitis), or it can become inflamed as a result of a nasal infection or allergy. A sore throat can also be a sign of irritation, polyps or growths, or cancer. If a sore throat persists or becomes worse, or if it is associated with symptoms other than those of the common cold, it should be examined.

DISORDERS

Problems in the ears, nose, and throat can be limited to one of these or can affect all of them. Diagnosis is focused on locating the exact source of the problem so treatment specific to the disorder can be given.

Ear Disorders

Disorders of the ear often share common symptoms of ringing in the ears (see "Tinnitus"), hearing loss, and sometimes vertigo or loss of balance. The tiny structures of the inner ear are very delicate and, although well protected by the skull, are susceptible to damage. Any noticeable change in hearing should be brought to the attention of a physician.

Infections

The most common infections of the ear canal are those in the external ear, called otitis externa, and the middle ear, called otitis media. The infections can be caused by bacteria or fungus.

Otitis externa causes severe earache, which becomes worse when the outside ear is moved or touched. Usually the external ear canal is red and swollen. It is generally caused by a bacterial infection of the lining of the ear canal. Treatment can include using antibiotic eardrops. If the canal is very swollen, a physician may place a wick in the ear to allow application of ear drops. Oral antibiotics also may be prescribed.

Swimmer's ear, a type of otitis externa, occurs when water remains trapped in the ear canal after swimming or showering. It may contain bacteria and fungus particles. Fungus trapped in the water grows and infects the lining of the canal. The ear feels blocked, and there may be discomfort and sometimes pain. It is diagnosed by looking into the ear with an otoscope, which may reveal a thick white substance or black fungal spores. Treatment is with antifungal ear drops. This condition can be prevented by shaking the water out of the ears after swimming and using alcohol-containing ear drops that will dry the canal. Earplugs can be used to prevent getting water in the ears.

Otitis media is an infection of the middle ear chamber behind the eardrum. Infection of the middle ear is usually secondary to an upper respiratory infection and is most often caused by bacteria. It causes severe pain and, if there is fluid in the chamber, hearing loss. In some cases, pressure builds up and ruptures the eardrum. At this point, there will be discharge from the ear canal and relief from the pain.

The diagnosis is confirmed by viewing the eardrum with an otoscope. It is inflamed and bulging, and sometimes there are blisters on it. Antibiotics are the usual treatment. Decongestants are also used to help open the eustachian tube so the middle ear can drain. Occasionally fluid will persist in the middle ear chamber. It usually responds to decongestants but may require corticosteroids to reduce swelling. Patients should remain under medical care until all symptoms, particularly impaired hearing, have disappeared.

Labyrinthitis

Inflammation of the labyrinth, the complex organ of the inner ear that is responsible for the sense of balance, can occur after a cold. This is called viral labyrinthitis. The main symptom is vertigo, a perception that the environment is moving, the room is spinning, or the floor is moving. A person with vertigo feels unsteady, which may lead to nausea and vomiting.

If vertigo occurs along with a feeling of pressure in the ears, tinnitus, and decreased hearing, it may be a sign of Ménière's disease (see Chapter 22). If this condition is suspected, special hearing tests should be done, and an otolaryngologist and a neurologist may need to be consulted. Otherwise, certain antihistamine-type drugs that are used to control motion sickness will relieve symptoms, usually within a few days.

Motion sickness is thought to be caused by the brain getting confusing messages from the inner ear. The three fluid-filled semicircular canals in the inner ear determine balance. The shifting of fluid in the ears, along with the eyes, monitors motion and sends messages to the brain. When the eyes send one message and the inner ear sends another, motion sickness can result. Boat rides are notorious for inducing motion sickness, especially when the water is choppy. Some individuals are unusually sensitive, and car and train rides also affect them. Taking anti-motion medicine ½–1 hour before traveling may prevent motion sickness. When exposure will be prolonged, as during a cruise, a drug called scopolamine may be given through a skin patch that is available by prescription.

Otosclerosis

This disease results in a gradual hearing loss in one or both ears. Otosclerosis occurs most frequently during the childbearing years and has been linked with pregnancy. Most cases of otosclerosis are due to calcium deposits and stiffening of the middle ear bones, specifically the stapes (the stirrup-shaped bone that vibrates to pass sound waves into the inner ear).

In most cases, otosclerosis can be treated successfully by surgery. The eardrum is lifted away from the stapes; the stapes is either removed and replaced with a tiny wire or stainless steel device, or is mobilized. Nonsurgical treatment involves the use of a hearing aid.

Eardrum perforation

The eardrum is a delicate membrane at the inner end of the ear canal. It can be perforated with toothpicks, bobby pins, or cotton-tipped swabs if they are used imprudently to clean the ears. The eardrum can also be ruptured by sudden pressure changes in an accident or a blow to the head, or during air travel. An eardrum can be perforated when an infection of the middle ear builds up pus that breaks through the thin drum. Symptoms include severe pain, loss of hearing, echoes in the head, dizziness, and nausea. Blood may be discharged from the ear canal.

Small perforations can be self-healing; large perforations require a complex procedure in which a graft of a vein or other material is used as a patch on the broken drum. Chronic perforation is a hole in the eardrum that usually is the result of an infection. It is important to be aware of having this condition because a perforated eardrum should be kept dry when showering, shampooing, and swimming. Earplugs or caps may be needed, but avoid eardrops unless prescribed by a physician.

Presbycusis

Gradual hearing loss that occurs with aging is called presbycusis. It affects up to 25 percent of adults in their sixties and seventies. The exact cause is not known. It could be related to changes associated with aging, or it could be linked to long-term exposure to noise or to circulatory problems that are common in the elderly. Damage to nerves that control centers for speech and hearing may also be a factor. The diagnosis is based on an ear examination that includes hearing tests.

Upper Respiratory Infections

Infections of the upper respiratory system can range from colds to inflammation of the sinuses, to chronic problems. In many cases, colds also involve a cough and symptoms in the rest of the respiratory system. A cold can lead to more serious conditions, such as bronchitis, pneumonia, and bacterial infection of the sinuses, ears, or throat. Although antibiotics will not help a cold, which is caused by a virus, they may be required for a secondary infection, necessitating a visit to your doctor.

Colds

The cold is probably the most prevalent of all human ailments. About 200 viruses can produce the common cold. It usually begins with an infection of the tissue behind the nose, resulting in a sore sensation high in the throat. The nose fills with mucus and runs, and there may be sneezing. The head feels congested, and the throat may be sore. Depending on the virus, there may be conjunctivitis, an inflammation of the eyes. Body aches and fever also may be present. Be-

cause of the congested nose, there is a loss of smell and taste, and the appetite may be depressed.

There is no quick cure for the common cold. The vast and confusing array of cold remedies in drugstores is convincing proof that there is no easy answer. A cold can be expected to last 1–2 weeks, longer if there are complications. There are medications, such as antihistamines, decongestants, and pain relievers, that can provide significant relief of symptoms. These medications can be used alone or taken in combination (see box).

The best course of action is to keep on hand a bottle of each type of medication and use what is needed to relieve symptoms. If combination medications are being used, the ingredients should be identified and precautions should be taken to avoid inadvertently "doubling up" on drugs (such as taking a combination drug with acetaminophen while also taking ibuprofen).

Although vitamin C probably does not prevent colds, it may help speed recovery. It aids in the healing process, and extra amounts are helpful in repairing injured membranes in the nose and throat.

Common bacteria normally found in the healthy nose or throat may grow and multiply because the cold makes the tissues more susceptible to infection. Complications include sinusitis, otitis, laryngitis, and bronchitis. Signs of bacterial infection include persistent yellow-green discharge from the nose or throat, fever, earache, aching over the cheeks or forehead, hoarseness, and a cough that produces yellow-green or brown phlegm.

Cough

A reflex that forces a rush of air from the respiratory tract through the throat at high speed, a cough clears the throat of irritating or obstructing debris, food, or mucus. Sometimes a cough can be lifesaving, although violent coughing can fracture ribs and rupture abdominal muscles.

A cough is a common symptom of a cold and usually goes away when the cold is over. If a cough lasts for several weeks, it should be checked and treated. A yellow or greenish mucus, or foul-smelling mucus, can indicate a complicating bacterial infection requiring antibiotics. "Postviral cough syndrome" is a long-lasting cough that occurs after a cold. It may respond to asthma medications. Persistent sinus inflammation may lead to postnasal drip and coughing. This cough may be worse in the morning and clear up during the day.

Sinusitis

Infection of the cavities draining into the nose is called sinusitis. It is usually caused by blockage of the opening that drains the sinus passage and can be due to nasal polyps (growths), allergies, or a cold. A bacterial infection develops within the blocked cavity.

Headache or facial discomfort often occurs with acute sinusitis. The pain is usually worse in the morning. It is located along the cheeks and upper teeth, about the eyes, and/or across the forehead, depending on which sinuses are involved. The pain is accompanied by greenish-yellow nasal discharge, sometimes blood streaked, or postnasal drip (coughed from the throat). There can be fever and achiness.

Chronic sinusitis occurs when there is persistent blockage of a sinus opening that does not clear up between infections. The lining of the sinus becomes thickened, and polyps project into the cavity.

In acute sinusitis, medications to open sinuses and permit drainage, and antibiotics to kill the infecting organisms are used. Decongestants like pseudoephedrine work well. Over-the-counter nasal sprays should be used for only 2–3 days.

For chronic sinusitis, it is important to control nasal swelling due to allergy and to see whether there is a specific blockage. The constant irritation of cigarette smoke worsens the problem. Surgery, which can be done through a nasal endoscope (see "Procedures"), can remove obstructing tissue and reestablish drainage. Blowing the nose should be done with care, one nostril at a time, with the mouth wide open, to avoid injecting infected material into the sinuses or the ear.

Throat Disorders

Cancer

Both the voice box (larynx) and the throat (pharynx) can develop cancer. Although less common in women, increasingly these cancers are being identified in women as the number of longtime women smokers continues to rise. The most common early symptom of laryngeal cancer is hoarseness. If the entire larynx is removed, alternate methods of speech production are implemented. One of these involves implanting a device to help produce an artificial voice.

The pharynx extends from the nasal cavity down the throat to the larynx and esophagus: it is in the pathway of both respiratory and digestive activity. Any cough, change in the voice, or pain on breathing or swallowing should not be ignored. It may be a sign of cancer. Treatment of cancer includes surgery, radiation therapy, or chemotherapy.

Laryngitis

An infection of the larynx (voice box) causes hoarseness. Laryngitis can be acute (coming on suddenly) and chronic. When the vocal cords of the larynx become irritated, they can become inflamed and swell. This swelling distorts sound produced by the air passing over them. This causes the voice to sound hoarse and husky.

Acute laryngitis is usually caused by a virus or, less often, a bacterial infection. It can also develop as a secondary illness due to a cold. Improper use of the voice or inhaling irritating gas may cause acute laryngitis. Chronic laryngitis can be due to chronic misuse of the voice, various growths, excessive consumption of alcohol, or inhalation of toxic gases.

If laryngitis is caused by a bacterial infection, antibiotics can be prescribed. Other treatments include resting the voice, inhaling steam, and drinking warm liquids. Chronic laryngitis caused by smoking or drinking alcoholic beverages is best cured by avoiding the use of these irritating substances.

Pharyngitis

Inflammation of the throat can be a component of an upper respiratory infection or occur by itself. Acute sore throats are most commonly due to infections caused by viruses or bacteria. "Strep throat" is characterized by extreme soreness, enlarged lymph glands in the neck, and yellow-white discharge on the tonsils (tonsillitis). It is important to identify the strep organism because some of the strains—group A beta hemolytic streptococcus—cause serious illnesses like rheumatic fever in susceptible individuals.

A culture of the discharge on the tonsils will identify the type of bacteria. If it is group A beta hemolytic strep, a 10-day course of antibiotics is recommended to eliminate the infection completely. The advent of antibiotics has led to a decrease in rheumatic heart disease as a long-term complication of strep infections.

Temporomandibular Joint Syndrome (TMJ Syndrome)

This abnormality of the joint in the jaw tends to affect more women than men. It may cause headache; pain in the ear, jaw, neck, back, shoulders, face, or throat; a clicking sound when eating; and grinding teeth during sleep. TMJ syndrome is often due to an imbalance in the working relationship of the jaw and skull with the muscles that are attached to and move these structures. It can be triggered by whiplash suffered in a car accident or a blow to the head. Although tension and stress may contribute to the syndrome, there is usually an underlying physical problem as well (See Figure 24.6).

Treatment is aimed at relaxing the muscles that are inflamed or in spasm. Anti-inflammatory drugs and moist heat are sometimes helpful. Dental splints or a bite plate may be needed to realign the joint. In very rare circumstances, surgery may be necessary.

HEARING AIDS

The concept of hearing aids dates back hundreds of years. The technology available today, although not perfect, can help most people with a hearing impairment. A certified audiologist is the most qualified professional to provide a hearing aid. If you live in an area where an audiologist is not readily available, the next best person is a certified hearing aid dispenser. The purchase of a hearing aid represents a significant commitment, both financially and in terms of the effort required to benefit from its use. It is important, therefore, to be well aware of the types of hearing aids and features that are available. There are three categories of hearing aids: behind the ear, in the ear, and in the canal. (See Fig. 24.5)

- A behind-the-ear (BTE) type consists of a curved plastic case that houses the electronic components and fits behind the ear. This type of hearing aid is used mostly by individuals with a severe hearing loss. The larger case can hold more circuitry and provide more power to the wearer. Although BTEs are usually very reliable and probably the easiest to use, they account for a small percentage of hearing aids sold. This is mostly because they are thought of as being too obvious. This is not necessarily so, however, because modern BTEs are quite small. In addition, the hair often covers the top of the ear so the device cannot be seen.

- In-the-ear (ITE) hearing aids consist of a custom molded shell containing all of the components. The hearing aid, the batteries required for its use, and the battery compartment and volume control are considerably smaller than in a BTE. These hearing aids are the most popular models sold today. They are effective in all but the most severe hearing losses, and they are moderately priced.

- In-the-canal (ITC) hearing aids are tinier versions of the ITE aids. They fit entirely in the ear canal and are hardly visible. One advantage of ITC

hearing aids is that because they come closer to the eardrum, they require less volume to be used. Some individuals report a more natural sound from this type of aid. There are some significant disadvantages to ITC devices: they cannot provide sufficient power to correct severe hearing losses, and the controls and batteries are very small and may prove to be difficult for some people to use. Also, ITC hearing aids tend to become clogged with ear wax. These devices are more costly than larger hearing aids.

Various features are available as extra options to standard hearing aids. Each of these features relates to how different types of sound are processed by the hearing aid. Your audiologist can offer advice regarding which, if any, of these features will benefit you.

The most technologically sophisticated hearing aids available today are programmed like computers. It is possible to have several settings that can be changed according to the wearer's changing environment. Although this type of hearing aid may enable the wearer to hear well in a number of settings, it is worthwhile to consider how often one's environment changes to determine whether this feature is worthwhile.

Hearing aid wearers often become discouraged with the results. Hearing aids will not restore normal hearing the way eyeglasses restore 20/20 vision. There is an adjustment period during which the wearer must relearn how to hear noises and speech that have not been heard in years. In addition, the sound of one's own voice is different when wearing a hearing aid, and this also takes some getting used to.

Techniques such as lipreading and concentration on speech sounds, as opposed to outside sounds, will improve the results obtained from hearing aids. Practice, perseverance, and patience, by both the hearing aid wearer and the dispenser, are essential to a positive experience.

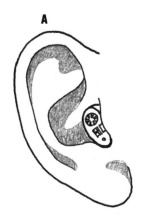 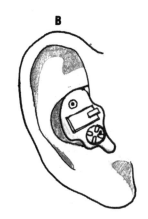 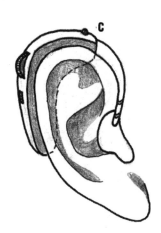

Figure 24.5. Types of Hearing Aids
A. In the canal (ITC).   B. In the ear (ITE).   C. Behind the ear (BTE).

Vocal cord lesions

These benign growths of the vocal cords vary in size and shape. Polyps are small, fluid-filled growths on the vocal cords. They cause hoarseness and other changes of the voice. Polyps develop from the misuse or overuse of the voice or from excessive smoking. Sometimes other growths occur that are called singer's nodules or teacher's nodules. Even very small nodules can affect the voices of singers and have been known to end a singer's career. They tend to occur on the

OVER-THE-COUNTER COLD REMEDIES MOST HELPFUL FOR COLDS

Antihistamines have limited usefulness for colds. They are very helpful for a runny nose, but this phase lasts for a limited period. If you continue to take antihistamines, you may find that your nasal passages get excessively dry and uncomfortable. If you experience the side effect of drowsiness, be aware that it can be not only annoying but even dangerous if you drive or use machinery.

Decongestants shrink the nasal and sinus membranes, decrease secretions, and make breathing easier. They may produce a dry sensation, but not to the same degree as antihistamines. They are related to adrenalin-like compounds and cannot be used by people with high blood pressure. They may cause wakefulness in some individuals. If they keep you awake, the last dose should be taken at least 4 hours before bedtime. Nasal sprays containing decongestants have limited usefulness. They can be used for 2–3 days but then should be discontinued, or they will cause rebound congestion. This is stuffiness of the nose caused by the drug itself, not the cold.

Pain relievers address fever, muscle aches, headache, and soreness in the nose and throat. People with peptic ulcer should not take aspirin or ibuprofen. Acetaminophen is safe to take.

Most combination drugs consist of decongestants, a pain reliever, and an antihistamine. Some contain two of these ingredients. It is best to determine what your needs are and use just the drugs that relieve your symptoms.

Type	Generic Names	Mechanism
Decongestants	Phenylpropanolamine Pseudoephedrine	Shrinks tissues, relieves congestion
Pain relievers	Acetaminophen Aspirin Ibuprofen Naproxen sodium	Decreases pain from headache, muscle aches, fever
Antihistamines	Chlorpheniramine Diphenhydramine	Stops secretions, dries tissues

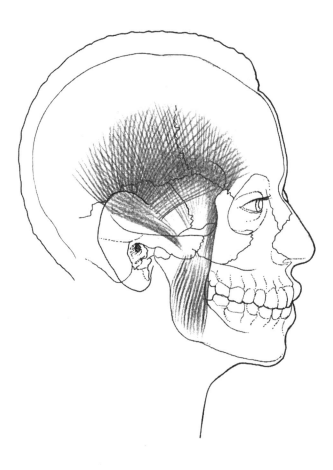

Figure 24.6. TMJ
Temporal mandibular joint syndrome can result from an inbalance in the muscles of this joint.

opposing surfaces of the vocal cords and prevent them from contacting each other. The air escapes through the defect and produces a raspy sound or hoarseness.

Treatment usually involves removal of the polyps by surgery. Nodules are treated with a course of voice therapy. Surgeons use a miniscope to allow the precise identification and removal of these tiny lesions, if necessary.

PROCEDURES

Otoscopy

The otoscope is designed to be used in examination of the ear; a light and a magnifying lens allow the physician to see in the ear canal. It is painless.

Endoscopy

More than 100 years ago, the first direct observation of the esophagus took place, via an open tube and a light. Since that time many small endoscopes, both flexible and rigid, have been developed to examine the nasal passages and the throat. They are tubes attached to a light source and a magnifying lens to allow viewing inside the body. These instruments allow a physician to identify areas where sinuses are blocked or view and biopsy tumors. Surgery on the sinuses can be performed with these instruments as well.

Hearing Tests

Tests to assess hearing are usually done in a soundproof room. To assess how well the eardrum and middle ear bones conduct sound, sounds at different frequencies are played in each ear through earphones. A probe with wires attached to it is inserted into the external canal of the ear to measure middle ear pressure. Air pressure is then varied at the same time that a tone is sounded through the probe tip. A machine attached to the probe records the movements of the eardrum and the middle ear bones, printing out the results on a graph called a tympanogram. The reflex to loud noise also may be tested. This is called an acoustic reflex test. These tests can take only a few moments and, because they involve automatic responses of the auditory system, can be done on anyone.

Other tests include measurement of the patient's hearing of two-syllable words and pure tones within a certain range. Wearing headphones, the patient indicates when sounds are detected, and the results are plotted on what is called an audiogram. The ability to discriminate speech is measured by having the patient repeat one-syllable words. Further tests may be conducted to determine the nature of the hearing loss. They involve altering tones and noises or using tape recordings to distort voice or sound signals.

Hearing also is assessed by recording the electrical activity of brain centers associated with hearing. Electrodes are attached to the head at various points. Clicks of varying intensities are transmitted to the patient through headphones. A computer analyzes the nerve cell activity in response to the clicks and shows the brain wave patterns on a screen. This is called auditory brain stem response, and it takes up to an hour.

EAR, NOSE, AND THROAT SPECIALISTS

Following are descriptions of health care professionals who treat disorders of the ears, nose, and throat. Because these organs and their functions relate directly to the nervous system, a neurologist, who specializes in the nervous system, may also be involved. In most cases, the first point of contact is the primary care physician, who may consult with the following specialists:

- Otolaryngologists—Physicians who have specialized education and training in disorders of the ears, nose, and throat. Their training prepares them for cosmetic facial reconstruction, head and neck tumor surgery, treatment of hearing and balance loss, and treatment of allergic, sinus, laryngeal, thyroid, and esophageal disorders.

- Otologists—Otolaryngologists who specialize in treatment of disorders of the ear.

- Audiologists—Licensed professionals with a master's degree-level education in the science of hearing and tests used to assess hearing. They also provide counseling and nonmedical rehabilitation for the hearing impaired, such as lipreading and hearing aid evaluation. The letters CCC-A after an audiologist's name stand for Certificate of Clinical Competence, indicating certification by the American Speech Language Hearing Association.

- Hearing aid dispensers—Professionals who are certified by the National Board for Certification of Hearing Instrument Sciences are indicated by the letters BC-HIS after their names. These individuals are certified to provide hearing aids.

For additional information or help in finding a physician near you, write or telephone American Academy of Otolaryngology, 200 First Street SW, Rochester, MN 55905; telephone 507-294-3410.

For further information on speech and hearing, write the National Association for Hearing and Speech Action, 10801 Rockville Pike, Rockville, MD 20852; call 800-638-8255.

For free information on hearing aids, contact the National Hearing Aid Society, 20361 Middlebelt, Livonia, MI 48152.

CHAPTER 25

The Breast

Janet Rose Osuch, M.D., F.A.C.S.

Breasts are an anatomic feature unique to a woman and her role as a mother. They are able to respond to stimulation—cold, sex, or a nursing baby. Because of the breasts' ability to be stimulated during sexual activity and because of the importance society has placed on them, the breasts are intimately tied to femininity.

The breasts serve a very important function—the feeding of a baby. Breast milk is the best food for a newborn. It's often been imitated but never equaled.

Of the various conditions that can affect the breasts, the most feared is breast cancer, the most common cancer in women. However, a woman has a number of ways to detect breast cancer early, when it can be treated with the most success.

This chapter describes the structure and function of the breasts, some common conditions that may occur, and the diagnosis and treatment of breast conditions. It also describes ways a woman can help keep her breasts healthy.

STRUCTURE AND FUNCTION OF BREASTS

The breast rests on the *pectoral* (chest) muscle. The interior of the breast is made up of fat, *stroma* (connective tissue), *lobules* (glands that produce milk),

ducts (the tubes to carry milk to the nipples), and blood vessels (See Fig. 25.1 A and B). The only muscles in the breast are the tiny ones near the nipple. You can see

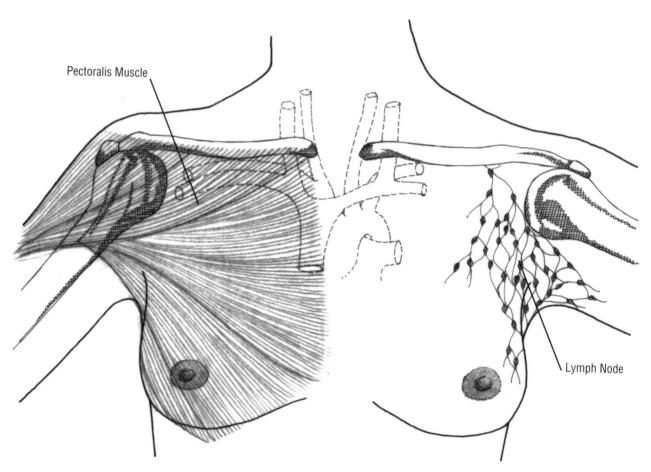

Figure 25.1A. The Breast
The breast is located on top of the pectoralis muscle of the chest (left). The tissue around the breast and under the arm contains clusters of lymph nodes, which are infection-fighting organs in the lymphatic system (right).

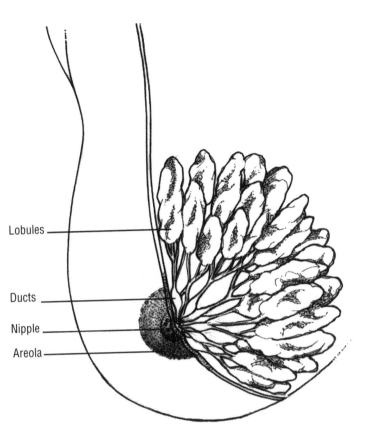

Figure 25.1B. Anatomy of the Breast
The breast is made up of lobules that are connected to ducts that lead to the nipple in the center of the areola.

Lobules

Ducts

Nipple

Areola

them at work when the nipple becomes erect from stimulation or cold; the purpose of this function is to make the nipple more prominent so a baby can nurse. The darkened area around the nipple is called the *areola*; it may be pink, brown, or black, depending on the woman's coloring. The areola contains small glands that lubricate the nipple during breast-feeding. Sometimes, quite normally, these appear as raised bumps on the areola.

Breast development and function depend on two major hormones, estrogen and progesterone, which are produced in a woman's ovaries. Estrogen elongates the ducts and causes them to create side branches. Progesterone increases the number and size of the lobules in order to ready the breast for its major function, nourishing a baby.

Each month, the hormonal environment in a woman's body changes according to the phase of her menstrual cycle. Between the first day of a woman's

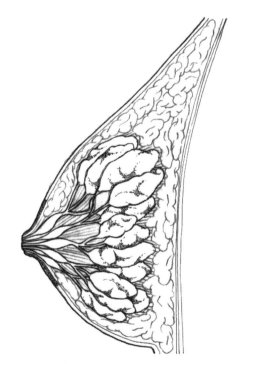
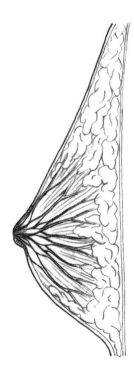

Figure 25.2. Effects of Pregnancy
During pregnancy (left), breasts become larger, and milk glands increase to prepare for breastfeeding.

menstrual period and about 14 days later, when an egg is released from her ovary (ovulation), the breasts are in a relatively dormant state. After ovulation, which occurs midcycle, progesterone makes the breast cells grow and the blood vessels enlarge and fill with blood. At this time, the breasts often become engorged with fluid and may be tender and swollen. This is especially true the week before menstruation.

LACTATION

The biological function of the breast is to feed a woman's offspring. When a woman becomes pregnant, her breasts grow larger and firmer as milk begins to form (See Fig. 25.2). This growth continues until the baby is delivered. If a woman nurses her baby, her breasts will remain firm and become engorged with milk throughout the day. When a woman stops breast-feeding, her breasts will sag and may become smaller than they were before pregnancy. Regardless of whether a woman nurses her baby, her breasts will become softer and more droopy as result of the pregnancy. All of these changes are normal.

CARE OF THE HEALTHY BREAST

A woman's day-to-day routine can include specific ways of supporting her breasts. Many women wear a bra for support and comfort. If a woman exercises, she may want to wear a special sports bra for comfort, to keep her breasts from moving around during exercise. There is no exercise, however, that will keep breasts from sagging, because this is a normal part of aging. Exercising can tone the chest muscles under the breasts, but there is no muscle in the breast itself to be toned, to grow, or to stop sagging. Exercising can help reduce overall body weight, and this in turn may reduce the size of breasts; in turn, weight gain often results in breast enlargement.

Some women use lotions on their breasts, but there is no need to treat breast skin differently from the skin of the rest of the body. Women who expose their breasts to the sun should always wear sun screen. The skin of the breasts is just as vulnerable to cancer as the skin on any other part of the body.

Cancer Screening

The single most important way to promote breast health is with regular breast cancer screening. Screening is looking for signs of disease in women with no symptoms. Some screening is done by the woman herself, and other screening is done by her health care professional. Both are important in finding cancer early, when it can be treated most successfully.

Compared with other cancers, breast cancers are quite slow growing in most women. On average it takes between eight and ten years for one breast cancer cell to grow and multiply to the point where it can be detected as an abnormal mammogram (8 years) or a lump in the breast (10 years).

Breast cancer screening involves self-examination, clinical breast examination (physical examination of the breast by a physician or nurse), and mammography (breast X-rays). Recommendations about the type and timing of screening by health care providers are hotly debated in the medical community, centering primarily on when routine mammography should begin and how often it should be done in women of specific ages. AMWA recommends the schedule shown in the box. These are the guidelines promulgated by the American Cancer Society. A woman and her doctor should decide together how often she should be screened.

One important consideration is a woman's family history. A woman with a first-degree relative (a mother, sister, or daughter) with breast cancer is at greater risk of developing breast cancer herself. She will need to be screened earlier and more often. Other factors that affect a woman's risk for cancer are shown in the box on risk factors. But 80 percent of women who develop breast cancer have no family history, so it is vital that all women undergo regular breast cancer screening. With early detection, breast cancer can be curable. Breast cancer screening could save your life.

Breast Self-Examination

If you don't already examine your breasts monthly, start now. If you examine yourself every month at the same time of the month, you can become familiar with

BREAST SCREENING GUIDELINES

Guidelines for breast screening depend on a woman's age. Recommendations for how often screening should be done are shown in the chart below. Clinical examination is an exam by a physician or nurse.

Age	Self-Examination	Clinical Examination	Mammography
20–39	Monthly	At least every three years	Not recommended
40–49	Monthly	Annually	Every year or every other year
50 and up	Monthly	Annually	Annually

RISK FACTORS FOR BREAST CANCER

Increased Risk

- Family history of breast cancer, especially in mother, daughter, or sister
- Older age (the older the woman, the higher the risk)
- No pregnancies or pregnancy after age 30
- Menstrual periods starting at a young age (under 10)
- Late menopause (over 52)

what your normal breast tissue feels like. If you are still menstruating, choose the week after your period for your self-exam. If you no longer menstruate, choose any time of the month (the first Saturday, for example, or your birth date) and follow that schedule. You may also want to examine your breasts soon after your health care provider does, since everything should be normal then.

Breast self-examination is simple to do. The basic steps are shown in the box below. Your doctor or nurse also can show you how.

At first, self-examination can be confusing. What should you expect to feel? The normal breast of a woman who has not gone through menopause feels bumpy. This is because the milk–producing cells form little "nests" between the fat cells. These nests increase in size at ovulation, which is why breasts are more bumpy at that time in the cycle. Following menopause, the nests of cells shrink and just the fat is left behind.

That's why normal breasts in postmenopausal women feel smoother.

One way to tell what's normal and what's not is to compare the two breasts side by side. For example, if you feel something "different" in the tissue near the underarm, examine the same spot by the opposite breast. If the areas feel the same, there is usually little need for worry. If the other side doesn't feel the same, however, there may be cause for concern. Call your doctor with any doubts or concerns.

Clinical Breast Examination

A clinical breast examination can be done by a woman's regular doctor or by a nurse in the doctor's office. The exam is most often done along with a routine pelvic exam and Pap test (the test for cervical cancer; see Chapter 37). If your doctor doesn't routinely examine your breasts, you should insist that she or he do so; if this isn't possible, find a different doctor.

The clinical breast exam is much like the breast self-exam you should do each month. It can vary a bit from doctor to doctor, however. A woman should try to schedule her breast exam for the week after her period, especially if she is worried about the results of her self-exam. This way, her breasts are less likely to be tender or swollen, and any abnormalities will be easier to notice.

Mammography

The third line of defense in maintaining breast health is mammography, or breast X-ray. It can be used for routine screening in women without symptoms or, if a problem is suspected, to aid in diagnosis. In mammography, the breasts are placed, one at a time, between two plastic plates. Pressure is applied to make the breast as thin as possible. Some women find this pres-

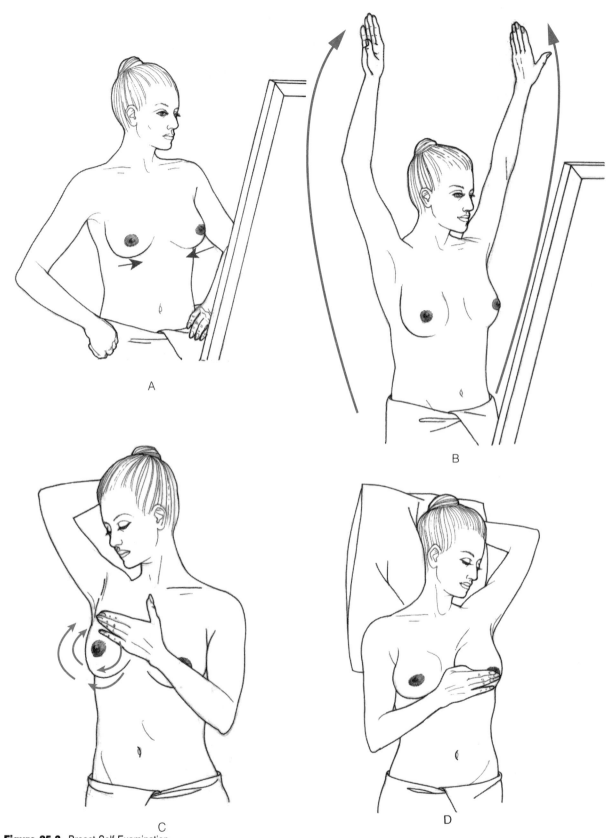

Figure 25.3. Breast Self-Examination
Breast self-examination should be performed monthly. In order to detect changes, a woman should become familiar with the normal shape and feel of her breasts. (See the box on the facing page—"Breast Self-Examination.")

sure painful, but it's necessary. The more the breast is compressed, the lower the radiation dose necessary and the better the image produced. (If you are still menstruating, it may be less painful if you have the exam right after your period.) Each breast is X-rayed in two views, a vertical view and a horizontal view. The X-ray that results from the exam—the mammogram—will be studied by a doctor for any signs of problems.

DETECTING AND PREVENTING BREAST CANCER

Having routine mammograms is critical. The test is capable of detecting breast cancer before it can be felt, when it is very small. The smaller breast cancer is when it is detected, the less chance it will have spread, and the greater the possibility of treatment that does not involve breast removal. Mammograms save lives; the death rate from breast cancer can be reduced 30 percent in women 50 and over who get mammograms at regular time periods.

Like any medical test, mammography has its limitations. It is less effective in young women who have what radiologists (physicians who specialize in use of X-rays) refer to as dense breasts. The breasts are normal, but they do not photograph well on the X-ray. When milk-producing cells and ducts are X-rayed, they appear white—the same color as an abnormality such as cancer cells. Therefore, the denser the woman's breasts, the less likely it is that a breast cancer will be detected by a mammogram. There is at least a 15 percent false-negative rate with mammography. This means the mammogram appears to show no abnormality when in fact there is a problem. In these cases, breast cancer will be diagnosed by physical examination alone.

BREAST SELF-EXAMINATION

1. Stand or sit in front of a mirror with your arms at your sides. Look for any changes in the breast, such as dimpling, redness, or different breast size or shape (A).

2. Look for the same signs with your hands on your hips (B) and then with your arms over your head (C).

3. Lying on your back, put your right arm over your head and use your left arm to examine your right breast. Palpate (press with the fingers), using dime-sized circles, moving in ever smaller circles from the outside of the breast toward the nipple. Cover the entire breast (D).

4. Feel the underarm area.

5. Switch to the other side and do steps 3–4 on that side. (See Fig. 25.3, A–D, facing page.)

Generally, mammogram results are classified into one of the following groups:

- Normal (no abnormalities on the X-ray)
- Benign abnormality (changes seen, but they are likely not cancer)
- Indeterminate (changes seen are probably benign but possibly cancerous)
- Suspicious
- Cancer until proven otherwise.

Depending on your results, there are a number of tests that may be done to diagnose the problem. You and your doctor will decide together what steps to take.

For a mammogram to be most accurate, it's critical that the X-ray equipment be of the best quality. Federal legislation in 1992 set laws on equipment quality. To find out about mammography machines in your area, call the American Cancer Society at 1–800–ACS–2345. The society can give you the names of mammography facilities in your area that are accredited by the American College of Radiology.

The need for breast cancer screening never stops. The chances of developing breast cancer rise as a woman ages. Therefore, it should always be a part of her life, just like Pap tests and trips to the dentist.

Cancer Prevention

While methods for detection are well studied, less is known about breast cancer prevention. Current research could take years to yield answers. One promising area is the use of the drug tamoxifen to prevent breast cancer. This synthetic hormone is also used to treat breast cancer. Researchers are also looking for a link between low-fat diet and lower rates of breast cancer. This is suggested from animal tests, but tests in women are not yet conclusive.

DISEASES AND CONDITIONS OF THE BREAST

Breast Cancer

The single greatest health concern regarding breasts is breast cancer. Here are some facts:

- Depending on how long a woman lives, her lifetime risk of getting breast cancer can be as high as 1 in 8.
- In the 1990s, almost 2 million women will be diagnosed with breast cancer.
- Breast cancer is the most common cancer in women.
- Breast cancer is the second leading cause of death from cancer, after lung cancer.
- Of women diagnosed with breast cancer, 80 percent have no family history or other risk factor except gender and age.

The good news is that early detection may mean cure. Regular breast exams and mammography, as recommended, can catch cancer early, when treatment is more likely to succeed.

Symptoms and Signs of Breast Cancer

There are a number of warning signs of breast problems, many of which are symptoms that a woman can detect herself (see box below). These symptoms do not necessarily mean cancer is present. They are warnings that further investigation is needed.

Breast lump

Most commonly a woman herself or her partner finds a lump, a hard area of breast tissue that stands out from the normal surrounding breast tissue when that spot is touched or examined. The lump can be as small as the size of a pea. The term "lump" refers to any firm tissue that is not present in the same location in the opposite breast, even if it feels like a thickening rather than an actual lump. Other than the lump, a woman generally will have no symptoms. In some cases, there may be some tenderness near the lump.

Nipple discharge

If discharge occurs only on nipple stimulation, it is normal. However, if discharge emerges on its own (staining underthings or bedsheets), a woman should see her doctor. A discharge from only one breast is more likely to be a symptom of cancer than if both breasts are involved.

Skin redness

Redness is always a cause for concern. It can mean an infection or cancer, especially when a woman is not breast-feeding. It should be checked by a doctor.

Breast pain

In very rare cases, breast pain may indicate cancer, especially when the pain is at the site of a lump or thickening. (See Fig. 25.4)

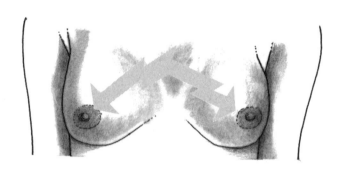

Figure 25.4. Lumps
Breast pain may occur at the site of a lump.

SYMPTOMS OF BREAST DISEASE

See your doctor if you have any of the following:

- Breast lump
- Nipple discharge that leaves a stain on clothing
- Breast pain
- Skin redness
- Nipple scaling
- Skin puckering or dimpling
- Any unexplained changes in how the breast feels or appears

Nipple scaling

If the nipple shows flaking or scaling, this can be a symptom of cancer even if no lump can be felt and the mammogram is normal. (See Fig. 25.5)

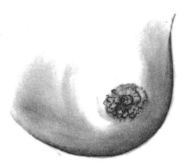

Figure 25.5. Scaling
Scaling of the nipple may be a sign of cancer.

Skin puckering or dimpling

If there is a growth in the breast, it may pull at the breast skin and cause puckers or dimples to appear.

In addition to these symptoms, abnormal results on a mammogram may be a sign that something is wrong. Mammography can sometimes find a tumor years before the woman herself would feel it. Not every abnormality is cancer; an abnormal mammogram usually suggests that further testing needs to be done. Mammograms will also miss some cancers that can be felt, which is why self-examination and clinical examination by a doctor or nurse are so important.

Diagnostic Procedures

If a woman has any symptoms of cancer or if she has had an abnormal mammogram, a number of procedures may be recommended to diagnose the problem. Some of the more common ones are described here.

Diagnostic mammography

This procedure uses the same technique as screening mammography. More views of the breast may be needed, so it may take longer. Mammography can also be used to assist with breast biopsy.

Ultrasound

Ultrasound, a diagnostic test that uses sound waves to make images of tissues, is most commonly done if a mammogram suggests there is a problem. It helps define whether an abnormality is a cyst (fluid-filled sac) or a solid mass.

Fine needle aspiration

A small needle is used to withdraw a sample from a breast lump. If the lump is a cyst (fluid-filled sac), aspiration of the fluid will cause the lump to disappear. If the lump is solid, cells can be smeared onto slides for examination in the laboratory. Aspiration does not remove solid lumps, it samples them. The test takes 30 to 60 seconds and can be performed in the doctor's office.

Core needle biopsy

This procedure is similar to fine needle aspiration. In it, a larger needle is used because actual breast tissue is removed, not just a few cells. A sample of the lump is obtained, but the whole lump is not removed. Core needle biopsies can be done when a mammogram detects a lump that cannot be felt; under these circumstances, a special machine is necessary to accurately locate the abnormality. This procedure is usually done by a surgeon or a radiologist. The area is numbed with local anesthetic, and the woman will feel some pressure.

Biopsy

In most breast biopsies, the entire lump is removed surgically. The tissue is then studied under a microscope. If a rim of normal breast tissue is taken all the way around a lump (lumpectomy), biopsy can also serve as part of breast cancer treatment. A breast biopsy is almost always done on an outpatient basis, under a local anesthetic. Some women are given a sedative as well. The procedure takes about an hour.

As a general rule, biopsies are done for these reasons:

- A solid mass persists after a menstrual cycle
- A solid mass is found in a woman who does not ovulate
- Cyst fluid contains blood
- A cyst does not completely disappear after aspiration
- A cyst comes back in the same spot on the breast within two to six weeks of an aspiration
- An asymmetrical abnormality persists.

In cases in which breast abnormalities must be removed but cannot be felt on physical examination, a special procedure called a needle localization will be done. During the localization the radiologist finds the abnormality with a needle, takes a mammogram, and repositions the needle as accurately as possible. A wire then replaces the needle, and the patient is sent to the operating room for the biopsy. Sometimes dye is used with the wire or instead of the wire.

Cancer staging

If the biopsy shows cancer, the pathologist will classify it. Cancer can arise in either of two basic breast parts: the lobules or the ducts.

Once the type of cancer is known, other tests—including lymph node removal in many cases—need to be done to determine if the cancer has spread, and if so, where. (See Fig. 25.6) Tests that may be used include blood tests, chest X-rays, and scans of the liver or bone. This process is called staging. It places the cancer in one of 5 groups, ranked 0 through 4. The higher the number, the more the disease has spread and the lower the chance for a cure. Staging helps the doctor decide on the type of treatment that has the best chance for a cure.

Stage 0 is also called cancer in situ. This means that the cancer is still in a strictly limited location. For example, stage 0 cancer of the duct cells is found only in duct cells and is confined to the inside of the duct. In stages 1–4, the cancer is invasive: it has spread outside its place of origin (for example, a cancer that started in the ducts is now in the surrounding tissue.)

Most breast cancer (88 percent) is invasive when detected. In stage 1 it is confined to the breast. In stages 2–4 it has spread to the adjacent lymph nodes in the armpit or metastasized (spread) to other parts of the body.

Treatment

The treatment for an individual woman will depend on what type of tumor she has (lobular or ductal), how large the tumor is, whether it is invasive or in situ, and, if it is invasive, whether it has spread to the lymph nodes or to distant parts of the body. Treatment for breast cancer usually begins with surgery to remove the tumor.

- *Breast Conservation.* The tumor and a surrounding ridge of tissue are removed. In case of invasive cancer, lymph nodes from under the arm are often removed for staging. Lumpectomy can be done if there is only one small tumor that has not spread. In many cases, lumpectomy plus radiation gives a woman the same chance for survival as the treatment formerly favored, mastectomy (removal of the breast).

- *Mastectomy.* Mastectomy involves removal of the breast.

  In a *modified radical mastectomy*, all of the breast and the adjacent lymph nodes in the armpit are removed. In a *radical mastectomy*, the chest muscles under the breast are also removed. Today, this is done only when the cancer involves the chest muscles and is rarely needed.

The decision about what type of surgery a woman should have can be a difficult one for a woman to make. Once a woman learns that she has cancer, she will usually be able to take time to discuss treatment options with her doctor and her family, and to begin to adjust to the idea of having breast cancer. Today, doctors know that there is no harm in waiting 2 weeks or so to reach a decision the woman prefers. In the past testing and treatment were done together. In this one-step approach, a woman would agree before her biopsy that if cancer were present, the breast would be removed right then, while she was still anesthetized. She had only one surgery, but she also didn't know whether she'd wake up minus a breast.

Following surgery, a woman often will have radiation therapy, especially if she had a lumpectomy. This is done to destroy any remaining cancer cells in the breast. The treatment is begun as soon as the wound from surgery heals. It usually lasts about 6 weeks. Radiation treatment is given by a type of radiologist called a radiation oncologist. Each treatment takes a few minutes. Radiation treatment is local—it is directed to the affected site. Side effects may include a skin reaction such as a sunburn effect or rash, fatigue, and a low white blood cell count (which increases a woman's risk of infection), especially toward the end of treatment. Most women are able to continue their normal routine.

A woman may also have chemotherapy or hormonal therapy, depending on the type of cancer and how far it has advanced. The purpose of these therapies is to treat any possible tumor cells that may have traveled from the tumor site, perhaps to other body parts. These treatments are systemic—they are circulated through the body in the bloodstream—so side effects can occur throughout the body.

Women who have no signs of cancer in their lymph

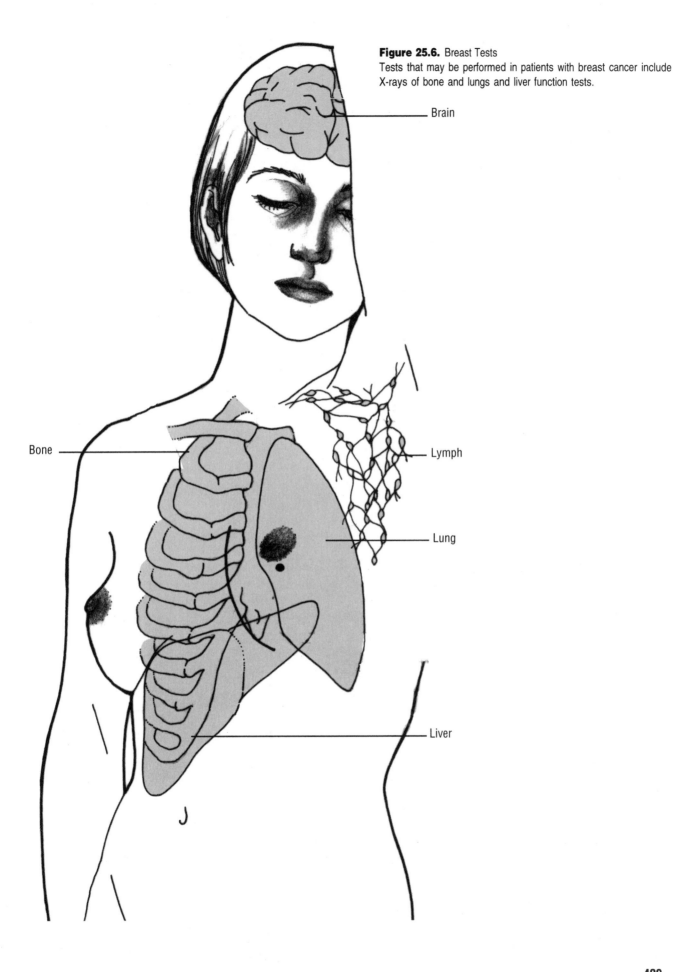

Figure 25.6. Breast Tests
Tests that may be performed in patients with breast cancer include X-rays of bone and lungs and liver function tests.

Brain

Bone

Lymph

Lung

Liver

nodes and women who have not gone through menopause will usually be given low doses of chemotherapy (anticancer drugs). Women who have cancer cells in their lymph nodes will get higher doses of chemotherapy. Chemotherapy works by poisoning the cancer cells, but it affects some normal cells, too, so there are side effects including hair loss, nausea, vomiting, and decreased numbers of cells made by the bone marrow (which increases a woman's risk of infection). Generally, chemotherapy is given by mouth or intravenously (into a vein) over the course of 3 to 6 months. The side effects almost always end when the course of treatment ends. There are differences of opinion regarding types of drugs to use, in what combinations, and in what dosages. Every case must be evaluated individually.

Before hormone therapy is offered, tests may be done to determine whether the cancer has estrogen and progesterone receptors. Having these receptors is a good sign: women with them are more likely to respond to hormone treatment and have an improved chance of survival. If a woman has this type of breast cancer, she will be offered a hormone, *tamoxifen.* It blocks the effects of estrogen on the breast and thus stops the growth of the cancer. The treatment may last for a number of years. Women treated with tamoxifen have a lower incidence of cancer in the other breast. Side effects include symptoms of menopause—hot flashes and vaginal dryness.

Some studies suggest that women who take tamoxifen have an increased risk of developing cancer in the lining of the uterus. For this reason, regular exams—and sometimes biopsies—of the lining of the uterus are usually done in women taking tamoxifen. There is now research being conducted to determine whether tamoxifen will prevent breast cancer in women who are at high risk, but who have not yet been diagnosed with breast cancer.

Breast Reconstruction

If a woman has had a breast removed because of cancer, she may want to consider breast reconstruction. A woman contemplating reconstructive surgery needs to make several choices; the most obvious one is whether to have the surgery. Only 30 percent of women who have mastectomies choose breast reconstruction. This choice shouldn't affect how they choose to have their cancer treated, although desire for reconstruction should be discussed with the surgeon treating the cancer. The way cancer surgery is done can affect whether and how reconstruction is done. The decision-making process should involve not only the patient and her

cancer surgeon but also the surgeon doing the reconstruction (a plastic and reconstructive surgeon).

Factors to consider in the decision about reconstructive surgery include the woman's medical condition and degree of tissue loss, the need for additional therapy, and her general health. Reconstruction can be more painful and difficult than the original cancer operation, so all factors should be carefully considered.

Psychological factors must be evaluated as well; some women feel that only reconstruction can put an end to the trauma of losing a breast. Women who choose reconstruction often experience profound improvement in their mental attitude afterward. But each woman will have to evaluate for herself whether reconstruction will help her get on with her life after breast cancer.

If a woman chooses not to have reconstructive surgery, she can use an external prosthesis (artificial breast) worn inside her clothing. A woman's appearance in clothes, as well as her level of physical activity, will influence how comfortable she'll be using a prosthesis.

If a woman chooses reconstructive surgery, it sometimes can be done at the same time as the surgery for cancer. (See Chapter 36). Other times, it will be done in a later operation. Some of the types of procedures that may be done include the following:

- Insertion of a saline or silicone implant, often after tissue expansion (but note new FDA restrictions on silicone implants)
- Use of the woman's own muscles (taken from the back, abdomen, or buttock) to reconstruct the breast
- Reconstruction of the nipple and areola.

These methods, how they are done, and their side effects are covered in Chapter 36.

Support for Women with Cancer

It's important that a woman who has breast cancer consider all the support services she can. A recent study showed that women who belonged to a support group had a higher rate of survival than women who had the same physical treatment but no support group. The American Cancer Society, the local hospital, physicians, and local therapists or counseling centers can help you find a support group. Some women are motivated to start a group. For many women this action not only helps them cope better but also may determine the extent of their physical recovery.

Diagnosis of Benign Lumps

To the touch, a cyst can feel like a solid lump, so much of the workup for a cyst will be the same as for a solid lump. Your doctor will take a history and examine you to confirm what you've found (if in fact the woman herself has detected a problem). Be sure to tell the doctor exactly where the lump is located, how long it has been present, how big it is, if it has changed during your monthly cycle, and if it is tender.

If you are age 30 or older, mammography will usually be done. An ultrasound exam may be done to see whether the lump is fluid filled (a cyst) or solid. If a lump can be felt, it is usually better to have a fine needle aspiration. If the lump is a cyst, it will disappear as a consequence of the aspiration and is thereby treated at the same time it's diagnosed. No further treatment is required. Because so few cysts contain abnormal cells, it's not routine to send fluid for laboratory examination unless it is bloody, which might indicate cancer. If the lump doesn't go away following aspiration, a biopsy should be performed.

Cosmetic Surgery

The decision to have breast surgery to alter appearance is a very personal one, involving complex issues of self-esteem, body image, even personal empowerment. It's a decision a woman needs to make carefully.

Breasts can be either enlarged or reduced. For either type of surgery, a woman should get complete information from her doctor about how the procedure is done, the risks, and what type of final appearance to expect. Because breast enlargement is a cosmetic procedure done on healthy breasts, it is not usually covered by health insurance. Breast enlargement and reduction are described in Chapter 36.

Breast Infections

The main symptom of breast infection is inflammation—redness and pain in the breast or any part of it. There are three possible causes.

- *Lactational mastitis.* This is a buildup of bacteria caused by a plugged milk duct in a woman who is breast-feeding. The diagnosis is usually based on the woman's history and physical exam findings; no special tests are needed. Treatment involves using hot compresses and hot showers in which the water is allowed to flow over the breast. If symptoms don't ease within 24 hours, antibiotics will be added. It's fine to continue nursing; neither the antibiotics nor the bacteria will harm the baby, and keeping the breasts emptied will ease the woman's discomfort.

- *Nonlactational mastitis.* Causes of this infection vary, but the symptoms resemble those of lactational mastitis. It is diagnosed and treated the same way.

- *Chronic subareolar abscess.* This is an uncommon infection in the oil glands around the nipple. It is difficult to treat; antibiotics may help, but usually surgical drainage becomes necessary. Since this is a chronic—or recurring—condition, the involved duct and tract are often removed; sometimes all of the ducts have to be removed. Very rarely, the entire nipple and areola have to be removed to control the infection. A woman should not have a mastectomy for this condition unless all previous measures have failed.

Noncancerous Breast Lumps

Not every breast lump is a sign of cancer. There are three common types of benign (noncancerous) breast lumps.

- *Fibrocystic changes.* Many women who have not yet gone through menopause have occasional pain or overall lumpiness in their breasts. These changes are called *fibrocystic changes.* It is natural for breast tissue to change in degree of "lumpiness" throughout a woman's hormonal cycle and also as she ages. The female hormones estrogen and progesterone are thought to be somehow involved in fibrocystic changes, but the cause is not known for sure. The tissue usually returns to normal after menstruation. After menopause, women's breasts become smoother in texture. Because these changes are so common and so little is known about their cause, they are hard to treat and cannot really be cured. Treatments that have been used include vitamins and advice to stay away from caffeine and chocolate. None of these has been a complete success. Breast pain can be treated by wearing a well-fitting bra, using pain medication, and limiting fluids, especially before the menstrual period. Fibrocystic changes do not increase the risk of cancer.

■ *Cyst.* This is a fluid-filled sac that usually occurs in women in their 40s and early 50s. It is caused by reabsorption of the breast lobules that occurs naturally as a woman approaches menopause. Cysts may be present on and off for several years; often they occur in groups. They are almost always harmless, but it is impossible to distinguish between a cyst or a

solid breast mass simply by feeling it, so aspiration or a biopsy will usually be recommended.

■ *Fibroadenoma.* This is a solid lump found mostly in women in their 20s and 30s. It results from excess formation of the lobules (milk-producing glands) and stroma (the connective tissue in the breast). The lump feels round and smooth, and often "shoots" to a different part of the breast when pushed upon. Such lumps are rarely cancerous, but usually should be biopsied just to be sure.

RESOURCES FOR MORE INFORMATION

The National Cancer Institute (NCI) is a good resource for information and publications about cancer-related subjects. Call the Cancer Information Service (800-4CANCER). The general public can receive information by fax as well; call 301-402-5874 from a Touch-Tone phone and follow the directions.

It a woman facing chemotherapy would like more information about individual drugs, she can call the NCI at 800-422-6237 and ask for "Anticancer Drug Information Sheets" for her particular drug.

Another source of information is the American Cancer Society (800-ACS-2345).

CHAPTER 26

The Respiratory System

Claudia S. Plottel, M.D., F.C.C.P

The respiratory system's functions include oxygen uptake, carbon dioxide removal, and balancing of the body's acid and base status. These functions occur through breathing, which is an automatic event. Diseases of the lung itself may affect breathing, and disorders in other organs can also express themselves in altered lung function.

STRUCTURE AND FUNCTION

The respiratory system is made up of the upper respiratory tract and the lower respiratory tract, along with the chest wall and its muscles. The upper respiratory tract consists of the nose, throat, sinuses, larynx (voice box), and vocal cords; it is described in Chapter 24. The lower respiratory tract is made up of the trachea (windpipe), bronchial tubes, the lungs and their covering called the pleura, and the diaphragm. (See Fig. 26.1)

The alveoli are highly specialized lung units that can be visualized as little air sacs encircled by a network of fine blood vessels called capillaries. Between the alveolus and the capillary blood network is a very fine membrane called the alveolar capillary membrane, an interface between the outside world we inhale and the internal milieu of the body. It is across this alveolar capillary membrane that respiration and gas exchange take place.

Organs

The basic function of the lungs is to exchange oxygen inhaled from the atmosphere for carbon dioxide, a metabolic waste product exhaled from the body. This process is called respiration.

Air is first inhaled through the nose, where it is warmed and where small hairlike structures called cilia filter out any impurities or particles. The air then passes through the structures of the upper airway, through the vocal cords, and into the trachea, which is the main breathing tube that leads to the lungs. The trachea divides at the carina into a right and a left branch, which are referred to as the right mainstem bronchus and the left mainstem bronchus. Each bronchus leads to its own lung.

After the trachea splits into right and left bronchi, those bronchi divide further, into divisions that lead to the various lobes of each lung. On the right there are three lobes: the upper, the middle, and the lower. The left lung has an upper division which splits into an upper lobe and into a lingula, and a lower lung division. Each mainstem bronchus splits into an upper, middle, and a lower division, and then into bronchioles. This system, often referred to as a branching tree, permits inhaled air that is oxygen rich to reach the lung alveoli.

Blood

Blood that bathes our bodies' organs is returned to the heart in an oxygen-poor, carbon dioxide-rich state. The carbon dioxide represents metabolic by-products. After the blood enters chambers of the right heart, it then passes into the lung through the capillary network. At the level of the alveolus, the oxygen-rich inhaled air comes into contact with this capillary blood supply. The oxygen from the inhaled air then passes into the capillary blood for distribution to the rest of the body, and carbon dioxide, which is a metabolic waste product, leaves the capillary blood and enters the alveolus. From there, the carbon dioxide within the alveolus is exhaled. The lungs' basic function is to exchange oxygen from the atmosphere that is inhaled for carbon dioxide, which is then excreted and removed from the body. This process is called respiration.

Along with the kidney, the lung is an effective organ for removing carbon dioxide; therefore, it plays a crucial role in maintaining the body's acid-base exchange. The body produces acids and bases in set quantities that must achieve a balance to maintain the body's homeostasis, or state of equilibrium. The kidneys and lungs regulate this delicate balance. In certain disease states, the body may produce an excess of acid

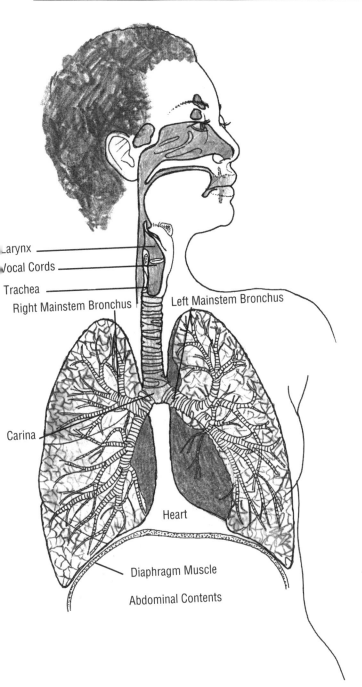

Larynx

Vocal Cords

Trachea

Right Mainstem Bronchus

Left Mainstem Bronchus

Carina

Heart

Diaphragm Muscle

Abdominal Contents

Figure 26.1 The Respiratory System

or base, disrupting the balance. The acid that is produced is chemically related to carbon dioxide. As the body produces more carbon dioxide from acid, the lungs excrete additional carbon dioxide. This is how the lungs help to maintain the acid-base balance (see Chapter 32 for more detail about this process).

Breathing

Respiration, or breathing, is an automatic event. We breathe during our sleep and, while healthy, we breathe without even being conscious or aware of it. Breathing is controlled by special centers in the brain; they are sensitive to messages from the body to increase or decrease respiration depending on the body's needs.

The chest wall and muscles move in and out as we breathe. The major muscle of respiration is the diaphragm, which is a large muscle that separates the chest cavity from the abdominal cavity. Other muscles playing an important part in respiration include the muscles between the ribs, called the intercostal muscles, as well as the muscles of the neck and shoulder area. Respiratory dysfunction can occur if the diaphragm is weakened or paralyzed, or if the nerve supply from the brain to the diaphragm or accessory muscles between the ribs is damaged or impaired.

The pleura is a very fine membrane that surrounds the lung. In fact, there are two pleura. The visceral pleura is closer to the lung than the parietal pleura, which is immediately adjacent to the visceral pleura. They are separated by a space. In certain disease states, the pleura can become inflamed, as in the case of pleurisy, and fluid can accumulate between the two pleural surfaces. This is often referred to as a pleural effusion or water on the lung. The integrity of the pleura is crucial for the maintenance of the lungs in a full or inflated state. If there is damage to the surface of the pleura, a pocket of air may collect in the pleural space, causing a collapsed lung (pneumothorax).

HEALTH PROFESSIONALS IN RESPIRATORY DISEASE

Internist—nonsurgical specialist
Pulmonologist—specialist in diseases of the lung
Thoracic surgeon—specialist in surgery of the chest
Oncologist—specialist in cancer
Infectious disease specialist
Intensive care specialist
Respiratory therapist—exercise and treatment specialist

KEEPING THE SYSTEM HEALTHY

We breathe an average of 15 times a minute during quiet breathing and more quickly during exertion and in the course of various illnesses. A normal individual exchanges approximately 6 liters of air in each minute, for 60 minutes an hour, 24 hours a day, 365 days a year. Substances that are inhaled could be absorbed via the alveoli into our bloodstream. The lungs, however, have a filtering system that allows only certain microscopic particles of defined size to actually reach the alveoli. Because of the lungs' capacity to absorb substances, we can administer medications by this route.

General health measures that maintain overall well-being benefit your respiratory system as well. Follow a balanced, healthy diet, exercise approximately three times a week, devote time to relaxation and leisure activities, and get adequate sleep. Always take any medications as prescribed and, of course, never take any medications that have been prescribed for others. If any respiratory symptoms develop and persist, do not hesitate to contact your doctor (see "Health Professionals in Respiratory Disease"). Early treatment is usually effective and, in many cases, can prevent more serious problems.

A common substance absorbed by the respiratory system is nicotine from cigarette smoking. Inhaling the products of tobacco smoke is harmful to the lungs. Cigarette smoking causes certain types of lung cancer and other respiratory diseases such as chronic bronchitis and emphysema. Smokers have upper respiratory tract infections more often and smoking increases the risk of cardiovascular disease and stroke.

Pregnant women who smoke have an increased risk of complications during pregnancy, and their babies are often small at birth and have problems. Children raised in smokers' homes are more likely to have asthma; even as nonsmoking adults, they have an increased risk of lung cancer years later as compared to those not exposed to passive cigarette smoke. Children raised in the home of smokers often smoke as adults.

It would be a major advance in public health if all cigarette smoking ceased. If you smoke you should stop, not only for your respiratory health but also for that of your family, close contacts, and children. Exposure to passive smoke has been shown to be carcinogenic. If you have children, raise them in a smokefree home and urge them not to smoke. (See Chapter 7).

Stopping smoking can be very difficult. Different programs and approaches to stopping smoking exist, yet no approach can be successful until the smoker herself truly wants to stop. Basically, she needs to decide herself that the time has come to quit. She should then enlist the assistance of loved ones and friends and should consult with her physician, who can help her achieve her goal and find the proper support resources.

Hazardous Substances

Substances such as radon, asbestos, and solvents also can be harmful if inhaled. Women should be aware of these agents and their effects and try to reduce or minimize exposure to them.

Radon has been known to be a potent lung carcinogen in exposed populations; historically these have been uranium miners. More recently we have discovered that homes constructed on top of areas contaminated with various radioactive substances may accumulate radon in doses high enough to prove harmful. If you are concerned about radon in your home, check your radon levels by comparing them to acceptable levels as defined by the Environmental Protection Agency.

Another substance known to cause respiratory disease is asbestos, a fiber highly valued for its insulating properties. When asbestos is in place it is not harmful. During the installation or removal of asbestos, however, workers disturb it, sending the fibers airborne where asbestos is inhaled and becomes harmful. Disease related to asbestos was first found in miners of the substance. Now we know that workers who installed asbestos are at risk for lung disease, as are their spouses who laundered the workers' clothing.

There is a long latent period between the exposure to asbestos and the development of disease. Exposed individuals often are free of symptoms for 20 to 40 years until lung disease develops. Lung problems related to asbestos include lung cancer, as well as a rare cancer of the lung lining called mesothelioma. Asbestos also causes noncancerous conditions such as pleural plaques, where calcium is deposited along the lung lining (pleura), and pleural effusions where fluid collects around the lung.

Not all exposure to asbestos leads to lung disease. Generally, disease-causing exposure must be either

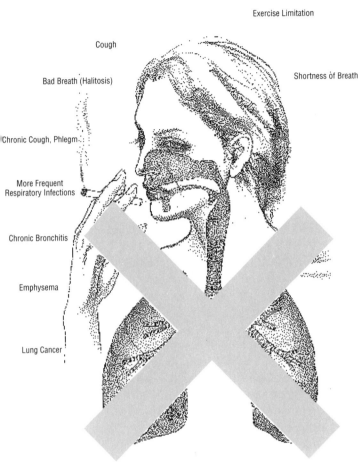

Exercise Limitation

Cough

Bad Breath (Halitosis)

Chronic Cough, Phlegm.

More Frequent
Respiratory Infections

Chronic Bronchitis

Emphysema

Lung Cancer

Shortness of Breath

Figure 26.2 Cigarette-Related Pulmonary Illnesses and Symptoms

very brief and intense or sustained at low levels over time. Much controversy has surrounded the issue of asbestos removal from older buildings. Many believe that asbestos in good condition should be left in place. If there is doubt that the asbestos is in good condition, however, or if it is breaking down and releasing particles into the environment, it should be removed. Asbestos must be removed in a particular way by a licensed contractor and disposed of according to state and local regulations.

Other inhaled substances that could damage your respiratory system include certain solvents, fumes, or chemicals. Some hobbies or professions may require special precautions. Electronic enthusiasts who solder, for example, should learn the proper technique. Jewelry makers, artists, sculptors, metal workers or sanders, painters, and do-it-yourself renovators should read product labels carefully and work in a well-ventilated space. We recommend wearing the respirator cup masks sold in hardware stores to protect your respiratory system.

Respiratory problems can result from rapid changes in atmospheric pressure. Scuba diving or deep-sea diving carries a risk. Precautions include proper training and technique, certification by a diving school, and common sense. Similarly, women who hike or trek at high altitudes should be familiar with the pulmonary edema and lung problems that can occur with rapid ascent and improper acclimatization. Gradual ascent and a medication called acetazolamide can help avoid serious problems, so you may wish to consult with your physician before your trip. (See Fig. 26.2)

HEALTH CONCERNS

Respiration is a vital function and anything that interferes with it can be potentially serious. Respiratory diseases can be acute, coming on suddenly, or they can be chronic, or long lasting.

Disorders in the respiratory system can affect its own function and that of other organs. They can be as minor as the flu or as major as diseases that can shut down the vital function of the heart as well as the lungs. Even seemingly minor disorders can become major, so it is important that symptoms, especially if they persist, be reported to a doctor.

Symptoms

A great many illnesses can affect the lungs—from cancers to infections to inherited problems—yet most have a limited number of symptoms that are often similar. Normally, none of these symptoms should be present. In health, we should have no awareness of our breathing and it should be completely automatic, quiet, and painless. When symptoms occur, their persistence over time warrants a visit to a physician.

Cough

Cough is a reflex and usually reflects a respiratory illness. It may be a manifestation of a simple cold or may indicate a potentially life-threatening disease such as cancer. Cough is not normal. It may be accompanied by sputum or phlegm, in which case it is called "productive," or it may be dry or "nonproductive." When blood is coughed up, hemoptysis is said to be present. A persistent cough, a change in cough, or a cough that awakens someone at night warrants a visit to the doctor.

The causes of cough are varied and include infections (such as pneumonia, influenza, bronchitis, or tuberculosis), cancer, asthma, and chronic obstructive lung disease, as well as sarcoidosis and others. Cough can also be due to illnesses of the heart and the gastrointestinal track.

Dyspnea

In health, we should have no awareness of breathing, which is an automatic event. Shortness of breath, at rest or during exercise, is a sign of lung or heart disease. This can occur with conditions such as asthma, emphysema, bronchitis, pneumonia or sarcoidosis.

Pain

A sharp severe pain in the chest that occurs during breathing may be caused by inflammation of the pleura, rib fractures, or muscles injuries.

Sounds

When examining the chest with a stethoscope the doctor is listening for abnormal sounds. Wheezes occur with asthma, crackles and squeaks with pneumonia, rubbing sounds with pleural disease.

Diagnosis

The physician must track down the cause of symptoms and can use a number of diagnostic tools to do so. The initial step is taking a complete and detailed history. The history includes events relating to the current symptom that brought the patient to the physician, any past medical or surgical illnesses, any present illnesses, smoking habits, and information on any relevant occupational and environment factors. Family history is very important to detect an inherited disease. History taking may take 45 minutes to an hour.

The next step is a physical examination. Vital signs, including heart rate and, in particular, breathing rate, are very important. Examination of the chest may include inspection of any sputum that the patient can produce, tapping on the back (percussion), as well as listening to the chest with a stethoscope while the patient breathes quietly and deeply (auscultation).

Examination of other parts of the body often yields clues to lung disease. For instance, a blue discoloration of the nails and sometimes of the lips, called cyanosis, can indicate lack of oxygen or severe anemia. Inspection of the nails can also reveal a deformity called clubbing that is seen in certain pulmonary diseases. For this reason, women should remove nail polish or false nails before they are examined.

Various radiologic evaluations help pinpoint the cause of a respiratory symptom. Such an evaluation may include a chest X-ray. It can be done from various views, straight on from the front or side, lying down, or on a slant. Sometimes a more precise picture of the anatomy is desired; a computed tomography (CT) scan of the chest gives a three-dimensional view of any abnormalities. Although magnetic resonance imaging, or MRI, usually does not provide additional information, it may help define problems that involve the chest wall or the blood vessels in the chest.

In addition to radiologic tests to evaluate anatomy, scans provide a view of the function of the lung. Two such tests are ventilation perfusion scanning and gallium scanning, which are often called nuclear medicine scans. For the test, a radioactive substance is injected intravenously. It concentrates in certain areas of the body and an image is created by a camera sensitive to the drug's effects. Ventilation perfusion scanning may be done when a pulmonary embolus or a clot lodged in the circulatory system of the lung is suspected. Gallium scanning gives information about the overall degree of inflammation within the lung. It is helpful in diagnosing certain infections.

A woman who is pregnant or thinks she is pregnant should inform the doctor and technician before undergoing a radiologic test. Chest X-rays may be performed safely during pregnancy. To guard the fetus, a special lead shield is placed over the woman's abdomen during the test. Except in extraordinary circumstances, nuclear medicine scans should not be performed during pregnancy.

Arterial blood sampling is a simple test that involves removing blood from an artery. Normally blood that has left the lung would be oxygen rich and carbon dioxide poor. Once the arterial blood sample is obtained, it is analyzed for acidity, or pH, and to assess oxygen and carbon dioxide content. This test determines if the patient suffers from lack of oxygen or if additional oxygen is needed.

Pulmonary function testing is a way to assess the dynamic lung as opposed to X-ray tests that provide a still image of the lung. Some pulmonary function tests include measurements of lung capacity, lung volumes, diffusion, compliance, exercise and bronchoprovocation studies, and polysomnography.

Other diagnostic tests involve entering the body while using local anesthesia to either view the inside of the lungs or to obtain a sample or both. These procedures include thoracentesis, pleural biopsy, or flexible fiberoptic bronchoscopy. Surgical procedures performed with general anesthesia include rigid bronchoscopy, mediastinoscopy, thoracoscopy, and open lung biopsy (see "Procedures").

Disorders

Among the most frequent illnesses in our society are respiratory ailments that are diseases of flow, sometimes referred to as diseases of the airways. Even though these illnesses are varied and diverse, they each cause a disturbance in the flow of air as it courses through the respiratory tree and bronchial passages. This disturbance of flow is usually seen on a pulmonary function test. These illnesses include asthma, bronchiectasis, cystic fibrosis, bronchitis, and emphysema; the latter two sometimes are called chronic obstructive pulmonary disease (COPD).

Another major category is diseases caused by infectious agents. These include influenza, various types of pneumonia, and infections of the lining of the lung. Infections of the lung can occur at any level, from the uppermost part of the lower respiratory tract, the trachea, down into the deepest part of the lungs. Vaccines can protect those at risk against certain disorders. (See Fig. 26.3)

Asthma

Asthma is a condition associated with episodes of difficult breathing and shortness of breath. The incidence of asthma is on the upswing in industrialized countries, and the death rate from asthma in large urban centers in these countries has increased despite the development of new and effective treatments. (See Fig. 26.4)

Symptoms

Asthma has a range of symptoms. The individual may be completely without symptoms when the dis-

ease is inactive. During attacks, the individual may have shortness of breath, cough, mucus production, chest tightness or discomfort, and wheezing. The symptoms often are provoked by a particular stimulus. A person with asthma whose symptoms are brought on by exercise might notice that after strenuous activity there is a brief period of shortness of breath followed by an attack 6–8 hours later.

The cause of asthma is unknown. It runs in some families, and often is associated with an allergy. Asthma is influenced by three separate mechanisms that affect each other and usually coexist:

1. Hyperresponsiveness of the airways to certain stimuli
2. Heightened constrictor response, causing narrowing of the airways and thus wheezing
3. Heightened inflammatory response within the lung itself that propagates the asthmatic attack

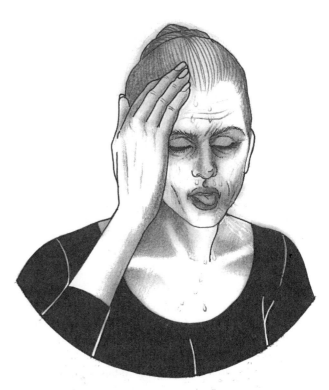

Figure 26.3 Infection

Symptoms of respiratory infection may include:
- cough
- sputum production
- generalized malaise
- unusual awareness of breathing

Different types of infections may exhibit similar symptoms.

Figure 26.4 Asthma
Asthma affects all age groups and
can have varied manifestations.

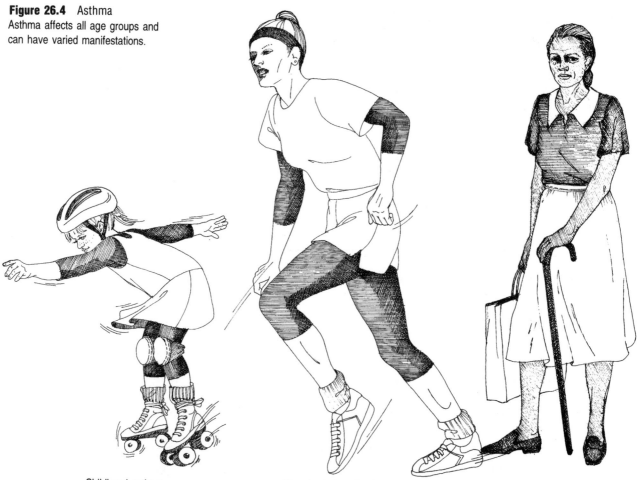

Childhood asthma
• is often associated with allergy,
eczema
• may become less severe as a
child grows into adulthood
• when treated properly allows for
participation in age-appropriate
activities, academic and recreational.

Exercise-induced asthma
• is symptomatic during and after
exercise
• may have as its only symptoms
cough and chest tightness after
exercise ends
• is easily treated, so there is no
need to give up sports
• tends to be diagnosed in
adolescents and young adults

Asthma in the elderly
• is a diagnosis frequently
overlooked, even though it is not
rare after age 65
• exhibits the same symptoms as in
younger age groups
• often requires daily use of
medication
• may be aggravated (along with
wheezing) by some prescriptions for
heart and eye conditions

Diagnosis

The diagnosis of asthma is based on the patient's
history and symptoms. Of special note are awakening
at night because of respiratory symptoms and symptoms following exertion, exposure to cold air, or to
certain irritants. In addition to auscultation of the lungs,
pulmonary function tests, particularly spirometry, are
often performed. These simple tests are painless. During an attack, spirometry shows clearcut signs that are
characteristic of asthma. In some cases, however, the
diagnosis may require more specialized pulmonary
function testing such as a bronchoprovocation challenge test. For this test, spirometry and pulmonary func-

tion tests are performed before and after the inhalation
of chilled room air. The patient exercises, for example,
pedaling a stationary bicycle, while inhaling the cold
air. Pulmonary function tests following the cold air and
exercise combination show a decrease in lung function
in a person with asthma.

Treatment

Once diagnosed, the patient and her physician
need to establish a treatment plan. Perhaps more than
any other disease, the patient with asthma must actively participate in her care because it requires a daily,
ongoing effort. Asthmatics should be able to participate

ASTHMA TRIGGERS

- Animal dander from cats, dogs, horses, rodents, etc.
- Pollens from trees, grasses, weeds, etc.
- Dust and dust mite droppings
- Molds
- Smoke
- Perfumes
- Chemicals like cleaning solutions, hair sprays, aerosols
- Change in weather or humidity
- Cold air
- Foods or food additives

fully in any activity they wish. The diagnosis of asthma should not be a barrier to sports or to professions that the woman wishes to pursue.

Medications for asthma are highly effective when taken as directed. Depending on the severity of the patient's asthma, her condition may be managed without daily standing medications, or she may consistently need as many as three inhaled medicines and perhaps two or three oral medications. In the period of a year, a woman with asthma may have several months when she requires no treatment or treatment daily, often several times a day.

Symptoms and medication effects can be monitored with a simple device called a peak flow meter. Asthmatics should test themselves at home on a regular basis. It takes approximately 5 minutes to measure one's peak flow. Testing can be done before and after a woman takes her medication. The peak flow meter monitoring done by a woman for herself or for her young child would indicate that the patient is relatively without symptoms, needs some medication, needs more medication, or needs to take it differently. Every asthmatic should know how to self-administer medications, when to increase the dose, and when it is safe to taper off medications based on their symptoms, their knowledge of the disease, and their peak flow measurements.

Medications used for the treatment of asthma fall into different groups based on their chemical class or their methods of administration. A stepwise approach to treatment is based on the patient's symptoms and pulmonary function tests. A person with mild to moderate asthma can be maintained in excellent health with inhaled medication alone. The advantage to an inhaled medication given by a little handheld puffer or by a nebulizer apparatus is that the medication enters the lung directly via the air passages and little or no medication enters the bloodstream. Because the medicine does not reach other organs such as the liver, brain, heart, or kidneys, side effects are minimal.

Of the inhaled agents the two broad categories include beta 2 agonists such as albuterol, bitolterol, pirbuterol, salmeterol, and metoproterenol, and anti-inflammatory agents such as inhaled steroid preparations, sodium cromolyn, and necrodomil sodium. The inhaled medications can be used on an as-needed basis or on a regularly programmed schedule at specific times as prescribed by a physician. Patients should learn the proper technique for self-administering these inhaled agents via a handheld canister metered dose inhaler (MDI). This device is easily carried in purse or pocket and is not difficult to use. Spacer devices help make inhalers easier to use. They reduce local side effects in the throat and should be used by children and patients with musculoskeletal limitations who may have difficulties using inhalers.

Medications also can be taken orally or intravenously. These include theophylline, steroids, and beta 2 agonists similar to the medications in the inhalers. Antibiotics may be prescribed if attacks are brought on or made worse by infection.

The long-term outlook for an asthmatic patient is excellent. With proper education, medical supervision, and a treatment that is closely coordinated with her physician, a woman with asthma should be able to continue the activities of daily living, including sports, work, leisure activities, childbearing, and raising a family.

Bronchiectasis

Bronchiectasis is an acquired condition characterized by the abnormal dilatation of portions of the bronchioles. These abnormalities increase the risk of recurrent infections in the affected area of the lung. Symptoms are chronic cough with sputum production and coughing up blood. Bronchiectasis is thought to result from a severe bacterial infection of the lungs that occurred many years earlier. With the increased use of antibiotics, the incidence of bronchiectasis in later life has decreased. Other causes of bronchiectasis include tuberculosis, as well as certain inherited diseases. De-

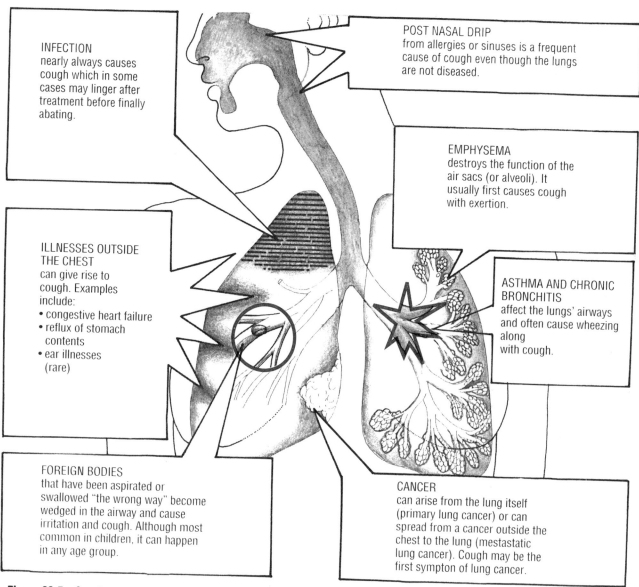

INFECTION
nearly always causes cough which in some cases may linger after treatment before finally abating.

POST NASAL DRIP
from allergies or sinuses is a frequent cause of cough even though the lungs are not diseased.

EMPHYSEMA
destroys the function of the air sacs (or alveoli). It usually first causes cough with exertion.

ILLNESSES OUTSIDE THE CHEST
can give rise to cough. Examples include:
• congestive heart failure
• reflux of stomach contents
• ear illnesses (rare)

ASTHMA AND CHRONIC BRONCHITIS
affect the lungs' airways and often cause wheezing along with cough.

FOREIGN BODIES
that have been aspirated or swallowed "the wrong way" become wedged in the airway and cause irritation and cough. Although most common in children, it can happen in any age group.

CANCER
can arise from the lung itself (primary lung cancer) or can spread from a cancer outside the chest to the lung (mestastatic lung cancer). Cough may be the first sympton of lung cancer.

Figure 26.5 Cough
Cough is a symptom of many different conditions

pending on the number of lung lobes affected and the severity of the condition, a patient may have a normal chest X-ray and no symptoms or her chest X-ray may show abnormalities and she may have severe symptoms, such as heavy respiratory secretions often mixed with blood.

Diagnosis

The diagnosis of bronchiectasis is suggested by the patient's history and by examining sputum to locate bacteria that indicate a more chronic and severe disorder. The diagnosis is best established by CT scanning of the chest. Previously, this condition was diagnosed by instilling special dyes through a bronchoscope di-

rectly into the bronchial tree. Although this technique, called bronchography, is no longer used routinely for diagnosis of bronchiectasis, it still has a place in certain specialized cases when surgery is contemplated.

Treatment

The treatment of bronchiectasis focuses on treatment of its complications. Once bronchiectasis has occurred and the bronchial tree is deformed, there is no way to reverse the process. Treatment with bronchodilators, antibiotics, and chest physiotherapy often cures the complicating infections, however, and permits the patient to become free of symptoms and not limited by the disease. In some cases—for example, when coughing up blood is life threatening—surgery may be performed to remove the affected area. Such patients should receive care by an experienced thoracic surgeon along with a pulmonary specialist.

Bronchitis

An inflammation of the major breathing passages, the bronchi, bronchitis can be a short-term acute infection or chronic, often associated with cigarette smoking. The main symptom is a productive cough of green or yellow sputum. The diagnosis of chronic bronchitis is made if the cough occurs on a daily or near-daily basis for at least 3 months out of the year for at least 2 successive years. Many patients who have chronic bronchitis also wheeze and have shortness of breath (dyspnea) often with exertion but occasionally at rest as the disease progresses. Currently, chronic bronchitis is less common in women than in men; however, as more and more women smoke cigarettes, there will be an increased incidence in women in the years to come.

The diagnosis of bronchitis rests primarily on the patient's history and the physical examination, which may disclose abnormal lung sounds. Treatment of the infection with antibiotics and control of wheezing with bronchodilators is most effective. Many patients who have chronic bronchitis also have emphysema. Cessation of cigarette smoking is mandatory to prevent further damage.

Cystic Fibrosis

An inherited disease, cystic fibrosis is mentioned in chapters 13 and 14. We mention it here, however, because this lung disease affects air flow. Patients with cystic fibrosis often have symptoms of bronchiectasis. The cause of death, at least in adults with cystic fibrosis, frequently is respiratory failure. Although it is an inherited disease often diagnosed in childhood, patients who are mildly affected may survive into their 20s and 30s before the disease is diagnosed. The diagnosis is based on symptoms and confirmed with tests.

Emphysema

In patients with emphysema, the delicate alveolar air spaces are broken down and replaced by large cystic cavities. There is less surface area for the lung's basic function of taking up oxygen and excreting carbon dioxide. The major cause of emphysema in the United States today is cigarette smoking. Although women are

currently affected less than men, the incidence of emphysema, as with chronic bronchitis and lung cancer, is increasing in women as more women smoke. An accelerated inherited form of emphysema is called alpha-1-antitrypsin deficiency. In this condition, patients lack a substance that protects them from emphysema. Patients who have alpha-1-antitrypsin deficiency and do not smoke are more prone to emphysema. If they smoke, their emphysema progresses very rapidly. Blood tests can detect alpha-1-antitrypsin deficiency.

Symptoms

Symptoms of emphysema include shortness of breath with exertion and, as disease progresses, at rest, along with a dry cough. A productive cough is not a feature of emphysema and usually suggests the presence of bronchitis as well. (See Fig. 26.5)

Diagnosis

The diagnosis is based on the patient's history, physical examination, pulmonary function testing, and chest X-ray. A CT scan discloses the extent of the disease and its distribution.

Treatment

Treatment of emphysema is directed to treatment of the symptoms. As in chronic bronchitis, cigarette smoking must cease to avoid further damage to the lungs. Treatment can involve both inhaled and oral medications. A new medication, called ipratroprium bromide, can be very effective in relieving shortness of breath. The lung damage in emphysema is permanent, however, and only the symptoms are helped by the medication.

In advanced stages, emphysema leads to respiratory failure. It is not uncommon for advanced emphysema to cause heart disease, a condition called cor pulmonale (heart made sick by lungs). When emphysema is very severe and heart failure ensues, the condition is critical. Some patients with accelerated emphysema who are young have undergone lung transplantation.

Goodpasture's Syndrome

An autoimmune disease in which antibodies to substances found in both the lungs and kidneys are produced in the body, Goodpasture's Syndrome is characterized by bleeding within the lung and renal disease. We mention it here because one of the first symptoms is coughing up blood.

Influenza

Influenza is a viral illness that can be complicated by pneumonia. The most common influenza viruses are types A and B. Influenza comes on suddenly and symptoms include fever, muscle aches and pains, a cough that is usually nonproductive, and headache. In most cases, the fever goes away in two or three days, the person feels better after five to seven days, and recovery is complete.

In some individuals, however, influenza can be more severe and complications, including death, can occur. In the United States, influenza has caused at least 10,000 deaths in each of seven epidemics between 1977 and 1988. Approximately 80–90 percent of these deaths were among individuals 65 years of age or older.

Groups considered to be at increased risk for complications from influenza include persons 65 years of age or older, especially if they are residents of nursing homes and chronic care facilities, as well as adults and children of any age with chronic cardiac or respiratory illnesses such as asthma, bronchiectasis, cystic fibrosis, emphysema, and bronchitis. Adults or children who have required medical care or hospitalization in the past year because of chronic conditions such as diabetes mellitus, renal disease, certain blood disorders called hemoglobinopathies, or use of immunosuppressive medications are also at risk of complications from influenza. The risk of complications from influenza is higher for pregnant women in the last three months of pregnancy than it is for women earlier in pregnancy or for those who are not pregnant. Influenza poses a serious threat to any individual who is infected with human immunodeficiency virus (HIV) or who has acquired immune deficiency syndrome (AIDS).

Fortunately, influenza often can be prevented or made less severe by immunization with the influenza vaccine. The influenza vaccine is a live viral vaccine produced from a purified virus that has been raised in eggs. The vaccine virus is noninfectious and it cannot cause influenza. Each year, a new vaccine is produced that offers protection against the three most common strains that occurred the previous winter.

About two weeks after immunization with the vaccine, an individual produces antibodies. These antibodies protect that person against the viral strains specific to that vaccine. After several months the antibody levels drop and the protection of the vaccine wears off. That is why influenza vaccines are given in the fall. In winter, when influenza tends to occur, a woman who has been vaccinated has good antibody levels that protect her against influenza so that she either does not become sick or, if she does, the illness is milder. A woman who receives an influenza vaccine one winter, no longer has antibodies to those strains the following winter and needs to be revaccinated.

Recent outbreaks of influenza in early winter have led some physicians to vaccinate as early as September. Those individuals who have been vaccinated in September, however, may lose their immunity too soon and be vulnerable to a late influenza outbreak in February or March. Those individuals who are high risk might discuss with their doctor the possibility of having one vaccine early in the fall with a second booster dose later.

Individuals who should be vaccinated fall into three categories (see the box). The first category includes those who are at risk for complications as described earlier. The second category is individuals who might transmit influenza to others who are at risk of complications. The third group is determined individually based on whether the vaccine would be of benefit.

A person who is allergic to eggs should not receive the vaccine. Most physicians will not immunize persons who are ill and have fevers. In adults, the vaccine is usually given in the arm, close to the shoulder in the deltoid muscle. Side effects are very unusual. The site of the injection may be sore for one or two days. Although the vaccine does not cause influenza, it may rarely be followed by one or two days of low-grade fever and aches. This does not occur often and when it does it is usually in children who have never been exposed to the virus in the vaccine. An immediate allergic reaction to the egg protein in the virus also may occur. In 1976 there was an outbreak of a serious neurologic disorder called Guillain-Barré syndrome in some people who had been vaccinated against swine flu. Subsequently, vaccines have been prepared from different viral strains and have not been associated with an increase in Guillain-Barré syndrome.

In addition to the influenza vaccine, an antiviral medication is effective against influenza A. The antiviral drug amantadine or its derivatives can lessen the severity of symptoms or prevent them if the medications are taken early enough after exposure to influenza A. Amantadine has prevented influenza type A. When given to young adults or children during an epidemic, for example, it is about 70-90 percent effective in preventing illness. Amantadine must be taken every day and, in many cases, needs to be continued during the winter months or as long as an epidemic lasts. The drug may be prescribed if there is an outbreak of influenza in a school or nursing home, or if a

ADULTS WHO SHOULD BE VACCINATED FOR INFLUENZA

Those at high risk of complications

- All adults 65 years or older
- Residents of chronic health care facilities
- People with respiratory illnesses, cardiac illness, certain metabolic illnesses such as diabetes, chronic renal disease or renal failure

Those who could transmit influenza to high-risk groups

- Physicians, nurses, hospital personnel, or other health care workers
- Nursing home workers and volunteer workers
- Household members

Other examples—discuss with your physician

- Women who are in the last three months of pregnancy during winter months
- Individuals who provide essential community service (such as firefighters and police)

person cannot tolerate the vaccine. When the influenza vaccine has been given late in the year, amantadine may be prescribed for the two weeks immediately after vaccination until enough protective antibodies are produced.

A woman who is at risk for complications from influenza should be vaccinated. If she can't take the vaccine or becomes ill with influenza, amantadine therapy can be considered. The influenza vaccine is very safe, well tolerated, and inexpensive. It can prevent illness, reduce its severity and complications, prevent hospitalization, and lower the death rate from influenza.

Neoplasms—Tumors and Cancers

Abnormal new growths are called neoplasms. They can be either benign (noncancerous) or malignant (cancerous). Benign neoplasms of the lung include adenomas. They are benign because they do not have the ability to grow unchecked and spread beyond the lung. They occur less frequently than malignant neoplasms of the lungs, which are cancers and have the ability to grow larger and to spread beyond the lung. Malignant neoplasms can arise within the lung, where they are called primary lung cancers, or they can arise in other organs and spread to the lungs via the bloodstream or lymph glands. Malignant neoplasms can first be diagnosed in the lung when, in fact, the primary cancer has arisen in another organ. Cancers of the breast, skin, lymphatic system, and kidney are known to spread to the lung and sometimes are diagnosed after this spread has occurred.

Neoplasms that are malignant also can arise from the pleura, or lining of the lung. The neoplasms of the pleura are called mesotheliomas. They are rare but occur more often in people who have been exposed to asbestos. The initial sign is usually fluid around the lung, often accompanied by weight loss, fever, and nearly always pain.

Primary lung cancer, often called bronchogenic carcinoma, has surpassed breast cancer as the number one cancer killer of American women. This is a direct consequence of the increased number of women who began to smoke during or after World War II. Before cigarette smoking was commonplace, lung cancer was extremely rare. Now that cigarette smoking is common, lung cancer is more prevalent and its incidence is rising. There has been very little improvement in the death rate from lung cancer despite advances in medicine. In addition to cigarette smoking, lung cancer is caused by exposure to radon and asbestos. As compared to nonsmokers who have not been exposed to asbestos, asbestos-exposed smokers have a 100-fold risk of developing lung cancer. Thus, cigarette smoking and asbestos work together to increase the risk of lung cancer. (See Fig. 26.6)

If untreated, lung cancer is a fatal disease; the rate of death is directly related to the extent of the disease at diagnosis. The best option for the treatment of lung cancer is surgery. Unfortunately, by the time a person seeks treatment for lung cancer it has often spread too far to be cured by surgery. The best chance of cure is with early detection, identification, and treatment, before the cancer has spread and while the patient is in good enough health to withstand surgery. The highest rate of cures is for those cancers found by accident before any symptoms have occurred, as when a chest X-ray is taken as a part of a physical examination, and it discloses an unsuspected lung cancer.

Symptoms

Symptoms of lung cancer are varied and depend on the location and size of the primary growth as well as any possible spread. A persistent cough, which may or may not be productive and show blood in the sputum, can be a symptom. Advanced signs of lung cancer include pain at bony sites not limited to the chest and weight loss.

Diagnosis

Cancer is detected on a chest X-ray or CT scan. The diagnosis is established by examining a sample of the cancerous tumor cells under a microscope. If the cancer has spread from the chest to another organ—for example, to a lymph gland in the neck—the lymph gland is sampled and the cancer identified within that gland. Once lung cancer is diagnosed, it is usually possible to classify the cancer by type (see "Types of Lung Cancer"). Small cell cancer must be distinguished from non-small-cell cancer (adenocarcinoma or bronchogenic carcinoma) because they are treated differently. (See Fig. 26.7)

Once the type of cancer is identified, the next step is to proceed with staging to identify how big the cancer is and how much it has spread, if at all. Staging is slightly different in the small cell variety than in non-small cell cancer. In small cell cancer, the disease is classified as limited or extensive disease depending on whether the brain and the bone marrow are involved. In non-small-cell lung cancer, staging is accomplished with X-rays, and CT scans of the brain, chest, abdomen, and pelvis. It also may include scanning of the bones and bronchoscopy.

Treatment

Once the lung cancer has been identified, the type defined, and staging completed, the next step is to proceed with treatment. Small cell cancer always is best

LUNG CANCER-NON-SMALL CELL TYPE
• Examples of various stages I-IV

Example of stage I cancer:

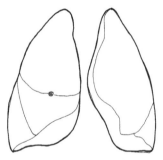

A small, single area of cancer without any spread.

Example of stage II cancer:

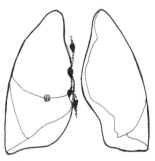

An area of cancer within the lung with cancerous involvment of a near-by lymph gland on the same side.

Example of stage III-A cancer:

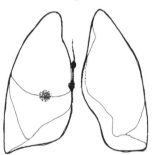

The cancer involves either chest wall, and/or lymph glands on the same side, within the chest.

Example of stage III-B cancer:

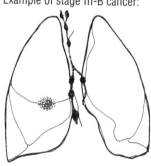

The cancer remains confined to the chest but there are cancerous lymph glands in the neck area.

Example of stage IV cancer:

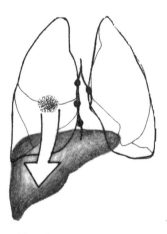

There is spread to organs outside the chest (for example, in liver, bone, brain).

Figure 26.6 The Spread of Non-Small-Cell Lung Cancer Examples of Stages I–IV

N.B. Stage III is separated into stage III-A and III-B based on which group of lymph glands are cancerous.

TYPES OF LUNG CANCER

Small cell (or oat cell) cancer

Non-small-cell cancer

- Squamous cell lung cancer
- Adenocarcinoma
- Large cell lung cancer
- Mixed cell lung cancer

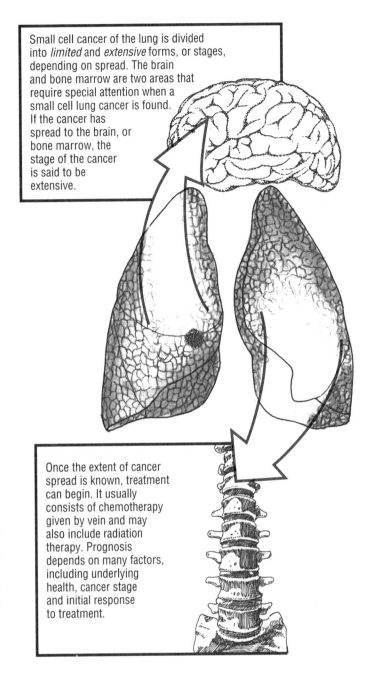

Small cell cancer of the lung is divided into *limited* and *extensive* forms, or stages, depending on spread. The brain and bone marrow are two areas that require special attention when a small cell lung cancer is found. If the cancer has spread to the brain, or bone marrow, the stage of the cancer is said to be extensive.

Once the extent of cancer spread is known, treatment can begin. It usually consists of chemotherapy given by vein and may also include radiation therapy. Prognosis depends on many factors, including underlying health, cancer stage and initial response to treatment.

Figure 26.7 Small Cell Cancer

treated with chemotherapy and sometimes radiation. Non-small-cell cancer is best treated with removal or surgical excision if the cancer is in an early stage. If the cancer is more advanced, chemotherapy or radiation or both are treatment options. The site of the cancer also guides therapy and affects the prognosis. Generally, the patient is treated by a cancer specialist called an oncologist.

The long-term outlook depends on many factors, including the patient's state of health, the type of lung cancer, the extent of disease or stage, and the response to therapy. Favorable factors include general well-being, less aggressive appearance of the tumor cells under the microscope, and early stage. Because lung cancer, when advanced, carries such a grave prognosis, attention has been directed to prevention and early detection. It is imperative that women who are concerned about their health not only stop smoking or never start but also encourage their loved ones not to smoke. Efforts at early detection have been disappointing and various studies attempting to identify early cancers in those who are heavy cigarette smokers have not positively affected disease or survival rates.

Obstructive Sleep Apnea Syndrome

A newly recognized condition characterized by brief periods of breathing cessation during sleep, obstructive sleep apnea syndrome is often first recognized by the bed partner of the afflicted person. Symptoms include a characteristic loud snoring while sleeping and excessive daytime sleepiness. A person affected with obstructive sleep apnea often falls asleep at inappropriate times, for example, during a meeting, while working or driving, or on a bus. The syndrome usually affects overweight males, but indirectly affects their spouses or bed partners; these women often find it so disturbing they insist the men seek medical attention.

The diagnosis is confirmed by a special study that documents the events during sleep. Referral is usually made to a specialist in polysomnography, and the patient spends the night in a sleep lab where breathing patterns can be monitored. Once the condition is diagnosed, treatment is very effective. It involves sleeping with a specially fitted nasal mask attached to a machine that provides support during breathing. This machine keeps the upper respiratory passages open during sleep. Usually patients who have obstructive sleep apnea immediately return to normal, restful, non-snoring sleep; they feel much more rested after the first night of sleep with this device. Other treatments for obstructive sleep apnea syndrome should not be used until the special mask is tried.

Pleural Infections

Pleurisy is an infection of the lining of the lung. These infections are usually viral and can be very painful. Symptoms are fever and pain that worsens during inhaling. The diagnosis usually is based on the patient's history, physical exam, and chest X-ray; treatment is directed toward making the patient more comfortable.

A condition called empyema occurs when infection begins in the lungs and spreads to the pleural space and infects it. Although pneumonia-causing bacteria such as pneumococcus are the most common causes of empyema, tuberculous empyema also occurs. Empyema is a serious medical condition; at its onset the patient has high fever and severe pain on breathing. The patient is very ill and requires admission to a hospital and aggressive treatment. If left untreated, empyema may require surgery to remove the infectious material that has gathered in the pleural space.

Pneumonia

An infection of the lower respiratory tract that involves the air sacs, or alveoli, is called pneumonia. Causes of pneumonia include bacteria, viruses (see "Influenza"), atypical organisms, fungi, rickettsia, and parasites. Two special kinds of pneumonia include hospital-acquired pneumonia, also called nosocomial pneumonia, and those pneumonias associated with HIV infection and AIDS.

Diagnosis

The diagnosis is based on a physical examination and chest X-ray. Bacterial pneumonia is treated with antibiotics that, depending on the particular type of pneumonia, may be given by mouth, by an injection in the muscle, or intravenously. Although the illness can be serious, even fatal, most people recover without long-term effects. Some types of bacteria cause more severe disease than others; usually the health of the person infected and the presence of other medical conditions determine the severity of the disease. Certain conditions increase the risk of pneumonia. These include preexisting lung disease like bronchiectasis or emphysema. Such patients should receive pneumococ-

cal vaccine to protect them against bacterial pneumonia. Vaccination to prevent pneumococcal infection and lessen its severity is recommended once in a lifetime and, for certain people, every 10 years. (See "Pneumococcal Vaccine").

Bacterial pneumonias run the gamut from the mildest of infections to severe, life-threatening infections. Classically, bacterial pneumonias produce symptoms of fever, cough, raising of discolored or odiferous sputum, and occasionally inspiratory chest pain. The patient generally feels ill. The pneumococus, also called *streptococcus pneumoniae*, is a common cause of bacterial pneumonia.

Atypical pneumonia is often seen in younger people, such as college students and military personnel. It can be self-limited. Symptoms include a moderate fever, nonproductive cough, headache, and body aches. The diagnosis is based on clinical signs and chest X-ray and blood tests. Antibiotics, such as erythromycin, clarithromycin, or tetracycline, often hasten recovery and make the patient more comfortable.

Fungal pneumonias occur in residents of areas of the United States where the fungus is common. This includes certain parts of California, for instance, and the Mississippi basin. Other fungal pneumonias occur sporadically in individuals with weakened immune systems that allow fungus to grow and cause disease. The diagnosis can be difficult and usually involves a patient history and physical examination, as well as blood tests and the recovery of a fungus from respiratory secretions or biopsy material.

Rickettsial and parasitic pneumonias are unusual in the United States. They are usually diagnosed by recovering the agent causing the infection from the respiratory system.

Hospital-acquired, or nosocomial, pneumonias are a modern problem. As hospitals care for larger numbers of elderly and ill patients, strains of bacteria that are resistant to many antibiotics have emerged. This type of pneumonia affects people who are hospitalized, often on ventilators, frail, and in a weakened state. They have fevers and abnormal chest X-rays. The treatment of hospital-acquired pneumonia generally requires further hospitalization and intravenous administration of antibiotics. Recovery depends on the health of the individual and the virulence of the strain of the infecting bacteria.

Infection with HIV increases the risk of bacterial pneumonia. The more advanced form of HIV infection, AIDS, incurs an additional risk of other forms of pneumonia that occur in patients with weakened immune systems. The most common of these pneumonias is called pneumocystis carinii pneumonia, or PCP. If untreated in an AIDS patient, PCP is fatal. The symptoms are progressive shortness of breath that begins with exertion and then occurs at rest, fever, and a nonproductive cough. Auscultation of the chest is usually normal. The diagnosis of PCP can be made by examination of lung secretions, but more often requires a procedure such as bronchoscopy, with or without biopsy of the lung.

Treatment

The first-line treatment of pneumocystis carinii pneumonia usually is a combination of trimethoprim and sulfamethoxazole or pentamidine. Much research is being directed toward combating this deadly pneumonia and to try to prevent it from occurring in AIDS patients.

Pulmonary Embolus

A pulmonary embolus occurs when a clot that has formed in the veins of the legs migrates to the blood vessels that feed the lungs. When it lodges in the lung circulation, the clot causes a blockage and blood cannot flow into that area of lung. If a large portion of the blood supply is blocked, as in a massive pulmonary embolus, the patient can lose consciousness and possibly die. In most cases, however, the embolus is not massive and symptoms can consist of pain in the chest, shortness of breath, or difficulty breathing, along with fever. (See Fig. 26.8)

Pulmonary embolus usually does not occur in normally healthy, active individuals. Some conditions that place a person at increased risk for pulmonary emboli include prolonged lack of movement of the lower extremities (which can occur postoperatively or with paralysis), cancers or malignancies, and abnormalities of blood clotting mechanisms. Birth control pills may promote the risk of clots and, therefore, the formation of pulmonary emboli, especially if a woman smokes.

The diagnosis of pulmonary emboli can be difficult. It is usually confirmed based on the patient's history, physical examination, and specialized scans. If the diagnosis is still not clear after these tests, an angiogram of the pulmonary vessels may be performed. A radiologist who specializes in angiograms performs this test by injecting dye into the blood vessels that feed the lungs to determine if there is a clot.

The treatment of pulmonary emboli may involve direct injection of clot-dissolving medication into the area of the emboli. If the embolus is not massive, it usually can be treated with a substance such as heparin

PNEUMOCCAL VACCINE

A vaccine is available to prevent pneumococcal pneumonia. It protects against 23 of the more than 80 strains of pneumococcus that can cause pneumonia. These 23 strains account for 85–90 percent of all pneumococcal illness, so by immunizing an individual with the vaccine, most cases of the disease can be prevented. Those who have a high risk of complications from pneumococcal pneumonia should receive the vaccine, including people who have the following conditions:

- Chronic disease, especially diseases of the heart and lung
- Absence of a spleen or a spleen that is not working properly
- Cancer such as Hodgkin's disease or multiple myeloma
- Diabetes or renal failure
- Organ transplant
- Infection with HIV or AIDS
- Alcoholism or liver dysfunction
- Age 65 or older

After vaccination, antibodies are produced that protect against the illness. It takes about 2–3 weeks for antibody production to begin and the protection appears to last anywhere from 5 to 10 years. In some cases, a physician may recommend a repeat vaccination after 10 or more years.

that prevents further clot formation followed by a pill called warfarin. When an individual is known to be at risk for the development of a pulmonary embolus, these drugs may be given in small doses to prevent clot formation in the legs in the first place and thereby prevent the embolus. Such patients might include those about to undergo certain types of surgery (for example, hip replacement or hip fracture surgery). A woman who has had a pulmonary embolus while taking birth control pills should stop taking them and change to another birth-control method. Repeated pulmonary emboli can be harmful to lung function and should be avoided.

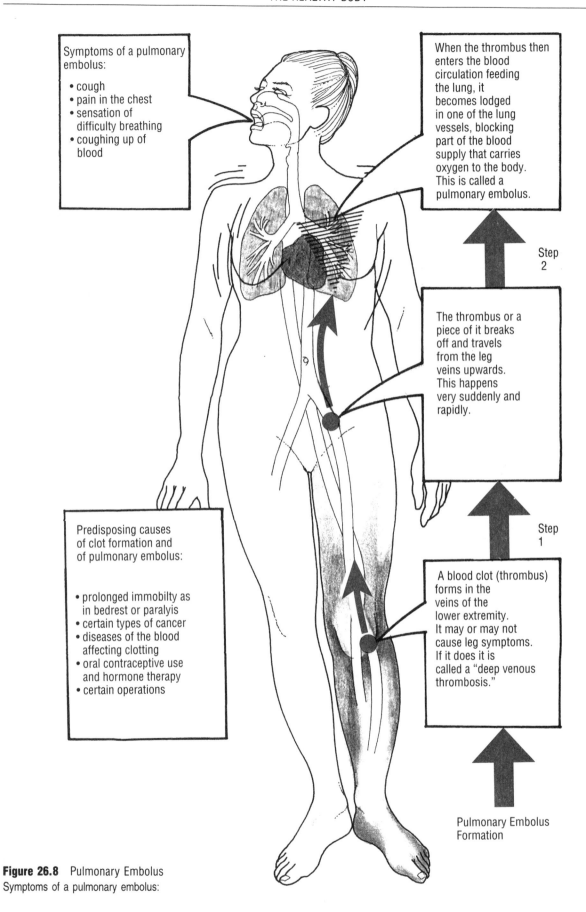

Symptoms of a pulmonary embolus:

• cough
• pain in the chest
• sensation of difficulty breathing
• coughing up of blood

When the thrombus then enters the blood circulation feeding the lung, it becomes lodged in one of the lung vessels, blocking part of the blood supply that carries oxygen to the body. This is called a pulmonary embolus.

Step 2

The thrombus or a piece of it breaks off and travels from the leg veins upwards. This happens very suddenly and rapidly.

Step 1

A blood clot (thrombus) forms in the veins of the lower extremity. It may or may not cause leg symptoms. If it does it is called a "deep venous thrombosis."

Predisposing causes of clot formation and of pulmonary embolus:

• prolonged immobilty as in bedrest or paralyis
• certain types of cancer
• diseases of the blood affecting clotting
• oral contraceptive use and hormone therapy
• certain operations

Pulmonary Embolus Formation

Figure 26.8   Pulmonary Embolus
Symptoms of a pulmonary embolus:

Pulmonary Fibrosis

Pulmonary fibrosis is a process in which normal lung tissue is replaced by diseased or fibrosed lung tissue that can no longer perform the functions of gas exchange. Some causes are unknown or idiopathic. Some nonpulmonary illnesses, such as rheumatoid arthritis, can lead to the condition. The symptoms of pulmonary fibrosis begin slowly and consist of shortness of breath with exertion and then possibly with rest and in some cases a dry cough. Certain causes of fibrosis cause the nails to look abnormal, a process referred to as clubbing.

The diagnosis of pulmonary fibrosis is based on specialized scans, such as a CT scan, and requires a biopsy of the lung. A large sample of tissue is required for study; usually this sample is obtained by a video-assisted thoracoscopic lung biopsy or by an open lung biopsy. The treatment of pulmonary fibrosis is usually not very effective because the fibrosis has already taken place and normal lung tissue cannot be regenerated. Often doctors try to slow the progress of the disease with steroid medication or other immunosuppressive drugs. If the disease progresses despite treatment, lung transplantation may be a valid option.

Sarcoidosis

A disease of unknown cause that affects women more than men, sarcoidosis is the abnormal collection of cells called granulomas in many different organs. The organs affected are most often the lungs but can include the eye, skin, liver, brain, and kidneys. The illness can be without symptoms and found on a routine chest X-ray done for a physical examination. Up to one-third of sarcoidosis cases are found this way and, in this situation, treatment may not be needed. Some patients have symptoms related to the respiratory system, the most common of which are cough and shortness of breath. Chest pain, sputum production, and coughing up of blood also can occur.

Sarcoidosis is diagnosed on the basis of clinical findings and the identification of granulomas in a sample of tissue obtained from an affected organ. The sample of tissue can be obtained from the lungs with a flexible fiberoptic bronchoscope. The procedure can be done with a mild sedative and does not necessarily involve a hospital stay.

Once the diagnosis is confirmed, sarcoidosis is treated based on the patient's symptoms and clinical findings. Some cases require no treatment, and the condition may go away on its own. In more advanced cases, it is treated with steroid medication and close monitoring.

Tuberculosis

Once thought to be nearly eradicated, tuberculosis is on the upswing in urban areas in this country. When active, tuberculosis has symptoms of chronic fatigue, cough that often produces blood, fever, and general malaise. It may be associated with an immune defect.

The diagnosis of tuberculosis can be very straightforward of very elusive. The definitive diagnosis is established by recovering the organisms causing the infection (*mycobacterium tuberculosis*) from the patient's respiratory tract. The way in which respiratory secretions are obtained varies. If an individual is coughing up secretions that contain the tuberculosis germ, a sample can be sent to a laboratory. If an individual is not coughing, however, bronchoscopy may be required to obtain a sample. The sample is then grown in a laboratory so the organism can be identified and the proper antimicrobial treatment for the particular strain of disease infecting the individual can be given.

Treatment of tuberculosis involves daily administration of pills. The pills usually consist of three, four, or more medications along with a vitamin supplement. They must be taken every day for a period of months to years (even after all symptoms have vanished) to ensure complete recovery. When the treatment is taken as prescribed, tuberculosis can be cured.

If antituberculous medication is not taken as prescribed, however, drug-resistant strains of tuberculosis can develop. Treatment of drug-resistant tuberculosis requires referral to a pulmonary specialist as well as an infectious disease specialist.

Wegener's Granulomatosis

Wegener's granulomatosis usually affects the kidneys, but we mention it here because it may cause the symptoms of runny nose and cough. This rare disease can be diagnosed by blood tests or by examining a tissue sample taken from the upper respiratory tract or sometimes the lung.

PROCEDURES

Arterial Blood Gas Sampling

Analyzing a sample of arterial blood can provide information on the oxygen content of the blood and the combination of acid and base that circulate in the bloodstream. A sample of arterial blood is obtained to measure (1) the partial pressure of oxygen, (2) the partial pressure of carbon dioxide, and (3) the pH.

This test permits assessment of the lung's functions of distributing oxygen to the other organs of the body and ensuring that the proper acid-base balance is maintained. If a woman has a symptom of shortness of breath when she exerts herself, the test may be performed to measure the oxygen content in the arterial blood and determine if the lungs are able to extract enough oxygen both at rest and during exertion. The measurement of oxygen content can be extremely important in the evaluation of patients with disorders such as emphysema and bronchitis. If a woman is found to have a low oxygen content, she may benefit from supplemental oxygen that can be provided by a mask or nasal cannula techniques. If the acid-base balance in the blood is found to be abnormal, certain medications or treatments can correct the balance.

Arterial blood gas sampling can be done in a doctor's office or in an outpatient setting. In hospitalized patients it is used for an acute respiratory problem, such as severe pneumonia, when the physician needs to know if extra oxygen is needed.

The blood sample is obtained from an artery, usually the radial artery in the wrist, which can be identified by feeling the pulse. The area is wiped clean with alcohol, a needle is inserted into the artery, and a small sample of blood is withdrawn. The amount may differ with the individual, but usually no more than one-fourth to one-half a teaspoon is required. The test is safe and simple and can be done in about one minute. Many laboratories perform arterial blood gas testing as a part of pulmonary function testing.

Pulmonary Function Testing

The many different pulmonary function tests—also referred to as PFTs—range from simple tests such as spirometry to complex measurements of lung function during exercise or after certain agents have been administered. The more common tests include spirome-try, measure of lung volumes, measurement of diffusion, as well as exercise or methacholine challenge testing. Arterial blood gas sampling and other procedures can be done as a part of pulmonary function testing.

Pulmonary function testing may be prescribed for a number of reasons. Often it is used in the evaluation of asthma, bronchitis, emphysema, as well as to assess symptoms such as wheezing and shortness of breath. Pulmonary function testing can be done to determine potential damage to the lungs or the severity of disease, such as from cigarette smoking or asbestos lung disease. It also can be performed prior to surgery that may include removal of a lung. For example, if a woman had lung cancer that would be treated with surgery involving removal of part or all of a lung, she would undergo pulmonary function testing to assess how well her remaining lung would function after surgery.

Certain medications, such as inhaled bronchodilators, should not be taken before pulmonary function testing is performed. This should be discussed with the doctor before the test. Various maneuvers must be performed during the test, so the patient should be as relaxed as possible and wearing comfortable clothing. For spirometry, a clip is placed on the woman's nose and she breathes through a mouthpiece while performing a series of maneuvers. Spirometry is a method of measuring how smoothly air flows through the lungs.

Measurement of lung volume shows how much air your lungs take in. It can be done with two different techniques. One technique involves breathing a helium mixture for approximately 5-10 minutes with the nose clipped. The other technique involves having the patient enter a box that resembles a phone booth where measurements are taken. These safe, painless tests require some effort and cooperation on the patient's part. Measurement of diffusion involves breathing through a circuit with a nose clip in place. It too is safe and requires some degree of cooperation.

Exercise tests are performed to evaluate symptoms that occur with exertion. The patient may be asked to run on a treadmill or pedal a stationary bicycle. Various medications can be prescribed to assess, for example, a response to therapy. If the results indicate that a person may have asthma, a brochodilating medication similar to those used in treatment of asthma may be administered to see if there is improvement with the medication. Another option is to have the test performed and then take medication for a period of days to weeks; the repeat test shows if there has been any change in the interval.

Bronchoscopy

Bronchoscopy allows inspection of the bronchi and the breathing passages as well as retrieving of any matter within the bronchi and obtaining a sample of tissue from inside the lungs. Areas that can be reached with the aid of a bronchoscope and be biopsied include the areas within the airways, where a lung cancer might occur, as well as air sacs or alveoli where there may be infections.

There are two types of bronchoscopes. The older variety is called a rigid bronchoscope, and the newer instrument is called the flexible fiberoptic bronchoscope. Rigid bronchoscopy is usually performed by a surgeon in an operating room using general anesthesia, whereas flexible bronchoscopy can be performed in an ambulatory surgery setting with the patient lightly sedated. The rigid bronchoscope is favored when a large foreign body must be retrieved or there is a massive amount of bleeding in the lung. Otherwise, the flexible bronchoscope is generally preferred.

Flexible bronchoscopy can be performed either on an inpatient basis or, for someone in generally good health, as same-day surgery. The patient fasts the night before, has the bronchoscopy the next day, and is observed for two hours before going home. Bronchoscopy is very safe and well tolerated. In addition to fasting the night before, special instructions may include discontinuation of medication before the procedure and having special blood tests and a chest X-ray performed.

The flexible bronchoscope is a thin tube containing a fiberoptic element that provides a light inside the lungs. The view is magnified so details of the lungs can be seen. It contains a channel through which medication can be directly instilled in the lung, secretions can be suctioned and removed, and biopsy forceps can be passed to obtain samples for further testing. Depending on the reason for performing bronchoscopy, this procedure may or may not be performed with X-ray guidance. Although the procedure can take between 20 and 30 minutes, depending on why the test is being done, additional time should be allowed for preoperative preparation. An important step prior to the procedure is to anesthetize the back of the patient's throat so she doesn't feel the urge to gag or cough.

Lung Biopsy

Sampling of an abnormal area of the lung may be useful in evaluating lung diseases. This sampling is called a biopsy. By removing a piece of the affected lung, it is possible to diagnose the disease entity and then treat it. The most common reason for performing a lung biopsy is finding an X-ray or CT scan abnormality in which cancer is suspected. This abnormality may be very small and contained, in which case it might be referred to as a coin lesion or it may be more extensive.

Different methods of lung biopsy may be used depending on the clinical setting and the appearance of the abnormality on the X-ray or CT scan. These methods include percutaneous fine needle aspiration of the lung, bronchoscopic lung biopsy, mediastinoscopy, thoracoscopy, or open lung biopsy. Patients and their doctors may choose to use the simplest technique, percutaneous needle aspiration, before proceeding to more invasive procedures.

A percutaneous fine needle aspiration of the lung is performed with the patient either lying under an X-ray camera or in a CT scan machine. These imaging devices provide guidance during the procedure. The patient is positioned, the abnormality is located either on the X-ray or the CT scanner, and a very thin needle is passed through the skin into the abnormal area. Cells are withdrawn through the needle's hollow core with a syringe device. This simple technique can be performed on an outpatient basis. Of all biopsy techniques, it yields clusters of cells with the smallest amount of tissue. The procedure is the least invasive; but there is an approximately 20 percent risk of pneumothorax, a buildup of air in the pleural space.

Sampling also can be done with bronchoscopy. Abnormal areas located within the bronchial passages are called endobronchial abnormalities; they are usually sampled with a bronchoscope using a special endobronchial forceps. Abnormalities near the air sacs can, if they are large enough to be seen on a chest X-ray, be located during bronchoscopy and biopsied. The procedure carries a risk of pneumothorax as well as possible bleeding.

Mediastinoscopy is a technique to biopsy the mediastinum, an area in the middle part of the chest behind the breastbone, where lymph glands that drain the lung can become enlarged. A lymph gland enlargement in that area may be related to an abnormality in the lung. The mediastinoscope is an instrument that is passed into the mediastinum at the top of the breastbone to obtain a sample of the abnormal lymph nodes. Mediastinoscopy provides large pieces of tissue and requires administration of a general anesthetic. Pneumothorax is not a complication, and bleeding is minimal or nonexistent.

Thoracoscopy is a newer technique used when large pieces of tissue are required for diagnosis. In the operating room while the patient is under general anesthesia, a surgeon makes a small incision between the ribs and passes a video camera into the area between the lung and chest wall. By looking inside with this camera, the surgeon manipulates the lung and obtains samples for analysis. Thoracoscopy requires general anesthesia and a hospital stay.

The most invasive measure for obtaining biopsies is open lung biopsy. It is done in an operating room while the patient is under general anesthesia. The surgeon makes a moderate incision between the ribs, spreads the ribs apart, inspects a piece of the lung, and takes a relatively large sample from that site. Because it yields a good-sized sample, open lung biopsy is said to be the "gold standard" that most often cinches a diagnosis.

Once a lung sample is obtained, it is submitted for analysis by a pathologist. Several days later the results are available and the diagnosis is known.

Ventilators and Life Support

When an individual develops respiratory failure—that is, if the lungs are unable to perform the work of breathing—death follows. Respiratory failure can be acute or chronic. The term *acute respiratory failure* implies that the individual's underlying lung health has been excellent. Acute respiratory failure might occur as a result of trauma, for example. The term *chronic respiratory failure* suggests that the patient's decline in lung function has occurred gradually over time: for example, a patient who has had progressive emphysema over 20–30 years and is no longer able to breathe without assistance.

Mechanical assistance, or life support, generally refers to a machine called a respirator or a ventilator. A relatively new technology, respirator or ventilator support requires a specialized team of doctors, nurses, and respiratory therapists. This therapy is given in an intensive care unit.

Respiratory support with ventilators can be lifesaving. It allows individuals to survive severe trauma and infections. Yet, this technology has created many ethical and moral dilemmas as patients, often aged and with fatal nonrespiratory conditions, have been placed on ventilators and their lives prolonged at no measurable benefit to themselves or to their families. Mechan-

ical ventilation is best used when it buys time for patients to receive therapy or allows them time to heal and to recover their own lung function and eventually resume breathing on their own.

When a patient develops a serious illness or a life-threatening illness or a chronic condition, it is appropriate for her to discuss issues of life support not only with her loved ones but also with her physician so that her wishes are known should there be an unexpected deterioration in her condition. Many states have guidelines to assist patients and their physicians in documenting the patients' wishes regarding life support.

A ventilator is a device that is programmed to give a patient a certain number of breaths per minute at a specific volume, depending on that patient's characteristics. It also enables the physician to administer varying amounts of oxygen as needed. Oxygen is given directly into the lung, either via an endotracheal tube which is passed in the back of the throat into the trachea, or through a tracheostomy, in which a tube is placed through an incision in the neck. If ventilator support is required for more than 1–2 weeks, it is generally advisable to provide it through a tracheostomy. Long-term survival is possible with ventilator technology, which should be instituted in consultation with the patient and the family.

Newer methods of delivering breathing assistance to individuals with chronic respiratory insufficiency are sometimes called noninvasive mechanical ventilation. Sometimes needed only at night during sleep, these machines are set up at the patient's bedside at home and the breaths and the oxygen are given through a face mask.

Lung Transplantation

Lung transplantation is a relatively new technique offered at specialized centers. Candidates for lung transplantation should be highly motivated patients who have a fatal illness of the lungs and are physically able to withstand the operation. An appropriate lung donor must be available. Currently, because of a lack of donors, there are many more patients waiting for lung transplantation than lungs available for transplantation. Conditions that lend themselves to transplantation include cystic fibrosis, where two lungs need to be transplanted, as well as certain forms of emphysema or pulmonary fibrosis, in which the patient may benefit from the transplantation of only one lung. Lung transplantation requires careful attention to detail and a system of ongoing care that is very sophisticated.

RESOURCES

Medic Alert: 800-ED-ALERT. A medic alert bracelet or necklace may be advisable for individuals who have severe allergies or chronic illnesses or are taking certain medications.

Allergy and Asthma Network/Mothers of Asthmatics, Inc. (3554 Chain Bridge Road, Suite 200; Fairfax, VA 22030; 800-874-4403). A good resource for any child or young adult with asthma, the network also serves people with allergies. A newsletter and helpful educational materials are available.

Further information on asthma is available through the National Asthma Educational Program (4733 Bethesda Avenue, Suite 530; Bethesda, MD 20814; 301-951-3260).

American Lung Association (1740 Broadway, New York, NY 10019-4374). The lung association provides informational brochures on many respiratory diseases. The association also may have lists of speakers available. Refer to your telephone directory for a local listing, or call 1-800-LUNG-USA (1-800-586-4872).

National Cancer Institute. Contact the National Cancer Institute for free informational brochures on asbestos, lung cancer, and smoking cessation in English and Spanish. The toll-free number for answers to your questions about cancer is 800-4-CANCER. Spanish-speaking staff members are also available to answer questions.

Asbestos Exposure. The Consumer Product Safety Commission (5401 West Bard Avenue, Bethesda, MD 20207, 800-638-CPSC) is responsible for the regulation of asbestos consumer products. Additional asbestos information can be obtained from a union or the International Association of Machinists and Aerospace Workers, Department of Occupational Safety, Health, and Community Service (1300 Connecticut Avenue, NW, Washington, DC 20036). For consumer information about asbestos contact the White Lung Association (1114 Cathedral Street, Baltimore, MD 21201); for industry information contact Asbestos Information Association of North America (1725 Jefferson Davis Highway, Arlington, VA 22202).

CHAPTER 27

The Cardiovascular System

Debra R. Judelson, M.D., F.A.C.P., F.A.C.C.

The cardiovascular system comprises the heart and blood vessels that circulate blood throughout the body (Figure 27.1). This system works continuously through a network of veins and arteries to ensure that oxygenated blood, needed for all vital functions, is distributed to organs and muscles. Any disruption in the flow of blood can cause damage to an organ, including the heart.

Cardiovascular disease is the number-one cause of death in both women and men. Coronary heart disease is the major cause of cardiovascular disease and leads to the death of approximately 236,000 women annually. Although the female hormone estrogen provides women with some protection against heart disease, after menopause, when they are no longer producing estrogen, the risk of coronary heart disease can exceed that in men. Almost all of the studies of cardiovascular disease have been conducted in men. It is known, however, that the disease affects women differently than men. Coronary heart disease occurs approximately 10 years later in women than in men, probably due to the effect of estrogen. Both diagnosis and treatment are often delayed in women, and women are referred for surgery and rehabilitation less often. This could be a factor of access to care, which is also affected by financial concerns, psychosocial stress, and family demands that could cause a woman to pay less attention to her own health care needs.

Heart disease develops with age. Risk factors can be identified, and some can be altered through a change in lifestyle. For instance, high blood pressure, which can be treated, increases the risk of heart disease. Other risk factors cannot be altered but can alert a woman to the need for special attention to the risk factors that are within her control.

STRUCTURE AND FUNCTION

The cardiovascular system circulates blood throughout the body, bringing oxygen and nutrients to muscles and organs, then returns it to the heart to be pumped again. The system of channels through which the blood flows is called the circulatory system. It includes the heart, lungs, and blood vessels. Arteries, arterioles (small arteries), and capillaries (tiny blood vessels) carry blood from the heart to the body. Veins and venules (small veins) return the blood from the body to the heart. The Latin term for the heart is *cor,* and the names of many of the parts of the circulatory system are derived from that word.

Normal Function

The circulatory system carries blood from the lungs, where it receives oxygen, to the left side of the heart, where it is pumped to the rest of the body through arteries. Blood that is rich in oxygen is bright red. After it circulates through the body and the oxygen and nutrients are used, blood is returned to the right side of the heart through veins. This deoxygenated blood is high in carbon dioxide, a waste product, and is dark and purplish blue. It passes from the right side of the heart back to the lungs.

In the lungs, air containing oxygen is inhaled and passes through the respiratory system until it reaches grape-like clusters of air sacs (alveoli) deep within the lungs. The alveoli are surrounded by a network of capillaries, tiny hair-like blood vessels. The air sacs and capillaries are separated by a membrane that transfers oxygen from the air into the blood and removes carbon dioxide from the blood to the lungs. The oxygenated blood is then returned to the heart to be pumped to the body. This process takes place with each breath. Deoxygenated blood flows over the air sacs, discards waste gases and becomes oxygenated, then moves on through larger and larger blood vessels to the heart and the rest of the body.

The heart is a muscle about the size of a person's fist in the middle of the chest, tilted toward the left side. The heart beat is an expansion and contraction of the muscle as it pumps. Each day the heart beats about 100,000 times and pumps about 2,000 gallons of blood.

It is made up of four chambers (Figure 27.2). There are two atria (right and left) and two ventricles (right and left). The atria are the upper chambers that receive the blood. The lower chambers, the ventricles, are thick-walled chambers made of muscle so they can pump the blood out of the heart. Four valves connecting the chambers and major arteries help pump and carry the blood:

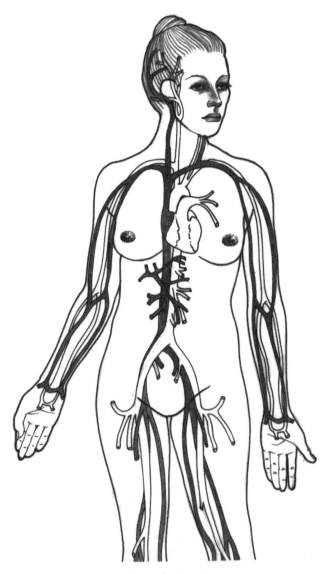

Figure 27.1   The Circulatory System
The heart circulates blood through the veins and arteries.

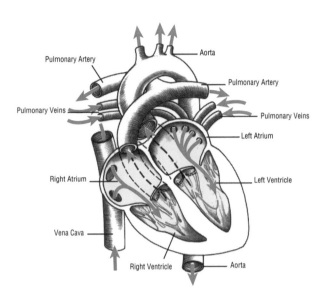

Figure 27.2   The Heart
Blood circulates through the four chambers of the heart. It enters the right atrium and flows to the right ventricle, where it is pumped to the lungs through pulmonary arteries. Blood returns from the lungs through the pulmonary veins to the left atrium. It flows to the left ventricle and is pumped to the rest of the body through the aorta. The vena cava carry blood back to the right atrium.

- the *tricuspid* valve, between the right atrium and the right ventricle;
- the *pulmonary* valve, between the right ventricle and the pulmonary artery;
- the *mitral* valve, between the left atrium and the left ventricle;
- the *aortic* valve, between the left ventricle and the aorta.

The valves open and close to move blood from an atrium to a ventricle or away from the heart through an artery. A change in pressure across the valves causes them to open and close. Each valve has a set of flaps called leaflets or cusps. The mitral value has two flaps and the other valves have three. The valves keep blood flowing in only one direction when the heart beats.

Blood is carried to and from the heart through the great vessels (see box). The blood moves into the heart, through it, and away from the heart into the body in a precise sequence:

- Blood low in oxygen returns to the right side of the heart through large veins (superior and inferior vena cavae) and drains into the right atrium, the first receiving chamber.
- The blood flows through the tricuspid valve into the first pumping chamber, the right ventricle.

THE GREAT VESSELS

The great vessels are the main channels to and from the heart and lungs:

- The *vena cavae* are the major veins that carry blood from the body back to the heart after the oxygen and nutrients have been removed. There are two vena cavae. The *superior vena cava* carries blood from the upper part of the body, and the *inferior vena cava* carries blood back from the lower part of the body.

- *Pulmonary arteries* carry unoxygenated blood from the right side of the heart to the lungs where it receives oxygen.

- *Pulmonary veins* carry oxygenated blood from the lungs back to the left side of the heart.

- The *aorta* is the major artery through which oxygen-rich blood is pumped from the heart to the rest of the body.

- The right ventricle pumps the blood through the pulmonary valve to the pulmonary artery, where it is carried to the lungs to receive oxygen.

- Oxygenated blood is returned to the heart via the pulmonary vein and enters the left atrium.

- Blood drains from the left atrium to the left ventricle through the mitral valve.

- The left ventricle pumps blood through the aortic valve to the aorta, the main artery that branches into smaller arteries to deliver blood to the body.

The heart needs a constant supply of blood to provide nutrients and oxygen for energy. The heart muscle is supplied with blood flow through branching blood vessels called the coronary arteries. The coronary arteries begin at the aorta. There are two major coronary arteries, right and left, whose work it is to supply freshly oxygenated blood to the muscles of all four chambers of the heart. The blood flow to each chamber is based on the amount of work it does; the blood supply to the left and right atria is relatively small because they do not work as hard as the ventricles, especially the left ventricle.

A chamber of the heart contracts when an electrical signal moves across it. The electrical signal starts in the right atrium in an area called the sinoatrial (SA) node. From there it spreads, causing the muscle in the atrium to contract and push blood into the ventricle. The signal moves through the right and left atria causing the muscles to contract. It then travels to the ventricles, causing them to contract together with a powerful force that squeezes blood from them through the valves. The heartbeat is the sound of the atria contracting and pushing blood into the ventricles and the ventricle contracting and pushing blood out into arteries. Once the heart-beat cycle is completed, it starts again in the SA node. When this cycle is repeated normally, the heart rhythm is called regular or normal sinus rhythm.

Dysfunction

The heart needs a steady blood supply to maintain pumping at normal levels of activity. Just as with any other type of exercise, the harder a muscle works, the more blood it requires. With exercise, the heart muscle pumps harder to increase the blood supply to the body's muscles. The coronary arteries dilate to increase blood flow, and the lungs work harder to bring oxygen to the blood. If the body's muscles receive an adequate supply of oxygen, a person can function at peak performance. If the muscles do not receive enough oxygen, however, pain and damage can occur.

The blood supply can be limited by a condition called atherosclerosis, which causes a buildup in the lining of the arteries that narrows their openings (Figure 27.3). Deposits of fatty substances, including cholesterol, calcium, and clotting factors in the blood called fibrin, build up into plaque and narrow the opening of the artery. As the condition progresses, it can lead to the vessel becoming narrowed enough to decrease blood flow. A small layer of deposit or narrowing does not affect blood flow, even at extreme amounts of exercise. The blood vessel needs to be narrowed by 70 percent in order to affect the heart muscle's blood supply. If more than 70 percent narrowing occurs, blood supply is even more limited and the amount of activity that triggers symptoms of chest pain is less and less. At normal levels of activity there may still be enough blood flow to allow the heart to work properly; however, problems may arise with vigorous exercise. The heart pumps faster and with more force, requiring more blood to travel through the arteries to keep up with the body's need. The coronary arteries dilate slightly but cannot open areas that have been narrowed. The heart muscle itself cannot get the additional blood flow and

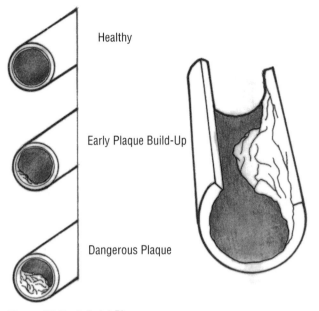

Figure 27.3 Arterial Plaque
The opening of the artery is narrowed when deposits build up and form plaque, blocking the blood supply.

Healthy

Early Plaque Build-Up

Dangerous Plaque

oxygen that it needs. As exercise continues, the muscle starts to cramp and pain occurs. If the heart's need for more blood is not reduced by immediate rest, the muscle will be damaged. This damage is called a myocardial infarction, or heart attack. Damage to the heart muscle due to atherosclerosis can occur at rest or with normal activities when the buildup nears total blockage. A partial blockage can become a total blockage in several ways:

- The cholesterol deposit or plaque may rupture because of bleeding in the blood vessel wall

that builds up under the plaque, raising it until the vessel is blocked.

- Blood cells called platelets can clump together and get caught on the narrowed area of the blood vessel and cause blockage.

- The vessel wall may go into spasm, constricting blood flow until it stops, even without narrowing of the artery.

Most heart attacks occur through a combination of these events. Once the blood flow is stopped or severely limited in a vessel, normal clotting occurs, just as it would in any other part of the body. The blood clot becomes more solid with each passing second and will fill the entire opening of the vessel. Once blood flow has been stopped for a few minutes, the clotted blood (thrombus) will prevent blood from passing through the vessel. If the initial cause of the blood vessel blockage is resolved—for instance, if spasm of the artery stops—the thrombus will prevent further blood flow to the heart muscle and a heart attack will still occur. If this clot can be broken up and blood flow reestablished, the heart attack can be halted or limited. This concept is the basis for the latest treatment of heart attack, "clotbusting" or thrombolysis.

Anything that irritates the wall of the blood vessel can trigger the development of deposits and lead to narrowing of the arteries. Possible causes include elevated cholesterol in the blood, high blood pressure (hypertension), and cigarette smoking. It is not known why certain areas of the arteries develop plaque and others do not. Atherosclerosis is a part of aging but can be worsened by diet, the presence of certain conditions, and family history.

KEEPING THE SYSTEM HEALTHY

About 40 percent of all coronary events in women are fatal, and most of these events occur without warning. The best way you can survive heart disease is to prevent it from occurring. The narrowing of the arteries that leads to coronary artery disease occurs slowly over time, and may begin as early as the teenage years. A healthy lifestyle can help you prevent heart disease.

Several factors increase the risk of coronary artery disease (see "Risk Factors"), and most of them are under your direct control. In addition to these factors, certain drugs, such as cocaine, can cause a heart attack

and should not be used. Some of the risks can be lessened by changes in lifestyle. Quitting smoking is the most important thing a person can do to reduce the risk of heart disease, cutting the risk by 50 percent. Diet and exercise can help lower cholesterol and hypertension, and the benefits of lowered blood pressure increase with age. Diabetes can be controlled by changes in weight and exercise. Hormone replacement therapy can lower a woman's risk of coronary artery disease by 40–50 percent.

Combinations of risk factors multiply rather than

add their individual effects to your likelihood of developing coronary artery disease. For example, the combination of hypertension, elevated cholesterol, and cigarette smoking will increase the risk of coronary artery disease by 10 times or more. A 40-year-old woman with diabetes who smokes is 10 times more likely than a nonsmoker to develop heart disease. A woman over the age of 35 who smokes and is taking oral contraceptives is 39 times more likely to develop coronary artery disease. These combinations point out the importance of changing those risk factors within your control.

Risk factor modification can be most effective when it is used to prevent heart disease. This is called primary prevention. The advantage is that coronary artery disease is prevented, delayed, or made less severe. The disadvantage is that there is no real certainty of the benefits. Once someone is proven to have heart disease, either by testing after showing symptoms or having a heart attack, the focus is on preventing the next cardiac event or heart attack. This is called secondary prevention. Every day that a person doesn't have another heart attack is viewed as progress, so the personal rewards are great.

Women should evaluate their risk of coronary artery disease, change those factors that can be changed, and reduce those risks that can be reduced so they can be as healthy and active as possible. They should also have their blood pressure and cholesterol levels checked on a regular basis so steps can be taken to lower them if they are elevated.

Lipids

Cholesterol

Cholesterol is a soft, fatlike substance that is found in all the body's cells. It is used to form certain tissues in the body, especially nerves. About one-third of blood cholesterol comes from the food we eat, and the body—primarily the liver—produces the rest. Foods from animals, especially egg yolks, meat, fish, poultry, and whole-milk dairy products contain it; most foods from plants do not. The body makes all the cholesterol it needs, so people do not need to consume it to maintain their health.

Cholesterol is made up of several major components called low-density lipoproteins (LDL) and high-density lipoproteins (HDL). LDL is considered bad cholesterol and HDL good cholesterol.

RISK FACTORS FOR CORONARY ARTERY DISEASE

- Diabetes
- Hypertension
- Tobacco smoking
- High LDL, low HDL, high triglycerides
- Family history of early heart disease
- Lack of exercise
- Obesity—waist predominance
- African-American heritage
- Age

Fat in food is digested in the body and taken to the liver, where it is processed into cholesterol. Thus, a diet high in fat, especially saturated fat, can lead to high cholesterol levels (see Chapter 3). Low-density lipoproteins carry fat from the liver to other parts of the body. They unload fat in the cells and circulate in the blood. The more LDL cholesterol in the blood, the greater the likelihood it will deposit within a blood vessel. LDL can push into the wall of a blood vessel, causing it to build up and narrow the opening.

High-density lipoprotein actually picks up LDL cholesterol deposits in the blood and carries them back to the liver to be discarded. Having low levels of HDL is a risk factor for heart disease because the LDL deposits are not picked up. In women, HDL cholesterol is especially important. For every 10-milligram increase in HDL there appears to be a 40 percent decrease in risk. The female hormone estrogen increases HDL and decreases LDL. The ratio of LDL to HDL rises substantially after menopause, which may contribute to the higher rates of coronary heart disease in postmenopausal women.

Triglyceride

Another lipid is triglyceride, a fat in the bloodstream that is a factor for heart disease in women, but not in men. Its levels increase with diabetes, high fat intake, alcohol consumption, obesity, and menopause. High triglyceride levels make LDL more likely to cause coronary lesions.

The levels of triglyceride and total cholesterol and their components in your body can be tested by lipid analysis. A young woman with no risk factors should have lipid analysis every 3 to 5 years to determine her levels. She should then try to maintain her levels within desirable ranges (Table 1). The lower the level of LDL and the higher the level of HDL the better. HDL can be increased by exercise, estrogen replacement, and a modest amount of alcohol (one glass of wine per day). Levels of LDL cholesterol can be lowered by a low-cholesterol diet, exercise, and weight control. Some people inherit a trait that causes the liver to make too much cholesterol. Such people need to take medications that act on the liver to lower LDL levels. Older women and women with risk factors should have their lipid analysis done every 1 to 3 years.

TABLE 1 CHOLESTEROL LEVELS

Cholesterol Level (mg/dl)	Classification[a]
Total	
Less than 200	Desirable
200–239	Borderline
Greater than or equal to 240	High
HDL cholesterol[b]	
Less than 35	Low
35–59	Normal
60 or more	High
LDL cholesterol	
Less than 130	Desirable
130–159	Borderline
160 or more	High

Source: Expert Panel on Detection, Evaluation, and Treatment of High Blood Cholesterol in Adults, "Summary of the Second Report of the National Cholesterol Education Program (NCEP) Expert Panel on Detection, Evaluation, and Treatment of High Blood Cholesterol in Adults (Adult Treatment Panel II)," *Journal of the American Medical Association* 269 (1993): 3015-3023.
[a] This classification is for people who do not already have established coronary artery disease.
[b] Women have a higher average HDL than men; therefore, an HDL below 50 may be considered low.

Hypertension

A woman with high blood pressure, or hypertension, has 2–10 times more risk of heart disease (See Chapter 37). Often the disease is not recognized until it is in later stages. With hypertension blood vessel walls become irritated by the increased pressure in the force of rushing blood. This irritation damages the vessel wall,

causing plaque to form. A woman should have her blood pressure checked regularly. If your blood pressure is high, take steps to lower it (see "Blood Pressure" box). Beginning at age 50, hypertension is more common in women than in men. High blood pressure can be lowered through weight reduction, exercise, salt restriction, and medications. Women with heart disease are more likely to have hypertension than men with heart disease.

Tobacco Smoking

There is no safe level of cigarette smoking in terms of risk of heart disease. A woman who smokes as few as 1–4 cigarettes per day is twice as likely to have heart disease as a woman who does not smoke, and that risk increases eleven-fold with 45 cigarettes a day. The risks are greater in premenopausal women who are older than 35 and taking oral contraceptives. Any woman who smokes risks facing a heart attack 19 years earlier than a nonsmoker.

Nicotine causes irritation of the coronary arteries, spasm of the muscles in the artery wall, clotting problems (which increase the risk of a clot developing), and high blood pressure. Smoking also increases the impact of coronary artery disease because carbon monoxide in the smoke reduces the oxygen level in the blood. The low oxygen level also irritates the vessel wall and triggers the development of plaque. Nicotine is a powerful spasm-producing substance and increases the likelihood that normal or only mildly narrowed

BLOOD PRESSURE

Blood pressure is measured in terms of systolic and diastolic pressures. Normal blood pressure is expressed as 140/85 mm Hg (millimeters of mercury). The first figure is the systolic pressure and the second figure is the diastolic pressure. Systolic pressure is the measurement taken when the heart contracts and pumps blood to the body. Diastolic pressure is the measurement taken when the heart is relaxed and the chambers are open and filling with blood. A sustained blood pressure greater than 140/90 requires treatment. Beginning at age 50, hypertension is more common in women than in men and more common in African-Americans.

vessels will develop spasms. Stopping smoking (or not starting to smoke) will help prevent heart disease from getting worse, regardless of other factors. It is the most effective way to prevent coronary artery disease.

Estrogen and Its Replacement

A woman with functioning ovaries produces the female hormone estrogen, which affects almost all of the body tissues, including the heart, blood vessels, and liver. It is thought that estrogen causes a woman to have a lower systolic blood pressure, a lower LDL cholesterol level, a lower triglyceride level, and a higher HDL cholesterol level. As a result, less cholesterol deposits build up in the arteries and less coronary artery disease develops. Spasm is also less likely in blood vessels that are exposed to estrogen, which helps maintain normal vessel function.

The average age of menopause is 51 years, but a woman's estrogen levels begin to decrease much earlier. As her ovaries produce less estrogen, a woman's level of LDL and triglyceride rises, her HDL falls, her blood pressure starts to rise, and she has a greater chance of spasm or irritation of a blood vessel. Over the next few years, a woman's lipid levels and blood vessel tone, as well as her risk of coronary artery disease, become similar to that of a man. The effects of the loss of estrogen are avoided in women who receive estrogen replacement around the time of menopause, whether natural or caused by surgery to remove the ovaries. In these women, HDL levels remain high because of increased production by the liver and LDL and triglyceride levels remain low. Blood pressure also remains low and vessels retain their good tone and tend not to spasm. Death rates are estimated to be reduced by 40–50 percent with estrogen replacement therapy.

However, estrogen taken alone is strongly linked to cancer of the uterus. This risk can be prevented by the addition of natural progesterone or artificial hormones called progestins. The disadvantage of progestin is that it reverses the benefits of estrogen on lipid levels. Although this was once thought to negate the benefits of hormone replacement therapy, studies have shown that the protection remains with combined therapy and is best with natural progesterone. Even without the lipid benefits, blood vessels retain good tone on progestin. All women approaching menopause should consider taking hormone replacement therapy unless they are at high risk of estrogen-related cancers or disorders. It not only protects against coronary artery disease, but also helps prevent bone loss (osteoporosis) that occurs during aging and may reduce the likelihood of developing Alzheimer's disease.

Oral Contraceptives

The hormones in oral contraceptives affect the levels of lipids in the blood. In the past, the higher doses of hormones that were used caused high cholesterol and blood pressure and led to heart attacks, particularly in women who smoked. The low-dose formulations used today carry little if any risk of coronary heart disease, but there is a slight risk of blood clots. Some of the newer types of oral contraceptives actually lower LDL and raise HDL. Because of the risk of blood clots in women who smoke, however, women who smoke should not use oral contraceptives, especially if they are over 35.

Diabetes

Women with diabetes are two to three times more likely to have a heart attack than women who do not have diabetes. Diabetes seems to nullify the protection provided by estrogen. A woman with diabetes has the same risk of coronary artery disease and heart attack as a nondiabetic man and almost as much as a man with diabetes. Women with heart disease are more likely to have diabetes than are men with heart disease.

Diabetes poses a risk in a variety of ways: it irritates vessel walls, increases LDL, increases triglyceride, lowers HDL, and raises blood pressure. People with diabetes often have other risk factors for coronary artery disease, including obesity. Careful treatment of diabetes may reduce the increased risk for coronary artery disease but cannot eliminate it. Measures to bring diabetes under control include weight reduction, strict diet, and exercise. Although the risk posed by diabetes may persist, these measures are also helpful in improving the health of the heart.

Obesity

Obesity increases the risks of other factors that contribute to coronary artery disease, such as high blood pressure, diabetes, and high cholesterol and triglyceride.

And weight gain alone is associated with increased LDL and total cholesterol and decreased HDL. The pattern of weight gain also can be a factor. Weight gained around the waist, called central obesity, increases the risk of heart disease. Weight gained around the hips, more typical of women, has less risk. For good health, women should maintain a weight that is suitable for their height. They should eat a variety of low-fat foods and follow an exercise program to help maintain their weight and reduce the risk of cardiovascular and other diseases (see chapters 3 and 4).

Sedentary Lifestyle

Lack of exercise is a risk factor for coronary artery disease. Exercise increases HDL and reduces LDL, helping to prevent heart disease. It also helps control weight gain and promotes cardiovascular fitness so the heart and lungs function at full capacity. Cardiovascular fitness increases as the body increases its ability to store oxygen. This increases a person's capacity for physical activity, giving her more energy. The heart must beat at a certain level in order for fitness to occur. This is called the target heart rate (see box). A woman should exercise at this level for 20 or more minutes at least three times a week.

Race

The African-American race is associated with an increased risk of coronary artery disease in women. Between the ages of 35 and 74, the death rate from heart attack in African-American women is twice that of white women. Death rates from coronary heart disease for African-American women is 33 percent higher than for white women.

Family History

A family history of heart disease, especially if it occurred at an early age, is a strong risk factor for cardiovascular disease. The cause appears to be related to a number of factors. Some medical problems, such as hypertension, diabetes, or high cholesterol, are inher-

TARGET HEART RATE

Your heart rate is a guide to how hard to exercise. To check your heart rate, count your pulse for the first 10 seconds after you stop exercising. Multiply this count by 6 to get the number of beats per minute. To get the best workout, you should exercise at your target heart rate. The target heart rate is 60–80 percent of your maximum heart rate, which is 220 minus your age. The following chart can help you find your target heart rate.

Age	Target Heart Rate	Avg. Maximum Heart Rate
(years)	(beats per minute)	(beats per minute)
20	120–160	200
25	117–156	195
30	114–152	190
35	111–148	185
40	108–144	180
45	105–140	175
50	102–136	170
55	99–132	165
60	96–128	160
65	93–124	155
70	90–120	150
75	87–116	145
80	84–112	140

CARDIOVASCULAR SPECIALISTS

Cardiologist—an internal medicine physician specializing in the diagnosis and treatment of ailments of the heart and other areas of the cardiovascular system

Clinical cardiologist—specializes in prevention, noninvasive diagnostic testing, and medication treatment.

Invasive cardiologist—specializes in cardiac catheterization, invasive testing, and treatment of the cardiovascular system using catheter techniques.

Electrophysiologist—specializes in diagnosis and treatment of heart rhythm disturbances.

Cardiovascular surgeon—a physician and surgeon specializing in the surgical treatment of the heart and cardiovascular system

ited. In families with these problems, cardiovascular disease at an early age is the result of these conditions. Families also tend to have similar habits, although habits can be changed. People often act, eat, and exercise as their parents and siblings do. The genes and habits that cause us to have central obesity, to be sedentary, to smoke, or to follow poor diets cluster in families.

A woman whose mother or father had a heart attack at an early age (before age 65 in her mother and 55 in her father) should be alert to her risk of cardiovascular disease. She should look at her risk factors and lifestyle and make the changes that are possible to avoid repeating her family history. If a woman has any symptoms of heart disease, she should seek medical care without delay, and may be referred to a specialist (see "Cardiovascular Specialists").

HEALTH CONCERNS

Early recognition of heart problems and prompt treatment can make a difference in the amount of damage done to the heart and overall recovery. Women without symptoms should have regular screening tests to detect any risk factors. Women with symptoms should see a doctor immediately and be especially alert to warning signs (see box). Women with symptoms are evaluated by personal and family histories, physical examination, and known risk factors and lifestyle. Diagnostic tests will be done to assess the symptoms and find their cause. These tests are also performed on women known to have coronary artery disease who notice a change in their symptoms.

During the exam, a woman's level of physical activity, particularly in relation to any symptoms, will be assessed. This is done to find out how much exercise she does on a regular basis and whether there are signs of symptoms during exertion. It is important for the doctor to know if chest tightness or shortness of breath occur with a certain level of activity, to identify that level, and to find out whether these sensations go away with rest.

One of the tests performed to assess heart problems is an electrocardiogram (ECG), which measures the electrical activity of the heart. A normal ECG exam does not exclude coronary artery disease, but it can suggest that a heart attack has not occurred. If a patient is having pain while the ECG is being done and the results are normal, the pain is probably not related to the heart. Any abnormalities shown by the ECG usually are caused by heart problems, although the test is not perfect and the results may be misleading. Other tests that may be used are stress testing and echocardiography (discussed later).

Once heart disease is diagnosed, several different medications may be used (see box). Some are designed to improve blood flow by dilating the coronary arteries or preventing spasm or by reducing the work of the heart. Other medications reduce blood clotting. Medications and treatments are aimed at treating risk factors as well as symptoms.

WARNING SIGNS OF HEART DISEASE

- *Angina*—a feeling of tightness, pressure, or pain that appears with exertion or stress and disappears with rest, usually in the chest, throat, upper abdomen, or arms.
- *Shortness of breath*—Difficulty breathing on exertion, when lying down, or while asleep.
- *Edema*—Swelling of ankles, usually at the end of the day.
- *Palpitations*—Forceful, rapid, or irregular heartbeat.
- *Fatigue*—Decreased ability to exercise, tiring easily.
- *Fainting*—Sudden loss of consciousness or lightheadedness.

Angina

The discomfort caused by a lack of blood flow through a blood vessel serving the heart is called angina. The heart muscle cries out in pain when its blood supply is limited. The chemical changes that occur as a result of this lack of blood flow are called ischemia. People with angina can have a variety of symptoms, including pres-

MEDICATIONS TO TREAT HEART DISEASE

- *Angiotensin converting enzyme (ACE inhibitors)* lower blood pressure and reduce the work of the heart in patients with congestive heart failure.

- *Antiarrhythmics* help prevent extra heart beats or repetitive arrhythmias. They work by suppressing the spontaneous electrical impulses that cause the irregular beating of the heart.

- *Antiplatelet* medications relieve angina by helping to prevent clumps of blood from forming and by reducing the risk of disrupting plaque on the wall of the blood vessel.

- *Beta-blockers* reduce or block the action of chemicals in the body that stimulate blood pressure and heart rate, lowering blood pressure and allowing the heart to work less and need less oxygen.

- *Calcium channel blockers* block calcium in muscle fiber cells, open the coronary arteries and other blood vessels, reduce the risk of spasm and, reduce the work of the heart.

- *Cholesterol-lowering medications* lower the LDL cholesterol level in blood when diet and exercise are not effective.

- *Diuretics* act on the kidneys to remove excess fluid from the body that occurs in congestive heart failure and, in low dosages, reduce blood pressure.

- *Nitrates* open coronary arteries and other vessels in the body, reducing the work of the heart and reducing spasm.

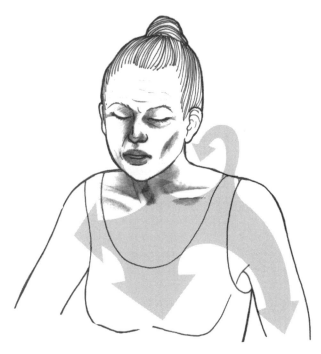

Figure 27.4 Chest Pain
Pain from a blocked blood vessel (angina or heart attack) can be felt in the chest, left arm, neck and jaw, and the abdomen.

sure, tightness, squeezing, burning, numbness, or heaviness located between the jaw and abdomen. The nerves that supply the heart send their signals to the chest area, causing discomfort. The pain occurs most often on the left side, but may also be felt in the arms, usually the left, or in the neck, jaw, lower chest, or abdomen (Figure 27.4). Some patients feel no discomfort or pay no attention to it when it occurs. This is called silent angina. Many patients, especially women, will not feel the typical left chest and left arm sensations that men do and instead will notice abdominal or jaw discomfort. Some patients who do not feel the discomfort will notice the changes associated with the chemical and heart reaction to the lack of blood flow. These changes include shortness of breath, extreme fatigue, nausea, sweating, or irregularity of heart beat. Each person is different in her response, but any discomfort or symptom that always comes on with exercise or stress and is relieved by rest may be your body's version of angina.

Angina can be stable or unstable. Stable angina is characterized by the episodes of discomfort occurring in a regular or predictable pattern, such as climbing two flights of stairs or after emotional upsets, and promptly being relieved at rest. Stable angina is usually treated by medications that reduce the work of the heart muscle. If the heart does not have to work as hard, it does not need as much blood supply and can function with the lesser flow it receives. Opening the coronary arteries and reducing the likelihood of clotting are the goals of treatment. Reducing other risk factors is also helpful, both for short-term improvement and long-term benefit in halting the progression of disease.

Unstable angina is more serious. It is discomfort that occurs without warning. It may come on with little or no exertion, even when awaking, or may suddenly develop with exertion when there were no prior symptoms. Unstable angina usually means the blockage of the vessel is large or has an irregular surface and that clotting or spasm is occurring. It is usually treated in the hospital because it often precedes a heart attack. The medications are given intravenously and include blood thinners such as heparin and aspirin, medications to reduce the work of the heart, and drugs that open the coronary arteries. If a patient does not respond to these medications, procedures such as coronary angiography and angioplasty may be performed to examine the coronary arteries and try to identify the location of the blockage and improve blood flow.

Angina can also be caused by spasm. This temporary squeezing or constriction of the muscular layer of a blood vessel will reduce the blood flow to an area of the heart muscle and cause angina. If the spasm continues, a blood clot can form and block the blood flow. Spasm is usually treated with medications that dilate the arteries. It can be given orally, under the tongue so it can be absorbed more rapidly, or intravenously.

A rupture in the plaque that builds up on the walls of the arteries also can cause angina. The blockage of blood flow will start the process of a clot forming. Even if the ruptured plaque is no longer blocking an artery, the clot that remains will continue to block blood flow through the blood vessel. Treatment consists of breaking up or preventing the blood clot.

persists in spite of resting or use of antacids could be symptoms of a heart attack, especially if they occur with sweating, shortness of breath, nausea, or palpitations. A person who is having a heart attack should get emergency help immediately (see box). A person who is already being treated for heart problems may have nitroglycerin tablets. These tablets are placed under the tongue and will relieve angina in 1–5 minutes. A second tablet can be used if the first is not effective. If two tablets do not provide relief, a third can be taken, but lightheadedness may occur because the medication lowers blood pressure. If two nitroglycerin tablets do not work, seek medical help.

Diagnosis

In the emergency room, all hospital personnel should be informed that the patient may be having a heart attack. Cardiac problems often are not diagnosed or treated promptly in women. While the patient's condition is being assessed, the heart will be monitored, blood samples will be taken for testing, oxygen will be given through the nose, and tubes will be inserted into the veins to give medications.

If the ECG results are normal but the symptoms are severe and persistent, the test should be repeated. It is not unusual for ECG results to be normal in the first hour after a heart attack and then to show abnormal

Myocardial Infarction

Sudden or progressive persistent blockage of blood flow or lack of adequate blood flow to any area of the heart causes the tissue served by that vessel to start to die. This process is called myocardial infarction, or heart attack. It starts after a few minutes, progresses after about an hour, then continues for the next 4–12 hours. During this time, the body responds to the failure of the heart to pump properly and to poisons that are released by the dying tissues, causing symptoms of sweating, nausea, racing heartbeat, and shortness of breath. The lack of blood flow and ischemia will cause areas of the heart muscle to become unstable, and irregular heartbeats (arrhythmias) can occur. The heart muscle closest to the blocked vessel dies first, and the damage spreads to affect any area of the heart muscle that is not served by other blood vessels.

Myocardial infarction occurs more often in the early morning hours or after exercise, exertion, emotional stress, or eating. Chest pain, pressure, or heaviness that

IF YOU THINK YOU ARE HAVING A HEART ATTACK

- Tell the people with you that you are ill and in need of emergency help.

- Sit or lie down and ask someone to call emergency services. Have the person calling indicate that it is a cardiac problem so the paramedics will respond appropriately.

- If you are alone, make sure the door is unlocked.

- If you are known to have a cardiac problem, chew two low-dose aspirin tablets.

- Do not try to drive yourself to the hospital or emergency room unless you do not have a telephone or a person who can help you.

results later. Results from blood tests do not become abnormal until approximately 6 hours after a heart attack.

Treatment

If it appears that a person is having a heart attack, aspirin will be given and treatment and other procedures will be explained. Thrombolysis may be offered as a treatment if the patient is not pregnant and has not had a recent stroke, surgery, or active bleeding. This treatment, nicknamed "clotbusting," does just that. Thrombolysis dissolves a blood clot that is blocking an artery. Used within 6 hours, it can reduce the risk of death and heart muscle damage significantly. However, this treatment also can cause bleeding elsewhere in the body and may require a transfusion. Bleeding can occur in the brain, causing a stroke. The risk of stroke is elevated in a heart attack, however, so the risks of treatment are not that much greater.

Timing of treatment is critical because heart muscle is lost with every minute of a heart attack. The doctor will try to begin thrombolysis as soon as possible, sometimes within 30 minutes. Treatment may begin in the emergency room or the cardiac care unit of the hospital. Other medications and procedures, such as cardiac catheterization and angioplasty, may be recommended, depending on the patient's condition and response to the thrombolysis.

Heart attack patients receive care in intensive care units or cardiac care units, where their conditions can be carefully monitored. Any symptoms or change in symptoms should be reported to the doctor or nurse in the unit. Medications can be given to treat any urgent problems and make the patient more comfortable. A patient who has had a heart attack may stay in the cardiac care unit for 2–3 days. The patient will notice an ache or discomfort in the chest area where the more severe pain had been. This is like the ache of a hurt muscle and is caused by the damage to the heart. Any damaged heart muscle will be soft and needs a few days to form a scar. Until then, the patient should avoid straining or being too active. As activity gradually increases, the patient is watched closely for further symptoms. Instruction is given on diet and lifestyle changes to help prevent further heart attacks, and an exercise program (cardiac rehabilitation) will be recommended to promote fitness. Before the patient leaves the hospital, tests may be done to assess whether the patient's condition is stable and to determine which blood vessels are narrowed and which ones need treatment. Medications may be given to reduce the work of the heart and improve blood flow to the heart muscle.

More women than men die in hospitals as a result of heart attacks, and women have a higher rate of complications after a heart attack. Approximately 5 percent of people who go to an emergency room with chest pain have a heart attack that is not diagnosed and are sent home. These people are at highest risk of dying from the heart attack. The likelihood of surviving a heart attack is much better with proper diagnosis and treatment in a hospital. Any person who is having symptoms of a heart attack and is sent home from an emergency room should have a clear understanding of what tests were done, the results, the diagnosis, and what should be done if the symptoms persist or get worse.

Arrhythmias

The regular heartbeat can be disturbed with racing or skipping, causing symptoms of palpitations or dizziness. This is called arrhythmia. It can be caused by a medical problem, such as an overactive thyroid, and made worse by alcohol or stimulants, such as caffeine. Some arrhythmias are more serious than others, depending on where they arise in the heart and what causes them. An arrhythmia can become serious enough to be life-threatening.

Symptoms

Arrhythmias can arise in the atria or the ventricles. The more serious forms arise in the ventricles, but sometimes an irregularity that arises in the atria can affect the beat in the ventricles. In the atrium, arrhythmias may take the form of an occasional extra beat. The extra beats may become repetitive, producing a rapid series of beats known as tachycardia. This may occur suddenly and cause dizziness or fainting but is rarely serious. The atria can become enlarged by high blood pressure or damaged by coronary artery disease or inflammation. When this occurs, they may start beating uncontrollably, which is called atrial fibrillation. A regular and rapid irregularity is called atrial flutter. Treatment is directed to any underlying medical problem, such as overactive thyroid. Avoiding caffeine, alcohol, and stimulants may help. Medications may be used to reduce the extra beats or return the heart to normal rhythm. If atrial fibrillation remains, there is an increased risk of stroke, and blood thinners may be used to reduce this risk.

Extra beats can also arise in the ventricles. If these beats become repetitive, they can cause ventricular tachycardia, which can be life-threatening. If the heart rate is too rapid, the heart does not have enough time to fill with blood between beats, which causes blood pressure to drop. This condition can worsen and turn into ventricular fibrillation, a fatal condition when the ventricles quiver and don't move blood at all. The treatment of ventricular arrhythmias is electrical shock, or defibrillation. This technique stops the heartbeat in the hope that the regular heart rhythm will take over. Medication can also be used, but many medications can have a bad effect on the heartbeat. Devices that are implanted in a person's body and produce small shocks can be used to correct the heart rhythm.

Treatment

Some heart rhythm problems are caused by damage to the electrical signal that starts or carries the heartbeat. This damage may be caused by heart attacks, illness, viruses, or medications. Very slow heart beats can occur causing dizziness, fainting, or congestive heart failure. Treatment is either removal of the medication or treatment of the underlying illness. If the problem remains, a pacemaker is needed to regulate the heartbeat.

A pacemaker uses a plastic tube (a lead) with a metal core and tip. If the pacemaker is being used only temporarily, the lead is placed into the heart through a vein, either through the side of the neck or in the leg. It is attached to a box with electrical circuits that constantly monitor the heartbeat. With each heartbeat, the system waits for the next beat. If no beat occurs within a second, it sends a tiny electric pulse down the wire lead. This stimulates the heart electrically at the tip of the lead and causes the heart to beat. If a permanent pacemaker is needed, the lead is passed through the large vein near the top of the chest wall, under the collarbone. A pacemaker the size of a book of matches is implanted under the skin through a small cut. This self-contained system will work for 5–10 years until the battery wears down, when it can be easily changed. Pacemakers can have one or two leads, stimulating the ventricle only or the atria and the ventricle.

Other causes of arrhythmias can be difficult to diagnose. Patients with difficult arrhythmias may need highly specialized testing by electrophysiologists and therapy to identify the area of heart muscle that is causing the trouble. This area can then be destroyed by high-frequency radio waves, curing the problem.

Congestive Heart Failure

Congestive heart failure is the result of damage to the heart from untreated hypertension, muscle disease, or myocardial infarction. When the heart is damaged, it can no longer pump effectively, and with each heartbeat it moves less blood out of the heart. Blood that doesn't move forward creates pressure on the rest of the body. In the lungs, this causes fluid to flood the air sacs that normally transfer only gases between the blood and the lungs. This fluid in the air sacs interferes with the ability of the lungs to provide the blood with oxygen.

Early symptoms of congestive heart failure include shortness of breath with exercise. As it worsens, congestion in the lungs and difficulty breathing develop. Patients may notice a wet sound while they are breathing, caused by the fluid in the air sacs. If the pressure is severe, fluid may build up in the legs, a condition that is made worse by gravity. Fluid that builds up in the legs during the day will be reabsorbed into the bloodstream at night and flood the lungs, causing the person to suddenly awaken short of breath. She may even need to sit up or stand to breath.

Treatment of congestive heart failure includes medications to reduce the work of the heart. Diuretics are used to help rid the body of fluid. Nitrates and angiotensin converting enzyme (ACE) inhibitors are used to help the body handle the fluid and reduce the work of the heart. Recent studies show that ACE inhibitors are more effective than originally thought, and some doctors recommend they be used to a greater extent. Congestive heart failure may improve if the problem is caused by very high blood pressure, a damaged heart valve, or recurrent angina that has not caused permanent damage. Once permanent damage is done, however, the problem can be treated but rarely cured. Congestive heart failure can also occur when the heart muscle is damaged by a toxin, such as alcohol, or a viral infection of the heart. This can happen suddenly, even in young people. When the damage is severe and does not respond well to treatment, a person's strength and breath, and thus their level of activity, are severely restricted. These patients are often hospitalized and may be referred for heart transplant.

Murmurs

Heart murmurs are abnormal sounds that the blood makes as it passes through the chambers of the heart.

The sounds of the heart valves are loudest directly over their location. Normally, the opening and closing of heart valves creates a "lub-dub" sound with each heart beat, and the blood flow itself is silent. If there is an abnormality in the opening or closing of the valves, or if there is an abnormal flow of blood within the heart, a swishing sound or murmur is audible. The timing of this sound, where it is heard, what makes it louder or softer, and other factors in the examination help to determine where the murmur is coming from and whether the condition is serious.

The most common cause of heart murmurs is valve disease. This can occur because of infection, unusual wear and tear on a valve, or a congenital problem. In some cases, weakened valves may be vulnerable to infection and may be treatable with antibiotics.

Infection

Rheumatic fever was once a common illness that caused damage to heart valves, although it is now relatively rare in the United States. Rheumatic fever is caused by bacterial infection in the blood stream, which usually starts with a strep throat infection and then spreads throughout the body. The use of antibiotics for strep throat has greatly reduced the occurrence of rheumatic fever and thus the development of new cases of damaged heart valves. This damage can still be seen, however, in older Americans and some immigrants. It most often affects the mitral and aortic valves. Other infections that can damage the heart valve include a bacterial infection among drug addicts caused by their use of needles for intravenous drug use.

The most commonly damaged valves are the tricuspid and pulmonary valves. Thick clumps of infection grow on the heart valve and cause mild to severe damage. If treated rapidly, the infection may be cured, but the valve damage will remain. When valves are damaged by infection, the leaflets of the valves can become thickened and have difficulty opening all the way. The narrowed opening reduces the amount of blood that can move across the valve with each heartbeat. Sometimes the thickened leaflets are frozen open, so blood flows backwards between beats. This is called regurgitation. These conditions can cause heart chambers to become enlarged and eventually cause increased pressure on the lungs, leading to shortness of breath and congestive heart failure. Swelling of the legs can also occur. The enlargement of heart chambers allows arrhythmias to occur more easily, increasing the risk of congestive heart failure.

Valve problems caused by infection are diagnosed by physical examination, EKG, chest X-ray, and cardiac echocardiography. Cardiac catheterization may be done if there is a question about the severity of the problem or leakage. Medications are used to control the heart rhythm and reduce swelling or fluid in the lungs. When the valve problem is so severe that the patient cannot function, open-heart surgery is performed to replace the valve. Coronary artery disease also may be corrected at the same time. The damaged heart valve is removed and replaced with an artificial valve or a valve taken from an animal or human donor.

Prevention of Infection

Valves can have minor thickening or wear and tear, resulting in soft murmurs. The abnormal blood flow causes an increased risk for infection of the heart valves. Even though the valves sit in the heart with blood all around them, their own blood supply is very limited. Any time bacteria enters the blood stream, the body's blood supply sends white cells to fight the bacteria and clear the infection. If the bacteria settle on the abnormal valves, the limited blood supply of the valve has a great deal of difficulty in fighting off the bacteria. Infection (bacterial endocarditis) can set in and cause damage to the heart valve.

Women with any type of valve abnormality are an increased risk of bacterial endocarditis. The most common source of bacteria in the blood stream is from dental work. The mouth is full of bacteria. When bleeding occurs during dental work, bacteria from the mouth can enter the bloodstream. If the bacteria settle on heart valves, infection can occur. This is extremely rare with normal valves, but occurs 10 to 100 times more often with abnormal, damaged, or artificial heart valves. To help prevent bacterial endocarditis, it is recommended that patients with abnormal heart valves take antibiotics before a procedure. Antibiotics taken before the bacteria enter the bloodstream and coat the bacteria and make them less "sticky" and less likely to stick to the heart valves and cause infection. The antibiotics also help kill the bacteria.

Mitral Valve Prolapse

A condition that is seen in up to 10–20 percent of women, mitral valve prolapse is caused by excessive wear and tear on the leaflets. Although the leaflets are normal when open, they become thickened and bulge into the atrium when they are closed. The prolapse, or bulge, is associated with extra heart sounds called clicks, as well as a regurgitation murmur if the closure is not firm. Patients with mitral valve prolapse may have chest pain that is not caused by coronary artery disease. They also may have palpitations and mild to severe arrhythmias, some requiring medication. Patients with mitral valve prolapse can expect a life of normal activity and expectancy. Mitral valve prolapse is diagnosed by examination and cardiac echocardiography. It is not known why some people develop prolapse, but it appears to run in families and occurs more often in thin women. If mitral regurgitation is present, antibiotics to prevent bacterial endocarditis are recommended. Patients with *mitral valve prolapse syndrome* have the symptoms seen with mitral valve prolapse, but do not have the actual valve prolapse.

Peripheral Vascular Disease

The same arteriosclerotic process that affects the blood vessels in the heart can affect the blood vessels in the legs. When the vessels of the leg are narrowed by cholesterol deposits and plaques, less blood is delivered to the leg muscles. There are no symptoms until the narrowing is severe enough to significantly reduce blood flow and cause discomfort in walking, usually felt as a cramp or pain in the thigh or calf. A few minutes rest relieves the pain.

As the leg artery continues to narrow, pain occurs more quickly or even at rest. This is a signal of damage or death of muscle in the leg (gangrene) and can lead to amputation.

The same risk factors are present as for coronary artery disease (see the box), and the same preventative and treatment measures apply. When a woman complains of leg pain, her physician examines her legs for reduced pulses or abnormal sounds. Blood pressures are often measured both before and after exercise, and there is often a duplex scan, using echo and doppler to image the blood vessels in the leg and assess blood flow. If significant narrowing is found, an angiogram can be done. Angioplasty can be used to open blocked blood vessels in the legs, or the vessels in the legs can be bypassed.

Other blood vessel complications can affect the aorta, which can suffer a thinning of the wall and ballooning (aneurysm). If the ballooning progresses, the vessel may rip or rupture. Since rupture is usually fatal, surgical repair of aneurysms at risk of rupture is recommended.

Congenital Defects

Murmurs may also be heard if blood flows through abnormal connections in the heart. The most common example is a hole in the heart between the two atria, called an atrial septal defect. The defect can be mild to severe and is often repaired in early childhood with surgery. A hole in the heart between the two ventricles, called ventricular septal defect, is more serious. Unless the opening is very tiny, this defect must be repaired. Ventricular septal defect may also occur as a complication of a heart attack. Although antibiotic protection against bacterial endocarditis may not be required for atrial septal defects, it is recommended for ventricular septal defects. Both conditions are diagnosed by examination and cardiac echocardiography.

Cardiac Disease during Pregnancy

The most common cardiac condition during pregnancy is palpitations. These are rarely dangerous. Hypertension can occur in pregnancy and requires close monitoring and treatment to avoid damage to the woman or fetus.

The most significant cardiac complication during pregnancy is caused by valvular heart defects. The work of the heart increases 30–50 percent by the middle of pregnancy. If this becomes a strain on a woman with a heart problem, she may need to make changes in her diet, activity level, or medication. Some of the drugs used to treat heart problems are harmful to the fetus, so it may be necessary for a woman to change her medication while she is pregnant or thinking about becoming pregnant. A woman who has heart disease should see a cardiologist before she becomes pregnant so her condition can be evaluated and stabilized before the changes of pregnancy occur. Rarely, congestive heart failure can occur because of pregnancy, requiring close monitoring.

Some of the physical changes of pregnancy are similar to those of heart disease, but certain symptoms could signal an underlying problem: limitation of physical activity due to shortness of breath, chest pain with exercise or increased activity, and dizziness preceded by palpitations or physical exertion. These problems should be assessed; echocardiography is the technique most often used in pregnant women. Although labor and delivery require the heart to work harder, a woman with a heart problem can give birth vaginally. Epidural anesthesia may be recommended. Special monitoring will be done throughout labor to check the heart rate and detect arrhythmias.

PROCEDURES

Tests and procedures are performed in patients with heart disease to assess the extent of the problem, to treat the condition or both. If the arteries are blocked, there are procedures to bypass those areas and reroute blood flow. In extreme cases, heart transplantation may be an option.

Electrocardiography

ECG records electrical signals in the heart that cause it to beat. For this test, electrodes are placed on the arms, legs, and across the chest wall, starting just to the right of the breastbone and running under the left breast to the armpit. These pads monitor heart activity as a series of electrical impulses, and the ECG machine records these data on paper. These readings can tell the physician whether the heart muscle is enlarged or thickened, whether part of the heart has been damaged by a heart attack, or if there is an irregularity in the heartbeat or angina. The test takes about 5–10 minutes to perform and does not require any special preparation.

Stress Testing

Stress testing uses ECG to show the heart's response to exercise. It is most useful when a patient has chest pain on exertion and normal ECG results at rest. No food should be eaten within 2 hours before the test, and comfortable clothing and shoes should be worn. The stress test is generally performed while the patient is walking on a treadmill or pedaling a stationary bicycle. The exercise level is very low to begin with, but it is increased every few minutes. As the person exercises harder, the heart beats faster and blood pressure increases. If the exercise causes angina, the electrical signals from the heart become abnormal.

The patient's blood pressure, heart rate, heartbeat, and ECG tracing are recorded in response to exercise and during the resting time after exercise. The exercise ends when angina occurs, when the person is exhausted, or when the target heart rate is reached. A maximal stress test is said to occur when the target heart rate is reached. If the maximal stress test results are normal, significant coronary artery disease is probably not present.

If chest symptoms do not occur with exercise testing and the ECG does not show changes, the test results are normal and the patient probably has a low risk of having serious coronary artery disease. Results may be misleading, however. A normal ECG at less than maximal stress levels may simply mean that the coronary artery disease is not apparent at the low exercise level. Abnormal results can be misleading as well: Women without symptoms often have ECG changes with exercise that do not reflect coronary artery disease. People with hypertension, those taking certain cardiac medications, and African-Americans often have falsely abnormal ECG changes with exercise that do not predict the presence of coronary artery disease. Stress testing is accurate about 60 percent of the time in women. Thus an abnormal ECG response is not reliable in women and more sensitive testing is often required.

Stress testing may be done after an injection of radioactive material (a tracer). This material attaches to the blood cells and traces where blood flow is able to go. The injection is usually given during maximal exercise. If there is narrowing of the coronary arteries, blood flow to that portion of the heart muscle is restricted. A picture of the radioactive material in the heart is obtained by a special camera positioned over the chest area. If blood supply to the heart is good, the radioactive material will be more obvious than if the flow is limited. After the patient has rested, the injection is repeated and the pictures are compared to the tests done during exercise. Blood flow will be better even in areas of narrowed blood vessels, while blood flow will still be restricted in areas of total blockage, such as those affected by a prior heart attack. The picture can be distorted, causing false results, if a woman has large breasts. Newer tests are now available to overcome this limitation and are especially helpful in women. Some patients are not comfortable with the use of radioactive material or the need for injections. In these patients, ultrasound of the heart can be used to show the movement of the heart muscle during exercise and at rest.

Echocardiography

This test uses harmless high-frequency sound waves, or ultrasound, to present a picture of the heart on a video monitor. A probe the size of a flashlight is placed against the chest wall and angled to allow sound waves to bounce off the structures of the heart. This creates an image of the size and movement of the heart muscle, chambers, and valves, which can be used to evaluate cardiac structure and function. The test can also be done with exercise to evaluate chest pain, imaging the the heart during exercise and at rest. If the exercise causes angina and restricted blood flow to an area of the heart, the muscle responds by reducing its ability to contract. This is seen on the monitor as a reduction in motion of an area of muscle. If this condition reverses at rest, it is a strong sign of coronary artery disease.

Sound waves will also bounce off moving blood cells and create an audio signal called doppler shift. The doppler shift will change depending on the direction the blood cells are moving. If a valve is leaking blood because it does not close properly, the doppler test will show it. Doppler testing can also detect if there is valve narrowing or a hole between chambers. The test takes about an hour to perform and requires no special preparation.

Holter Monitoring

A holter test monitors the heartbeat over a period of time, usually 24 hours, during which time a diary of activity or symptoms is maintained. Electrodes or pads similar to those used for an ECG are attached to the patient to record heart activity with a portable box. Every heartbeat cycle is recorded by the equipment, usually on a cassette tape. After 24 hours, the equipment is removed and the tape examined. The rate and rhythm of the heartbeat, frequency and type of irregular beats, and palpitations or skipped beats can be assessed and cross-referenced with the patient's diary. All usual activities, except showering or bathing can be performed while wearing the monitor.

Cardiac Catheterization

The chambers and blood vessels of the heart can be examined by the use of specialized X-ray studies called cardiac catheterization. This test is done to evaluate coronary artery blockages. A catheter is inserted into the large artery in the leg or arm and moved through the artery, across the aortic valve, and into the left ventricle, where it can measure the pressures in the heart chamber. X-ray contrast material can be injected

into the left ventricle to outline the size and shape of the chamber on X-ray photographs and show how well the chamber moves. The catheter can be moved to the coronary arteries, and the same X-ray methods can be used to show any blockage in the coronary artery. After the test is completed, the catheter is removed from the artery.

Cardiac catheterization is a sophisticated test done by specialists and may require an overnight stay the night after. The patient is awake for the procedure, and a local anesthetic is used where the catheter enters the artery. The test is usually over in an hour, and the patient should rest for a day and try not to bend where the artery was punctured. Most people experience no pain with this procedure, although it can cause angina. The results are available within a few minutes, and the patient can usually watch the procedure on a video monitor. As with any procedure, there are risks. Serious risks such as stroke or heart attack occur less than 1 percent of the time. Bleeding or clotting, damage to the blood vessel or heart chambers, or allergic reactions can occur. The most common side effect is a reaction to the X-ray contrast material, which contains iodine. Most people feel hot when the material is injected, and some may experience rash, hives, nausea, or vomiting. Although this test requires specialized equipment, it is commonly done at many institutions. Because the images of any blockages of the coronary arteries are so clear, this test is the standard for evaluating the severity of coronary artery disease. The test is also used to assess valve disease and whether valves require treatment. Many treatment decisions are made based on the results of this test.

Angioplasty

When severe blockages are found in the coronary arteries, attempts are often made to open the blood vessel. Angioplasty is the procedure used to reshape the coronary arteries. It is done after cardiac catheterization, using specialized catheters through the artery. The specialized catheter is inserted into the artery in the leg through a sheath that holds the artery hole open. The catheter has a deflated balloon at its tip. After it has been positioned to lie across the most severe area of narrowing, the balloon is inflated and deflated several times. The pressure of the expanded balloon sqeezes the cholesterol deposit against the wall of the coronary artery. Most patients experience angina when this occurs. Afterwards the balloon is deflated and the catheter removed. X-rays of the reshaped arteries are taken to see if there is an improvement in blood flow. After the procedure the sheath usually remains in the artery for several hours while the patient is given blood thinners to reduce clotting in the coronary artery. The most serious risk is sudden closure of the reshaped artery. If this occurs the catheter can be reinserted through the sheath. If no problems arise, the sheath is removed. Pressure is maintained over the hole in the artery, and the patient is usually allowed to go home the next day.

An increased risk of closure of the coronary artery remains for several weeks. Medication will be used to reduce clotting and the likelihood of spasm. A stress test is given and repeated every 3–6 months after the procedure to identify further coronary artery narrowing before symptoms develop. Most important, risk factors are evaluated and recommendations made about lifestyle changes to reduce the chance of coronary artery disease progressing. Although this procedure has a success rate of 90 percent and the rate of major complications is low, improvement in the opening of the blood vessel is variable and continued benefit depends on a number of factors.

Other Procedures

Other studies, although investigational, may be appropriate when angioplasty alone has not been effective in opening the vessel or in keeping it open. Most of these techniques are less effective or have higher complication rates in women and in older patients because of their average smaller vessel size. In development are new techniques that will improve the ability to reach narrowed areas in the coronary artery and to manage complications that can arise with current procedures.

Stents

Stents are metallic coils or meshes implanted within the coronary artery to line the inner layer of the vessel. They create a smooth vessel wall and keep the vessel open when there is spasm or closure of the coronary artery after angioplasty. Stents are very effective at keeping the vessel open (success rate approaches 90 percent), but they require extensive blood thinners to reduce the risk of clotting, which can cause heart attack. Their long-term effect is not known.

Atherectomy

This procedure consists of using cutting blades located at the end of a catheter to enlarge the opening of the

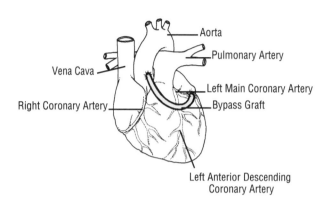

Figure 27.5 Coronary Bypass
With coronary artery bypass surgery, a piece of healthy vein is used to reroute the blood supply around a blocked artery.

coronary artery. Small amounts of plaque are chipped away, then a balloon catheter is passed through the catheter and angioplasty performed. Atherectomy devices are used when an artery is too narrowed to allow the balloon catheter to be inserted in it. Other types of devices include a rotating burr that smashes plaque instead of cutting it. These devices are useful only in large vessels and usually need to be followed by balloon angioplasty. Their risk of damage to the wall of the vessel is limited but real. The most common complication is spasm of the coronary artery or injury to the leg artery, where the device is inserted, because the device is so large.

Laser

With laser therapy a pulsed energy source can be directed inside the coronary arteries to destroy plaque on contact. This technique can have a success rate of up to 90 percent with a 6 percent complication rate. It is used to create a small channel opening, especially in blocked or nearly blocked vessels, so angioplasty can be performed. It is especially useful in vessels that are too small for the atherectomy devices. The greatest risk of this procedure is perforation of the vessel or closure of the vessel by clotting. Blood thinners are used in high dosages to reduce the risk of clotting.

Coronary Artery Bypass Surgery

Patients with angina may not be candidates for angioplasty or other procedures because the vessels of the heart may have atherosclerosis at several sites. When several vessels are involved, coronary artery bypass surgery (CABG) may be recommended. This surgery creates a new route for blood around the blocked part of each vessel, usually consisting of healthy veins taken from the legs during surgery. These vein grafts are attached from the aorta to the area of the coronary artery downstream from the blockage (Figure 27.5). In this way, fresh oxygenated blood will enter the coronary artery and provide blood flow to the heart muscle. The arteries within the chest wall can also be pulled away from the chest wall and attached to the vessel to reroute blood flow around blocked arteries. They do not need to be attached to the aorta because they are already receiving oxygenated blood. When more than one blockage is present, more than one graft is needed. The veins from the legs and the chest are extra vessels that usually are not missed when they are used and their flow is diverted. Coronary bypass surgery can be performed as an elective or emergency procedure.

Patients may put off having CABG until they are faced with a heart attack, but then the risks of the procedure are greater. Women are more likely than men to decline CABG, perhaps because their physicians do not stress strongly enough the importance of the procedure or the need to have it done when they are not seriously ill. Even when the procedure is recommended strongly, however, many women will refuse it because of the risks, hoping that medical therapy will continue to be effective. This may be because of fear of the procedure, desire to avoid an operation or having their body image changed, responsibilities that cannot be turned over to others, and the higher mortality rate in women with the procedure. Also, because women have heart disease later than men, they often do not have a spouse to help them after the procedure. All of these factors often lead women to postpone cardiac catheterization and CABG until a crisis arises. This causes a higher rate of complications and death after surgery, even when other factors are taken into account.

Whether surgery is done on an elective or emergency basis, it will take time to heal. Moderate recovery occurs at 1 month, and full recovery is usual by 6 months. Although patients have trouble sleeping for a while, the improvement in cardiac symptoms will be dramatic.

CHAPTER 28

Hypertension

Lois Anne Katz, M.D., F.A.C.P.

At least 50 million people, or about 15 to 20 percent of the population, have high blood pressure or hypertension. It's the most common reason for visits to the doctor, and more prescriptions are written for antihypertensive drugs than for drugs for any other medical condition. Left untreated, hypertension can lead to stroke, kidney disease, heart attack, and heart failure.

The overwhelming majority of people with high blood pressure have *no* symptoms—that's why it's often called the "silent killer." There are few clues, so it's important to have your blood pressure checked periodically.

In a sense, having high blood pressure is a little like having termites in your house: You may not see the bugs in the system, but they can still do great damage.

WHAT IS BLOOD PRESSURE?

Blood pressure is a measure of the amount of force the blood exerts against the walls of the arteries, the blood vessels that carry blood away from the heart. Blood pressure must be maintained at a certain level to ensure that blood, which carries nutrients and oxygen, is pumped to vital organs.

The level of blood pressure is determined by two factors: (1) the pumping action of the heart, or cardiac output, and (2) the resistance in the arteries. With each heartbeat, the heart contracts and pumps blood out; this contraction is called *systole*, and the blood pressure rises; this measurement is called the systolic blood pressure. When the heart relaxes during *diastole* and the heart is filling with blood, the blood pressure falls—this is called the diastolic blood pressure. This pressure is a measure of the tone of the small arteries throughout the body.

Blood pressure is routinely described by two numbers: the systolic blood pressure over the diastolic blood pressure. If blood pressure is 120/80—described verbally as "one hundred twenty over eighty"—the systolic blood pressure is 120 and the diastolic is 80. Blood pressure, which is measured in millimeters of mercury (mm Hg), is determined using a device called a sphygmomanometer, which consists of an inflatable balloon inside a loose cuff that is secured with Velcro. The balloon is attached to a column of mercury or other means to register the reading. The blood pressure cuff is placed on the upper arm at the level of the heart; to gauge the blood pressure a stethoscope is placed over the artery just below the cuff. The cuff is

BLOOD PRESSURE MEASUREMENTS

The diagnosis of hypertension is usually made after at least three readings have been taken several days apart. The *Fifth Report of the Joint National Committee on Detection, Evaluation, and Treatment of High Blood Pressure* (JNC V) released in January 1993, has classified blood pressure in the following way.

Classification	Systolic Blood Pressure (mm Hg)	Diastolic Blood Pressure (mm Hg)
Normal	130	85
High normal (borderline)*	130–139	85–89
Hypertension		
Stage 1 (mild)	140–159	90–99
Stage 2 (moderate)	160–179	100–109
Stage 3 (severe)	180–209	110–119
Stage 4 (very severe)	210	120

* *Note:* About 80 percent of people with hypertension fall in the mild category.

inflated, cutting off the pressure completely. The doctor listens for the noise of the blood when it first flows into the vessel (systolic pressure) and then notes the pressure at which the noise stops (diastolic pressure).

WHAT IS HIGH BLOOD PRESSURE?

There is some controversy about what level of blood pressure is normal and what level should be classified as "high." In adults, systolic blood pressures of 140

mm Hg or higher and diastolic blood pressures of 90 mm Hg or higher, are generally considered high blood pressure, or hypertension. Individuals may have high diastolic and systolic blood pressure, only high diastolic blood pressure (diastolic hypertension), or high systolic blood pressure with normal diastolic blood pressure (isolated systolic hypertension). Isolated systolic hypertension is most common in people over 55; when it occurs in younger people it is often a predictor for later diastolic hypertension.

Until recently, most doctors paid more attention to the diastolic blood pressure. It is now thought that systolic pressure is important, too.

TAKING A READING

Because hypertension is basically an asymptomatic condition (you don't know you have it), it can be detected only by directly measuring the blood pressure. It's recommended that healthy women have their blood pressure checked once every 2 years, and if you are in any risk category, then you should be checked at least annually.

Caution: Do not rely only on the blood pressure machines available at drugstores and malls or on free blood pressure tests offered in many communities. High blood pressure is more than just determining the numbers. Unlike measuring height and weight, blood pressure is variable, and the numbers require interpretation by someone who knows your complete health history.

Determining whether or not someone has hypertension is not based on a single blood pressure reading. Some individuals develop hypertension that is related to the anxiety of seeing a health care provider; their blood pressure can be as much as 30 points higher than normal when measured in the doctor's office. This phenomenon is known as "white coat hypertension." It has also been observed that blood pressure is sometimes higher when taken by a doctor rather than by a nurse. Blood pressure may also vary with time of day, your activity level, and your emotional state.

Most commonly, blood pressure is measured in the sitting position, but it may also be measured when you are lying down or even standing. Blood pressure should

TAKING BLOOD PRESSURE AT HOME

It is important to follow these guidelines when measuring or monitoring your blood pressure at home. Rest for 5 minutes before taking your blood pressure, and sit with your arm out at chest height. Carefully follow the instructions included with your blood pressure kit, and make sure you get a cuff that fits your arm. Take at least two readings separated by 2 minutes and record your measurements. Consult your physician about the device that is reliable and best for you.

be measured after 5 minutes of rest. Both smoking and drinking caffeinated beverages should be avoided for at least 30 minutes before the blood pressure is measured, because both activities may temporarily raise pressure. If a blood pressure reading is high on one visit, repeat measurements should be done on at least two subsequent visits. How soon these following visits should be scheduled will depend on the initial blood pressure reading. If the blood pressure is only mildly elevated, repeat measurements can be done over several months; higher levels should be rechecked within 1 or 2 weeks. If there is very severe hypertension (210/120), immediate further evaluation and treatment is indicated.

HYPERTENSION AS A RISK FACTOR

The classification of hypertension is based on how the level of blood pressure affects an individual's risk of disease. Below the age of 65 the risks of hypertension appear to be somewhat lower for women than for men. However, women between the ages of 45 and 74 with elevated diastolic pressure have twice the risk of developing heart disease as women with normal pressure. In elderly women, hypertension is the major risk factor for both cardiovascular disease and mortality. If individuals with hypertension have other cardiac risk factors—such as smoking, high cholesterol levels, or diabetes mellitus—these add up to even *more* risk.

Numerous studies have demonstrated that reduction of blood pressure in hypertensive individuals reduces the risk of heart attacks and stroke. Until recently, most of these studies were done in men. It is not clear whether there are equal benefits of treating hypertension in women. But there are data that support the benefits of treating certain groups of hypertensive women, particularly African-American women and women with more severe levels of hypertension.

TYPES AND CAUSES OF HIGH BLOOD PRESSURE

There are two types of high blood pressure: primary and secondary.

Primary Hypertension

The overwhelming majority of patients who have hypertension have *essential,* or *primary, hypertension,* which means there is no single, definable cause. We do know, however, that there are many environmental and lifestyle factors that seem to contribute or interact to cause high blood pressure. It has sometimes been called the "disease of civilization," because blood pressure is lower in nonindustrialized countries.

Known Contributing Factors

There is evidence suggesting that eating certain foods, being physically inactive, being overweight, and using alcohol chronically are major contributors to high blood pressure. People who are 20 percent above their ideal body weight are more prone to hypertension. In women, those whose fat is distributed around the waist rather than on the hips are more at risk. Societies that consume high amounts of salt also have a greater percentage of people with high blood pressure.

Doctors have long noted the connection between *stress* and high blood pressure. In response to stress, the sympathetic nervous system causes the heart to pump harder and faster and constrict the small arteries, resulting in higher blood pressure.

The relationship between stress and high blood pressure may be particularly important for women who routinely juggle multiple roles on a daily basis. In a recent study, 120 working women had their blood pressures analyzed around the clock. Blood pressure

PROFILE: WHO DEVELOPS HIGH BLOOD PRESSURE?

In young adulthood and early middle age, men are more likely to be hypertensive than women. By age 55, however, women are as likely as men to have high blood pressure. As the population ages, men and women develop hypertension at about the same rate, but by age 65 women are even more likely to be hypertensive.

African-Americans particularly tend to develop hypertension at younger ages and often have higher blood pressure levels than whites. The cause is thought to be related to environmental factors, such as diet and stress, as well as genetics.

While blood pressure tends to rise progressively with increasing age—older people are vulnerable because their arteries have become less elastic—many older individuals have normal blood pressures. Hypertension is no longer considered an expected consequence of aging.

High blood pressure tends to run in families; many hypertensive people have parents, siblings, or other relatives with the same problem. If one or both of your parents is hypertensive, you are twice as likely to be. This suggests that genetic factors may determine who gets hypertension. There does not appear to be one specific gene, however, that causes hypertension and that is directly passed on from parent to child.

was observed to rise whenever a woman was in a situation she felt to be particularly stressful. Working mothers seemed the most vulnerable—their blood pressures often remained elevated a good part of the time.

Secondary Hypertension

About 5 percent of individuals have high blood pressure that is the result of some other disease. This condition is called *secondary hypertension* and is cured if the primary condition is diagnosed and treated. The most common underlying causes are kidney disease, renovascular disease (diseases of the arteries supplying blood to the kidneys), endocrine disease such as hyperaldosteronism, pheochromocytoma, or Cushing's disease (see Chapter 30). Renovascular disease may be due to either atherosclerotic (cholesterol deposits) or fibroplastic (increased fibrous tissue) lesions. One type of fibroplastic lesion, medial hyperplasia, usually occurs in young women and may be surgically correctible.

FACTORS THAT CONTRIBUTE TO HYPERTENSION

- Stress
- Obesity
- High salt intake
- Heavy drinking
- Family history of hypertension

Some medications can cause hypertension. In young women, the birth control pill is a common cause.

HYPERTENSIVE EMERGENCIES

Hypertensive emergencies occur when someone's blood pressure is so high that it must be reduced within hours. *Malignant hypertension* is a severe form of hypertension; if left untreated it can result in kidney damage or stroke. *Hypertensive encephalopathy* is the term for brain symptoms resulting from very high blood pressure or rapid rises in blood pressure. Patients may develop headaches, visual difficulties, mental confusion, seizures, stupor, or even lapse into a coma. These conditions require immediate treatment.

DIAGNOSIS OF HYPERTENSION

If you are found to have high blood pressure, you should expect a comprehensive evaluation. Your doctor will take a complete medical history from you, asking specific questions about previous high blood pressure, kidney disease, hypertension during pregnancy, family history of hypertension, and cardiovascular risk factors. Your doctor will ask for a list of all the drugs and medications you are taking, whether prescription or not. Even over-the-counter nose drops, cold remedies, and NSAIDs such as Advil and Motrin can elevate blood pressure.

An evaluation should also be done to determine whether the hypertension is essential or secondary and to look for evidence of any damage to other organs such as the heart, kidneys, or eyes.

During the physical examination, the doctor will look for abdominal masses (which could be evidence of polycystic kidney disease, a type of inherited kidney disease) and will listen for bruits, or abnormal sounds caused by irregularties in the artery walls, over the renal arteries, which might suggest renovascular disease. Pulses will be checked in the neck, arms, and legs, and arteries will be examined for bruits. The eyes will be examined with an ophthalmoscope to allow the physician to see the retina (the inside of the eye). Patients with hypertension can develop abnormalities in the retinal blood vessels known as *hypertensive retinopathy*.

In addition to the physical exam, the following other tests are likely to be done:

- A urinalysis, or examination of the urine, for blood, protein, and glucose (sugar)
- Blood count to look for anemia
- Blood chemistries to check blood urea nitrogen (BUN) and creatinine (which tests whether the

kidneys are clearing waste products), sodium, potassium and other electrolytes, calcium, cholesterol, uric acid, and glucose

■ An electrocardiogram (ECG) and chest X-ray to look for enlargement of the heart

If there are any abnormalities detected with these routine tests, some additional tests may be ordered, such as an echocardiogram of the heart. This test uses ultrasound (high-frequency sound waves) to detect car-diac enlargement. Similarly, X-ray or an echo examination of the kidneys may be done to evaluate function and to determine the size and condition of the kidneys. In selected patients, plasma renin (a hormone produced by the kidney) levels, urinary sodium excretion, and other hormone levels may be measured. More complex diagnostic studies such as arteriograms and computerized tomography (CT) scans are necessary only for patients thought to have renovascular disease or endocrine tumors causing their hypertension.

TREATMENT OF HYPERTENSION

Because there is no one cause for hypertension, there is no standard, uniform treatment—and certainly no magic pill to cure it. If the hypertension is secondary to another disease, your doctor will treat the condition causing the hypertension, while continuing to monitor your blood pressure. If the hypertension is primary or essential, treatment depends on the severity of the hypertension, the presence of other factors or diseases (such as obesity and diabetes), and on the extent of organ damage. Your doctor will develop an individualized plan to control your blood pressure indefinitely.

For mild hypertension, the first step is lifestyle modification. In most cases, treatment includes both lifestyle modification (non-drug treatment) and drug therapy.

Lifestyle Modification

The goal of lifestyle modification is to eliminate as many environmental and physical risk factors as possible to see if blood pressure will drop to normal levels. These guidelines are a good prescription for everyone, by the way, whether or not you have high blood pressure.

■ *Nutrition.* Diet change is one of the most important factors in treating hypertension. It is recommended that everyone with hypertension restrict salt intake by avoiding processed foods and table salt. You should consume no more than 1 teaspoonful (or 5 to 6 grams) of salt a day. If your cholesterol is high, too, your diet should be modified to a lower fat intake.

■ *Weight Maintenance.* Studies have shown that if you are significantly overweight, you increase your chances of developing hypertension. (Being thin isn't a guarantee you won't develop hypertension, however.) Obesity stimulates an increase in insulin production, which may be a factor in causing hypertension. If you lose weight, you may be able to reverse your high blood pressure. In one study, 75 percent of overweight people who lost 20 or more pounds achieved normal blood pressure through weight loss alone. However, not everyone with obesity and hypertension responds to weight loss with a decrease in blood pressure. As you can see, it makes sense to use dietary therapy—a combination of nutrition and weight maintenance—as the first line in the battle against hypertension.

■ *Alcohol.* Drinking moderate to large amounts of alcohol daily may cause hypertension; even drinking small amounts may raise blood pressure in some people. People with high blood pressure should drink no more than 1 ounce of "absolute alcohol" daily—that means 2 ounces of 100-proof whisky, 8 ounces of wine, or 24 ounces of beer. Alcohol should also be avoided because it has lots of empty calories. Abstaining from alcohol consumption is the healthiest choice.

■ *Exercise.* Regular aerobic exercise is good medicine for your heart. Fast walking, jogging, and bicycling also may lower blood pressure. (*Caution:* It may be wise to have a physical exam and a cardiac stress test before beginning any exercise program. See Chapter 27.) Avoid exercises like wrestling and weightlifting, however, where you may clamp down on muscles and raise your blood pressure even higher.

- *Smoking.* Don't: within minutes of inhaling, blood pressure goes up. Smoking injures blood vessel walls and may contribute to hardening of the arteries. Smoking speeds up the pulse and increases the work of the heart.

- *Reduce the Stress in Your Life.* Easier said than done, but biofeedback, meditation, relaxation therapy, and yoga can all help lower tension and stress, with no side effects. Relaxation techniques lower blood pressure by directly reducing, or quieting, sympathetic arousal. Biofeedback studies show healthy individuals can lower their blood pressure as much as 10 or 20 points in response to different biofeedback cues. Studies on patients with hypertension show that blood pressure can be lowered by 6 or 8 points.

Drug Therapy

Is there a specific high blood pressure above which drug treatment is necessary? In general, if your diastolic number is above 95, some drug therapy is usually prescribed. If you have moderate or severe hypertension, you'll be routinely started on drug therapy along with a lifestyle modification program. Your blood pressure will then be checked at frequent intervals until it is normal.

The goal of drug therapy is to lower blood pressure using the lowest dosages with the fewest side effects. Your doctor will probably try to control your blood pressure with a single drug taken once a day. You may be given several different drugs until your physician identifies the right treatment for you. If a drug causes an undesirable side effect or an allergic reaction, inform your physician immediately. The doctor will discontinue the drug and try another medication. Antihypertensive drugs can also interact with other drugs, so your doctor *must* be aware of *any* other medications (prescription or otherwise) you may be taking.

Up until the 1950s the drug cupboard was practically bare; today physicians have a full arsenal of drugs to choose from. The many different classes of hypertensive drugs include diuretics, converting enzyme inhibitors, calcium-channel blockers, sympatholytics, and vasodilators.

Diuretics

Often called "water pills," diuretics are the traditional medications prescribed for high blood pressure and probably the best known. They lower blood pressure by increasing urinary output of salt and water and by reducing the volume of the body's fluids. Diuretics usually increase urination, at least initially. The most common diuretics used are the thiazides. Relatively inexpensive and very effective, they can, unfortunately, have various side effects, including

- Loss of potassium, which can result in fatigue and cramps
- Elevation of blood sugar or cholesterol levels
- Elevation of uric acid levels
- Generalized weakness or reduced libido

Using low doses or minidoses of diuretics often avoids these side effects while maintaining their antihypertensive effects. The loss of potassium may be corrected by increasing dietary intake of high potassium foods (bananas, orange juice).

Angiotensin Converting Enzyme Inhibitors

Angiotensin converting enzyme inhibitors (ACE inhibitors) are a relatively new class of antihypertensives that are now being widely used. They work by inhibiting or reducing the production of angiotensin, a hormone that increases blood pressure. Captopril was the first drug in this class; other ACE inhibitors are enalapril, lisinopril, and benazepril. Although these drugs tend to be costly, side effects are uncommon. Some possible side effects include loss of taste, rashes, and coughs. ACE inhibitors must not be given to pregnant women.

Calcium-Channel Blockers

Calcium-channel drugs interfere with the cellular intake of calcium and lead to the relaxation of the blood vessel walls. (Limiting calcium uptake reduces the vessels' ability to contract.) Examples of these drugs are nifedipine, diltiazem, and verapamil. This newer class of drugs is expensive; it has relatively few side effects, but they include swelling of the ankles because of fluid retention, constipation, dizziness, and either a fast or slow heart beat.

Sympatholytics

Sympatholytics act on different parts of the sympathetic nervous system to lower blood pressure. Sympatholytics include beta-blockers, alpha-blockers, and central acting drugs such as alpha-methyldopa and clonidine. Beta-blockers such as propranolol and atenolol reduce the heart rate and the amount of blood the heart pumps; they also indirectly relax the blood vessels by blocking signals from the nervous system that would normally make the blood vessels contract. Possible side effects include depression, fatigue, nightmares, and impotence in men. They are not usually prescribed during pregnancy.

Direct Vasodilators

Direct vasodilators cause blood vessels to relax. Side effects include a rapid heart beat that may cause palpitations, fluid retention, and sometimes headaches and rashes. Vasodilators are usually not given alone, but in a combination with beta-blockers and/or diuretics. They tend to be used for more severe hypertension, but not for mild or moderate cases. Vasodilators include hydralazine and minoxidil. Since minoxidil can cause increased hair growth, it is rarely prescribed for women.

Women and Hypertension

Unfortunately hypertension research has rarely focused specifically on women. Many antihypertensive drugs have not been studied in women. It's known that treatment of hypertension in men reduces the possibility of heart disease, but the evidence for women is inconclusive. We also know that certain drugs—particularly the sympatholytics—have detrimental side effects on male sexuality. As a result, sexual side effects associated with hypertensive drugs are almost always discussed in male terms. It is possible that medications that cause sexual dysfunction in men may also cause sexual dysfunction in women, but this question has rarely been addressed.

Oral Contraceptives

Many women taking oral contraceptives have a small increase in blood pressure, but it usually remains within the normal range. About 5 percent of all women who use oral contraceptives develop hypertension: Some women develop mild to moderate hypertension, and a very small number may develop the accelerated form. Patients receiving oral contraceptive preparations with high doses of estrogen and progesterone are more likely to develop hypertension, but all pills containing estrogen may cause a rise in blood pressure. (Newer pills have lower doses of both hormones.) The exact mechanism for the development of hypertension through the use of oral contraceptives is unknown. If you develop hypertension on oral contraceptives, your physician may advise you to discontinue taking birth control pills. Your blood pressure will return to normal within a few months after stopping the pill.

Pregnancy

About 1 out of 10 pregnant women will suffer from some form of hypertension (see Chapter 17). Some women enter pregnancy already diagnosed with hypertension. The good news is that 85 percent of all women with chronic hypertension can have normal pregnancies, free of complication. Each drug a pregnant woman takes, however, must be carefully evaluated for its effect on the fetus. Women with high blood pressure, who are contemplating pregnancy, should consult their doctor first about switching to safe medication. The same advice holds true for a woman who wants to breast-feed, because every medicine enters breast milk to some degree.

Blood pressure usually decreases during the first 6 months of a normal pregnancy. However, in the last 3 months, pregnancy-induced hypertension may develop. A diagnosis of hypertension is made if the systolic blood pressure increases more than 30 points and/or the diastolic increases 15 points. This measurement is compared with the woman's average blood pressure before she reached her 20th week of gestation. The management of hypertension in pregnancy is complex. Your physician will decide which therapy is best for you.

THE LIMITATIONS OF DRUG THERAPY

There are some inherent concerns with all drug therapy. For one, it's expensive—some drugs cost as much as $75 a month. In general, medication must be taken daily and for a long period of time—at least 1 year, but often forever. If you lose a large amount of weight, however, or modify your lifestyle significantly, it may be possible to reduce or withdraw drug treatment.

A continuing problem with drug therapy is noncompliance: People often feel they are "cured" and discontinue their medication. They stop taking their medicine because they "don't feel so bad" or because they don't like the side effects of the drugs.

Menopause

Hypertension is not part of the menopausal syndrome. Some women may develop increased blood pressure, possibly related to increased body weight.

Estrogen-Replacement Therapy

Hypertension does not contraindicate postmenopausal estrogen-replacement therapy (ERT). Some women may develop a rise in blood pressure secondary to estrogen therapy, so blood pressure should be monitored after estrogen-replacement therapy has begun. The chemical nature of the hormone used in ERT and its effects are different from the hormone used in oral contraceptives.

The Benefits of Follow-up Treatment

The goal of any hypertension treatment program is to lower blood pressure; in fact, *any* lowering is viewed as a partial victory. Regular checkups are essential. If you are undergoing treatment, your doctor will schedule periodic return visits. It is possible to monitor yourself at home, in addition to keeping office appointments.

If your blood pressure is controlled for at least 1 year, you may be able to reduce the amount or dosage of drugs in slow progressive steps while maintaining a healthy lifestyle.

You are not cured, however. Your blood pressure can rise again weeks or months later. For this reason, your blood pressure must be carefully monitored whenever drug treatment is reduced or withdrawn.

Hypertension may be a silent killer, but today's arsenal of drug remedies and the knowledge we have about the role of lifestyle changes can help you win the battle—or at least reach a peaceful truce with your condition.

CHAPTER 29

The Blood and Lymphatic Systems

Marjorie S. Sirridge, M.D., M.A.C.P.

The blood and lymphatic systems are responsible for the formation and development of blood cells. This process is called hematopoiesis. It controls the continued production and circulation of cells that perform the vital functions of blood. Just like other cells in the body, the characteristics of blood cells are determined by heredity. The blood type, as well as certain disorders, can be inherited. Other disorders can arise that interfere with the number and function of the cells. Blood and lymph circulate through the body, serving major organs and providing protection from disease. Their function, both normal and abnormal, can have a major impact on a person's overall health.

STRUCTURE AND FUNCTION

The average healthy woman has three to five liters (about 6–10 pints) of blood in her body that form about 7–8 percent of her weight. Blood carries out several important functions as it circulates through the body.

Oxygen is brought to organs and muscles and waste products are removed in the blood. In the lungs, inhaled oxygen is picked up in the blood and delivered by the arteries to tissues throughout the body. At the same time, blood removes carbon dioxide, a waste material, from the tissues and returns it, through veins, to the lungs where it is exhaled. The blood circulates continuously through the heart and lungs, renewing its oxygen supply and carrying oxygen and nutrients to the rest of the body. The oxygen-rich blood in arteries is thick and bright red. In the veins, after the oxygen has been removed, it is dark purplish red.

Blood also carries nutrients from the digestive system to the cells in the body. Waste products from these cells are then transported to the kidneys and liver where they can be filtered and excreted.

The lymphatic system and the blood work together with the immune system to help the body combat disease. Certain blood cells fight infection and set up a system to protect the body from invaders. Other blood cells help to stop bleeding and promote healing.

Blood helps the various parts of the body communicate by sending messages to other parts of the body to coordinate and regulate its functions. The hormones of the endocrine system and the antibodies of the immune system are carried by the blood. Blood also helps to regulate body temperature by removing the heat produced in the muscles through the skin. When the air temperature is cold, blood moves away from the extremities to protect the internal organs and keep them warm. This results in a chilling effect in hands and feet.

Blood cells are produced in the bone marrow and various parts of the lymphatic system. This system includes, in addition to bone marrow, the thymus gland, the spleen, lymph nodes, and the channels that con-

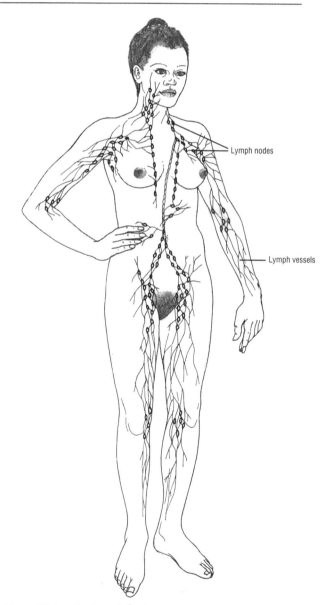

Figure 29.1 The Lymph System
The lymph system, made up of *lymph vessels* and small filtering organs called *lymph nodes*, assists the veins in returning blood and other fluids to the heart.

nect these organs to the bloodstream and to each other. The process of hematopoiesis—the formation and development of blood cells—involves a complex interplay between blood, bone marrow, and the lymphatic system.

The lymphatic system is made up of a network of thin tubes that branch out to all areas of the body. A clear fluid called lymph flows through these channels from the tissues to the heart. This fluid also contains infection-fighting white blood cells called lymphocytes. The lymph vessels are connected to small round organs, called lymph nodes. Lymph nodes filter lymph as it passes through the system. They are found in the neck, underarm, chest, groin, and abdomen. Lymph nodes are the main places where lymphocytes multiply, interact, and ready themselves to attack invading organisms. The thymus is a gland in the chest that influences the development of one kind of lymphocyte.

The spleen is a large lymphoid organ located in the upper left quarter portion of the abdomen, behind the stomach. (See Figure 29.1)

About 60% of women's blood is plasma, the fluid part of blood, and the other 40% is blood cells. There are three types of blood cells: red blood cells, white blood cells, and platelets (see Figure 29.2). The red blood cells are the most numerous, followed by platelets and white blood cells. All three blood cell types begin from a single stem cell and then mature to perform different functions. Most blood cells are produced in the bone marrow, a material in cavities inside many of the bones in the body. Some blood cells begin in the bone marrow and then mature in the thymus, spleen, or lymph nodes.

Red blood cells are called erythrocytes. They make up over 99 percent of all blood cells. These cells contain hemoglobin, a red substance that gives red blood

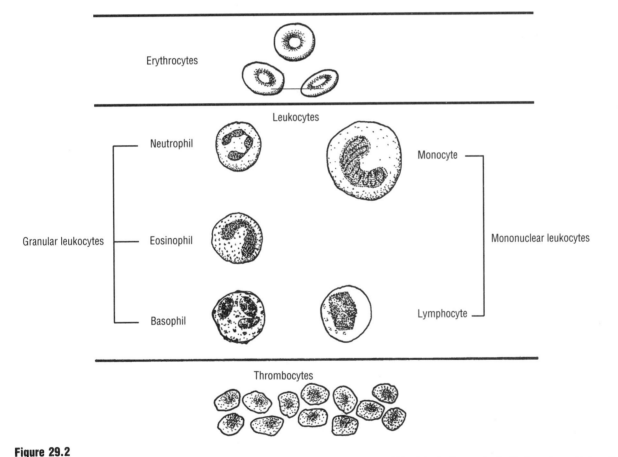

Figure 29.2

About 4-5 million red blood cells, or *erythrocytes* (top), occupy each cubic millimeter of blood in the human body. Erythrocytes, which make up the chief component of human blood, transport oxygen and carbon dioxide to and from body tissues. Five types of white blood cells, or *leukocytes* (middle), protect against infection by microorganisms. They number about 5,000-10,000 per cubic millimeter of blood. The *granular leukocytes* comprise *neutrophils* and *basophils*, which attack and destroy invading microorganisms, and *eosinophils*, which help to detoxify foreign substances and to dissolve clots. The *agranular leukocytes* are instrumental in the body's immune response against foreign substances. *Thrombocytes*, also called platelets, number about 130,000-360,000 per cubic millimeter of blood. They play an important role in blood clotting.

cells their color. Hemoglobin is made up of a heme molecule, which contains iron, and four different amino acid chains, called globin. Hemoglobin binds easily to oxygen, carrying it from the lungs and delivering it to the rest of the body.

White blood cells are called leukocytes. The three types of white blood cells—granulocytes, monocytes, and lymphocytes—all combat disease in one way or another.

Granulocytes are the most common form of white blood cell. They get their name because their cytoplasm—the jellylike substance that surrounds the nucleus of all cells—contains granules. When the body is infected with bacteria, the number of granulocytes circulating in the blood increases; when infected by viruses, the number usually decreases.

Monocytes, the largest of all leukocytes, are two to four times the diameter of red blood cells. Monocytes ingest foreign particles, such as bacteria and tissue debris that may occur during the healing process. When infection or inflammation occurs, monocytes leave the circulation to go to the site to function.

Lymphocytes react specifically to infecting agents. They memorize the infecting agents, called antigens, and some of them create antibodies that combat the infection. The antibodies then remain in the body to continue their protection. There are two types of lymphocytes: B cells and T cells. B lymphocytes produce antibodies and T lymphocytes combat infection more directly.

Platelets, also known as thrombocytes, are the smallest of the cells circulating in the blood. They prevent and control bleeding by helping to repair injured blood vessels. They do so by forming plugs in these vessels, called clots, and are aided in this function by certain proteins, known as clotting factors. However, a thrombus, or blood clot, can also form in uninjured veins or arteries, which is potentialy dangerous.

The blood cells float in a fluid called plasma. This yellowish fluid contains clotting factors and other substances, including albumin (a protein), glucose (blood sugar), fats, minerals, immunoglobins (antibodies formed by the immune system), and hormones. Plasma also carries waste products to the lungs, kidneys, and liver for excretion. Plasma is about 95 percent water and is salty.

Blood cells must be renewed constantly to perform their functions. For each cell that dies a new one must be made to replace it. Only the number of cells that die must be replaced, however. This balance is maintained by substances that regulate cell production and keep the numbers of cells at constant levels. They monitor the blood cells in the body to detect deficits and trigger production of new cells as needed. The substance that regulates the production of red blood cells is a hormone produced in the kidneys called erythropoietin. White blood cells are regulated by a group of substances called colony-stimulating factors.

The marrow of bones is the site of the production and maturation of all of the red blood cells and most of the white blood cells. In adult women it is found in the ribs, vertebrae, and pelvis.

Red blood cells (RBC's) grow in the bone marrow and are then released for circulation in the blood when they mature. A red blood cell lives for 120 days. The cell slowly wears out as it performs its function of circulating in the blood, getting oxygen from the lungs, and delivering it to the heart and the rest of the body. The red blood cell works with every heartbeat, every breath. When it has reached the end of its life, the red blood cell is broken down in the spleen. The iron from the hemoglobin is returned to the bone marrow and used to produce more red blood cells. A product of the breakdown of hemoglobin is bilirubin, an orange-yellow compound that is excreted by the liver into the bile. When a large number of red blood cells are destroyed at one time, thus overwhelming the capacity of the liver to excrete bilirubin, jaundice, a yellow discoloration of the skin and eyes, may result. The increased rate of destruction of RBC's is called hemolysis.

Some white blood cells live only a few hours, so they are replenished rapidly. Some white blood cells begin in the bone marrow and are then sent to other parts of the lymphatic system to mature and develop their special functions. Each of these types of white blood cells fights infection in a different way.

The granulocytes are released from the bone marrow. They circulate in the blood only about six to eight hours. When infection occurs, the granulocyte rushes to the part of the body where it is needed and ingests the invader. It basically eats itself to death and begins to fall apart, with pieces scavenged by phagocytic cells at the site of infection.

Lymphocytes multiply in the spleen and lymph nodes. These cells leave the lymph nodes and are eventually returned to the blood. After circulating in the blood, the lymphocytes may return to the lymph and circulate there. The B lymphocytes create antibodies to infectious agents that circulate through the body and call the immune system to action.

Sometimes the immune system can malfunction and form antibodies against a person's own body cells and attack them. This is called an autoimmune disorder. Some types of arthritis are examples of autoimmune diseases. Certain disorders can disable the immune system. For instance, infection with human immunodeficiency virus damages the T lymphocytes, leaving a person open to infections.

Blood is divided by types or groups (see box on ''Blood Types''). A woman's blood type is determined by her parents. Each cell in the body, including red blood cells, is coated with proteins called antigens that can induce an immune response. An antigen stimulates the manufacture of antibodies that interact only with that antigen. The blood type is based on the presence or absence on the red blood cells of such antigens and, like other physical characteristics, is controlled through genes inherited from parents. If a person receives blood group antigens of a different type, antibodies can attack the cells that carry these antigens.

The four major blood types are further divided into two other antigen types known as Rh positive and Rh negative. About 15 percent of the white population of the United States has Rh-negative blood; the trait is slightly less common in other races. If a woman has Rh-negative blood, her red blood cells do not carry the Rh antigen. If a woman has Rh-positive blood, her red blood cells do carry it.

The Rh factor causes problems when an Rh-negative person's blood receives Rh-positive blood. The person with Rh-negative blood then produces antibodies to fight the Rh factor as if it were a harmful substance. This can occur if a Rh-negative woman becomes pregnant with a Rh-positive fetus. The mother's body then produces antibodies that attack the Rh-positive red blood cells of the fetus. This can be prevented by giving the mother a blood product that prevents her from producing antibodies against Rh-positive red blood cells.

KEEPING THE SYSTEM HEALTHY

To ensure that her blood can conduct its many important functions, a woman must provide her body with enough essential nutritional building blocks to produce healthy blood cells. She also should protect herself against harmful substances and organisms that may damage her blood cells or the organs that make them.

Three nutrients—iron, vitamin B_{12}, and folic acid—are required by bone marrow to produce healthy blood cells. Vitamin B_{12} and folic acid are necessary for the division of cells in the bone marrow. Without sufficient B_{12} and folic acid, bone marrow is unable to produce enough red blood cells. Without sufficient iron, the body cannot produce enough hemoglobin to deliver the oxygen needed to keep every cell nourished with oxygen. The lack of sufficient red blood cells and hemoglobin results in anemia, the most widespread blood disorder among women.

Women are especially at risk of iron-deficiency anemia because they lose blood on a regular basis through menstruation. Women who are pregnant require additional iron for the red blood cells of the fetus and usually are advised to take iron supplements.

You can protect yourself against anemia caused by a vitamin or mineral deficiency by eating a balanced diet that includes foods rich in iron, folic acid, and vitamin B_{12} (see Chapter 3, Nutrition). Because animal products, particularly liver and other organ meats, are important sources of these nutrients, women who are vegetarians or who follow certain macrobiotic diets are at special risk. These women need to make a special effort to compensate for the lack of animal products by eating plenty of leafy green vegetables (such as kale and spinach), as well as lima beans and kidney beans.

Although supplements in the form of vitamins are available, you should get your daily requirements from the food you eat. In particular, do not take iron supplements unless your doctor has recommended them. There are several inherited abnormalities of hemoglobin production in which iron is not helpful and can even be harmful.

You can take advantage of the power of the white blood cells to protect yourself from infections through immunizations. Vaccines against tetanus, measles, and flu cause your body to produce antibodies that protect you from these diseases (see ''Adult Immunization'' in Chapter 2). There is no vaccination to prevent human immunodeficiency virus (HIV) infection, which causes AIDS. Infection with HIV causes the destruction of T lymphocytes that are essential for normal functioning of the immune system (see "AIDS: Women" in Chapter 20).

Harmful Substances

There are several substances that could damage either blood cells or the organs that make them. These include both drugs you may be taking to treat other conditions and chemicals with which you may come in contact in your job and at home. Drugs used to treat rheumatoid arthritis, such as gold compounds, are especially dangerous to the developing blood cells of those who are sensitive to them. In addition, certain antibiotics can cause severe damage to the bone marrow. Even commonly used over-the-counter drugs, such as aspirin and nonsteroidal anti-inflammatory drugs (such as ibuprofen) may play a role in blood disorders. They can cause irritation of the stomach lining and gastrointestinal bleeding. To lessen irritation, these drugs should be taken with food and should not be taken in combination. If you are taking a medication and suffer any adverse reaction such as fever, rash, or unusual bleeding, you should discontinue the drug immediately and notify your physician.

Cancer can pose a risk to blood cells, either by involving blood-forming organs or by the effects of treatment for cancer. The treatment for cancer often includes radiation and chemotherapy, both of which kill blood cells as well as other cells. Exposure to radiation damages blood cells and cell production. This is why people who work around radiation equipment wear badges to record the amount of exposure. Chemotherapeutic drugs used to treat cancer and related disorders affect the bone marrow, and dosages must be carefully adjusted to avoid severe damage.

Toxic chemicals such as benzene and related compounds (solvents, rubber cement, some insecticides) can destroy very young blood cells. Immature cells, that would normally develop into mature blood cells, can be killed in the bone marrow of people exposed to these harmful chemicals.

Early Detection

You must be aware of the types of substances with which you work and how they may affect your health. If you work in the agricultural industry, for instance,

BLOOD TYPES

Antigens and antibodies are specific to blood types.

Blood Type	Antigen on Blood Cells	Antibody in Blood
A	A	Against B antigen
B	B	Against A antigen
AB	A and B	None
O	None	Against A and B antigens

you may come into contact with insecticides that could damage your bone marrow. Jobs that use certain chemicals also may put you at risk (for more information about occupational hazards, see Chapter 6).

Many blood disorders do not cause symptoms until they are very far advanced. Women often learn that they have anemia and even certain cancers through routine physical examinations. Because many of these disorders are more easily and successfully treated early, periodic checkups that include a complete blood count, urinalysis, and certain blood tests are recommended. Blood chemistry tests can sometimes provide information about less common blood disorders.

Some blood disorders are inherited. If there is a history of a blood disorder in your family, you should be aware of your risk of having the same disorder. Women who have blood disorders in their families may consider preconceptional testing if they are thinking about having a baby. Some disorders, or the trait that underlies the disorder, can be detected in the blood of the prospective mother or father or, if a woman is pregnant, in the fetus. Certain disorders occur predominantly in certain populations, so people in these groups are offered prenatal testing routinely.

If your doctor thinks you have a blood disorder, you may be referred to a hematologist, a physician who specializes in diseases of the blood. Some hematologists also specialize in oncology; in addition to treating patients with blood disorders, they treat those with cancer.

HEALTH CONCERNS

The blood and lymphatic system reach every tissue of the body and help maintain its overall health. As a result, the first sign of a blood disorder may appear in another organ. Conversely, the first sign of a disorder in an organ may appear in the blood because the blood comes in contact with all parts of the body. Thus a patient may have signs and symptoms of one disorder when the cause is another source. For this reason, a careful patient history and physical examination are important parts of the evaluation in any disorder relating to the blood and its production. Symptoms of a blood disorder should be evaluated, especially if they persist (see box on "Major Symptoms and Signs of Blood Disorders").

Cancer can occur in blood-forming tissues just as it does in other cells of the body. All cells in the body reproduce by dividing. Normal growth and repair of body tissues take place in this manner. Cancer occurs when cell division is not orderly, when it becomes abnormal and cell growth is out of control. This can occur in leukemia, when white blood cells multiply. Lymphomas are cancers that develop in the lymphatic system. Another form of cancer is multiple myeloma, in which plasma cells proliferate. Most of these cancers have symptoms of anemia.

As one of the most common disorders of the blood, anemia can occur in many forms. Anemia can be a symptom of a disorder, or it can be caused by a deficiency in vital nutrients. When anemia occurs, the cause must be found and treatment determined based on the cause.

Other disorders of the blood may relate to a problem in one of the factors that cause clotting. There are 12 or more factors that participate in the blood clotting mechanism. A deficiency in any one of these factors may interfere with blood clotting. This can occur with inherited disorders such as hemophilia or von Willebrand's disease. Bleeding disorders can also arise when the platelets are decreased or are not functioning normally, such as in leukemia.

Anemia

Hemoglobin, the main component of red blood cells, combines with oxygen in the lungs and carries it throughout the body. When a person lacks hemoglobin, the cells in the body do not receive the oxygen they need to function properly. Anemia is a condition in which the hemoglobin content of the blood falls below the normal level. This can be because of a decrease in the number of red blood cells or a decrease in the amount of hemoglobin in each cell or both.

A person who has anemia may feel more tired than usual or become fatigued by only mild exertion. Often, if anemia is mild, there may be no symptoms. When the condition is more severe, symptoms include pale skin (particularly under the eyelids and the fingernails where blood vessels are close to the surface), weakness, faintness, and an increased heart rate. The heart, in trying to compensate for anemia, pumps blood faster than normal to get oxygen to all the cells of the body.

There are several types of anemia (see box on "Types of Anemia"). Anemia can be a disorder in and of itself, or it can be a symptom of another disorder. Anemia can occur as a result of deficiencies, be an inherited condition, or be acquired as a disorder. The most common types of anemia are those that occur

MAJOR SYMPTOMS AND SIGNS OF BLOOD DISORDERS

Condition	Symptom or Sign
Anemia	Pallor, palpitations, fatigue, shortness of breath
Leukemia	Fever, weakness, bleeding problems, enlarged lymph nodes, enlarged spleen
Lymphoma	Swollen lymph nodes, enlarged spleen, loss of appetite, fever, night sweats
Bleeding disorders	Tiny red spots under the skin that indicate bleeding, increased bruising, nosebleeds, heavy menses, bleeding after trauma or surgery
Deep vein thombosis	Swelling and pain in legs, shortnesss of breath, chest pain

TYPES OF ANEMIA

Iron deficiency anemia
Anemia of chronic disorders (associated with cancer, chronic inflammations, autoimmune diseases, kidney disease)
Anemia due to invasion of bone marrow (leukemia, cancer)
Thalassemia
Hemoglobinopathies
Vitamin B_{12} deficiency and folic acid deficiency
Acquired hemolytic anemia
Aplastic anemia
Anemia with multiple causes

when one or more elements essential for building red blood cells or hemoglobin are missing. Different forms of anemia can arise from deficiencies in iron, vitamin B_{12}, and folic acid.

Blood loss for any reason—including injury, trauma, menstruation, or gastrointestinal problems such as an ulcer or cancer—is an important cause of anemia. Bleeding also can be caused by aspirin and other painkillers that irritate the lining of the stomach. A small amount of blood is found in the stools of as many as 70 percent of the users of these medications. When large numbers of red blood cells are lost at once, the bone marrow is unable to produce enough to replace them immediately. When blood loss is slow and steady, a woman may not be able to absorb enough iron from her diet, and iron deficiency occurs.

Other types of anemia are caused by abnormalities in the production or function of red blood cells. When red blood cells are broken down (hemolyzed) at a faster rate than they can be replaced, hemolytic anemia results. This may be due to an inherited condition such as sickle cell anemia and thalassemia. Another type of inherited anemia is known as G6PD enzyme deficiency that results in anemia when certain drugs are taken. About 10 percent of African-American men have this problem, but it is rare in women. Hemolysis also may be caused by the presence of antibodies in the blood that attack the red cells or by drugs taken for other conditions.

Anemia can result from the failure of bone marrow to manufacture red blood cells, a condition known as aplastic anemia. Aplastic anemia may follow exposure to large amounts of radiation or contact with one of many substances that destroy the bone marrow's ability to produce red blood cells. A type of anemia can also occur with chronic diseases.

Anemia is diagnosed by a laboratory analysis of the blood called a complete blood count. If red blood cells make up less than 36 percent of the total blood volume, or the blood's hemoglobin value is below 12 grams per 100 cc. of blood, a woman is said to be anemic. A stained smear of the blood examined under a microscope may provide more information about the cause from the appearance of the blood cells. Depending on the results of these tests, other tests to detect abnormalities in iron, B_{12}, folic acid, or the structure of hemoglobin may be done. If iron is found to be low, particularly in a postmenopausal woman, a stool sample is checked for the presence of blood. If blood in the stool is found, other tests may be needed to evaluate the gastrointestinal tract. A bone marrow biopsy may, rarely, be required.

The goal of treatment for anemia is to restore the body's ability to make healthy red blood cells able to carry oxygen to tissues throughout the body. Each type of anemia requires a different therapy to correct it.

Deficiency Anemia

Iron-Deficiency Anemia

If red blood cells do not have an adequate supply of iron to make hemoglobin, they are unable to carry oxygen to the body. Of all the iron present in each adult, 70 percent can be found in hemoglobin. Blood loss, either chronic or acute, is a common cause of iron-deficiency anemia. Acute loss of blood, such as hemorrhage that occurs with injury, decreases the number of red blood cells in the body. In chronic loss, such as during heavy menstrual periods or chronic gastrointestinal bleeding, the bone marrow can usually keep up red blood cell production until the body runs short of iron or another essential building block of healthy red blood cells.

Iron deficiency anemia is often a symptom of another disorder, such as an ulcer or cancer. Because of this relationship, the cause of blood loss should be found in addition to treating iron deficiency.

Women in particular are apt to suffer from iron-deficiency anemia. The slow, intermittent loss of blood during monthly menstruation puts a woman at risk for iron-deficiency anemia, as does the use of intrauterine devices (IUD) that can cause abnormally heavy menstrual flow. Pregnancy makes heavy nutritional demands on the body. Pregnant women must have sufficient iron to cover the requirements of the fetus, the placenta that nourishes the fetus in the uterus, their own expanded blood volume, and the blood loss that occurs during childbirth. It is estimated that 1 out of every 10–15 menstruating and pregnant women have some degree of iron deficiency. In the United States, menstruating women have only one-fourth to one-half the stored iron men have. Iron deficiency in most postmenopausal women is usually due to blood loss from the gastrointestinal tract and must be evaluated by a physician.

Diagnosis

On a blood smear, the red cells may be small and deformed. A substance called serum ferritin is measured to confirm the diagnosis. Ferritin is a protein that stores iron in the tissues, and the amount in blood provides an indirect measure of the total amount of iron stored in the body. There is almost a total lack of stored iron before anemia develops. Another test used to diagnose iron-deficiency anemia is transferrin saturation. Transferrin is a protein that takes iron absorbed from foods as well as iron from broken down red blood cells and carries it to developing red blood cells in the bone marrow. If very little transferrin is saturated with the mineral, iron stores may be deficient or there may not be enough iron to make hemoglobin or both.

Treatment

If anemia is the result of a nutritional deficiency, the daily intake of iron-rich foods should be increased. The recommended dietary allowance (RDA) for iron for men and postmenopausal women is 10 milligrams. For menstruating women, the RDA is 15 milligrams. A balanced diet consisting of an average of from 3 to 6 ounces of meat, poultry, or fish a day, along with five servings of vegetables and fruits provides the body with all the iron it needs. Animal sources of iron, including beef, poultry, and fish, contain a form of iron known as heme iron that the body absorbs better than it does other forms. Fruits, vegetables, and beans contain non-heme iron, which is more difficult for the body to process. Eating foods that contain nonheme iron with foods containing vitamin C enhances iron absorption. For instance, adding some tomato slices, which contain vitamin C, to a salad that has beans allows the body to absorb a greater amount of the iron from beans. The presence of heme iron has the same effect: The body absorbs nonheme iron in potatoes when they are combined with some heme-containing beef.

Iron supplements may be prescribed for iron-deficiency anemia. They should be taken only if prescribed and, even then, use should be carefully monitored to ensure that what might be a need for short-term supplementation does not turn into unnecessary long-term iron therapy. Iron supplements can cause unpleasant side effects, including constipation, diarrhea, and stomach upset. They also can cause nutrient imbalances. Too much iron can interfere with your body's ability to use the essential nutrients copper, manganese, and zinc. Iron overload can cause liver damage as well as damage to other organs.

Hemochromatosis is a condition that occurs when the body absorbs and stores too much iron. It is an hereditary disease estimated to afflict about a million Americans. Hemochromatosis is diagnosed by a serum ferritin or transferrin saturation test or both. It is treated by periodically withdrawing blood from a vein to get rid of excess iron stores.

Vitamin B_{12}-Deficiency Anemia

In addition to being essential to the normal division of developing red blood cells, vitamin B_{12} is vital to the maintenance of the nervous system. If vitamin B_{12} is inadequate, red blood cell production falls and those cells that are formed are large and defective. Symptoms of vitamin B_{12} deficiency include those of other types of anemia and may involve balance and memory problems related to brain and spinal cord damage caused by this deficiency.

In the United States, diets generally contain sufficient amounts of B_{12}, although those on some macrobiotic diets may suffer from a nutritional deficiency. In most cases, however, vitamin B_{12} deficiency anemia occurs because a person's body is unable to absorb the vitamin from foods eaten. Normally, the vitamin attaches to a substance called intrinsic factor, which is manufactured by special cells in the stomach. Intrinsic factor is necessary for vitamin B_{12} to be absorbed into the bloodstream from the lower portion of the small intestine.

The most common type of vitamin B_{12} deficiency is called pernicious anemia. Pernicious anemia results when intrinsic factor is not available in the stomach because the lining cells that secrete it have been destroyed. This occurs more often in older people, and may be related to an autoimmune process in which antibodies to the cells or the intrinsic factor are present and can be detected in the blood. In other cases the body may not be able to absorb vitamin B_{12} because of abnormalities of the digestive tract. Because of disease or surgery of either the stomach or the last part of the small intestine, the body's ability to absorb the vitamin may be reduced significantly. The liver can store about a 4-year supply of vitamin B_{12}, so the anemia and the signs of deficiency develop long after B_{12} absorption has been compromised.

Diagnosis

A workup to detect vitamin B_{12} deficiency usually includes evaluation of the complete blood count and examination of a blood smear. The size of red blood cells is large, and in addition to vitamin B_{12} levels, folic acid blood levels should be checked since the cells can also be enlarged in folic acid-deficiency anemia. Other tests may measure absorption.

Treatment

Once the ability to absorb vitamin B_{12} through the digestive tract has been lost, it is rarely regained. Treatment of pernicious anemia and most other types of B_{12} deficiency consists of lifelong B_{12} injections, which are usually given monthly. Vitamin B_{12} injections should not be taken unless the deficiency is due to an inability to absorb the vitamin. If the condition is due to poor diet, foods rich in vitamin B_{12} or oral supplements can be used to correct the deficiency.

Folic Acid-Deficiency Anemia

Anemia can result from a lack of sufficient folic acid; along with vitamin B_{12}, this nutrient is essential for the normal division of developing red blood cells. Because a person's body cannot build large reserves of this vitamin, a deficiency can show up within a few months as a form of anemia. Folic acid deficiency often occurs in pregnant women who need extra supplies of the vitamin for the developing baby. It is particularly common in people with severe alcoholism because alcoholics often do not eat properly and alcohol interferes with the the body's absorption and use of folic acid. Rarely, diseases of the digestive tract decrease the body's ability to absorb the vitamin. The symptoms of folic acid deficiency anemia are like those of other types of anemia.

The diagnosis of folic acid anemia includes evaluation of the complete blood count and examination of a blood smear. Measurements of levels of vitamin B_{12} and folic acid in the blood are both done. If the folic acid level is found to be low, careful consideration is given to diet, malabsorption, and alcohol abuse as possible causes. Folic acid can be given orally to treat the deficiency and replace the reserves.

Inherited Anemia

Some diseases that result in anemia are inherited. Inherited disorders that cause the production of abnormal forms of hemoglobin are called hemoglobinopathies. Conditions in which inherited abnormalities occur include sickle cell anemia, hereditary spherocytosis, and thalassemia. They can result in hemolytic anemia, the premature destruction of red blood cells. Hemolytic anemia may be hereditary—in which case it is present at birth or soon afterward—or it can be acquired (see "Acquired Anemia").

Hemoglobinopathies affect certain populations. Genetic counseling can help inform a woman of the chance that her offspring may be affected by a disease. In some cases, prenatal testing can be done during pregnancy to detect the disorder in the fetus.

Thalassemia

An inherited disorder that occurs most often in people of Mediterranean, African, and Asian descent, thalassemia results in insufficient formation of hemoglobin A, the type of hemoglobin that is normally found in the red blood cells after the first months of life. There are several types of thalassemia. Thalassemia major is the name given to the most severe form of the disease. A milder form is called thalassemia minor. Since thalassemia is inherited as an autosomal dominant trait, it is mild when it is inherited from only one parent. The severe form occurs when both parents pass on the abnormality.

Diagnosis

Many people with thalassemia minor have only mild symptoms that mirror those of other types of anemia. When the anemia is severe, symptoms include pallor, fatigue, and palpitations.

The diagnosis is based on examination of the blood count, the blood smear, and special tests to detect the composition of the hemoglobin. The red cells may appear small in thalassemia, as they do in iron-deficiency anemia. It is important that the thalassemia is diagnosed correctly because iron therapy should not be taken by people with this condition.

Treatment

With the severe form of the disease, regular lifelong blood transfusions are required to relieve the symptoms of anemia. Drugs also are prescribed that help eliminate excess iron. Those with the milder forms of thalassemia may require no specific treatment at all.

Sickle Cell Anemia

One type of hemoglobinopathy is sickle cell anemia, which is caused by the presence of an abnormal form of hemoglobin called hemoglobin S. It is an inherited autosomal recessive disorder. As many as 12 percent of African-Americans may carry the trait that can result in this disorder. If both parents have the sickle cell gene, they have a 25 percent chance of producing a child with sickle cell anemia.

The hemoglobin abnormality in sickle cell anemia causes the early destruction of red blood cells. In parts of the body where the amount of oxygen is relatively low, red blood cells also can become deformed, or sickled (see Figure 29.3). These abnormal cells do not flow smoothly through small blood vessels, cause an obstruction, and impair delivery of oxygen and nutrients. Such events related to sickle cell disease are called sickle cell crisis and are quite painful. Sickled cells can occur in the bone marrow, lungs, kidneys, brain, and other organs. People with this disorder also have frequent infections that require prompt treatment.

The disease usually appears during a baby's first year. There is no cure. Victims rarely survive beyond age 50 and many die earlier. Women with sickle cell anemia have special concerns. They should not take oral contraceptives, which appear to speed up the tendency to form blood clots. They should also never have a saline abortion because of the danger of the stimu-

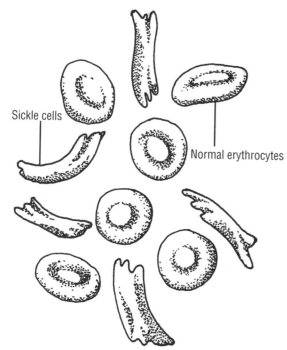

Figure 29.3 Sickle Cell Anemia
Sickle cell anemia is caused by an abnormal form of the protein hemoglobin, which is a key factor in oxygen transport by red blood cells. The abnormal protein causes red blood cells to become sickle shaped, which interferes with the circulation and transport of oxygen and nutrients.

lation of clotting that may occur. Pregnancy is a serious burden for women with sickle cell anemia. Usually, the anemia becomes worse and the attacks of pain more frequent. There is also significant risk to the infant: About one-third to one-half of babies with mothers who have the disease die in miscarriage, stillbirth, or shortly after birth. The greatest danger to the mother is blood clots, that often occur in the lungs and can be fatal.

Spherocytosis

In spherocytosis, an inherited type of hemolytic anemia, the red blood cells are spheroidal and appear round, and their membranes are weak so the cell cannot survive normally. Spherocytosis is an autosomal dominant disorder that is usually inherited from only one parent. Most people with the disorder are mildly anemic and some have slight jaundice (yellow discoloration of the skin and white of the eye). Symptoms become worse when they have infections. They also have enlarged spleens; the usual treatment is removal of the spleen.

Acquired Anemia

Hemolytic Anemia

In hemolytic anemia, which may be hereditary or acquired (see "Inherited Anemia"), red blood cells are prematurely destroyed by the body. One type of acquired hemolytic anemia occurs when a person's body produces antibodies like those that normally protect against infections. Such antibodies can attach themselves to red blood cells and prevent them from surviving for the usual life span of 120 days. Acquired hemolytic anemia can also be caused by drugs.

Symptoms common to other types of anemia result. In addition, jaundice may occur, with the skin becoming yellow and urine darker than usual. In hemolytic anemia, jaundice is due to a buildup of bilirubin, an orange-red pigment formed from the breakdown of hemoglobin.

Diagnosis

The diagnosis of hemolytic anemia is usually evident from abnormalities in the complete blood count, additional blood tests, and a test to detect the presence of antibodies. When acquired hemolytic anemia is caused by drugs, it is treated by discontinuing the drugs. When the disease is an autoimmune disorder, drugs to suppress the immune response and treat the underlying disorder are usually effective.

Aplastic Anemia

The bone marrow's production of blood cells decreases with aplastic anemia, reducing the total number of cells in the bloodstream. This may occur suddenly or develop gradually for a variety of reasons.

In many cases, the cause of the problem cannot be identified. In others, the cause can be traced to exposure to a toxic substance such as benzene (a chemical used in solvents and dyes) or to exposure to certain kinds of radiation. In sensitive individuals, certain drugs, including some used to treat epilepsy as well as anti-inflammatory medications, may cause aplastic anemia to develop. In some women, pregnancy may trigger this condition.

Diagnosis

The symptoms of aplastic anemia are those common to other types of anemia—fatigue, pallor, and rapid heartbeat. Because production of all types of blood cells is often affected, a person is more susceptible to infection due to the lack of white blood cells. A lack of sufficient numbers of platelets can lead to bruising or spontaneous bleeding from the nose or mouth.

Laboratory blood tests to detect other forms of anemia are performed. If these tests point to a diagnosis of aplastic anemia, bone marrow examination may confirm the diagnosis.

Treatment

In cases where the disease is caused by a drug being taken for another problem, the drug may be stopped or another drug substituted. If the condition has been caused by exposure to a toxic chemical, that exposure should be removed immediately. When the disorder is caused by an immune system response, it may respond to drugs that suppress this response. Initially, the anemia is treated with transfusions of red blood cells. Antibiotics also may be prescribed to protect against infection. As many as 80 percent of less severe cases may respond to a combination of drugs that suppress the immune system, a treatment preferred in patients over 40 years of age. In younger patients, or in those in whom the disease is particularly severe, a bone marrow transplant offers the best hope of recovery. Bone marrow transplant has an overall success rate of about 60–70 percent.

Anemia of Chronic Disorders

Diseases that bring on this type of anemia include rheumatoid arthritis and related autoimmune disorders, as well as infections such as tuberculosis and AIDS. The symptoms of anemia are combined with those of the underlying disease. Severe cases of this anemia can be treated only with transfusion, but the condition should improve if the underlying cause can be treated. People who have chronic kidney disease often become anemic, in part because their kidneys do not make the hormone erythropoietin, which stimulates the production of red blood cells. Because erythropoietin now is manufactured, synthetic forms can be used to treat this condition. It is also used for patients with AIDS.

Bleeding and Bruising

Bleeding occurs when blood vessels are damaged. If damaged vessels are beneath the skin surface, blood seeps into surrounding tissue and a bruise forms. Where delicate blood vessels are very near the surface of tissue, as they are on the inside of the nose, for example, a very slight injury or irritation may cause external bleeding.

For most people, bleeding causes no harm because the body soon stops it by a process called hemostasis. This is a complex process requiring the presence of platelets (tiny, disk-shaped cell fragments) and other substances called clotting factors. To stop bleeding, the body's blood vessels close to restrict the flow of blood from the wound. The platelets in the blood then build up where the blood vessel is damaged and stick to the vessel walls and to each other to form a plug. Then interweaving strands of a material called fibrin form in the damaged area. Blood cells are then trapped in a fibrin mesh and they form a clot that seals the break.

In diseases that cause or result in abnormal bleeding, one or more of the mechanisms that halt bleeding do not work properly. In some disorders, including thrombocytopenia, leukemia, and other conditions that affect the bone marrow, the body produces fewer platelets than are required to stop bleeding. Other diseases that have bleeding and bruising as primary symptoms include some hereditary disorders. In hemophilia, crucial clotting factors are deficient; in von Willebrand's disease, both clotting and platelet function factors are involved.

Petechiae are small, bright red and dark red dots, and purpura is larger areas of bleeding just under the skin. Petechiae and purpura are symptoms of bleeding disorders, particularly thrombocytopenia and disorders of small blood vessels.

Thrombocytopenia

Thrombocytopenia is a bleeding disorder caused by a lack of platelets, the blood cell fragments involved in blood coagulation. When there are not enough platelets, the body is unable to properly control bleeding. As a result, people with this disorder bleed more and longer than usual when injured. In addition, episodes of spontaneous bleeding may occur.

Any kind of drug or disease causing a decrease in the number of cells in the marrow that normally develop into mature blood cells can result in a low platelet count. Thrombocytopenia is more often caused when the body forms antibodies that attack its own platelets. Healthy platelets are coated by the antibodies and then removed from the bloodstream at an increased rate. This type of thrombocytopenia is known as idiopathic thrombocytopenic purpura (ITP). Thrombocytopenia also may occur because of a drug taken for an unrelated purpose, or as a part of treatment for other blood disorders, such as leukemia.

Diagnosis

A complete blood count shows the platelet level and may indicate whether the thrombocytopenia is an isolated finding or a sign of another disease. A measurement of platelet-associated antibodies is useful in determining the cause. It also may be helpful to test for certain autoimmune disorders. Sometimes, a bone marrow examination is required to determine if there are enough cells in the marrow.

Treatment

Because a number of drugs can produce thrombocytopenia in sensitive individuals, most or all drugs are stopped as primary treatment. If the cause appears to be an antibody, a cortico-steroid drug may be prescribed to slow the destruction caused by antibodies. This allows the level of platelets in the blood to rise. Often, the disease resolves itself after several weeks with or without treatment. If not, removal of the spleen may be required. Although the spleen normally destroys only worn out red blood cells, it also can destroy platelets. When thrombocytopenia is caused by underproduction of platelets by the bone marrow and a serious bleeding problem is present, a transfusion of platelets may provide temporary relief.

von Willebrand's Disease

The most common inherited bleeding disorder in women is due to the lack of a clotting factor that controls the ability of platelets to stick to the wall of an injured vessel and to each other. This inability results in nosebleeds, excessive bleeding from tooth removal and other surgical procedures, and heavy menstrual periods.

The diagnosis of von Willebrand's disease requires special tests that are usually done when a person has a suggestive history of bleeding and suggestive laboratory tests. The drug desmopressin may be prescribed to prevent or stop bleeding in this condition. It works to stimulate the release of the missing clotting factor from blood vessel walls. Medication that might worsen bleeding, such as aspirin, should be avoided.

Hemophilia

Hemophilia is a hereditary bleeding disorder due to a deficiency in certain blood clotting factors. There are two types of hemophilia, due to deficiencies of different clotting factors: type A and type B. Type A, or classic hemophilia, is the most common severe inherited coagulation disorder and accounts for more than three-quarters of all cases in the United States. Both types are sex-linked recessive genetic disorders passed by mothers to their sons. Complications may appear shortly after birth and increase in severity and fre-

quency with age and activity. In severe cases, bleeding can occur in the joints, most commonly the knees, as well as other parts of the body. Bleeding can be brought on by mild trauma or can occur spontaneously. In milder cases, bleeding episodes usually do not occur spontaneously but instead result from trauma or surgery. Bleeding is treated by giving transfusions of concentrated material that contains the missing clotting factors.

Blood Clots

Thrombosis is the medical term to describe the formation of a thrombus, or blood clot, which may partially or completely block a blood vessel. Thrombosis in a vein near the surface of the skin may cause an inflammatory response. This response is referred to as superficial thrombophlebitis. When clots form in deeper veins, the condition is called deep-vein thrombosis.

There may be changes in the blood that result in increased stickiness of platelets and increased tendency to form clots. Women who take estrogen, either in the form of birth control pills or as postmenopausal therapy, may have a slightly higher risk of blood clots. A woman who smokes cigarettes and takes estrogen increases her risks significantly.

Thrombosis in the legs often develops after long periods of being inactive, especially after surgery or during recovery from an illness. This is because the blood flow becomes sluggish. When a vein in the leg is clogged, the leg usually becomes swollen and painful. The major danger of deep-vein thrombosis is that a piece or pieces of the clot will break off, enter the bloodstream, and flow through the heart and into the lungs, resulting in a pulmonary embolus. Heart attacks occur when clots form in the coronary arteries, and strokes occur when vessels supplying the brain are blocked (see Chapters 22 and 27).

Leukemia

Leukemia is a form of cancer of the blood. As with any cancer, certain cells grow and multiply in an abnormal manner. The term *leukemia* refers to a group of diseases in which there are too many white blood cells formed in the bone marrow and/or lymphatic system. Normally, the number of white blood cells that are produced equals the number that die off as part of the natural process of cell turnover in the body. With leukemia, excess white blood cells are produced which can interfere with the manufacture of normal blood cells.

Leukemia can be either acute—developing suddenly—or it can be chronic and develop slowly over time. It is further defined by the type of white blood cell involved: myeloid leukemia involves white blood cells that would have matured into granulocytes; lymphoid leukemia involves cells that would have matured into lymphocytes.

Although leukemia is the most common of the childhood cancers, it occurs more often in adults. Approximately 25,000 new cases of leukemia are diagnosed annually in the United States. Women are affected by leukemia 30 percent less often than men.

Since the 1930s, there has been an increase in leukemia in industrialized nations. Although there is no accepted theory about the cause of leukemia, its rising incidence is assumed to result from increased exposure to toxic substances in the environment: industrial pollution, food contaminants, or radiation. Leukemia also can occur as a result of the breakdown of the body's immune system, such as that which accompanies AIDS.

Symptoms of leukemia include unexplained weight loss, low energy, fever, unusual bleeding or bruising, and lowered resistance to infection. All of these symptoms can be present as well as swelling of lymph nodes and the spleen.

The initial diagnosis is based on abnormalities in the white blood cells. There may be either increased or decreased total numbers, but the most important finding is abnormalities in the kinds of white cells. Mainly immature cells are seen in acute leukemia, while more mature cells are present in chronic leukemia. Bone marrow biopsy is usually required to confirm the diagnosis. The treatment depends on the type of leukemia involved.

Acute Lymphoblastic Leukemia

Although acute lymphoblastic leukemia (ALL) is most common in children under the age of 5, it occasionally affects adolescents and adults. It involves the overproduction of immature blood cells that would otherwise develop into healthy mature lymphocytes. The overgrowth of these cells in the bone marrow crowds out normal production of red blood cells and platelets. Without sufficient red blood cells the person becomes anemic, and without sufficient platelets there are problems with bruising and bleeding (including nose-

bleeds). Fever and infection are common because the body lacks normal white blood cells to destroy bacteria and viruses and to mount an immune response.

Modern medical therapy—usually involving combination chemotherapy and, if the leukemia resists chemotherapy, bone marrow transplantation—allows more than 70 percent of children to survive more than five years after diagnosis, indicating that the disease has been cured. The prognosis for adults, however, is less optimistic: Current statistics show that only about 20 percent achieve long-term survival.

Acute Myelogenous Leukemia

Acute myelogenous leukemia (AML) is rapidly progressive and usually fatal. It accounts for less than 1 percent of all leukemia and affects slightly fewer women than men. Although AML occurs at all ages, it usually affects people between 30 and 60 years of age, with frequency increasing with age. This form of leukemia involves the overproduction and lack of maturation of blood cells that normally would develop into white blood cells called granulocytes. As their numbers increase, the leukemic cells fill the bone marrow. This invasion results in a decrease in the production of normal granulocytes, red blood cells, and platelets. Leukemic cells also can grow in other organs and tissues, particularly the spleen and liver. The disease usually occurs suddenly, with the symptoms of leukemia and anemia becoming pronounced over a few weeks. If AML is not treated promptly, it can be fatal, sometimes within only a few weeks.

Treatment with transfusions of red blood cells and platelets, as well as with antibiotics to reduce the chance of infection, is usually given. Chemotherapeutic drugs can eliminate most of the leukemia cells from the blood and bone marrow, but after treatment is completed the disease frequently recurs. A bone marrow transplant to replace diseased blood-forming cells with healthy cells offers the best chance of a cure in most cases; a significant number of patients with AML treated in this way survive for at least five years after transplant.

Chronic Lymphocytic Leukemia

Slow growing chronic lymphocytic leukemia is most common in people over 50 and is two to three times less common in women than men. It involves an overproduction of lymphocytes. After some time, perhaps several years, the leukemia cells gradually crowd out normal white blood cells in the bone marrow, lymph glands, and spleen. The ability of the remaining healthy cells to fight infection is then reduced. The normal cells also overflow from the lymphatic system and bone marrow into the bloodstream. As the number of abnormal cells in the bone marrow increases, they interfere more and more with the production of other types of blood cells. This leads to a number of other problems, including anemia, risk of infections, and bleeding and bruising.

Often, people with chronic lymphocytic leukemia have no symptoms at all and the condition is diagnosed only when a complete blood count or other blood tests are done during a regular examination. The course of this type of leukemia varies widely; people with it can survive for decades without treatment, although progress is much more rapid in some than in others.

Chronic Myelogenous Leukemia

Chronic myelogenous leukemia involves the overproduction of granulocytes, blood cells that are produced normally in the bone marrow. It is relatively rare and occurs most commonly in people between the ages of 20 and 50. In more than 90 percent of those who have chronic myelogenous leukemia, an abnormal chromosome is present and thought to be the cause of the disorder.

More than one-third of the patients have no symptoms at the time of diagnosis. When symptoms are present, they include those common to other types of leukemia, such as anemia and enlargement of the spleen.

Although this disease usually has a short-term response to chemotherapy, it is chronic and progressive and cannot be cured except by bone marrow transplant. The course of chronic myelogenous leukemia is often marked by a medical emergency, called a blast crisis, which usually develops within 3–4 years of onset. The blast crisis signals the advance of the disease to a kind of acute leukemia that is extremely difficult to treat. Death often quickly follows a blast crisis.

Lymphoma

Malignancies of the lymphatic system involve an abnormal proliferation of lymphocytes, or white blood cells, in the lymph nodes and spleen. Sometimes, the bone marrow and other parts of the body also are involved. As with most malignancies, the cause is not definitely known. The two general types of lymphomas are Hodgkin's disease and non-Hodgkin's lymphoma.

Hodgkin's Disease

Hodgkin's disease is a disorder of the lymphatic system that usually attacks young adults and about half as many women as men. Symptoms are those common to other lymphomas, including swollen glands, usually in the neck, armpit, or groin. There are often other symptoms such as periodic fever, night sweats, weight loss, and itching.

Diagnosis is based on blood tests, X-rays, and biopsies. A sample taken from an enlarged lymph node is examined for signs of lymphoma. If it is found, the stage of the disease must be determined to guide treatment.

Recent medical advances have resulted in improvements in the long-term outlook of most patients with Hodgkin's disease. If the disease has not spread, a 95 percent cure rate can be expected with radiation therapy alone. If the disease is discovered at an advanced stage, treatment includes multiple chemotherapeutic drugs, sometimes in combination with radiation.

Non-Hodgkin's Lymphoma

In non-Hodgkin's lymphoma, cells of the lymphatic organs begin growing abnormally and multiplying rapidly, usually forming a palpable tumor and spreading to other parts of the body. The first symptom is usually a swollen gland, most often in the neck, armpit, or groin. Other possible symptoms include a general sense of not feeling well, loss of appetite, fever, and night sweats. The initial diagnosis usually depends on a biopsy of an affected lymph gland. If a lymphoma is diagnosed, special studies on the tissue may further define its specific type.

Treatment depends on information about the extent of the disease, so X-rays, CT scans, and bone marrow examination are usually necessary. It is often possible to assign a stage to lymphomas of from I to IV, with I showing involvement of a single group of lymph glands and IV indicating spread beyond the lymphatic system into other tissues. If the disease is localized to a single part of the body, such as the neck, treatment may be radiation therapy alone or radiation therapy with chemotherapy. Treatment may require a short hospital stay, followed by injections of drugs in an outpatient setting.

Multiple Myeloma

Multiple myeloma is a rare, serious disease of plasma cells, which are derivatives of the B-lymphocytes and normally produce antibodies that help destroy bacteria, viruses, and other infectious agents. In this disease, plasma cells begin to multiply out of control. The cells usually produce excessive amounts of an abnormal protein, which can cause symptoms. As the number of plasma cells increase, the production of red blood cells, platelets, and granulocytes (a type of white blood cell) is decreased, often leading to anemia and thrombocytopenia.

The first symptoms of myeloma are often those of anemia (fatigue, rapid heart rate) as well as some bruising and bleeding. Another early symptom of this disease is bone pain. The pain is caused by the plasma cells proliferating in the bone marrow and destroying bone. There is an increased risk of infection because the normal plasma cells produce fewer antibodies to fight against bacteria and viruses that enter the body. Patients may also have kidney failure.

Treatment consists of chemotherapy to destroy the malignant cells. Although the course of the disease varies, drug treatment can help patients with myeloma have good health for a time. More recently, bone marrow transplants have been used with some success.

Polycythemia

The cause of polycythemia vera (or true polycythemia) is unknown. This disease of the bone marrow cells results in the overproduction of all types of blood cells, particularly red blood cells. In polycythemia vera, red blood cells, granulocytes, and platelets are overproduced, and this condition must be differentiated from secondary polycythemia, which occurs as a result of an underlying cause, such as severe lung disease, certain kinds of congenital heart disease, tobacco smoking, and living at high altitudes. Such conditions prevent the red blood cells from obtaining enough oxygen to pass on to the body's tissues. This results in increased amounts of erythropoietin, the hormone that stimulates production of red blood cells. Tumors and other lesions of the kidney may also result in the formation of increased amounts of erythropoietin and cause secondary polycythemia.

COMPLETE BLOOD COUNT

The complete blood count (CBC) determines how many of each type of blood cell are in a given volume of blood and examines the cells for any abnormalities in structure. The red blood count hemoglobin and hematocrit values of the CBC measure the quantity of red blood cells; the white blood count (WBC) measures the number of white cells. A differential count compares the relative numbers of the various white cells.

Blood counts are reported according to the number of cells in one cubic millimeter. Following is the approximate number of cells in one cubic millimeter, which is one small drop:

Red blood cells	5 million
White blood cells	7,000
Granulocytes (50–70 percent)	
Lymphocytes (20–40 percent)	
Monocytes (2–7 percent)	
Platelets	300,000

The symptoms of polycythemia include recurrent headaches, dizziness, and a ruddy complexion due to the increased blood volume. Sometimes there is severe itching. Although many people with the disorder live without symptoms for many years, the increased number of red blood cells may lead to serious complications, including stroke, heart attack, gout, and eventually acute myelogenous leukemia.

The diagnosis is based on an increase in the total volume of red blood cells in the body (total red cell mass). If the total red cell mass is increased, it is necessary to determine the cause. Studies of oxygen saturation of the arterial blood and the level of erythropoietin in the blood are helpful in determining the type of polycythemia.

To lower the number of red blood cells, blood can be taken from a vein in the arm. In some cases, this treatment may need to be repeated periodically. With polycythemia vera, drugs may also be needed to control the overproduction of blood cells. With secondary polycythemia, the underlying cause must be treated as well.

TESTS AND PROCEDURES

Most of the procedures used to evaluate disorders of the blood and lymphatic system are laboratory tests. The tests measure the numbers of various types of blood cells as well as their sizes and shapes. The most routine test is the complete blood count (see box on "Complete Blood Count"). Many diseases have a direct effect on blood cells which is often not detected until a routine complete blood count is performed. One way to assess the production of blood cells is to sample the bone marrow. Blood transfusions can be given to relieve symptoms and replace valuable blood components. If the disorder is chronic, a bone marrow transplant may be considered.

Laboratory Tests

Blood is the easiest tissue to obtain for study. Evaluation of the blood cell components is a key part of an examination. The assessment includes determination of hemoglobin, red and white blood cell counts, platelet count, and a description of the blood cells as seen in a blood smear studied under a microscope. Tests also may be performed to detect antibodies and to assess bleeding and clotting times.

A blood test may be done to measure the total red blood cell mass: In this test, a small volume of red blood cells is marked with a radioactive material and injected into the vein of one arm. Later, a blood sample is taken from the other arm. By determining the number of cells marked by the radioactive material cells, it is possible to estimate the total volume of red blood cells.

Blood Transfusions

Patients who are hemorrhaging or who have chronic anemia or clotting disorders may be treated with transfusions of blood components. A transfusion can consist of whole blood or of concentrations of specific blood components, such as red blood cells, plasma, platelets, and a variety of factors that promote blood clotting (see Figure 29.4). A person who receives a blood transfu-

sion is given blood from a donor whose blood has been matched to that person's own blood type.

Blood transfusions are generally quite safe and painless. They involve infusing blood or blood products into the body through a needle in a vein. Depending on the circumstances under which the transfusion is required, treatment may be given in the hospital or on an outpatient basis.

Rarely, despite all precautions, transfusions can cause bad reactions or result in infection. Such instances usually occur in patients with rare blood types. They also can result from human error on the part of the health care professional who is determining the type, matching it with a donor, and transfusing the blood. If a person is given the wrong blood type, the body's immune system develops a kind of allergic reaction. Fever,

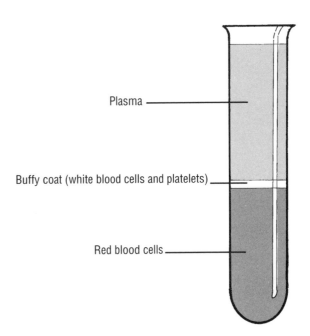

Figure 29-4 Whole Blood
Whole blood is made up of three distinct components that can be seen when it is spun at high speed in a centrifuge. Red blood cells become packed at the bottom of a test tube, leaving the fluid portion of blood, or *plasma*, at the top. White blood cells and platelets form a "buffy coat" in the middle that separates the other two components. Whole blood is separated in this way so that specific components can be used for blood transfusions.

BLOOD TRANSFUSIONS IN THE AGE OF AIDS

There are always dangers associated with the transfusion of blood. Viral infections such as hepatitis and AIDS have been transferred this way in the past. Since 1984, however, all donated blood has undergone careful screening of donors and extensive laboratory testing, which has greatly decreased the likelihood of such events. However, blood transfusions should be given only when absolutely necessary.

Since there is always a need for blood of all types, all healthy women should donate blood regularly if possible. This is in no way harmful as long as the donor follows the instructions of the blood bank and takes some additional oral iron medication for a few weeks following each donation.

It is also a good idea to donate blood in advance for elective surgery. A person's own blood can be retained for use in the event it is needed.

chills, chest pain, hives, nausea, and shock may occur. Blood products that have not been carefully screened and treated have also spread infections such as hepatitis, cytomegalovirus, and AIDS (see box on "Blood Transfusions in the Age of AIDS").

Bone Marrow Aspiration and Biopsy

Bone marrow aspiration and biopsy involves the removal of a sample of tissue for laboratory study. Bone marrow is removed for examination by bone marrow aspiration or biopsy or both ways. Bone marrow aspiration involves the use of a needle inserted through the skin to the bone. The needle is long enough to penetrate the bone and reach the bone marrow. A syringe is then attached and creates a vacuum to suck up a sample of bone marrow.

Bone marrow biopsy is performed in a similar way, except that a solid core of marrow tissue is removed intact with a hollow needle. Aspiration allows the physician to see the mixture of cells that the marrow is producing, while a biopsy allows the study of the actual structure of the marrow.

Both methods of bone marrow examination can be painful. The patient is given a local anesthetic at the site from which the bone marrow sample is to be taken. This is usually the breast bone or the back of the pelvic bone. There may be some pressure as the biopsy needle is inserted and many patients feel pain as the marrow is aspirated. Fortunately, that part of the procedure takes only a few seconds. The site may be tender for a few days following the biopsy.

Bone Marrow Transplantation and Donation

A routine treatment for some forms of leukemia, bone marrow transplantation also is used more and more to replace malfunctioning bone marrow in some nonmalignant disorders, such as aplastic anemia. It involves removing bone marrow from a compatible donor and inserting it in a person whose bone marrow is not functioning properly. This major procedure involves a certain amount of pain or risk for both donor and recipient. Transplants have been found effective in the treatment of leukemia, Hodgkin's disease, aplastic anemia, and other forms of cancer such as breast and ovarian cancer.

The potential donor's marrow is measured by a human leukocyte antigen (HLA) test that examines antigens found on the surface of white blood cells to determine if they are compatible with the recipient's.

There are three main types of bone marrow transplants:

- Syngeneic transplants are those that take place between identical twins. Because the HLAs of identical twins are the same, there is no risk of graft versus host disease.

- Allogeneic transplantation is usually done from siblings or parents of the patient. It is also done from unrelated donors who have similar HLA antigens.

- Autologous transplantation involves removing the patient's own marrow, treating it to remove abnormal cells if necessary, storing it, and then returning it to the patient who has received intensive chemotherapy.

When there is no family donor, patients who require bone marrow transplants can attempt to find unrelated donors with similar HLA types. A national bone marrow registry has been established to help patients find compatible donors.

The transplant operation involves two main procedures. First, the diseased or abnormal marrow of the recipient is destroyed by radiation and chemotherapy. The donor is given anesthesia, and marrow is withdrawn from the pelvic bones by a syringe. Second, the marrow is processed and stored or infused promptly into the recipient.

Throughout the transplant process, the recipient usually stays in a special hospital room ventilated with filtered air to minimize the risk of infection and receives therapy with antibiotics. Patients require transfusions of red blood cells, platelets, and special

stimulating factors to stimulate the growth of transplanted marrow cells. Once the new marrow begins to produce cells in adequate quantities—which can take as long as 4–6 weeks if there is no major complication—these special precautions are no longer necessary and the patient can usually leave the hospital. The donor may have considerable discomfort after the procedure, but it should not be permanent.

One major risk to the recipient of a bone marrow transplant is graft versus host disease. It results from incompatibility of the bone marrow of the donor with that of the recipient. Some of the cells of the implanted marrow may attack the host cells. This reaction is controlled with immunosuppressive medication.

CHAPTER 30

The Endocrine System

Doris Gorka Bartuska, M.D., F.A.C.P. and
Joan A. Lit, M.D.

The endocrine system acts as a control mechanism for the entire body. Complex and finely tuned, it coordinates the body's activities and its responses to changes in the environment, both internal and external. The endocrine system affects height, weight, metabolism, growth, sexual development, menstruation, hair and bone growth, fertility, pregnancy, and breast milk production, as well as some aspects of personality and behavior.

The endocrine system (Figure 30.1) consists of glands that work interdependently: the two *adrenal glands,* located on the top of each kidney; the *pancreas,* found in the abdominal cavity behind the stomach; the *parathyroid* and *thyroid,* located at the base of the neck; the *pituitary,* located at the base of the brain; and the *ovaries* and *testes,* the female and male sex glands (see Chapter 15).

The endocrine glands produce hormones, chemicals released into the bloodstream that regulate the activity of various organs, tissues, and body functions. (Other organs and systems, such as the kidneys and the gastrointestinal system, also produce hormones, which affect the body; see Chapters 32 and 33.) Each gland produces different hormones that are targeted to a particular area of the body. The endocrine glands work in tandem with the organ, efficiently controlling the ebb and flow of hormones so that the body's glandular activity remains constant, much the way that a thermostat turns off a heater when the temperature reaches the appropriate level. Occasionally, an endocrine gland may produce too much or too little of a hormone and upset the balance.

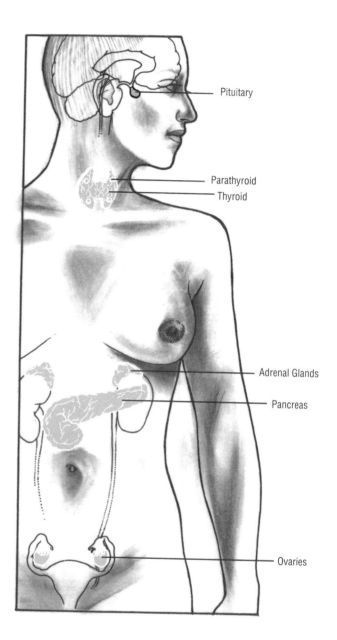

Figure 30.1 The glands of the endocrine system produce hormones that regulate body functions.

KEEPING THE ENDOCRINE SYSTEM HEALTHY

When the delicate hormonal balance that the endocrine system controls is maintained, your body efficiently performs many vital functions. Because the endocrine system is so complex and carefully calibrated, however, a variety of problems, both great and small, can result if it malfunctions. Women experience endocrine system abnormalities much more commonly than men, including thyroid diseases and osteoporosis,

and must therefore be more alert to the prevention, early diagnosis, and appropriate treatment of this type of disorder.

Some endocrine disorders are related to diet, so the single most effective preventive measure a woman can take is to eat nutritious, healthy meals. Calcium intake is especially important, as a lack of sufficient dietary calcium—the mineral that gives bones their strength and density—and a low estrogen level are the most common causes of osteoporosis. Osteoporosis, the loss of bone density, is found in one in every four older women in the United States today. Sufficient calcium intake throughout your life is, therefore, essential.

Another diet-related endocrine disorder is goiter, or enlargement of the thyroid, which can result from lack of iodine in the diet. After the introduction of iodized table salt, however, goiter became uncommon in the United States.

Keeping your body at a healthy weight will greatly diminish your risk of developing type II diabetes mellitus, the most common endocrine disorder in the United States. Diabetes affects almost 10 million people, about half of them women, and type II diabetes accounts for more than 85 percent of all cases. Obesity is believed to increase the body's resistance to the action of insulin, the hormone that stimulates cells and tissues to use the energy produced by the food we eat.

Maintaining a healthy weight is vital to preventing and controlling this condition.

Knowing your family medical history is also important. Among the familial endocrine disorders are diabetes and hypothyroidism. Some genetically linked disorders involve more than one gland. If one member of the family has hypothyroidism, for instance, then others may be at risk for other endocrine disorders (polyglandular autoimmune diseases). Although you cannot change your genes, recognizing that you are at risk, taking preventive measures, and seeking early diagnosis and treatment can greatly limit the effects of the condition.

If you are at risk for developing an endocrine disorder, or are currently suffering from one, you may be referred to an endocrinologist. An endocrinologist is a specialist in internal medicine, with additional training in endocrinology, diabetes, and metabolism.

THE ENDOCRINE SYSTEM AT WORK: PROBLEMS AND TREATMENTS

In the following pages, we discuss the glands and hormones of the endocrine system, as well as the problems that result when these glands malfunction.

The Adrenal Glands

The two adrenal glands are each located on top of a kidney. About the size of the end section of your thumb, each gland consists of two basic parts. The central portion, or medulla, is made up of cells that secrete hormones called catecholamines, the most important of which is adrenaline, also called epinephrine. The outer layer, or cortex, surrounding the medulla is responsible for producing several groups of steroid hormones, including glucocorticoids, mineralocorticoids, and the sex steroids.

The cortex portion of the adrenal gland is controlled by a pituitary gland hormone called adrenocorticotropin or ACTH. ACTH stimulates the conversion of cholesterol to cortisol.

Congenital Adrenal Hyperplasia

This condition occurs when there is a blockage in the process that converts cholesterol to cortisol. The pituitary gland, sensing the low cortisol level caused by the

blockage, then produces more of the hormone ACTH to stimulate the adrenal glands so they can produce a normal amount of cortisol. But the increased stimulation causes an excess of other hormones, including androstenedione, DHEA, and DHEA-S, which are androgen, or male, hormones.

Most forms of congenital hyperplasia are discovered in infancy or in childhood because of the symptoms that result from low cortisol levels or high androgen levels. If your blockage is only partial and the hormone levels are normal or only slightly elevated, you may not have problems in childhood.

Symptoms
Growth of hair in areas that are typically associated with males, including the upper lip, chin, breast bone, and below the navel. Acne is common. Irregular menstruation and infertility may occur.

Diagnosis
After a medical history and physical examination, diagnosis is made through blood studies, specifically tests of testosterone, androstenedione, LH and FSH, DHEA-S, and 17-hydroxyprogesterone levels. A cosyntropin stimulation test may confirm the diagnosis.

Treatment

Treatment depends on the severity of the hormonal disturbance as well as the symptoms. If your symptoms are not severe and infertility is not a problem, then no treatment may be necessary. If the symptoms are severe or if conceiving a child is an issue, treatment would include small oral doses of steroid hormones such as hydrocortisone, prednisone, or dexamethasone. By ingesting the hormones rather than stimulating the adrenal glands to produce cortisol, fewer androgens will accumulate and symptoms may improve. When congenital adrenal hyperplasia is diagnosed in infancy or childhood, lifelong treatment with supplements to replace missing hormones is necessary.

Addison's Disease

Also known as adrenocortical insufficiency, this condition occurs when the adrenal gland stops producing the steroid-based hormones, especially cortisol.

Adrenal insufficiency is often considered an autoimmune disease as it most commonly occurs as a result of the body reacting to the adrenal gland as foreign matter and producing antibodies to attack and destroy it. The adrenal gland can be attacked independently in this way or in association with other autoimmune disorders such as Graves' disease, and Hashimoto's thyroiditis, rheumatoid arthritis, and pernicious anemia, to name a few. The gland can also be destroyed by an infection, such as tuberculosis.

The secretion of adrenal hormones could also be blocked if the gland is affected by pituitary injury, surgery, radiation treatment, or bleeding into the pituitary gland. In addition, symptoms of adrenal insufficiency can occur if a glucocorticoid steroid hormone medication, such as prednisone, is administered for a long period of time in high doses and is then stopped abruptly.

Symptoms

The physical examination may reveal low blood pressure, darkening of the skin, weakness and lethargy, and abdominal pains. The pain may be accompanied by nausea, indigestion, diarrhea, and vomiting. Laboratory evaluation may discover low sodium and high potassium levels in the blood.

Diagnosis

The symptoms of Addison's disease usually develop slowly over a period of months. Sometimes the disorder appears suddenly. For a diagnosis, your physician will conduct a series of tests, including a cosyntropin stimulation test. This test, which measures adrenal gland function, consists of two separate tests. The first measures hormone levels as they normally occur in the bloodstream; the second—taken 30 to 60 minutes after an injection of an artificial adrenal gland stimulator called cosyntropin—establishes whether the adrenal gland is functioning normally. Sometimes the test is not fully informative and a longer test, requiring a 48-hour continuous infusion of cosyntropin, is required. The longer test is also indicated if a pituitary disorder is suspected.

Treatment

If you suffer from an adrenal insufficiency, you will have to take an oral replacement of the deficient hormones, usually synthetic hormones such as hydrocortisone or prednisone. If your blood pressure or sodium levels drop, a second drug, fludrocortisone (Florinef), is necessary as well. These medications are vital to your continued health and well being and you will have to take them on a regular basis to avoid acute adrenal failure. Acute adrenal failure includes dehydration from severe diarrhea and vomiting, shock, and loss of consciousness.

Cushing's Syndrome

Cushing's syndrome, also known as adrenocortical excess, is the opposite of Addison's disease. This disorder results from excess cortisol or other glucocorticoid hormone levels in the body, which leads to breakdown of protein and the depositing of fat in the tissues. Elevation of other hormones, particularly androgens, may accompany the increase in the cortisol levels.

Adrenocortical excess has a number of different causes: The adrenal gland can produce too much cortisol because of an adrenal-stimulating tumor in the pituitary gland or the lung. The adrenal gland can develop benign tumors called adrenal adenomas, which can produce the cortisol. Adrenal carcinomas can also cause the syndrome. Finally, the extended use of medications that contain glucocorticoid hormones, including cortisone, prednisone, and dexamethasone—commonly used in the treatment of asthma, rheumatoid arthritis, and systemic lupus erythematosus—can also result in Cushing's syndrome.

CAUSES OF ADDISON'S DISEASE

Autoimmunity
Tuberculosis
Fungal disorders (histoplasmosis)
Drugs (ketoconazole, rifampin, anticoagulants)
Congenital defects (inability to produce cortisol)
Surgery (bilateral adrenalectomy)
Acquired Immuno-Deficiency Syndrome (AIDS)

Symptoms

The most common symptom is unexplained weight gain, especially in the abdomen, above the collar bone, or behind the neck. The face may appear rounded (Figure 30.2), and the complexion is typically ruddy. Increased facial hair may also develop. There may be wide, dark purple stripes (striae) on the abdomen, buttocks, or near the armpits. Because of the breakdown of muscle tissue, you may feel weakness, especially when getting out of a chair or climbing steps. Thinning of the skin may result in easy bruising and poor wound healing. Skin often darkens, menstrual periods may change, and the sexual drive may decrease.

Diagnosis

A medical history and a physical examination are often enough to raise the question of Cushing's syndrome. A thorough history will reveal whether medications might be the cause. Tests must be done to confirm elevated cortisol levels under normal conditions and after medical manipulation to suppress the production of this hormone. One test is the dexamethasone suppression test: A dose of dexamethasone is administered

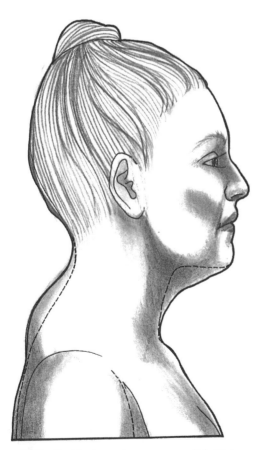

Figure 30.2 Cushing's syndrome can result from a malfunction in a gland or the use of certain medications, resulting in a characteristic weight gain behind the neck, rounding of the face, and a ruddy complexion.

CAUSES OF CUSHING'S SYNDROME

Pituitary tumor
Hypothalamus (over-production of ACTH-releasing hormone)
Adrenal adenoma or carcinoma
Too much glucocorticoid medication
Other cancer (not adrenal or pituitary) that produces ACTH

at 11:00 P.M. to try to turn off the adrenal gland's production of cortisol. Blood cortisol levels are measured at 8:00 A.M. A series of urine specimens is then collected over a 24-hour period. The first collection is considered the baseline and reflects the amount of cortisol eliminated in the urine over a one-day period (the more cortisol present in the blood, the more that will be present in the urine). The next step is to try to suppress the body's cortisol production with a small amount of another glucocorticoid hormone called dexamethasone, taken every six hours for two days. The dose of dexamethasone is increased and the process is repeated. Some doctors prefer to do the suppression testing by giving the medication and then measuring the levels of cortisol in the blood. The information gathered from the test helps the doctors decide among different causes of Cushing's syndrome. Once the characteristics of the cortisol level are established, then further radiologic studies, or a CAT scan or MRI, may be necessary to localize the problem.

Treatment

If the syndrome is due to a pituitary or adrenal tumor, then surgery is indicated. If it is the result of medication used in treatment of another illness, the dosage should be decreased to the lowest amount possible for adequate treatment of that illness.

Hirsutism

Hirsutism is the name given to male-patterned hair growth in a woman. The hair may grow on the face, chest, and abdomen. Hirsutism occurs when the fine hair follicles are stimulated by the male hormone testosterone to become coarse, or terminal, hairs. Hair on the chin, upper lip, chest, and abdomen contain hair follicles that are especially sensitive to the growth-promoting effect of testosterone.

Every woman has low levels of testosterone in her body. The testosterone comes from the ovaries and from precursor hormones that originate in the adrenal glands. Some women have hair follicles that are very

ALL ABOUT HORMONES

The key mechanism of the endocrine system is the hormone. The following hormones—together with your nervous system—help keep your metabolism working efficiently.

- *Adrenocorticotropin (ACTH)* is a hormone synthesized and stored in the pituitary gland. Large amounts are released in response to any form of stress. ACTH controls the adrenal gland's secretion of the corticosteroid hormones.

- *Catecholamines* are a group of hormones produced by the adrenal gland, the most important of which are adrenaline (epinephrine) and norepinephrine. Produced in the central or medullary portion of the adrenal gland, these hormones are secreted in larger amounts in response to stressful situations.

- *Follicle-stimulating* hormone is produced and released by the pituitary gland. It stimulates the ripening follicles (eggs) in the ovary and the sperm in the testes.

- *Glucocorticoids* are a group of hormones produced by the adrenal gland. The name refers to the ability of these hormones to increase the level of sugar in the blood. Synthetic glucocorticoids include prednisone, dexamethasone, and hydrocortisone (cortisol), all of which are used in the treatment of many disorders, including severe arthritis and asthma.

- *Insulin* is one of the hormones produced by the pancreas. As soon as your body converts carbohydrates into glucose—this normally occurs shortly after you eat a meal—insulin makes it possible for the cells to tap into this most basic source of fuel necessary for energy. When there is a shortage of insulin, the sugar stays in your bloodstream, causing the disorder known as diabetes mellitus.

- *Luteinizing hormone (LH)* is made and released by the pituitary gland. It stimulates ovulation. *Prolactin*, another pituitary hormone, stimulates milk production after childbirth and stimulates the production of progesterone by the ovaries.

- *Mineralocorticoids* are hormones produced by the adrenal glands that help keep blood volume normal. An excess of these hormones causes fluid retention, high blood pressure, loss of potassium, and a slight increase of salt in the body. A lack of these hormones results in low blood pressure, excess potassium, heavy salt loss, and a collapse of blood circulation.

- *Sex steroids* are hormones produced by the cortical parts of the adrenal glands. They contribute to normal sexual development prior to and during puberty, and include progesterone, DHEA, DHEA-S, and androstenedione. After puberty, the main source of these hormones is the ovaries in women and the testes in men.

- *Thyroxine* is the hormone secreted by the thyroid gland. It controls the pace of chemical activity in your body and helps determine how fast you burn up calories.

---

sensitive even to normal female testosterone levels and develop some coarse hair as they age. In others, the problem stems from excess testosterone produced by the ovaries or adrenal glands, the result of polycystic ovarian syndrome or ovarian tumors (see Chapter 15).

Excess androgen hormones can also be produced by the adrenal glands, often from uncontrolled stimulation of the adrenal glands by a pituitary tumor. A blockage in the process through which cholesterol is converted to cortisol can lead to a build-up of androgens that the body can convert to testosterone. Adrenal gland tumors can also cause hirsutism.

Symptoms
Development of coarse hair on the upper lip, chin, breast bone, or abdomen. (Some women naturally have a layer of dark, fine hair over the upper lip. This visible hair may be cosmeticaly annoying, but it is not necessarily a symptom of hormonal abnormality. Hair around the areola [nipple area of the breast] is also normal.) Excess testosterone can also interfere with the body's normal hormonal functions, so menstrual irregularities, infertility, and acne can occur.

Diagnosis
The first step in diagnosing the underlying problem is a medical history and a complete physical examination. Blood tests will be done to measure the amounts of the adrenal hormones. If there is a high suspicion that the hair growth is the result of a blockage of the adrenal hormone production pathway, then a cosyntropin stimulation test is performed. If the work-up suggests there is an adrenal or ovarian tumor, then you

may have to have an abdominal CAT scan to locate the tumor.

Treatment

Treatment depends on the cause of the hair growth. If the problem is a tumor of the adrenal gland or ovary, then surgery is the treatment of choice. If the hair growth is due to a block in the normal hormonal pathways of the adrenal gland, the treatment might include hormonal supplements such as hydrocortisone, prednisone, or dexamethasone. Ovarian causes can sometimes be treated with estrogen/progesterone medications such as the birth controll pill (see Chapter 15).

Unfortunately, these treatments only address the source of the excess testosterone. If the hormonal problem is mild and uncomplicated by infertility, then medications that block testosterone's action on the hair follicle, such as Spironolactone, are helpful. Eliminating the source of the testosterone or blocking its effects will only prevent new follicle development, not cure the current problem. The hair follicles that have already been stimulated may require years to turn off. In that case, electrolysis, which destroys the follicle and prevents further growth, is recommended. Despite popular belief, shaving does not make hair grow thicker and darker; therefore, if hair growth is slow, this also can be a simple but effective method to get rid of excess hair.

Pheochromocytoma

Tumors that typically develop in the central portion (medulla) of the adrenal gland are called pheochromocytomas. Tumors of this type prooduce symptoms that are related to the secretion of the hormones adrenaline and norepinephrine. Usually solitary (although they can develop in both adrenal glands [multiple endocrine neoplasia]), these tumors are most often benign. Pheochromocytomas may develop in association with other endocrine tumors, and in neurofibromatosis. These tumors run in families and occur in individuals with hypertension.

Symptoms

Episodes of palpitations, fainting, and severe headaches are the classic symptoms associated with pheochromocytomas. Blood pressure that is erratically elevated and/or difficult to control may also indicate the presence of an adrenal tumor. Other symptoms include anxiety attacks, increased sweating, tremor, and weight loss.

Diagnosis

The first step in diagnosing a pheochromocytoma is a medical history and physical examination. The physical exam should include measurements of pulse and blood pressure both lying down and standing up. Diagnosis is made by documenting elevated adrenal medulla hormones (epinephrine, norepinephrine, and dopamine) or their breakdown products in a 24-hour urine collection. Sometimes more than one urine collection is required to identify the abnormality. If there is an increase in the level of hormones in the urine, the next test is an MRI of the abdomen to locate the tumor. Ninety percent of tumors are found in the adrenal gland; of that numer, 10 percent will be present in both adrenal glands. Another 10 percent will be located elsewhere in the abdomen. If the MRI is unable to locate the tumor, then a body or MIBG scan (see Appendix), which uses a small amount of radioactive material, can be performed.

Treatment

Once identified, pheochromocytomas should be surgically removed. Prior to any operation, you will need to take medications that block the effects of a sudden release of adrenaline that may occur under the stress of surgery.

The Pancreas

Located behind the stomach, the pancreas is a long, thin organ, approximately the length of the hand. Playing a key role in the digestive process, the pancreas produces enzymes essential to the digestion of food and also hormones that enable your body to metabolize the food you eat. These hormones regulate your body's use of glucose, a simple form of sugar that is an energy source for the daily activity of all your cells.

Three hormones are produced by the pancreas:

- *Insulin* is produced when the concentration of glucose in the body increases, such as after eating. Muscle and fat cells are stimulated by insulin to absorb the glucose they need as fuel for their activities. Surplus glucose is stored by the liver in the form of a starch called glycogen.

- *Glucagon* breaks down the stored glycogen and raises the concentration of sugar in the blood when needed by the body.

- *Somatostatin* is thought to be a factor in regulating the production and release of both insulin and glucagon. It also inhibits release of growth hormones.

Diabetes Mellitus

Diabetes occurs when the body cannot efficiently use food as energy because of a lack of the hormone insulin or as a result of a blockage in the function of insulin. (Contrary to what some people believe, diabetes is not caused by consuming too much sugar.) The most common endocrine disorder in the United States, diabetes occurs in about 3 percent of the population, or 10 million people. Diabetes mellitus is a serious disorder. In the United States, 5,000 patients with diabetes each year will develop blindness from the disease, 4,000 will develop severe kidney disease, and uncontrolled diabetes accounts for 80 percent of medically amputated legs and toes. In addition, people with diabetes are at risk for heart disease, heart attacks, nerve damage, infections, and strokes.

Symptoms

The symptoms of both types of diabetes are similar, because both result from the body's inability to metabolize carbohydrates.

There are two types of diabetes mellitus. About 10 or 15 percent of diabetics have type I diabetes. Usually occurring in childhood, type I diabetes results when the pancreas makes little or no insulin. Type II diabetes, also known as insulin-resistant diabetes, is far more common, accounting for 85 to 90 percent of all diabetes cases. Type II occurs when there is interference with the body's ability to use the insulin produced by the pancreas. Type II is seen in older people and is frequently associated with obesity.

Types of Diabetes

Type I diabetes occurs when the pancreas is unable to make insulin. About one in ten people with diabetes, or about 800,000 Americans, have type I diabetes. The exact cause of type I diabetes is not known, but it is considered to be an autoimmune disease in which antibodies destroy the cells in the pancreas that make insulin. It is more common in families with a history of type I diabetes. If the pancreas has been injured by a viral infection, type I diabetes may also result.

Treatment consists of daily insulin injections as well as the maintenance of a balanced diet and regular exercise regime. The number of daily insulin injections depends on the patient's weight, height, level of physical activity, and food intake. Most people with type I diabetes require two or more insulin shots a day. Insulin injections and meals should be taken at the same time. It is also important not to use other medicines that may increase blood sugar to treat infections and to avoid stress.

ALL ABOUT INSULIN

Insulin, a hormone that lowers sugar levels in the blood, also enables the sugar to pass into the cells of the body. Insulin can be made from the pancreas of cows (beef insulin), pigs (pork insulin), or from a mixture of the two. It can also be made synthetically. There are many types of injectable insulin: Some lower blood sugar more quickly, others keep blood sugar lower for a longer period of time.

Type II diabetes results from insulin resistance, interference with the ability of insulin to lower blood sugar. The exact cause of type II diabetes is not known, but the condition is more likely to develop if you:

- are overweight
- have a family history of diabetes
- have high blood sugar levels when pregnant
- had a newborn baby weighing more than 9 pounds
- are over 40 years of age
- have high blood pressure
- are African-American, Hispanic, or Native American.

If you have type II diabetes or have a family history of the disease, the keystone of treatment includes eating nutritious, low-fat foods and maintaining a healthy weight.

TYPES OF INSULIN

Name	Action
R insulin (regular)	Acts quickly in a short time.
N insulin (NPH or Lente)	Acts slowly but lasts longer.
70-30 insulin (a mixture of N and R)	The 70% acts slowly for a long time; the 30% acts quickly for a short time.
BR insulin (buffered regular)	Meant to be used with an insulin pump; infused into the body through a needle inserted into the skin of the abdomen.
U insulin (Ultralene)	Long-acting
P-PZI insulin	Long-acting

SYMPTOMS OF DIABETES MELLITUS

Type I	Type II	Both
drowsiness	increased weight gain	extreme fatigue
fruity breath	frequent urination	blurred vision
severe thirst	itchy skin	increase in hunger
sudden weight loss	frequent infections (vaginitis/boils)	
increased passing of urine/bedwetting	slow healing of cuts/sores	
	numbness in extremities	

If you cannot control the disease through diet and exercise alone, you will probably be required to take oral hypoglycemic agents, drugs that will lower your blood sugar. Not to be confused with insulin, oral hypoglycemic agents help the pancreas put out more insulin and aid the insulin in moving sugar from the bloodstream into the cells of the body. Take the oral hypoglycemic once or twice a day, about 30 minutes before a meal. The medication may need to be changed as you age or if you alter your eating habits.

Type I and type II diabetes have different symptoms, as well as some effects in common.

Diagnosis

When diagnosed by a blood test, diabetes is present if fasting blood sugar is above 140 mg/dl on two occasions (the normal blood sugar is about 115 mg/dl) or if fasting blood sugar is over 200 mg/dl two hours after a meal (normal is less than 140 mg/dl). If you have borderline readings, you will be encouraged to take a glucose tolerance test. In a glucose tolerance test, a large amount of sugar, usually in a sweet drink, is given by mouth. Your blood will be tested at periodic intervals over three hours to see if the glucose levels rise into the diabetic range.

Treatment

For both types of diabetes, the goal of treatment is to keep blood sugar normal or as near to normal as possible. Treatment also consists in preventing the condition from affecting the eyes, kidneys, heart, or nerves, and decreasing the incidence of infection. A combination of diet, exercise, and medication is usually prescribed.

A healthy diet for a person with diabetes is high in starches and fiber and low in sugar, fats, and salt.

Regular physical activity also helps to decrease blood sugar and is an important part of controlling diabetes. Exercise:

- uses up sugar in the body;
- burns off extra body fat;
- improves muscle strength and blood flow;
- improves physical appearance;
- improves energy and sense of well being.

Many type II diabetics who eat a healthy diet, maintain a healthy weight, and exercise can avoid the need for medication.

If you have diabetes, schedule regular appointments with your physician to check your blood sugar levels, as well as to diagnose and treat any complications. If you take insulin or oral hypoglycemic agents, notify your doctor if you contract a virus or another infection so that your medication can be adjusted. It is also recommended that anyone with diabetes have an annual eye examination, regular blood and urine tests to check kidney function, and a regular examination of the feet to check for sores that may indicate the development of circulatory problems.

TREATMENT GOALS FOR PEOPLE WITH DIABETES

- Keep blood sugar in the normal range.
- Keep cholesterol and other blood fats in the normal range.
- Keep blood pressure normal.
- Lose weight if necessary.
- Maintain target range weight.
- Eat a balanced diet with appropriate vitamins, minerals, and fiber.

Complications of Diabetes

Two immediate health problems may arise from poorly controlled diabetes: diabetic coma and hypoglycemia (low blood sugar). Both conditions can cause a diabetic to become suddenly unconscious. If you are on medication for diabetes, always carry identification that includes your medical history so that the problem can be quickly recognized and treated.

Diabetic coma: Also known as ketoacidosis, this condition is a medical emergency requiring immediate attention. A relatively common complication of diabetes mellitus (usually type I), diabetic coma occurs when there is little or no insulin in the body, causing blood sugar levels to soar. Without insulin, the body cannot burn sugar and begins to burn fat, producing by-products called ketones. Ketones acidify the blood, causing widespread metabolic abnormalities that can result in coma and, eventually, death.

Most often, failure to receive scheduled insulin injections is the cause of ketoacidosis. An accidental injury resulting in unconsciousness, acute infection, or loss of fluids through vomiting or diarrhea may precipitate the coma. Symptoms of impending coma are increased urination and an unquenchable thirst developing over the course of several hours. Weakness and drowsiness follows, along with vomiting, diarrhea, and abdominal pain. The breath often begins to smell fruity, a symptom that may be mistaken for alcohol consumption. At a more advanced stage, breathing becomes deeper and more rapid. Unconsciousness soon ensues.

Treatment

This condition requires immediate administration of insulin and an intravenous infusion to replace lost body fluids. Blood glucose levels and fluid status must be closely monitored.

Hypoglycemia: This condition results when the concentration of glucose in the blood falls below normal, less than 60 mg/dl. When too little glucose circulates to the nervous system and other cells, they become starved for energy.

Hypoglycemia is a symptom, not a disease. Too often, people are erroneously diagnosed with hypoglycemia when the source of their problem lies elsewhere. Most cases of hypoglycemia occur in people who are taking insulin or oral hypoglycemic drugs. In rare cases, low blood sugar may result from liver or kidney disease, drug reactions, too much alcohol, or malnutrition. Hormonal imbalances, such as a lack of cortisol or overproduction of insulin due to a pancreatic tumor, may also cause hypoglycemia.

Symptoms

Common symptoms of hypoglycemia include sweating, nervousness, inability to concentrate, fast

---

COMMON CAUSES OF LOW BLOOD SUGAR IN DIABETICS

- Taking too much insulin or oral hypoglycemic medication.
- Skipping or not finishing meals or snacks.
- Failure to adequately coordinate meals and insulin injections.
- Overdoing exercise.
- Experiencing prolonged vomiting and diarrhea.

---

heartbeat, dizziness, blurred vision, weakness, fatigue, headache, irritability, hunger, abdominal pain, sudden drowsiness, confusion, and tingling or numbness of the mouth, hands, or body. When hypoglycemia is severe (when glucose levels fall below 20–30 mg/dl), it can lead to convulsions and unconsciousness (coma).

Treatment

Immediately ingest a source of sugar, such as ½ cup of orange juice, apple juice, or soda, three teaspoons of sugar, a cup of milk, several hard candies, or a tablespoon of honey. You can also take glucose tablets or gel, or glucagon (an injection to raise blood sugar).

If the symptoms persist after 15–20 minutes, repeat the same dosage of sugar. If it will be more than an hour until regular meal time, eat a sandwich or some other snack to prevent a further decrease in blood sugar. If symptoms continue, go to the nearest emergency room, with an escort if possible. Later, discuss the hypoglycemic reaction with your physician. You may need to change your medication to prevent further episodes.

Diabetes in Pregnancy

The health of your baby depends on your having normal blood sugar levels before conception and during pregnancy. High blood sugar crosses the placenta, and your baby may run the risk of having birth defects. For that reason, an experienced health care team is required to care for pregnant diabetic women. The team includes an obstetrician, a diabetologist, a pediatrician, a diabetes educator, and a nutritionist. All pregnant women with diabetes must have their blood sugar checked frequently and receive counseling about nutrition, diet, and adjustment of insulin doses. Type II diabetics taking oral hypoglycemic agents should switch to insulin injections before conceiving.

Gestational Diabetes

This is a type of functional diabetes that appears during pregnancy and then vanishes immediately upon delivery. Unless your blood glucose is checked periodically, the diabetes may go unnoticed. The disease still poses a risk to the fetus, however, so every attempt should be made to regulate and maintain normal blood glucose. Women at risk for gestational diabetes are most commonly over 35, overweight, have had big babies, and have a family history of high blood sugar.

The Thyroid Gland

Located at the base of the neck, the thyroid gland helps set the rate at which your body functions. It produces thyroid hormone, which helps regulate important aspects of your body's metabolism and determines how fast you burn up calories.

Hyperthyroidism

Also known as an overactive thyroid, hyperthyroidism occurs when the thyroid gland produces excessive amounts of thyroid hormone, causing an increase in the body's normal expenditure of energy, or its basal metabolic rate. Two forms of hyperthyroidism are Graves' disease, which is most common in women, and Plummer's disease. In Graves' disease, the thyroid gland is stimulated excessively by an abnormal antibody instead of by the normal thyroid-stimulating hormone (TSH) from the pituitary gland. In older women, the disease can be caused by a thyroid nodule producing too much thyroid hormone.

Symptoms

Hyperthyroidism causes increased appetite, rapid heart rate, weight loss, tremor of the hands, sweaty palms, protruding eyes, difficulty in sleeping, and muscle weakness. The excessive stimulation of the thyroid also may lead to a goiter, an enlargement of the thyroid gland.

Treatment

The first line of treatment is antithyroid medication to suppress the excessive amounts of thyroid hormone. In many cases, this drug can completely relieve the symptoms. The signs of hyperthyroidism often return, however, when the drug is discontinued. If that happens, radioactive iodine is administered by mouth. The radioiodine is absorbed by the thyroid cells and the gland slows down its production of the hormone.

Hypothyroidism

The reverse of hyperthyroidism, this condition is the result of an underactive thyroid. The gland fails to produce enough hormone, causing the body's basal metabolic rate to slow down. Hypothyroidism can occur at any age, but it most commonly affects middle-aged women. The symptoms of hypothyroidism often go unrecognized in older people and can be mistaken for the normal signs of aging.

In some cases, hypothyroidism results from the failure of the pituitary gland to produce enough thyroid-stimulating hormone. The cause is commonly an autoimmune disorder known as Hashimoto's thyroiditis, in which antibodies attack and destroy the thyroid. Hypothyroidism may also stem from the medical treatment given to those suffering from hyperthyroidism, when the drugs work too well, causing the reverse symptoms.

Symptoms

The first signs of hypothyroidism are a constant fatigue, muscle aches, and weakness. More advanced symptoms are a slowed heart rate, weight gain, intolerance to cold, constipation, dry skin and hair, and heavy prolonged menstrual periods.

Diagnosis

Hypothyroidism usually develops slowly over the months and even years. The most effective way to diagnose the condition is through laboratory tests, particularly blood tests, to measure the amounts of hormone being produced in the thyroid, TSH, and thyroid antibodies.

Treatment

If you have a thyroid deficiency, your doctor will prescribe a thyroid replacement supplement. In most cases, the condition improves noticeably within a week or so after therapy is begun; all symptoms disappear in a few months. You will probably have to continue the treatment for the rest of your life.

The Parathyroid Gland

The parathyroid glands are found in the neck behind or near the thyroid gland. The four glands produce parathyroid hormone (PTH), which regulates the amount of calcium in the blood. When the calcium level goes down, more PTH is secreted; when the calcium level is elevated (hypercalcemia), the amount of PTH decreases. PTH causes calcium to be released from bone, increases calcium absorption in the intestines, and stimulates the kidney to make a very potent form of vitamin D, which enhances calcium absorption from the gastrointestinal tract.

Hypercalcemia, or mild elevations of calcium in the blood, may be caused by hyperparathyroidism, other endocrine disorders, drugs, cancer, and diseases such as tuberculosis, sarcoidosis, and AIDS.

Hyperparathyroidism

Hyperparathyroidism results when one or more of the parathyroid glands produce an excess of PTH, the hormone that increases the amount of calcium and decreases the amount of phosphorous in the bloodstream. Hyperparathyroidism is more common in women than in men, and most patients are over 50 when the disease is discovered. About 85 percent of hyperparathyroidism is caused by a benign parathyroid tumor. Other causes are enlargement of the parathyroid glands (hyperplasia) and, rarely, multiple endocrine neoplasia syndromes, called MEN I and MEN II.

Symptoms

Patients with mild elevations of calcium known as hypercalcemia may experience no symptoms at all or feel only mild fatigue. Lethargy, apathy, nausea, personality changes, muscle weakness, abdominal pain, increased urination, and constipation are other symptoms. Severe hypercalcemia is associated with nausea, vomiting, kidney stones, peptic ulcer, pancreatitis, stupor, and coma.

Diagnosis

If elevated calcium levels are found in routine blood tests, hyperparathyroidism may be suspected. To confirm the diagnosis, physicians will take blood tests to measure serum calcium, phosphorous, total proteins, 24-hour urine calcium, and parathyroid hormone. During the evaluation, other causes of hypercalcemia must also be considered.

Treatment

Parathyroid surgery, called parathyroidectomy, is the treatment of choice to prevent the development of severe hypercalcemia, bone pain, severe osteoporosis, kidney disease, kidney stones, or peptic ulcers. More conservative treatment such as increased water intake, nonthiazide diuretics, estrogen, and increased physical activity may be helpful if the patient is older, is asymptomatic, or has other illnesses that make surgery inadvisable.

Hypoparathyroidism

When the parathyroid glands produce too little PTH, preventing the body from making proper use of calcium, hypoparathyroidism results. This is a rare condition, however, and is far less common than hyperparathyroidism.

The most common cause of hypoparathyroidism is damage to the parathyroids during surgery to treat hyperthyroidism, neck cancer, and, less commonly, hyperparathyroidism. Because most people with hyperthyroidism are now treated with drugs or radioactive iodine rather than surgery, consequent postsurgical hypoparathyroidism is now also rare.

Symptoms

Numbness and tingling of the hands, feet, and mouth, muscle cramps, and spasms are common. Cataracts may also develop.

Treatment

Calcium and vitamin D supplements can help alleviate the symptoms. Calcium carbonate is particularly recommended as it has a high calcium content (40 percent). Usually 1 to 2 grams are taken in divided doses (one chewable tablet three or four times a day). Calcium levels are retested after four to six weeks and medications are readjusted accordingly. After appropriate doses are established, calcium blood levels should be checked about four times each year.

Osteoporosis

A disease that causes the bones to become more porous and the skeleton to weaken, osteoporosis is most common in postmenopausal women. One out of every four women over 45 and nine out of ten women over 75 have some degree of osteoporosis. This common type of osteoporosis is called primary osteoporosis. Excessive loss of bone after menopause occurs when certain hormones essential for bone formation and maintenance decrease substantially. Secondary osteoporosis is much more rare and usually accompanies other endocrine disorders such as acromegaly and Cushing's syndrome and can result from excessive use of corticosteroid drugs.

The endocrine system keeps the correct level of calcium circulating in the bloodstream; if your body does not receive enough dietary calcium to meet its needs, it takes calcium from the bones to make up the difference. The sex hormone estrogen protects bones from being robbed of calcium by other demands of the body and helps produce and maintain collagen, an important component of bone. Another hormone, calcitonin, may help facilitate the uptake of calcium from the blood into the bone and, at the same time, inhibit the loss of calcium from the bone.

Risk factors for osteoporosis include a family history of the disease, early menopause, a lack of physical activity, cigarette smoking, alcoholism, and some medications. A high dosage of thyroid medication, for example, can lead to bone weakness in the hips and wrists. Caucasians are most at risk, as are thin, small-boned women.

Preventing osteoporosis and limiting bone loss after menopause are vital. Once bone mass is lost, it is difficult or impossible to replace. Preventive measures include maintaining adequate levels of calcium and vitamin D and exercising regularly. High intake of calcium after menopause will also help reduce age-related bone loss. Estrogen replacement therapy helps prevent bone thinning.

Estrogen replacement therapy (ERT): ERT relieves most menopausal symptoms (hot flashes, sweating, vaginal dryness) as well as other side effects of estrogen loss, including coronary artery disease and osteoporosis. ERT is usually advised for women who experience early menopause (before age 40) or who have had their ovaries removed. In addition, women who have had a spine fracture due to low bone mass or have low bone mass as measured by a bone density test should also consider taking ERT. Women who have other risk factors for osteoporosis may want to consider taking ERT as well. (For further information on osteoporosis, see Chapter 11.)

The Pituitary Gland

Although small in size, the pituitary gland is the most important of all the endocrine glands, because it acts as a control center for the body's long-term growth, daily functioning, and reproductive capabilities. Located at the base of the brain behind the nasal passages, the pituitary is stimulated by hormones from the part of the brain called the hypothalamus. The pituitary secretes hormones necessary for growth, reproduction, and sexual development, as well as for thyroid and adrenal function. The hormones are luteinizing hormone (LH), follicle-stimulating hormone (FSH), prolactin, growth hormone (GH), adrenocorticotropin (ACTH), and thyroid-stimulating hormone (TSH).

Pituitary disorders in adult women are caused by one of two types of tumors: a craniopharyngioma, which exerts pressure on the pituitary as it grows and results in decreased hormone production; or an adenoma, a benign pituitary tumor that can result in increased hormone production.

Symptoms

A pituitary disorder can cause severe headaches, changes in vision, too rapid or too slow growth and/or sexual development, changes in menstruation, fatigue, weight gain or loss, dizziness, increase or decrease of body hair, and sometimes the production of breast milk not related to pregnancy (galactorrhea).

Diagnosis

The examining physician will take a thorough history. Special blood and urine tests can determine the amounts of hormones circulating in the bloodstream and being excreted. If abnormal amounts are found, a CAT or MRI scan may be done to determine if a pituitary tumor is present.

Acromegaly

The overproduction of growth hormone by the pituitary can affect the limbs and internal organs. The cause is usually a tumor on the pituitary. In children, this condition is known as gigantism and leads to abnormal skeleton growth. In adults, the overproduction of growth hormone after normal growth has been completed results in the gradual overgrowth of certain bones in the body and a thickening of the skeleton. This condition is called acromegaly.

Symptoms

When acromegaly occurs after puberty, the bones of the hands, feet, and head enlarge. Increased shoe, glove, ring, and hat sizes are common. The chin may get larger and spaces between the lower front teeth may appear. The skin becomes coarse and thick, and sweating increases.

Diagnosis

Blood tests can determine whether growth hormone and somatomedin C levels are elevated. An MRI will reveal an enlarged pituitary.

Treatment

Surgery and/or X-ray treatment is usually recommended. Post-treatment blood tests can confirm the removal of the tumor. New drugs, specifically bromocriptine and octreotide, are being developed for patients who continue to have elevated growth hormone after surgery.

Cushing's Syndrome

This syndrome results from a tumor of the pituitary which causes overproduction of ACTH and stimulates the adrenal glands to make increased amounts of cortisol.

Diabetes Insipidus

Diabetes insipidus is a disease that develops when too little antidiuretic hormone (ADH), which controls the balance of water in the body, is produced by the posterior pituitary gland. This condition should not be confused with diabetes mellitus, which is the result of an insulin deficiency.

A pituitary tumor is the most common identified cause of this condition. Other causes include damage to the pituitary from a head injury or from surgery for pituitary tumors. In more than half of the cases, the cause is unknown.

Symptoms

Excessive urination and severe thirst are the main signs of this disease.

Diagnosis

If diabetes insipidus is suspected, your physician will probably conduct a water deprivation test as well as blood tests to determine salt and water balance.

Treatment

Increased fluid intake and the administration of an antidiuretic hormone, available as an injection or a nasal spray, is usually the treatment of choice. You may have to adopt a salt-restricted diet. If a tumor is present, surgery should be performed to remove it.

Hypopituitarism

A disorder in which the pituitary gland produces insufficient quantities of one or more of the pituitary hormones, hypopituitarism is usually the result of a tumor on the pituitary gland. It also can develop after a serious head injury. Some women experience hypopituitarism after childbirth (Sheehan's syndrome, see below).

Symptoms

Depending on which hormones are deficient, symptoms may include cessation of menses, infertility, the inability to lactate after childbirth, fatigue, depression, loss of pubic hair, and decreased appetite. Because the pituitary gland also produces hormones that activate other glands, conditions such as hypothyroidism and adrenal insufficiency can result.

Diagnosis

Blood tests are performed to measure levels of TSH, ACTH, GH, thyroid, cortisone, and estrogen.

Treatment

The deficient hormone can be replaced by a synthetic version.

Prolactinoma

The overproduction of the hormone prolactin, which stimulates milk production after childbirth, is most commonly caused by an adenoma, a benign tumor. Other causes of elevated prolactin include the use of certain oral contraceptives, tranquilizers, and hypothyroidism.

Symptoms

Irregular or lack of menstrual periods, infertility, and the appearance of breast milk not related to pregnancy (galactorrhea) are common signs of this condition. Visual disturbances, indicating the presence of a large tumor compressing the optic nerve, may also occur.

Diagnosis

Blood tests can establish prolactin and thyroid hormone levels. If prolactin levels are high, thyroid function is normal, and you are not taking any of the drugs listed above, then a picture of your pituitary will be made with an MRI. In addition, a complete eye examination will be made for acuity and fields of vision.

Treatment

Tumors can be treated with drugs, surgery, or both. Certain drugs can decrease prolactin levels and lead to normal menstrual periods. If a large tumor is causing visual problems, neurosurgical removal is recommended. Very small tumors (microadenomas) can be monitored with careful follow-up, repeated blood tests measuring prolactin levels, and an MRI, unless the patient wants to become pregnant. If conception is desired, it is necessary to decrease prolactin levels so that ovulation and regular menstrual cycles can be established.

Sheehan's Syndrome

This is a type of hypopituitarism that occurs after childbirth. The pituitary gland, which normally increases in size during pregnancy, grows so large that the body is unable to provide it with oxygen and the other nutrients it needs, causing some or all of the gland to die. It can also occur if heavy bleeding and a sharp drop in blood pressure cause the pituitary to lose its blood supply, causing a decrease in pituitary hormones. Symptoms of Sheehan's syndrome include the failure to have breast milk, no menstrual periods, loss of body hair in the axilla and pubic regions, and depression.

CHAPTER 31

The Immune System and Allergies

Leslie Carroll Grammer, M.D., F.A.C.P.

The immune system is a network of cells and organs that work together to defend the body against "foreign" invaders. These are primarily viruses, bacteria, fungi, and parasites. The word "immune" comes from the Latin word *immunis,* meaning "release from an obligation." Today, in medical terms, immune means "exempt from a disease." The immune system does just that—it keeps the body free from disease.

Because the human body provides an ideal environment for the growth of many organisms, they try to break into it. The immune system's job is to keep them out or, failing that, to seek them out within the body and destroy them.

Certain chemicals can provoke a response from the immune system. Allergic reactions occur when an otherwise harmless substance is identified as an invader. Cells from another person in blood transfusions or organ transplants are recognized as foreign and trigger a response. Finally, there are certain diseases, the "autoimmune" diseases, in which the immune system attacks normal cells of the body.

STRUCTURE AND FUNCTION

The immune system is able to recognize cells and substances that are not a part of the body. It can tell the difference between normal, healthy cells and cells that are foreign. The function of the immune system depends on an elaborate network of communications among millions of cells throughout the body. (See Fig. 31.1) For more details about the role of blood cells in keeping the body healthy, see Chapter 29.

Components

The body has numerous ways of protecting itself from disease. Mucus in the nasal passages, filters in the respiratory system, and fluids that circulate through the tissues of the body are designed to keep out offending agents. When they fail, the lymphatic system takes charge. Unlike other systems in the body, which are made up of groups of organs, the immune system cells are all over the body, in the tissues and circulating in the blood. They are concentrated in the thymus gland (located at the base of the throat, behind the breastbone), the lymph nodes, the spleen (an organ located in the upper left abdomen), and the lymphatic channels. (See Fig. 31.2)

The lymphatic system is a circulatory system that works in concert with the veins. It collects fluid from the tissue spaces in the body and returns it to the heart through a series of vessels called lymphatics. At various points in this network of vessels are nodules of tissue called lymph nodes. Lymph nodes contain concentrations of lymphocytes, a special type of white blood cell. When germs are carried through the system into the lymph nodes, the lymphocytes kill or contain them.

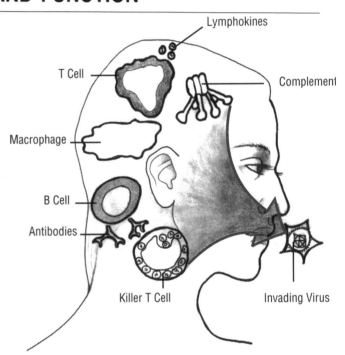

Figure 31.1 The Immune System
The immune system comprises a variety of defenses that come into play when the body is threatened by an invading organism. *T cells* are stimulated to release several different types of *lymphokines* when confronted with a disease-causing organism. Lymphokines act in different ways to directly or indirectly destroy the invader. *Macrophages* are derived from certain types of white blood cells called *monocytes*, engulf invading organisms, and digest them in a process known as *phagocytosis*. *B cells* produce *antibodies* to fight off specific invading organisms. *Killer cells* (also called killer T lymphocytes) help defend against viral and fungal infections. Unlike B cells, which can attack from a distance by releasing antibodies, killer cells must be in close proximity to their target in order to attack. *Complements* are made up of proteins that target specific invaders identified by antibodies.

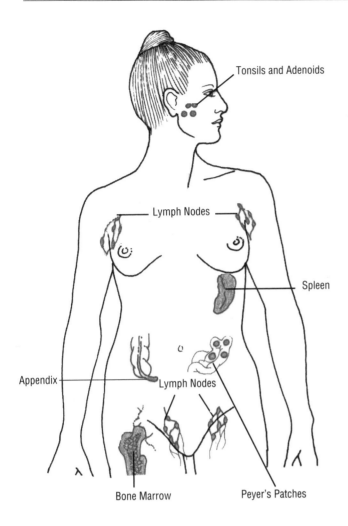

Figure 31.2 Immune Defenses
Numerous organs and structures play important roles in immune defense. The *tonsils* and *adenoids* are small organs located in the back of the throat. They are sources of *phagocytes*, special cells that destroy bacteria entering the mouth. The *thymus*, located at the base of the throat, and the *spleen* produce cells that aid in destroying foreign invaders. *Lymph nodes* are small blood-filtering organs that occur in clusters in specific regions of the body. Infection-fighters include *Peyer's patches*, specialized cells in the small intestine lining; the *appendix*, a fingerlike projection at the base of the large intestine, containing lymphatic tissue; and *bone marrow*, which produces some white blood cells.

Lymphocytes coordinate much of the immune system's function. In addition to helping destroy an organism, lymphocytes can remember the invader and react to protect the body if it returns. There are two types of lymphocytes: B cells and T cells. Although they work in different ways, both B and T cells are programmed to respond to a particular antigen, which is a substance that triggers an immune response.

The Immune Response

The body's immune system is called into action when it is exposed to an antigen. The antigen can be a protein on the surface of a cell or a substance like pollen grains or the oil in poison ivy plants. An allergen is an antigen that provokes an allergic response.

Antigens cause the immune system to form antibodies that protect against disease. Some antibodies give lifelong immunity, whereas others give short-term immunity, depending on the type of antigen, the amount of antigen, and the route by which it enters the body. Immunity can also be influenced by the genes a person inherits.

There are two kinds of immune responses to antigens. One type is brought about by B lymphocytes through the production of antibodies. The other is carried out by the T lymphocytes.

B-Cell Immunity

The presence of an antigen prompts the B cells to make antibodies to fight it. Each B cell is programmed to make a specific antibody. When a new antigen is recognized, the B cell forms an antibody against that antigen. These antibodies are able to react only with the antigen that caused them to be produced. For example, a flu antibody will attack only antigens on the surface of the virus causing the flu. (See Fig. 31.3)

The purpose of antibodies is to make antigens unable to harm the body. Antibodies directly correspond to an antigen as precisely as a key fits into a lock. (Fig. 31.4) Once the key is in the lock, they are bound together. When an antigen-antibody complex is formed (the key is in the lock), the antibody proceeds to disable the antigen.

If the invading organism produces a toxin, the toxin will usually have antigens. The antibody can lock onto the antigen on the toxin and neutralize it (render it harmless). Antibodies also can force the organisms containing antigens together into a clump, allowing other immune system cells to destroy them. Some very strong antibodies can attack the foreign substance directly and rupture its cells.

After an infection, antibody levels decrease. At the same time that B cells produced the antibodies, however, they also produced memory cells. Stored in the

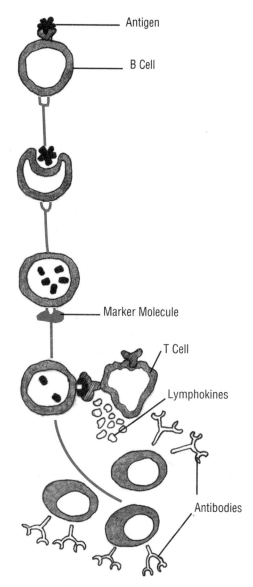

Antigen

B Cell

Marker Molecule

T Cell

Lymphokines

Antibodies

Figure 31.3 B Cells
When an antigen comes into contact with a B cell, it is recognized by receptors on the B cell's surface. The B cell then engulfs the antigen and produces marker molecules that attract a T cell. This interaction stimulates the release of lymphokines, specialized molecules that allow the B cell to divide and mature into plasma cells. These plasma cells go on to produce antibodies against that specific antigen.

lymph nodes, memory cells are able to recognize the specific antigens. When any one of these antigens is reintroduced into the body, the memory cells quickly respond and release antibodies.

Because of this cellular memory, many diseases occur once in a lifetime, after which a person is immune to them. A good example is mumps, which occurs in childhood and makes the person immune in adult life.

For some of these childhood diseases, like measles, scientists have discovered ways to imitate cellular memory through vaccines. The vaccine that is given prompts the body to make antibodies, so that the illness need not occur.

T-Cell Immunity

The T cells contribute to the immune defenses in two major ways: some direct and regulate the immune responses, whereas others attack cells that are infected or cancerous. Because transplanted organs are recognized as "foreign," the T cells also attack them. (See Fig. 31.4)

Like B cells, each T cell recognizes and responds to a particular antigen. When the T cell is exposed to this antigen, it becomes attached to the invading agent and destroys it. Once T cells have been activated, they multiply and form four different types:

- *T-memory cells* recognize invading antigens.
- *T-killer cells* destroy antigens.
- *T-helper cells* stimulate antibody production.
- *T-suppressor cells* suppress killer and helper T cells to stop the response once the danger has passed.

System Malfunctions

Not all immune reactions protect the body from invaders. In some cases, the immune system may malfunction and harm the body rather than protect it.

The immune system can make antibodies that work against you. They act as though there is a threat to the body when none actually exists. The most common example of this is an allergy. If a person has an allergy, a normally harmless material—such as nuts or ragweed—is mistaken for a threat. The immune system attacks it, causing the discomfort of allergies. Another example is autoimmune diseases, such as lupus erythematosus, scleroderma, and rheumatoid arthritis (see Chapter 34). For reasons not yet completely understood, the immune system malfunctions and targets healthy cells (normal parts of the body) as foreign invaders.

With some infections, the immune system may win the first battle against the organism, but it is only a temporary victory. For instance, chickenpox is caused by a virus that can lie dormant in the body and reemerge during adulthood as shingles. Another example is herpes simplex, caused by a virus that can be dor-

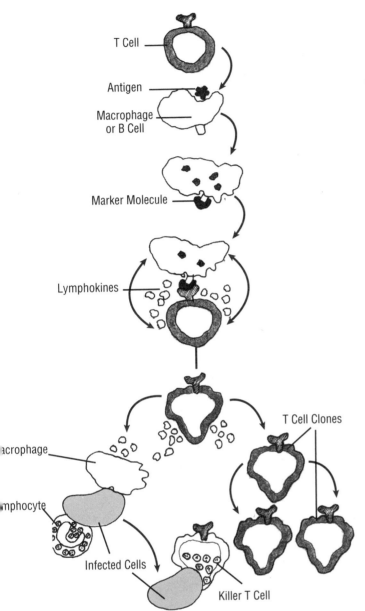

T Cell

Antigen

Macrophage or B Cell

Marker Molecule

Lymphokines

acrophage

mphocyte

Infected Cells

Killer T Cell

T Cell Clones

mant in the nerves and reappear as an outbreak after the initial infection. These outbreaks are more likely to occur when the immune system is weakened.

When part or all of the immune system is unable to function properly, the body is said to be immunodeficient. Some children are born without a functional immune system as the result of a genetic defect. Without treatment they can live only in a germfree environment. Other immunodeficiencies are acquired later in life and are caused by infection or certain diseases that disrupt the immune system and impair immune response. This leaves the body without defense against infections and diseases. The best-known example of this is AIDS, in which the crucial T lymphocytes are destroyed by a virus (see Chapter 20).

Other things known to interfere with function of the immune system are trauma (including surgery), poor nutrition, illness, and lack of rest. The immune system and the nervous system are linked in several ways. When the body is under stress, the brain directs the body to release certain hormones that can alter the effects of antibodies and lymphocytes.

Figure 31.4 T Cells
Unlike B cells, which can attack invading organisms from a distance by producing antibodies, T cells must be in close contact with their target in order to destroy it. This process starts when a T cell encounters a macrophage or a B cell that has ingested an antigen and is displaying specific marker molecules on its surface. The T cell recognizes the marker molecule and produces lymphokines, which in turn stimulate the T cell to mature and to divide into more T cells. Some of these new T cells are clones that go on to attach to additional B cells or macrophages; some attract macrophages or lymphocytes to the infected cells to aid in their destruction; and still others become what is known as killer T cells, which track down and destroy antigens.

KEEPING THE IMMUNE SYSTEM HEALTHY

The immune system is your main protection against infectious diseases. You can help keep this system healthy and working well by avoiding potential hazards, keeping up to date on recommended adult immunizations, and protecting yourself against allergies. Women who have allergies can take steps to prevent serious allergic reactions. There are various health care professionals who can help you in these efforts.

Lifestyle

The most important step you can take to protect your immune system is to protect yourself from contracting the human immunodeficiency virus (HIV)—the cause of AIDS. AIDS destroys the immune system and leaves the body open to fatal disease. It is passed in two main ways: sharing needles used to inject drugs and having unprotected sex with someone who is infected.

The best ways to avoid getting AIDS from a dirty needle are not to inject drugs and not to have sex with someone who does. If you need help to kick a habit, many social service groups are there for you (see Chapter 7).

Having "safe sex" will help to protect you from AIDS. Sexually active women should limit their relationships to mutually monogamous ones and insist that a condom always be used.

Infant Feeding

Mothers can give their babies a good start in life by breast-feeding. The mother's antibodies are passed through the breast milk to her baby. They provide the

WHO TREATS THE IMMUNE SYSTEM?

Many different physicians specialize in treating diseases of the immune system. The doctor you will see will depend on the condition you have.

Allergists focus on diagnosing and treating allergies. They are specialists in internal medicine or pediatrics who have advanced training in the field of allergy and immunology, and have been certified in the field by passing a specialty board exam. To identify a qualified allergist, ask your internist or your local or state medical society for a referral.

Rheumatologists are internists or pediatricians with advanced training and certification in diseases of the musculoskeletal system, particularly autoimmune diseases. They treat people with lupus, scleroderma, and rheumatoid arthritis.

Infectious disease specialists are internists or pediatricians with advanced training in diseases caused by infections. They have particular expertise in treating AIDS and the many opportunistic infections that can complicate AIDS.

Oncologists are internists or pediatricians who have advanced training in the treatment of cancer, including that of the immune system. They also have expertise in treating the complications of immune system suppression that occur as a result of the chemotherapy given for many types of cancer.

baby with protection against disease until the baby can develop antibodies. Breast-feeding alone, delaying the introduction of new foods, may decrease allergy development in susceptible infants (see Chapter 18).

Immunizations

Childhood immunizations provide immunity against common yet potentially serious infections. Some of these immunizations—such as tetanus shots—need to be repeated from time to time to boost the immunity. Immunity to rubella (German measles) is very important to women of child-bearing age. Others, such as immunizations for the flu and pneumococcal pneumonia, need to be added as a woman ages or develops respiratory diseases such as asthma. Recommended immunizations are included in Chapter 2.

If you are traveling outside the United States, you may be at risk for illnesses not covered by routinely recommended immunizations. They include cholera, hepatitis A, typhoid fever, and some types of meningitis and encephalitis. The Centers for Disease Control and Prevention offer an excellent service that supplies up-to-date information, by fax or telephone, for disease prevention in all areas of the world. You can reach the International Travelers' Hotline by calling 404-332-4559.

Allergies

People can be allergic to foods or drugs, substances in foods, or things in the atmosphere. Some allergens are easier to avoid than others. If you know you are allergic to a particular substance, the best course is to avoid it completely. If you are allergic to a food, ask how unfamiliar dishes are prepared and whether they contain the food that provokes your symptoms. If you are allergic to any drugs, be sure that you inform any doctor or other medical professional who may be treating you. This is especially important if you are seeing someone other than your regular doctor—for example, if you have to use an emergency room or need medical care while you are traveling.

It is not possible to avoid most allergens completely. After all, house dust mites and pollen are all around. There are many medications available without a prescription that can ease the symptoms of allergies (see

"Specific Allergies"). There are various ways to minimize your exposure.

- *Pollen allergies* are seasonal. You may be allergic to many types of pollen or just one. Pollen counts are lowest in the middle of the day, on cool days, and after it rains.

- *Animal dander,* dry flakes of shed skin, contains proteins that can provoke an allergic response. Keeping pets outdoors prevents their dander from clinging to carpets and upholstered furniture. Try to keep at least one room, such as the bedroom, pet free. Regularly bathing your pets may limit the amount of dander.

- *Dust allergies* are usually due to dust mites, microscopic organisms that live in dust. They thrive on carpets, on upholstery, in mattresses, and in pillows. Try to make at least one room, such as the bedroom, dust free. Take up the carpet, use furniture without upholstery, and use blinds instead of curtains. The box springs, mattress, and pillows should be encased in special dustproof zippered covers. Wash bedding in hot water once a week.

- *Mold allergies* result from exposure to mold and spores. You can reduce exposure by discarding all old or damp furniture. Dehumidifiers can support mold growth if they are not emptied and cleaned regularly. Use antimildew sprays in damp areas of your home.

Special Warning!

If you have had a severe allergic reaction, called anaphylaxis, to a food, a drug, or a biting insect, be prepared at all times to act quickly if you become exposed. You should have protective emergency medication in your home and with you when you travel.

CONDITIONS OF THE IMMUNE SYSTEM

AIDS

AIDS is covered in detail in Chapter 20. It is caused by infection with HIV. The virus seeks out T-cells that have a specific antigen, known as CD4. After a period when HIV has been present with no symptoms, the virus begins to kill the body's T-helper cells, and the immune system becomes severely impaired. A woman with AIDS has a lowered resistance to certain infections and diseases that are called *opportunistic infections* because they take advantage of the opportunity the weak immune system gives them. Ultimately, one of these opportunistic infections proves fatal.

Although there are some treatments for the opportunistic infections, there is as yet no drug that removes the AIDS virus. For now, the best course is to avoid becoming infected with the virus.

Allergy

Allergies are examples of the immune system gone wrong. A substance that is not normally harmful, like pollen, is perceived as an infectious agent by the immune system. Antibodies or sensitized cells develop. As part of its defense system, the body releases histamine and other chemicals, which produce the symptoms of an allergic reaction.

Not everyone has allergies. The combination of a genetic tendency and exposure to potential allergens increases the risk of developing an allergy. Babies may develop allergies early in infancy because their gastrointestinal tract is immature and admits more proteins (potential allergens) into the body than a mature tract. Breast-feeding and strictly limiting food types offered for the first six months of life may lower the risk of developing allergies in those who may be susceptible.

People with allergies are commonly allergic to more than one thing. This is because all allergies have one root cause: a hyperreactive immune system that perceives innocuous substances as infectious agents.

Types of Allergic Reactions

Allergic reactions can be immediate or delayed. Immediate reactions can occur in localized groups of sensitized cells, as in the nose with pollen allergy or in the bronchial tubes with allergic asthma. Fluid is released from the blood vessels into the tissue spaces and swelling occurs. This is due to release of histamine and other mediators from sensitized cells. A typical example of delayed allergic reactions mediated by T cells is the skin rash due to poison ivy. There are also delayed respiratory hypersensitivities.

Hives (Urticaria)

Hives are slightly raised white or pink wheals (bumps) or swellings of the skin that are very itchy. In fact, the itching may be noticed before the bumps. They tend to appear on the chest, the arms, and the trunk, but they can be more widespread. Hives are usually triggered by allergy to a substance that is eaten or drunk—medications or food. They also can be seen with viral illnesses, such as mononucleosis, and are sometimes caused by histamine release due to exercise. They are treated with antihistamine medications. It is helpful to pinpoint the cause so that the triggering substance can be avoided. In the case of chronic hives (more than 6 weeks), a specific cause is unlikely to be identified.

Angioedema

Angioedema is marked by swelling. It tends to affect the face, throat, hands, feet, and genitals. It usually occurs episodically. It may be caused by an allergy, but often a specific allergen cannot be found. The usual treatment is antihistamines.

Anaphylaxis

Anaphylaxis is a severe allergic reaction. It is a medical emergency that requires immediate treatment. Anaphylaxis is caused by a sudden release of histamine and other body chemicals that participate in immune reactions. As with hives and angioedema, fluid moves from the blood vessels into the open tissue spaces. With anaphylaxis, however, so much fluid moves that it decreases the blood pressure and swells the bronchial tubes, passages critical to breathing. The most common causes of anaphylaxis are bee stings, penicillin, nuts, and fish. A rare form of anaphylaxis is triggered by physical exercise.

Anaphylaxis includes one or more of the following life-threatening symptoms:

- Faintness or loss of consciousness due to low blood pressure
- Swelling of the throat, larynx, or vocal cords, resulting in the feeling of not getting enough air
- Spasms in the bronchial tubes (asthma), resulting in coughing, shortness of breath, or wheezing.

People experiencing anaphylaxis describe having a feeling of impending doom. They often appear very fearful and in great distress.

Anyone with the symptoms of anaphylaxis should be transported immediately to a medical facility. The initial treatment is an injection of epinephrine (adrenaline). If the airway is constricted or the person's blood pressure is low, oxygen and intravenous fluids will be given. Antihistamines and corticosteroids are also used.

If you have had an anaphylactic reaction, you should be thoroughly examined to find the cause of it. If a cause is found, avoidance is the treatment of choice. Because of the seriousness of anaphylaxis, it is wise to have available a kit containing epinephrine that can be self-injected, which can be prescribed by your doctor.

Specific Allergies

Asthma

Asthma is a condition of the lungs that causes wheezing. It is covered in detail in Chapter 26. The wheezing is caused by airway inflammation and abnormal contraction of the smooth muscle in the bronchioles (small airway tubes).

It is now thought that the bronchioles become hyperreactive and that an important treatment should include anti-inflammatory medications that counteract immune responses. Some of these medications can be inhaled into the lungs so that they cause minimal side effects in the rest of the body. Bronchodilators, drugs that widen the airways by relaxing the surrounding muscles, are also used.

Bee Stings

Stings from bees, wasps, and hornets can cause severe local reactions such as itching and swelling in everyone. People who are allergic to the venom of these insects develop a more pronounced immediate hypersensitivity reaction: hives, angioedema, or anaphylaxis. Appropriate emergency treatment must be given.

Cats and Dogs

Cats and dogs shed dry skin, called dander, that contains various proteins. When dander gets in the air and is inhaled, it can provoke an allergic response. Cats tend to be a particular problem for people with allergies. This is because, as they groom themselves, they spread the dander from their skin to their fur, where it can be more easily released into the air. Cats are not fond of baths, but if you can manage it once a week, your exposure to dander may be reduced.

Drug Allergies

Some drugs can act as allergens in some people. After a susceptible person is exposed to such a drug, if he or she is exposed to it again, an allergic reaction occurs. The reaction can be a rash, hives, or anaphylaxis. Allergies to penicillin and sulfa are the most common, at least partly because they are very frequently used. Other types of drug allergy may occur. They are caused by different immune mechanisms and may affect specific organs. For instance, the liver may develop hypersensitivity hepatitis from drugs that are commonly used to treat high blood pressure, tuberculosis, high cholesterol levels, or seizures. In other cases, an immune reaction may be triggered that resembles an autoimmune disease.

Drug allergies are not the same thing as side effects. A drug side effect is an unwanted pharmacologic effect that has nothing to do with the immune system. For example, an asthma attack due to taking penicillin is an allergic reaction; stomach discomfort from taking penicillin is a side effect. If you have an allergy to a drug, you should not take it again. Tell your doctor about your allergy. You should avoid not only the drug that causes the allergy but also any drugs that are related to it or derived from it.

The best course of action when dealing with any reactions to medication is to report them to your doctor. Together, you can decide what type of reaction occurred and what to do about it in the future.

Dust and Mold

In dust allergies, the allergen prompting the symptoms is not the dust itself but tiny organisms called dust mites that live in dust. They thrive in carpets, pillows, and upholstery. In mold allergies, the cause is exposure to mold spores. Ways that you can minimize dust and mold allergies are covered in the ''Keeping the Immune System Healthy'' section of this chapter.

Food Allergies

Many people think that the reactions they have after eating certain foods are allergies. Actually, less than 1 percent of the adult population suffers from food allergies, and they usually have other allergic problems, such as asthma or eczema (a skin condition). The foods that most commonly cause severe allergic reactions in adults are peanuts, tree nuts, shellfish, and fish.

There are ways to tell whether food is causing your reaction. Food allergy symptoms typically occur within an hour of eating. The ''oral allergy'' reaction is a feeling of itching in the mouth and around the lips. It is often caused by fresh fruits and vegetables—tomatoes, melons, or strawberries. Cooking these foods can change the protein structure of the allergen and may eliminate the reaction. Other allergic symptoms from food include skin rashes, abdominal cramps, pain, and diarrhea. The most serious reactions are hives, asthma, and anaphylaxis.

People who have cramps, pain, and diarrhea may have another medical problem—food intolerance. This occurs when the body cannot digest the food, often because it lacks a vital enzyme. For example, people who get symptoms from drinking milk may have lactose intolerance. In this condition, the body does not have enough lactase, the enzyme needed to digest lactose (milk sugar). (See Chapter 33).

A whole body of myths has been built up around food allergies. A particular food cannot cause depression or fatigue. There is no evidence for a "systemic yeast infection" that causes fatigue and other symptoms. Specific food allergies and intolerances can be treated by eliminating offending foods from the diet.

Hay Fever

Hay fever, or allergic rhinitis and conjunctivitis, is the most common allergy, affecting 40 million people in the United States. It is also the most annoying allergy. It generally develops between the ages of 3 and 45. People who have other allergic conditions, such as asthma or dermatitis, are particularly susceptible.

There are two types of hay fever: seasonal and perennial. Seasonal hay fever occurs only when allergens, such as pollen, are in the air. (See Fig. 31.5) Perennial hay fever occurs all year because it is caused by allergens that are always around (for example, animal dander and house dust mites).

The most common symptoms of hay fever are frequent sneezing and a runny nose. Some people also have red, itchy, watery eyes. Rubbing the eyes seems to make the condition worse. A person may wheeze and have a dry throat. Symptoms tend to be most severe for 15- to 30-minute periods called allergy attacks.

The best way to treat hay fever is to avoid the allergen that brings on the symptoms. Nonprescription and prescription drugs can be taken to alleviate symptoms, and immunotherapy can significantly reduce allergies affecting the eye or nose.

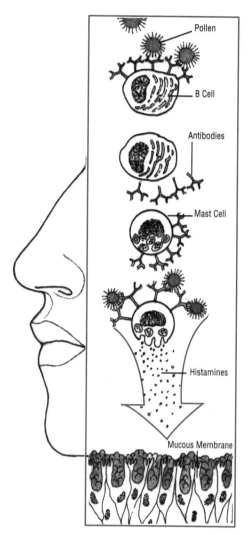

Figure 31.5   An Allergic Reaction
An allergic reaction occurs in some people when a harmless
substance, such as pollen, is perceived as a threat by the immune
system. B cells that encounter the pollen produce antibodies against
it. When specialized *mast cells*, which have receptors for
these antibodies, afterward come into contact with the
pollen, they release a flood of chemicals, such as
histamines, that trigger allergic symptoms like sneezing
and runny nose.

Treating Allergies

The main types of medications used to treat hay
fever are antihistamines and decongestants. Under
some circumstances, a special desensitizing procedure
called immunotherapy can be helpful.

Antihistamines

The mainstays for treating allergic symptoms are
antihistamines. As the name suggests, antihistamines
counteract histamine, the most important chemical released in allergic reactions. Although most types of

antihistamines are taken in pill form, eye drops are also
available to treat allergic conjunctivitis (inflammation
of the eyes).

There are two types of antihistamines: short acting,
like diphenhydramine, and long acting, like terfena-
dine. Short-acting antihistamines are most useful in
countering the immediate effects of an allergy—hives
and itching. They are used in emergency treatment of
allergic reactions. One drawback is that they may
cause drowsiness, to which tolerance usually develops. When you are taking these drugs, do not drink
alcohol—it causes drowsiness, too, and the combined
effect is dangerous. Do not operate machinery or drive
while you use this medication. Long-acting antihistamines do not cause drowsiness. They are a good choice
when day-in, day-out relief is needed, as with hay fever. They are taken once or twice a day.

Decongestants

Decongestants work by constricting blood vessels.
This helps to shrink swollen membranes in the nose and
sinuses and to clear those passages. They come in pill
form, as with pseudoephedrine and phenylpropanola-
mine, or as nasal sprays or eye drops. Because they are
related to epinephrine, they may stimulate the heart and
raise the blood pressure. They can cause insomnia.
They should not be used by women who have high
blood pressure, heart disease, an overactive thyroid, or
diabetes. Use of decongestant nasal sprays for more
than a week can actually cause nasal congestion.

Immunotherapy

Immunotherapy is the process of desensitizing an
allergic person to an allergen. It is most effective for
allergic rhinitis and conjunctivitis, and can also be used
in people with severe allergies, such as to bee stings.

Doses of the allergen are given as shots, weekly,
biweekly, or monthly. Slowly, the amount of allergen is
increased. Giving the allergen reduces the reaction to
it. The goal is to reduce the allergic reaction to the
antigen. If this therapy is successful, the reaction to the
allergen should steadily decrease. After 3–5 years, the
therapy can be stopped.

Unfortunately, immunotherapy does not work for
everyone. Also, it requires an investment of time and
money to get the shots over a long period, and not
everyone can make this investment. People with seasonal allergies that are relieved by medications may
not want to bother with immunotherapy. On the other
hand, someone with perennial allergies might be
strongly motivated to try it.

Autoimmune Disease

The immune system's method of recognizing foreign substances can become confused. When that happens, the body manufactures T cells and antibodies directed against the body's own cells and organs. The misguided T cells and autoantibodies contribute to many diseases. For instance, T cells that attack pancreas islet cells contribute to diabetes, and an autoantibody known as rheumatoid factor is common in persons with rheumatoid arthritis. Women with systemic lupus erythematosus (SLE) have antibodies to many types of cells and cell components.

Exactly what starts the process that results in an autoimmune disease is not known, but multiple factors are likely to be involved. These include elements in the environment, viruses, and certain drugs. Also, sunlight can damage or alter normal body cells. Hormones and heredity are suspected of playing roles. Most autoimmune conditions are more common in women than in men.

Cancer

The immune system provides one of the body's main defenses against cancer. When normal cells turn into cancer cells, some of the antigens on their surface may change. These new or altered antigens activate the immune system. According to one theory, the immune system is constantly on the lookout for cancerous cells, which it then seeks to eliminate. Tumors are known to occur when the immune system is impaired (see Chapter 37).

Several types of treatment using the immune system to fight cancer are being explored. One approach is to use cytokines (immunoregulatory substances) to boost the natural immune responses. Another is to develop specific cells or antibodies that will attack cancer cells throughout the body.

Chronic Fatigue Syndrome

Chronic fatigue syndrome (CFS) is an exhausting fatigue that comes on suddenly and is relentless or relapsing. It causes debilitating tiredness for no apparent reason and a profound weakness that lasts for months. The cause of CFS is not known, but it may involve the immune system.

The symptoms of CFS may come on suddenly. They are usually not alarming because many of them—headache, sore throat, low-grade fever, fatigue and weakness, tender lymph glands, muscle and joint aches, and inability to concentrate—mimic the symptoms of a viral illness. However, these symptoms do not go away. They can continue for 6 months or longer.

CFS was first reported in well-educated women in their 30s, but the syndrome affects all ages and socioeconomic groups. It affects more women than men.

Currently no effective treatment exists for CFS. Limited success has been reported with antiviral drugs, antidepressants, and drugs that boost the immune system. People with CFS may benefit from maintaining a healthy lifestyle: eating a balanced diet, getting enough rest, and exercising regularly. CFS is not a progressive disease, and it does not appear to worsen with time.

PROCEDURES

Various procedures can be done if a person is suspected of having an immune system problem, especially allergies. Because the immune system is linked with the rest of the body, procedures done on other parts of the body—such as organ transplants—can involve the immune system.

Allergy Testing

All allergy testing should be done under the supervision of a qualified allergist. The different types of tests that can be used to determine what substance is triggering an allergy include those discussed below.

- *Skin or skin prick test*—A small amount of the allergen is injected under the skin. The skin is then observed for swelling and redness. If this happens, this means that the person has allergic antibodies to the substance tested.

- *Patch test*—The suspected substance is placed directly on the skin and covered by a bandage. The site is examined later to see if a reaction has occurred. This test is useful in identifying substances causing a skin reaction.

- *RAST test*—The RAST test (radioallergosorbent test) is done on a person's blood to determine if a substance in the blood (immunoglobulin E, or IgE) reacts with a specific allergen. In general, skin tests are more sensitive and specific than RAST.

- *Elimination or exclusion diet*—In an elimination test, the diet is restricted to certain foods. As new foods are introduced, the doctor and patient watch for signs that these foods cause allergic symptoms. In the exclusion test, the suspected food is excluded from the diet for two weeks, and the effect on the allergic symptoms is evaluated.

Transplantation

If the cells of one person are introduced into another person's body, an immune response will result. The new cells are perceived as disease, and immune cells are sensitized to attack them. In some cases, this response can be suppressed so vital organs can be transplanted. The closer the match of cells between donor and recipient, the better the chance of acceptance of the transplant.

Tissue and Organ Transplants

Thousands of women have had their lives prolonged by transplanted organs. Kidney, heart, lung, liver, and pancreas transplants are now being done. For a transplant to be successful, the body's natural tendency to rid itself of foreign tissue must be lessened. One way this is done is by selecting a donor whose tissue is as similar as possible to that of the recipient. Studies are done on both the donor and the recipient to identify what type of antigens they carry. This is done through a complex set of tests on tissue. The chances of people having identical transplant antigens is about 1 in 100,000. The chances are highest in identical twins and next highest in other family members.

Another way is to suppress the recipient's immune system. This can be done with powerful immunosuppressive drugs such as corticosteroids and cyclosporine A or by using laboratory-made antibodies that attack T cells.

Bone Marrow Transplants

Bone marrow transplants are used to treat leukemia (cancer of the blood) and tumors that have invaded the bone. As with other transplants, transplants of bone marrow require a close match with the donor. Not only is there a danger that the body will reject the transplanted bone marrow cells, but mature T cells from the bone marrow transplant may counterattack and destroy the cells of the recipient ("graft vs. host" reaction). To prevent this, physicians use drugs or antibodies to rid the donor marrow of potentially dangerous T cells. Until a bone marrow transplant "takes," the person has very little immunity.

FUTURE RESEARCH

Even the most advanced researchers do not have all the answers on how the immune system works, but more is learned every day. Some areas of current research are discussed below.

- Scientists are now able to mass-produce immune cells for many diseases. The ability to create antibodies and specialized immune cells furthers their research and improves their understanding of the immune system.

- Monoclonal antibodies are antibodies made by cloning (multiplying a single cell). When these cells are grown in tissue culture or injected into research animals (mice), they will secrete the made-to-order antibodies over a long period of time.

- Genetic engineering allows scientists to remove genes (segments of DNA, the material that is the body's genetic blueprint) from one type of organism and combine them with a gene of another organism. These organisms are used to make large quantities of human proteins, such as insulin. The process has also helped scientists to manufacture proteins from hepatitis, AIDS, or cancer cells. These disease proteins can be used to develop vaccines. This has been done for hepatitis; vaccines for AIDS and cancer are not yet available.

■ Gene therapies for a variety of disorders are being developed. Cancer-fighting cells are taken from the patient's tumor, a gene that boosts the cells' ability to fight cancer is inserted into them, and the new cells are reinjected into the patient to battle the cancer.

■ Research studying the suppression of a sometimes overactive immune system is under way.

CHAPTER 32

The Kidneys and the Urinary System

Tamara G. Bavendam, M.D., F.A.C.S. and
Sandra P. Levison, M.D., F.A.C.P

The urinary system eliminates waste products while saving materials needed by the body. It does this by producing and excreting urine, a watery substance made up of excess fluid, waste products, and toxins. The body produces urine continually. No conscious effort is needed to produce urine, but excreting it does require being aware of when the bladder is full and getting to the toilet to urinate.

The urinary system includes the kidneys, the ureters, the bladder, and the urethra. Together, these structures are called the urinary tract.

HOW THE URINARY SYSTEM WORKS

The kidneys are a pair of bean-shaped organs that lie in the upper part of the abdomen, next to the spine at the base of the lower ribs (see Fig. 32.1). Human beings need only one functioning kidney, so an individual born with just one kidney can still live a normal life.

The kidneys work as filters, retaining materials the body needs from the blood and putting them back in the body's circulation. Wastes and harmful products like toxins are passed out as urine and excreted by the body. The kidneys also monitor the body's need for water and *electrolytes,* such as sodium, potassium, chloride, and bicarbonate. Electrolytes help keep the body's systems balanced. By saving or excreting electrolytes and other materials as needed, the kidneys play a valuable role in maintaining a constant healthy environment for the body.

The main functioning unit of the kidney is the *nephron* which acts as a filtering system for the body. Each kidney is made up of about 1 million nephrons, each consisting of a group of blood vessels formed into a cuplike structure, the glomerulus. The glomerulus is attached to a structure called a tubule; together, one glomerulus and one tubule form one nephron.

Blood is filtered in the capillaries (tiny arteries) of the glomerulus, and red blood cells and proteins are retained. The fluid that remains passes through the tubule, where sodium, potassium, and water are secreted or reabsorbed, depending on the body's needs. This

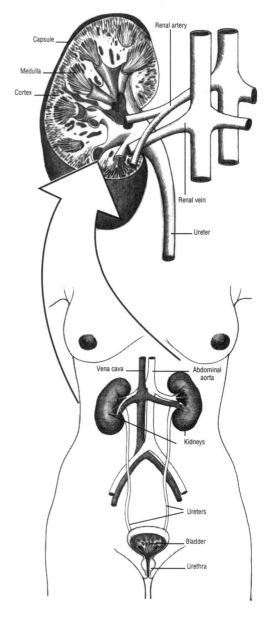

Figure 32.1 The Urinary System
The urinary system is composed of the *kidneys,* two fist-sized organs on either side of the body; the *ureters,* tubes that lead from the kidneys to the *bladder,* where urine is stored; and the *urethra,* through which urine is passed to the outside of the body. The kidneys play a vital role in filtering waste products and maintaining chemical and electrical balances within the body. Each kidney is covered with an outer *capsule* made up of strong fibrous tissue. Inside the capsule, the *cortex* and the *medulla* contain specialized structures that collect and process fluids, waste, and metabolic products. Blood is supplied from the *renal artery,* which branches off from the central *abdominal aorta,* and drained by the *renal vein,* which joins the *vena cava* before returning to the heart.

small tubule joins with other tubules, which lead to larger and larger tubules. Eventually, the large tubules empty into the ureter.

The amount of fluid taken in or lost (through vomiting or diarrhea, for example), type of diet, any medications taken, and exposure to extreme temperatures all affect the amount and type of urine produced. The urine is then transported to the urinary bladder through the ureters. The bladder is a sac of muscle located in the middle of the lower abdomen behind the pubic bone. The bladder's main function is to act as a storage bin for urine. The amount the bladder can hold varies from person to person. Once the bladder has reached its capacity, the urine passes into the urethra, a tube which is 2 to 3 inches long in women. Then, it exits the body from a small opening above the vagina.

Urination is a two-step process: First, the walls of your bladder begin to stretch because it is full. This stretching sends signals to the brain that it is time to urinate. Second, when you are ready to urinate, you relax the urinary sphincter muscle at the base of the bladder around the urethra. This allows urine to pass. The amount of urine varies anywhere from less than an ounce to a cup or more.

The muscles that provide support for the pelvic organs (the bladder, uterus, and rectum) also assist the workings of the urinary tract. Although they are a part of the musculoskeletal system, they are important in maintaining bladder control. If these muscles weaken and sag, incontinence, or loss of urinary control, can result.

In women, the urinary and reproductive pathways are separate. In men, the urethra transports not only urine but also semen. The urethra in women is shorter than that in men, which means women are more likely to have some urinary problems, such as infections.

KEEPING THE URINARY SYSTEM HEALTHY

To keep your urinary system healthy, drink plenty of water. Water plays many important roles in the healthy functioning of your urinary tract. The amount of water in your body helps the urinary system determine whether more electrolytes, such as sodium, should be retained or excreted. When the concentration of electrolytes is too high, your body releases a hormone that causes water retention and stimulates your feelings of thirst. The kidney then gets rid of the excess electrolytes and water.

Drinking enough water allows you to produce a large quantity of urine. You should drink enough fluids, particularly water, to allow emptying the bladder every 3 to 4 hours during the day. At least half of the fluid each day should be noncarbonated water. (Carbonation can worsen some urinary conditions.) Although the urinary tract is usually sterile, producing large amounts of urine helps wash harmful bacteria out of the urinary system if they should enter.

Usually, if your kidneys work well, you do not need to limit your diet. If, however, you have high blood pressure—which is linked with some kinds of kidney disease—a salt-restricted diet may be prescribed. If you are prone to developing kidney stones, you may need to limit the amount of calcium and oxalate, two main components of stones, in your diet. Calcium is found in milk and other diary products, as well as some leafy, green vegetables and fish with bones. Oxalate is found in large amounts in tea, dark colas, and green leafy vegetables.

Research has shown that cranberry juice can help prevent recurrent urinary tract infections, particularly in older women. There is usually no harm in drinking moderate quantities of cranberry juice. Since it is a good source of vitamin C—one of the essential vitamins—it can be a part of a good diet. If you already have an infection, however, drinking large amounts of cranberry juice or other acidic juices may aggravate the pain and should be avoided.

A condition called "irritable bladder" may be brought on by drinking a lot of coffee or carbonated beverages or by eating acidic, spicy foods. If you tend to have this problem, alter your diet accordingly. Also, be careful with medications, even over-the-counter products. Medications as well as toxins are filtered by the kidneys. This generally allows safe use of drugs without high levels building up in the blood. Even so, large amounts of drugs can build up in the kidneys. This is particularly true of the pain medications known as *nonsteroidal anti-inflammatory drugs* (NSAIDS), which include ibuprofen and naproxen. If you take these drugs for a long time, you may damage your kidneys.

Good hygiene is also helpful. Because a woman's urethra is very close to the vagina and fairly close to the rectum, infections can be passed from one of these openings to the others. Wiping from the front to back after defecating helps prevent infecting the urethra with bacteria that are normally present in the vagina or rectum. For the same reason, women who are prone to infections should avoid tub baths and douches.

Good hygiene after intercourse is also important. During intercourse, bacteria from the vagina or from the man's penis can enter the urethra. Cleansing the genital area after having sex helps prevent this. Urinating after intercourse helps to flush bacteria out of the bladder and urethra before they can build up and cause an infection. This is most helpful when the quantity of urine is large enough to create a good stream to wash out the bladder.

Smoking tobacco increases the risk of some urinary tract conditions. Tobacco smoking is also associated with atherosclerosis, including the blood vessels, that go to the kidney. This can cause high blood pressure and loss of kidney function. Smoking tends to cause chronic coughing, which can add to problems with bladder control. It also increases the risk of bladder cancer—which can occur even years after a woman has quit smoking. The best thing is not to start smoking in the first place. If you do smoke, quit.

COMMON URINARY PROBLEMS

Problems affecting the urinary system are common. Certain symptoms are related to specific problems. Recognizing symptoms can help you decide whether or not you need to see a doctor. Your regular doctor can treat some problems, but others may require referral to a specialist (see "Who Treats the Urinary System?").

WHO TREATS THE URINARY SYSTEM?

If you have such urinary symptoms as pain, bloody urine, or frequent urination, you can be treated by any one of several kinds of doctors. An internist or a family physician can diagnose and treat simple problems, such as infections, and refer you to a nephrologist or a urologist for more specialized care if needed.

A *nephrologist* is a medical doctor who specializes in problems affecting the kidney. She or he is a specialist in internal medicine with advanced training in kidney disease, unbalanced electrolytes, kidney failure, and other problems connected to the kidneys, such as high blood pressure or swelling. A *urologist* is a surgeon who specializes in the structure of the urinary system, the drainage of the kidneys, and the function of the bladder. If the kidneys fail, nephrologists and urologists both can be involved with diagnosis and treatment. If artificially filtering the blood (dialysis) is needed, a nephrologist supervises the whole process.

Some urinary problems, such as infection and bladder control, can be treated by your gynecologist as well.

Some urinary tract symptoms affect just the urine. For example, the urine may be bloody or unusually colored, or you may feel you need to urinate right away (urgency) or more often than usual (frequency). In other cases, urination is painful. Some symptoms affect other parts of the body: high blood pressure, fever and chills, back pain, or puffy hands, feet, or eyes. Some women have no symptoms at all, even if a kidney is slowly beginning to fail. When this happens, the body has adjusted to the failing kidney and so there are no symptoms. Other women may have severe symptoms caused by relatively minor problems that are easily treated. The severity of the symptoms is not always a good indication of the seriousness of disease.

Symptoms

Bloody Urine

Normal urine is pale to medium yellow. Blood in the urine (hematuria) is a sign that a serious condition may be present. It should prompt you to see a doctor as soon as possible. The urine may be bright red with clots, a light pink, gray, or dark brown like tea or cola. The color depends on the amount of blood, how "old" the urine is, and how acidic. Even if the urine is not an unusual color, small amounts of blood can be present. Although invisible to the naked eye, the blood can be seen if the urine is examined with special paper (dipstick) or under a microscope.

An infection of the urinary tract is the most common cause of hematuria. Fever and urinary pain, frequency and urgency of urination also are common with infection. Other causes of bloody urine include trauma and injury, kidney diseases, such as glomerulonephritis, stones, and tumors (mostly cancers). Blood in the urine also can be caused by very strenuous exercise, such as jogging (particularly very long distances). It is important to have a further evaluation to determine the cause. In some cases, no cause can be found.

Because a woman's urethra is close to her vagina and rectum, bloody urine can sometimes reflect blood from these structures rather than blood from the urinary system. Finally, the red or brown colored urine may be caused by medication, some forms of liver disease, or even, in some people, a recent serving of beets.

Pain

One frequent cause of pain is a urinary tract infection. When a kidney is infected, the pain is felt in the upper back or side, and fever and chills may occur. If the pain is low and in front and occurs mostly when you are urinating, it is more likely to be a bladder infection.

Another bladder condition, called interstitial cystitis, can cause pain. If you have pain when you urinate and chronic pain in the genital area (for example, the clitoris, the labia, and the vagina) or the thighs or lower back, you may be suffering from this condition.

Stones in the urinary tract are another cause of pain. Such pain is spasmodic and can travel from the back down the side into the vaginal lips. Although stones in the kidneys do not usually cause pain, when stones leave the kidneys and pass down the ureter, they can cause severe pain that has been described as worse than labor pains. This is called renal colic.

Urinary Urgency and Frequency

A strong feeling that you must urinate is called urinary urgency. Urinary frequency is the need to void often. Both are common symptoms of a urinary tract infection or interstitial cystitis. Urgency and frequency are not always linked to disease, however. In cold weather it is common for people to void often. Pregnant women typically experience an increased need to urinate as the uterus grows, causing pressure on the bladder.

COMMON CONDITIONS AFFECTING THE URINARY TRACT

Some urinary tract conditions are minor problems that can be easily treated. Others can seriously harm the body's ability to function and can even be life-threatening if they are not caught in time.

Urinary system conditions can be grouped into the following types:

- Infections
- Irritations or inflammations
- Stones
- Urinary incontinence
- Kidney failure
- Nephrotic syndrome
- Inherited kidney disease
- Tumors
- Systemic disorders

INFECTIONS

Bacteria are normally present in some parts of the body, such as the vagina and rectum, but not in the urine. When bacteria invade a part of the urinary system, infections can occur. Women are more likely to have urinary tract infections than men, because a woman's urethra, vagina, and rectum are all close together and her urethra is fairly short. It is relatively easy for bacteria from the vagina or rectum to travel up the urethra into the bladder and then to the kidneys.

Since common symptoms of frequency and painful urination can occur with other urinary conditions, a diagnosis of infection cannot be made on the basis of symptoms alone. Diagnosis depends on examination of a urine specimen and obtaining a urine culture. If pus cells are seen in the urine and bacteria can be grown in the urine culture, then infection is likely the cause.

Usually, infections that are not complicated by

other problems can be easily treated with antibiotics. The antibiotic needed for treatment can be determined by studying the urine culture. When medicine is prescribed, take all the pills, even if symptoms disappear before all the medication has been taken. Stopping antibiotics too soon increases the chance that the infection will recur.

Bladder Infection

Cystitis or bladder infection is the most common urinary tract infection. Because of the proximity of the vagina and the urethra, it is not unusual for bladder infections to begin when a woman becomes sexually active. Some women are particularly prone to these infections. They may have more aggressive bacteria, or they may lack needed defense mechanisms to fight off the infection.

Sexual intercourse itself may prompt a bladder infection. Sometimes you can have symptoms within hours of having sex, sometimes days later. The typical symptoms of a bladder infection are frequency, urgency, and pain with urination. The urine may be bloody or cloudy, or it may have an unusual odor.

A bladder infection is diagnosed by examining a urine sample and obtaining a urine culture. Most bladder infections not associated with a kidney infection can be cured within 3 to 5 days by using antibiotics. You can help the process by increasing the amount of water you drink and urinating often.

Kidney Infection

Kidney infections often start with bacteria in the bladder. The bacteria travel up the ureters to the kidney and cause the infection. When kidney infections recur, the cause may be reflux, the backing up of urine from the bladder to the kidneys. This is caused by a faulty valve mechanism where the bladder and the ureter join. Other causes of recurrent kidney infections are stones, diabetes mellitus, and previous scarring.

Kidney infection is also called *pyelonephritis* and is much less common than bladder infection. If you have a kidney infection, you may first experience urinary urgency and frequency. Later symptoms are fever and chills, pain in the upper back or side, nausea, and sometimes vomiting.

Diagnosis

A clean catch urine specimen and urine culture are examined to make the diagnosis. An X-ray or ultrasound of the kidney can help determine if an obstruction exists that could make the infection more serious. Also, a special X-ray of the bladder can identify infections caused by reflux.

Treatment

Sometimes, a kidney infection disappears spontaneously. However, because complications may occur if it doesn't, all kidney infections should be treated by a physician with antibiotics. Drinking large amounts of water, although helpful for other reasons, cannot flush infection out of the kidney. Antibiotics should be taken for 7–14 days to prevent complications. If you are too ill to take pills or if the infection is severe, you will be treated in the hospital with intravenous medication.

Hospital treatment is usually required if a woman has both a serious kidney infection and a urinary obstruction caused, for example, by stones. While most kidney infections heal with proper treatment, complications such as shock, bloodstream infection, and abscess formation may occur. The kidneys may become scarred and may fail to function properly. When stones or other obstructions occur along with infection, both intravenous antibiotics and relief of the blockage by surgery are needed.

IRRITATIONS AND INFLAMMATIONS

Bladder infections are only one type of cystitis. The symptoms of urinary frequency, urgency, and painful urination can also be caused by other types of cystitis, including irritation, or inflammation, of the bladder. These conditions are not caused by bacterial infection.

Irritable Bladder

Irritable bladder refers to an irritation of the lining of the bladder that is not caused by bacteria. It is also known as cystitis, chronic urethritis, trigonitis, or urethral syndrome.

Certain foods and beverages can cause the symptoms of irritable bladder; for example, too much coffee, carbonated beverages, or foods and beverages that are acidic or spicy. Some women also find their symptoms made worse by sex, emotional stress, and changes in their hormones that occur just before their menstrual periods. When irritable bladder is suspected, you should have a pelvic exam in addition to the usual urine studies.

For doctors and patients alike, irritable bladder can be a frustrating condition. The symptoms are similar to those of a bacterial infection. It is not unusual for symptoms to improve while you are taking antibiotics and then become worse when you stop. Antibiotics may seem to improve the condition because they are usually taken with extra water. When the course of antibiotics is completed, most people return to their normal drinking habits—often not enough water—and symptoms return. Antibiotics, however, do not usually provide a lasting cure and can be harmful. Taking antibiotics for weeks to months can lead to the development of recurrent yeast infections in the vagina.

More water intake is the best treatment. Increase your water intake whenever you begin to have symptoms of bladder irritability. Self-treatment begins with drinking 8 ounces of water every 20–30 minutes for 2–3 hours. This usually promotes a good washout of bacteria or other irritants. You may also find it helpful to keep a diary indicating when symptoms occur and what seems to cause them. Once the cause has been identified, often it can be avoided. Warm baths to relax the pelvic muscles may be soothing, too.

If increased water intake does not eliminate the symptoms, pills can be prescribed (phenazopyridine hydrochloride) that make the inside of the bladder numb. This medication changes the color of the urine to orange. Physical therapy may also help.

Interstitial Cystitis

Women who have interstitial cystitis have not only urinary frequency, urgency, and pain with urination but also chronic pelvic pain. When symptoms are severe,

you may urinate every 10–15 minutes, day and night, trying to eliminate the pain and the intense need to urinate. The intense pain is often temporarily relieved by urination. Because of the pain, this condition is also referred to as painful bladder syndrome.

The cause of interstitial cystitis is not known, but it occurs more often in women than in men. Like irritable bladder, stress and changes in hormone levels both seem to initiate the symptoms.

Diagnosis

The diagnosis of interstitial cystitis begins with a taking of your medical history. You may have a history of recurrent bladder infections. The evaluation includes urine studies and a pelvic exam. When a cystoscopy (a look inside the bladder with a special instrument) is done, its findings are usually normal. Your symptoms and the negative cystoscopy confirm the diagnosis.

Treatment

The symptoms can be minimized or controlled by a variety of treatments. Options include the increased water intake described for irritable bladder. For some women, medications may be effective, including:

- Phenazopyridine hydrochloride
- Tricyclic antidepressants (amitriptylline, doxepin, nortriptylline)
- Antihistamines
- Calcium channel blockers

Placing medications directly in the bladder helps more than half of women with this condition. Medications used this way include:

- Dimethyl sulfoxide
- Steroids
- Heparin

Because changes in hormone levels seem to provoke symptoms, medications that change hormone levels—such as birth control pills—can be an important part of treatment. After you go through menopause, you stop producing the female hormone estrogen. Replacing this hormone with medication is generally helpful. Counseling or biofeedback therapy to improve stress management can help, too.

STONES

Stones are composed of substances normally found in the urine (for example, calcium, oxalate, and uric acid) which have built up in high concentration. Although

they are produced in the kidneys, stones can be found anywhere in the urinary tract. Stones in the kidneys usually do not cause symptoms, however. Stones are more commonly found in the bladder or the ureter, where they can cause great pain.

Stones in the urinary tract can be present for a long time and not cause pain until they obstruct excretion. A stone in the ureter can prevent the passage of urine. When this happens, urine continues to be produced and the part of the urinary tract above the stone dilates (expands) with the urine that cannot escape. This expansion of the urinary tract causes severe pain, which may radiate into the groin and vulva. Nausea, vomiting, and fever can occur as well. (See Fig. 32.2).

Pain from kidney stones is worse when they are being passed; therefore, the pain seems to come and go intermittently. The stone temporarily blocks off the ureter, causing pain, then moves slightly, allowing urine to pass. This gives temporary relief until the stone lodges again in a position that blocks the ureter.

The type and location of the stone may be linked to the cause. Some stones are commonly associated with infection and certain bacteria. The tendency to form certain types of stones may be inherited, as in the case of the uric acid stones and cysteine stones. Still other stones are formed as a result of another medical condition, such as calcium stones in patients with overactive parathyroid glands, or as a complication of leukemia or chemotherapy for lymphoma.

Risk factors for stone formation are dehydration (not drinking enough water), excessive sweating, excessive calcium intake, and prolonged bed rest. Individuals who have had a severe injury and need long periods of bed rest are prone to having stones. For unknown reasons, men are more likely to form stones than women.

Diagnosis

Stones can be suspected on the basis of intermittent sharp, knifelike pains. To diagnose stones, doctors use X-rays of the urinary tract or methods that allow them to view the urinary tract directly. Stone composition can be determined by analysis of the urine and the stone.

Treatment

Most stones eventually pass into the bladder and require no treatment except pain medication. Stones smaller than one-quarter inch usually pass on their own; stones larger than one-half inch often require treatment. Treatment may include methods to dissolve or remove stones as well as drugs to prevent them from forming again. The treatment depends on the size and composition of the stone.

Often stones can be broken or crushed into sand inside the body without surgery. This procedure is re-

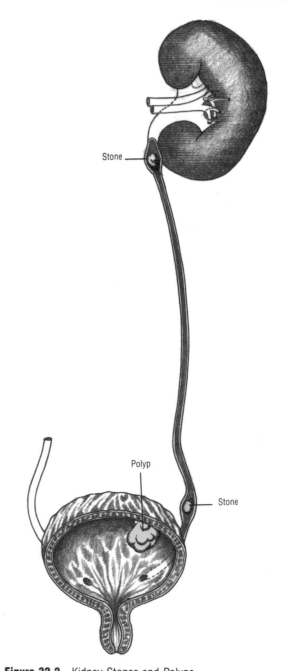

Figure 32.2 Kidney Stones and Polyps
Stones in the urinary tract can result from infections or disorders that cause excessive excretion of certain types of waste products that may begin to crystallize and form granules and eventually larger stones. Stones in the ureter can cause a great deal of pain as the ureter contracts in an attempt to pass them. Polyps are usually benign masses of tissue that form inside the bladder.

ferred to as lithotripsy. Different forms of lithotripsy are available, many of which can be done under local anesthesia in a doctor's office or an ambulatory care center. Once the stone is broken into smaller pieces, these pieces pass without further assistance into the bladder. Some pain may be experienced passing these fragments. Once the stone fragments are in the bladder, though, they can be passed through the urethra with minimal discomfort. After lithotripsy is performed, the urine passed from the body contains the dust and fragments from the stones, which can be collected for studies. Knowing the composition of the stone helps doctors to understand why the stone formed and how future stones can be prevented.

Stones also can be treated with small instruments that are passed through the urinary tract. No outside incisions are needed. With this technique, the stones can be removed or fragmented by lithotripsy or by means of a laser (strong, highly focused beams of light). With the treatment options available today, few women need major surgery to have stones removed.

Once stones have been treated, you can take steps to prevent a recurrence. Again, the best way to prevent stone formation is to drink plenty of water. It is hard to know exactly how much you need to drink to prevent stones, but a general rule is to drink enough water and other fluids to produce about 2 quarts of urine a day. Medication and special diet can help prevent stones.

URINARY INCONTINENCE

Urinary incontinence is the involuntary excretion of urine. The amount of urine may be as little as a few drops or as much as the entire contents of the bladder. Although urinary incontinence can happen at any age, it is more likely in women after they have had children and after menopause.

Our aging population means that incontinence is a concern for many women today. Adult diaper and other types of pads are a growing business. These products help prevent embarrassment from leaks, but they do not cure the problem. Many ways to improve or cure bladder problems exist, however. Most women can free themselves from relying on pads with appropriate treatment.

To maintain control of your bladder, a balance must be struck between the bladder and the bladder outlet. The bladder outlet consists of the urethra plus the pelvic muscles that surround the urethra. These muscles are also called the pelvic floor muscles. When the bladder contracts, it allows the urine to empty. When the bladder outlet contracts, it prevents urine from passing. To prevent urine from leaking, the bladder outlet keeps up a high pressure as the bladder is filling and at times of stress (for example, coughing, lifting, or bending). Any time the bladder's contractions exceed those of the bladder outlet, urine leaks.

There are several types of urinary incontinence:

■ *Stress* incontinence is urine loss that occurs when the bladder outlet's pressure is exceeded. Coughing, sneezing, bending, and lifting are some actions that can cause this form of incontinence.

■ *Urge* incontinence is linked with having a strong urge to urinate and being unable to get to the toilet in time.

■ *Spontaneous* incontinence involves urine loss for no identifiable reason. There is no sense of urgency or specific activity linked to the leakage.

■ *Enuresis, or bedwetting,* is common in children, but it tends to resolve with age. When enuresis occurs in an adult, there is generally some neurological problem causing the loss of bladder control.

The common causes of urinary incontinence are weak pelvic floor muscles, an overactive bladder muscle, inability to completely empty the bladder, and neurological diseases such as strokes, multiple sclerosis, or Parkinson's disease. In older women, restricted mobility, low levels of estrogen after menopause, inability to recognize that the bladder is full, and multiple medications are important causes. (See Fig. 32.3)

Diagnosis
The diagnosis of incontinence begins with the taking of your medical history. You may be asked to complete a diary that shows when you drank fluids, when you urinated, whether urine was leaked (and if so, how much), and what you were doing when the urine leaked. A urine sample is examined for blood or signs of infection. When blood is found, a kidney X-ray and cystoscopy are needed to rule out other problems.

A pelvic exam is done to allow the doctor to look for signs in the tissues that too little estrogen is being produced. (Lack of estrogen can weaken the pelvic floor muscles.) The doctor can also check the pelvic floor muscles and determine whether they are providing enough support to the base of the bladder and the

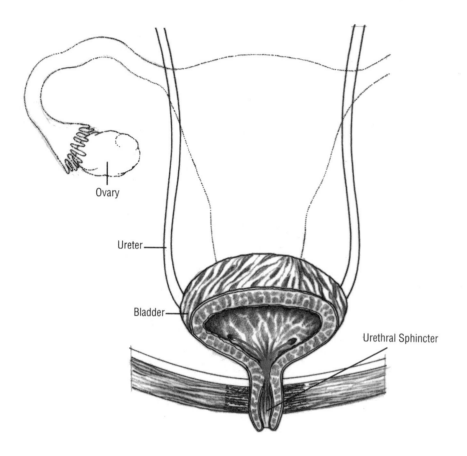

Ovary

Ureter

Bladder

Urethral Sphincter

Figure 32.3 Incontinence
One cause of urinary incontinence in older women is decreased production of estrogen at menopause. This decrease can cause the muscular wall of the bladder to thicken, which makes it able to hold less urine and can cause leakage of urine.

urethra. Weakness in the pelvic floor muscles can allow the bladder and urethra to sag into the vaginal space. Sagging of just the bladder is called a cystocele, while sagging of both the bladder and the urethra is called a cystourethrocele.

Even if blood is not found in the urine, cystoscopy may be done to look at the lining of the bladder and to examine the position and function of the urethra. Often, special studies of bladder function called urodynamics are done to check bladder sensation, bladder capacity, presence of abnormal bladder contractions, and ability of the bladder to empty.

Treatment

The first step in treating urinary incontinence is to see a physician. Many women suffer with this problem needlessly because they are either embarrassed or do not want to have surgery, which they think is the only cure. In fact, there are many methods of treatment other than operations (see "Where to Get More Information.")

If you have problems with bladder control, you may wish to begin by changing your diet. As with irritable bladder, coffee, tea, carbonated drinks, and acidic spicy food and drinks can increase bladder irritability and add to incontinence. Many women tend to cut back on the amount of water they drink, thinking that this will help prevent leakage. On the contrary, this makes the problem worse. The concentrated urine that forms when not enough water is drunk is more irritating to the bladder than diluted urine. Therefore, slowly increasing the amount of water drunk each day is a good idea. You can expect that urinary frequency may increase until the bladder becomes used to the extra water.

You can make other changes to ease problems with incontinence and improve the chance that any treatment will succeed. Chronic coughing and constipation strain the system and should be avoided. Also, try to become aware of any habits you have in sports or at work that can affect the delicate balance of bladder control. For example, don't strain to lift heavy weights.

Bladder training is also important. In bladder training, you go to the bathroom on a regular schedule whether or not you feel the need to urinate. You start off with a schedule of urinating every hour, and gradually increase the intervals between urinating.

Doing special exercises can help you strengthen your pelvic floor muscles. These exercises, sometimes called Kegel exercises, require you to identify and squeeze a certain group of muscles. A doctor or nurse can explain how the exercises are to be done and check that they are being performed correctly. A positive effect is usually seen after 6 weeks of performing 10–20 10-second contractions 4 times a day. (You may only be able to hold the contractions 2–3 seconds at first but can gradually work up to 10 seconds.) Biofeedback can also help with pelvic muscle exercises. A small device is placed in the vagina to measure the contractions of the muscles and give you immediate feedback when you are squeezing the right muscle.

Small weights, called vaginal cones, can be used with the exercises. They help you learn which muscles to contract and can increase the strength of the pelvic floor muscles. You insert a weight into your vagina and then use your pelvic muscles to prevent it from falling out. Hold the weight in for 15 minutes at a time and do the exercise twice a day. These weights are available without a prescription, but they work best after you have learned how to use them properly from a doctor or nurse.

If you have problems with bladder control because your pelvic organs sag, it can be helpful to use a contraceptive diaphragm when you are doing a physically stressful activity like jogging or playing volleyball or tennis. The diaphragm helps give the urethra the support the pelvic muscles lack. The use of the diaphragm should be combined with pelvic muscle exercises to strengthen the muscles.

The newest form of treatment is electrical stimulation of the pelvic muscles. Although its use is fairly common in Europe, it is just becoming available in the United States.

Medications can also improve urinary control. Some drugs relax the bladder muscle, allowing it to store large volumes of urine and prevent uncontrollable bladder contractions. Common examples are oxybutynin chloride, propantheline, hyoscyamine, and imipramine. If you take these medications, be alert for constipation, a side effect that can make urinary incontinence worse. Other medications work by increasing the strength of the bladder outlet. This type is commonly found in over-the-counter cold medications whose active ingredients are pseudoephedrine and phenylpropnolamine.

Estrogen replacement therapy may also help. Estrogen helps the bladder and urethra to function normally and improves the strength of the pelvic muscles. Estrogen creams placed in the vagina probably provide the most immediate improvement in the urinary tract, but pills and patches are available, too. Use the medications along with a bladder training program and pelvic muscle exercises.

When bladder training, exercises, and medications are not successful, surgery is usually needed. Surgery can be performed regardless of age. The goal of surgery is to lift the bladder and urethra back to their normal position and prevent them from sagging into the vagina. The surgery does not strengthen the pelvic floor muscles, however.

Many types of surgery may be done, and the selection depends on the surgeon's experience and preference as well as factors individual to the woman. In general, 50–60 percent of women remain dry, with good bladder control, 5 years after the operation.

A new option is injection of material around the urethra to support it. A relatively minor operation compared to some other types of surgical treatment, it can be done with local anesthesia.

After treatment, try to adopt healthy habits that do not strain the muscles and bladder:

- Quit smoking.
- Get treatment for chronic respiratory conditions.
- Avoid heavy lifting when possible.
- Avoid becoming constipated.

You can prevent having urinary incontinence if you perform routine pelvic muscle exercises throughout your life. Once learned, these exercises can easily be made a part of your daily routine. They can be performed while driving, waiting in line at the grocery store, or brushing your teeth. Taking estrogen at menopause, if recommended by a doctor, can also help prevent incontinence.

KIDNEY FAILURE (RENAL FAILURE)

Acute Kidney Failure (Acute Renal Failure)

In acute renal failure the kidneys stop functioning suddenly. This almost never occurs in otherwise healthy women. The most common causes are shock due to infection, bleeding, severe dehydration, exposure to toxins, drugs, or abnormalities in the arteries in the kidneys. Acute renal failure can occur in pregnant women who have severe high blood pressure.

In some cases, acute kidney failure can be reversed if the correct diagnosis is made and the right therapy is promptly started. In other cases, kidney failure lasts for about 10 days before recovery begins. Rarely, women do not recover and develop end-stage kidney disease.

Kidney failure is usually part of a long, continuous process. The initial damage may be slight but progress until all the nephrons are damaged. Or, healthy nephrons may work harder to compensate for the damaged nephrons, and after years they become damaged from overwork. This leads to further decline in function, so a vicious cycle is established, leading to chronic renal failure.

Chronic Kidney Failure (Chronic Renal Failure)

The rate at which kidney function declines varies from person to person. In conditions like polycystic kidney

DIALYSIS—THE ARTIFICIAL KIDNEY

In dialysis, filtering that is normally done by the kidneys is done by an artificial method. There are two types: hemodialysis and peritoneal dialysis. Dialysis is started when serious or uncomfortable symptoms cannot be managed by more conservative methods. It is a chronic form of treatment. Once it is begun, it must be continued to prevent uremia. The effectiveness of dialysis usually depends on your general health and your willingness to cooperate with this chronic therapy. If you receive a kidney transplant, dialysis is no longer needed.

HEMODIALYSIS

If hemodialysis is selected, a minor operation is performed to create permanent access to the blood system. Blood can then be pumped into the dialysis machine for filtering and purification and then back to the patient. Treatments usually last 4–5 hours and are needed three times a week, but this depends on your size and other factors. Although you can be taught to perform dialysis at home, most people go to dialysis centers for treatment. (See Fig. 32.4)

The chronic and time-consuming nature of dialysis requires careful planning and scheduling and often requires you to make changes in your life. It may interfere with working unless your schedule is very

flexible. It is necessary, for example, to plan in advance for trips away from home. Usually a temporary referral to another dialysis center can be arranged.

PERITONEAL DIALYSIS

Peritoneal dialysis, sometimes called continuous ambulatory peritoneal dialysis (CAPD), also requires a point of access to the body. In this case, a catheter is placed surgically in the abdomen so sterile dialysis fluid can flow in and out. The fluid is allowed to remain there for 6–8 hours. When it is drained out, excess fluids and toxins are drained out with it. The patient needs to perform 4 such exchanges a day. (See Fig. 32.5)

This type of dialysis can be taught easily so that you can do it at home. If you live far from a dialysis center, this may be the only practical way you can receive dialysis. Because infection is a risk of this method, you must carefully follow the procedures described by your doctor. As long as you are in a clean environment, you can perform this technique at home, at work, or on vacation.

While the fluid is in the abdomen, it causes some slight abdominal distension but no discomfort. The swelling is not noticeable, and the presence of the catheter tube does not interfere with sexual activity.

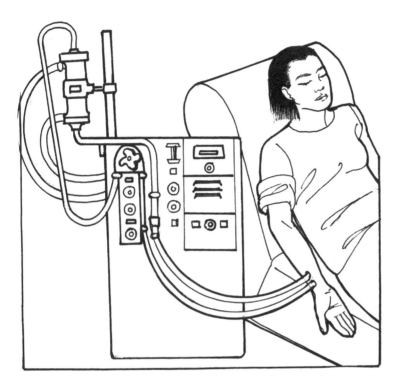

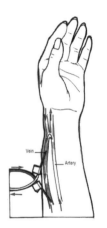

Figure 32.4 Dialysis
Dialysis allows the filtering of bodily fluids that is normally done by the kidneys to be done artificially (left). In hemodialysis, blood is pumped from an artery through a machine, where it is cleansed and then returned to the body through a vein (below). Waste products are filtered out of the blood through a membrane, while substances needed by the body remain in the blood.

disease or diabetes the process is protracted over decades. Rapid kidney failure, of months to a few years, occurs in HIV-associated kidney disease and some patients with lupus.

Women with failing kidneys usually show no symptoms until the failure is well advanced. The only signs may be high blood pressure or abnormal laboratory results if blood and urine are examined. Once the kidneys are working at only 15–20 percent of normal capacity, however, most women begin to develop symptoms. As the kidneys continue to fail, symptoms worsen and can include fatigue, increasing shortness of breath, nausea, vomiting, diarrhea, problems thinking clearly, poor memory, muscle weakness, abnormal

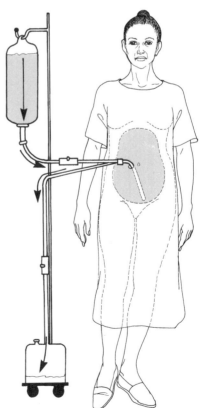

Figure 32.5 CAPD
Continuous ambulatory peritoneal dialysis (CAPD) allows the filtering of excess fluid and waste when this function cannot be done efficiently by the kidneys. Dialysis fluid flows in and out of the abdomen through a catheter that is placed surgically. The fluid must be replaced every 6-8 hours.

muscle twitching, anemia, easy bruising, itching, and bleeding from the gums, stomach, and intestines. There may also be dehydration or swelling. Menstruation can become irregular and eventually stop. Sex drive diminishes. Although conception can take place, pregnancy in patients with chronic kidney disease is very risky for the mother. Live births occur in women with renal transplants, but rarely in women treated with dialysis. Without treatment, such as dialysis or transplant, women with severe symptoms eventually develop seizures, coma and death.

Today, there are effective treatments for kidney failure, all of which require professional care with a nephrologist. If your kidneys are not functioning well, your daily fluid intake may be limited so you don't drink more fluids than your kidneys can process, and you may be asked to weigh yourself daily. Amounts of sodium and potassium in the diet are often restricted for the same reasons. If too much protein is eaten, the symptoms of uremia are worsened. The nephrologist will recommend a renal dietician to work with you to plan a diet.

Recent research suggests that early in kidney failure, medication (angiotensin-converting enzyme [ACE] inhibitors) can delay the development of kidney failure and end-stage renal disease (ESRD). The main treatments for ESRD are dialysis and transplantation (see "Dialysis—The Artificial Kidney").

End-Stage Renal Disease (ESRD)

End-stage kidney disease occurs when kidney function is so poor that a person cannot survive without aggressive treatment. The severe symptoms are known as uremia and include

- Malaise
- Fatigue and disturbed sleep
- Nausea, vomiting, and diarrhea
- Loss of appetite and sex drive
- Inability to concentrate
- Itching
- Swelling
- Shortness of breath

In more advanced cases (rarely seen today, due to early treatment), uremia causes twitching, muscle jerks, increased skin color, chest pains, seizures, bleeding and bruising, or coma. Patients with uremia appear wasted (overly thin), and their skin may be pale or yellow. Their breath smells like wine, with a distinctively bad odor. In advanced cases, the skin may be covered with a white frost, and the person may exhibit a flapping tremor when the hands are raised. Fortunately, aggressive early treatment with dialysis or a transplant can prevent these types of severe symptoms.

NEPHROTIC SYNDROME

In nephrotic syndrome, serum proteins pass into the urine because of damage to the glomerulus of the nephron. This condition, formerly known as nephrosis, is associated with swelling and abnormal laboratory test results. Along with treatment for the specific causes of nephrotic syndrome, alterations in diet can help in managing this condition. Low salt intake can help control the swelling, and the amount of protein in the diet must be increased to make up for that lost in the urine.

The most common causes of nephrotic syndrome are various forms of glomerulonephritis, diabetes, lupus, and multiple myeloma.

Diagnosis

Glomerulonephritis, or inflammation of the glomerulus, occurs when protein leaks into the urine. Red blood cells appear in the urine. Diagnosis and identification of the type of glomerulonephritis requires a kidney biopsy. In some cases, glomerulonephritis causes rapid decline in kidney function over weeks to months. This is known as rapidly progressive glomerulonephritis. Uncommon but severe, it is linked to conditions such as AIDS, other forms of glomerulonephritis, high blood pressure in pregnancy, and lupus. A kidney biopsy is nearly always needed to make a quick, accurate diagnosis. Prompt treatment is needed to prevent irreversible damage to the kidneys.

Treatment

Common types of glomerulonephritis are post-streptoccal glomerulonephritis, membranous glomeru-

TRANSPLANTATION—THE GIFT OF LIFE

The successful transplantation of a kidney restores normal function. With a transplant, a woman does not need dialysis or any restrictions to the diet.

Special tests are done prior to a transplantation to match the patient with the kidney least likely to be rejected. Blood from the donor and the patient is tested for tissue type, the presence of antibodies, and other factors that affect the likelihood of rejection.

The best match is a kidney donated by an identical twin. Women who are identical twins share the same immune systems, which makes them likely to accept each other's organs. A kidney from another family member may succeed as well, especially if both the donor and the recipient have the same tissue types. Blood-related (true) brothers or sisters are the best match after an identical twin, followed by parents or children. A living kidney donor must have two normal kidneys (since only one healthy kidney is needed by the body) and be in good health, with no signs of disease, psychological problems, or infection. If no match is available in the family, a kidney from an unrelated, deceased donor (cadaver donor) can be used. Cadaver donation is the most common form.

The body's immune system responds to a transplanted organ as it would to any foreign material. It would destroy the new kidney if there were not some way to suppress the immune system. To do this, medications must be taken that suppress the immune system enough to prevent rejection of the organ, but not completely. Complete suppression of the immune system would leave the person open to disease. Those taking immunosuppressive drugs are more likely to have problems with infection since the immune system is less able to fight off the invader.

Your nephrologist will help you select a transplant center. The center should do at least 40 kidney transplants each year. The United Network of Organ Sharing (see "Where to Get More Information") can help provide assistance.

Some people are not candidates for a transplant. They include those who:

- Are unable to tolerate the operation
- Have an infection that cannot be treated
- Are infected with HIV or have AIDS
- Are likely to have recurrent kidney disease in the transplanted kidney
- Are unable to take the needed immunosuppressive medication
- Have incurable cancers
- Have debilitating diseases that severely limit their life expectancy
- Have severe, disabling psychiatric disease

lonephritis, minimal change disease, and focal glomerulosclerosis (FGS). Post-streptoccal glomerulonephritis can follow a strep sore throat or skin infection. Once thought to be a disease of children, it is now diagnosed in adults and the elderly. Membranous glomerulonephritis does not usually cause microscopic blood in the urine, but it can still cause protein to be lost in the urine and nephrotic syndrome to occur. A kidney biopsy can distinguish this condition from minimal change disease. Membranous glomerulonephritis may be treated with steroids or immunosuppression. These therapies help reduce the amount of protein passed in the urine and prevent kidney failure from occurring. However, up to 40 percent of people with this condition improve even without treatment. If no other cause is found, membranous glomerulonephritis may be linked with cancer, such as lung cancer or cancer of the stomach or intestines. Focal glomerulo-

nephritis is one of the most common causes of glomerulonephritis, and it is increasing in frequency. It responds poorly to treatment with immunosuppression, and renal failure generally occurs after some years. FGS behaves differently in patients with HIV, being associated with rapidly developing renal failure.

Those who have swelling, abnormal amounts of protein in their urine, and nephrotic syndrome have minimal change disease if a standard kidney biopsy appears to be normal. When the same kidney tissue sampled is examined under an electron microscope, changes are seen. This condition also can be treated with steroids or immunosuppressants. While it sometimes disappears without treatment, it may recur even after successful therapy. Although repeated treatment may be meeded, it rarely leads to kidney failure. Sometimes, minimal change disease is linked to lymphomas.

INHERITED KIDNEY DISEASE

The most common type of inherited kidney disease is autosomal dominant polycystic kidney disease (ADP-KD). In this condition, one parent affected with the condition passes it to his or her children. This condition rarely develops without an affected parent. Men and women are equally affected.

With this polycystic kidney disease, the kidneys are a normal size at birth; then they begin to expand due to multiple cysts (fluid-filled sacs) developing in both organs. (See Fig. 32.6) The cysts grow, multiply, and eventually replace healthy kidney tissue. As the number and size of the cysts grows, kidney function declines. Cysts also may appear in other organs, such as the liver, spleen, and uterus. These other cysts rarely cause symptoms or affect body function.

Symptoms

Some with this condition do not have symptoms, and they can expect a normal life span. Others will eventually have kidney failure. Symptoms occur at different times in various people; many do not need dialysis to support their kidneys until they are around 55 years of age. The age of onset of symptoms is usually similar within families.

When symptoms do occur, the most common ones are back and abdominal pain, bloody urine, recurrent urinary tract infections, high blood pressure, or kidney stones. ADPKD is also associated with weakness in the wall of the blood vessels in the brain called cerebral aneurysm. If these aneurysms rupture, it is life-threatening and can be fatal. However, with special X-ray studies, aneurysms usually can be detected before rupture occurs.

Diagnosis

Diagnosis of ADPKD usually depends on detection of the cysts in those who have a family history of the disease. In adults, the enlarged kidneys can be felt on physical exam; other, nonsurgical methods of detection, such as ultrasound, can also detect them. If an

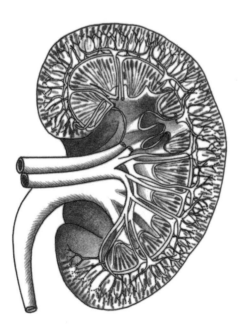
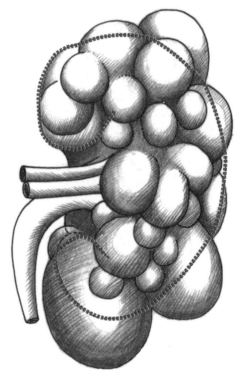

Figure 32.6 Polycystic Kidney Disease
In polycystic kidney disease, the kidneys are normal at birth (left); but as the individual grows older, they begin to become enlarged and deformed (right) with fluid-filled sacs, or cysts, that begin to multiply and eventually replace healthy tissue in the kidney.

ultrasound is done after the age of 30 and cysts are absent, ADPKD is not present. Genetic testing is available to detect the disease even before cysts begin forming, if blood can be obtained from a family member with the disease.

Treatment

People with autosomal dominant polycystic kidney disease should be alert to medical problems, such as high blood pressure and urinary tract infections, that can go along with the disorder and make it worse. Aggressive treatment of these other medical problems may slow the decline in kidney function. Bleeding into the cysts can occur and can be painful. The pain should be treated with painkillers.

Since autosomal dominant polycystic kidney disease is a genetic condition, it can be passed on by either parent to the children. If you have this condition or you have a family history of it, you may want to have genetic counseling (see Chapter 14).

TUMORS OF THE URINARY SYSTEM

Kidney Tumors

Tumors, or growths, on the kidney can be cystic (fluid-filled) or solid, cancerous or noncancerous. Most kidney tumors do not cause symptoms. When they do, blood may appear in the urine.

Kidney tumors are detected by imaging techniques that allow examining the kidney without surgery. Several examinations may be needed to determine the size of the tumor and whether it has spread outside the kidney or not.

Although a kidney tumor is serious, it can be treated. When a tumor is suspected of being a cancer, the whole kidney can be removed by surgery. (You can live a normal life with just one kidney.) Chemotherapy may be required. With the increased use of imaging techniques today, many kidney tumors are discovered when they are small and have not yet caused symptoms.

Bladder Tumors

Bladder tumors often cause symptoms of urinary frequency or urgency. There also may be visible blood in the urine or blood seen during a microscopic examination of the urine. Most bladder tumors are cancerous; usually they can be easily treated if caught in time. Smoking increases the risk of bladder cancer, sometimes for years after the habit has been stopped.

Most bladder cancers grow from the lining of the bladder and not below the surface of the bladder. These tumors can be treated through a cystoscope; once inserted into the bladder, this small instrument scrapes the tumor off the lining of the bladder. Unfortunately, bladder cancers tend to recur, either at a different place on the bladder lining or along the ureters or in the kidneys. Long-term follow-up care is needed to be sure the cancer has not reappeared. When new tumors are detected early, continued scraping of the bladder lining eventually cures the cancer. If tumors recur often, medication to prevent this can be placed in the bladder through a catheter tube.

If tumors have grown into the wall of the bladder, additional treatment is needed. This may include partial or total removal of the bladder, radiation, or chemotherapy.

SYSTEMIC DISORDERS

Systemic disorders affect the body as a whole. Some have a particular effect on the kidneys and urinary tract. They include diabetes, high blood pressure, sickle cell disease, lupus, and sexually transmitted diseases.

Diabetes Mellitus

Diabetes is a complex metabolic disorder in which the body cannot process glucose. Normally, the pancreas produces insulin to help with the utilization of dietary sugars. If it does not produce enough insulin or if the insulin is ineffective, levels of sugar in the blood increase. Some need insulin injections to keep their blood sugar levels stable, while others can control them by diet, exercise, and pills.

Diabetes also affects other organs such as the heart, brain, nerves, eyes, bladder, and kidneys. Women with diabetes who must take insulin have a substantial risk of developing kidney disease, usually 15–20 years after diabetes starts.

Kidney disease in people with diabetes usually results from the high blood glucose level, causing the nephrons to work too hard (hyperfiltration). Later, increased amounts of protein appear in the urine, and in time the kidneys lose the ability to function. Eventually, kidney failure occurs. In fact, kidney disease due to diabetes is one of the most common causes of end-stage renal disease. Diabetics are also much more likely to have other problems with the urinary system, such as urinary tract infections. Additionally, they may have high blood pressure, poor vision, and heart disease.

Keeping blood glucose at a normal level can help prevent damage to the kidneys as well as other organs. Diabetics can help prevent problems by seeking early care from a specialist, following their doctor's recommendations, and being alert to symptoms and infections. Because women with diabetes often have hypertension, lowering the blood pressure is very important. Taking medications such as ACE inhibitors may delay the development of ESRD, as these medications prevent the kidneys from working too hard and losing their ability to function.

Although dialysis or transplantation can correct many of the complications of kidney failure caused by diabetes, neither can prevent the effects of diabetes on other organs. A transplant may help with kidney function, but diabetes will recur in the transplanted kidney. Pancreas transplants are now in an early stage of development. Successful pancreas transplants remove the need for insulin injections and eliminate the complications of diabetes in other organs.

High Blood Pressure

Kidney disease is often associated with high blood pressure. Diseases of the kidney, such as renal artery stenosis and glomerulonephritis, can cause high blood pressure. Conversely, high blood pressure itself can cause ongoing kidney damage. Detection and treatment of high blood pressure, which may have no symp-

toms in its early phases, can prevent kidney damage and preserve kidney function.

Sickle Cell Disease

Sickle cell disease is an inherited condition that predominantly affects African-Americans. It also can occur in people of Mediterranean descent. It occurs in two forms, SA (sickle cell trait) and SS (sickle cell disease). SS disease tends to be more severe but less common. Sickle cell disease results when a component of the red blood cells, hemoglobin, is formed abnormally. This causes the red blood cells to curve or "sickle." Sickled cells may block the blood vessels, prevent normal blood circulation, and cause great pain. If the sickled cells become lodged inside the kidneys, they can damage kidney function.

Sickle cell disease can produce severe bleeding in the kidneys, due to the poor blood supply, as well as death of kidney tissue. Glomerulonephritis may also occur, or pieces of kidney tissue may actually break off and be passed like a stone (see Chapter 29).

Lupus

Systemic lupus erythematosus, or lupus, is more common in women than in men. In this autoimmune disease, the body forms antibodies against its own tissues. It can affect many organs in the body, including the kidneys.

Diagnosis of kidney problems in a woman who has lupus begins with examination of a urine sample. The urine can be completely normal, or there can be protein or red blood cells in it. (Even if a woman has no symptoms and her urine tests are normal, a kidney biopsy can find mild changes.)

There are several types of kidney disease in lupus. Its mildest form may show up as only minimal change in the patient's urinalysis, and is rarely progressive. Some lupus patients develop nephrotic syndrome, and hypertension is common. In its most dangerous form, kidney disease due to lupus causes kidney damage at an accelerated rate.

The treatment of lupus with kidney involvement is complex, often requiring treatment with intravenous steroids and immunosuppressants. Results are variable, so treatment should be started early by an experienced nephrologist (see also Chapters 31 and 34).

Sexually Transmitted Diseases

Sexually transmitted diseases (STDs) are infections passed on during sexual intercourse. Some STDs affect the kidneys.

Syphilis

Syphilis has existed for a long time. As with many other STDs, its rates of infection have increased dramatically, especially among African-American women.

Syphilis is caused by infection with an organism known as Treponema pallidum. Its early effects include painless sores around the genitals, fever, sore throat, headache, and a rash. If it is not treated, it can affect many body systems, including the kidneys. When the immune system tries to fight off syphilis, the nephrotic syndrome may result. All patients with the nephrotic syndrome should be tested for both syphilis and HIV. Syphilis can be treated with penicillin (see Chapter 19).

HIV and AIDS

Infection with human immunodeficiency virus (HIV) usually leads to AIDS, which is a fatal disease, months to years later. Some people infected with HIV develop kidney problems such as nephrotic syndrome or kidney failure. When HIV causes the nephrotic syndrome, it is often associated with focal glomerulonephritis, which in turn tends to cause a rapid form of renal failure. A kidney biopsy can identify this problem.

An infected woman who has kidney failure but has not yet developed AIDS may be a candidate for dialysis. Some women with HIV are well enough so that dialysis can be performed at home, and some who are otherwise well can continue on dialysis for years.

Unfortunately, AIDS-associated kidney disease is more severe and harder to treat than other causes. Uremia usually develops in 3–6 months. General treatment depends largely on the woman's health. If her condition is fairly stable and her quality of life is acceptable to her, she may wish to use dialysis. When AIDS is very advanced, a woman's quality of life is poor and dialysis is unlikely to prolong her life.

Receiving a kidney transplant is not an option for a woman who has either HIV infection or AIDS. Transplantation requires suppressing the immune system so that the kidney is not rejected. This is too risky in someone whose immune system already functions poorly (see also Chapter 20 and Chapter 31).

PREGNANCY AND THE URINARY TRACT

Although some changes in kidney function normally happen throughout a woman's menstrual cycle—such as premenstrual bloating from fluid retention—the major concern is pregnancy. Many of the changes in the body during pregnancy can affect the kidneys and the rest of the urinary tract. Some of these changes are normal, but others bear careful watching and may require treatment.

Normal Pregnancy

During pregnancy,, your body must produce enough blood to circulate through your own body and also that of the fetus. To do this, the kidneys must work harder and increase in size, and there is salt and water retention due to hormonal changes. Blood pressure frequently drops slightly in the first trimester of pregnancy and goes back to normal closer to the time of the infant's birth.

The effects of hormones produced in pregnancy and the growing fetus cause the ureters to expand and remain that way for up to 4 months after the baby is born. Although this is a normal development, it can be mistaken for hydronephrosis—a sign of urinary obstruction in women who are not pregnant.

As the uterus grows in pregnancy, it puts pressure on the bladder. For this reason, early in the pregnancy you feel the need to urinate more often. As pregnancy progresses and the uterus sits higher in the abdomen, the pressure on the bladder is eased slightly.

Gradual swelling of the extremities due to fluid retention often occurs in pregnancy, particularly in the last trimester. You may need to buy larger shoes or find that your rings are too tight. This usually disappears soon after the baby is born. Minor swelling is not usually a concern, but swelling that causes substantial weight gain of more than 1 pound per week or rising blood pressure is dangerous and should be treated.

Urinary Tract Conditions in Pregnancy

Some conditions that affect the urinary tract are more common in pregnancy. Others can affect the pregnancy and endanger the fetus if they are not carefully monitored and treated.

Urinary Tract Infections

Women are at greater risk for developing a urinary tract infection when they are pregnant. Even if you have never had such an infection before, you may develop one when pregnant. The exact reason for this is unknown, but it is thought that hormonal changes and the effect of the uterus pressing on the urinary tract are responsible.

If a urinary tract infection in pregnancy goes untreated, it can cause several problems, including severe infection, premature labor, and fetal death. For this reason, visits to an obstetrician include tests for detecting urinary tract infections. If infection does occur, it should be treated promptly with antibiotics.

High Blood Pressure

Normally, blood pressure drops somewhat in pregnancy. If blood pressure rises instead, it causes risks for the woman and fetus alike. In fact, high blood pressure is the second largest cause of maternal deaths in pregnancy. The fetus may be born too early, may be too small, or may be stillborn. Proper care of high blood pressure in pregnancy is essential.

If you had high blood pressure before you became pregnant, you need special care by both an obstetrician specializing in high-risk care and a hypertension specialist. Some medications used for treating blood pressure can harm the fetus, and so treatment should be selected carefully. For example, ACE inhibitors should not be used by pregnant women. If you suffer from mild hypertension, you may find the dip in blood pressure early in pregnancy beneficial. Your doctor may be able to taper off your medication, but careful monitoring is still required. Blood pressure may rise late in pregnancy and require treatment again.

High blood pressure can occur in pregnancy even if a woman did not have it before. Pregnancy-induced hypertension, preeclampsia and eclampsia, is more likely to occur in:

- Women with kidney disease
- Women with a family history of the condition

- Older women who have not had children before
- Teenagers who are pregnant
- Women carrying twins
- Women with an immune system disorder, such as lupus

When pregnant women with high blood pressure excrete too much protein in their urine, particularly in the latter half of pregnancy, it is called preeclampsia. A woman with preeclampsia can develop kidney failure, bleeding, and a complication called eclampsia, in which the brain is affected and seizures occur. This is very dangerous and may cause death.

If blood pressure reaches dangerous levels late in pregnancy, when the fetus is mature and healthy enough to live on its own, prompt delivery of the baby can save both mother and child. When blood pressure increases earlier in pregnancy, before the fetus can survive on its own, treatment depends on how high the blood pressure is. Small increases can generally be monitored by the doctor without treatment. More severe increases may need to be treated with antihypertensive drugs. If the increase is very high, the baby may have to be delivered to save the mother's life.

After delivery, a woman's blood pressure usually returns to normal. In some hypertensive women, however, it may remain high, requiring drugs. Since antihypertensive medication is excreted in breast milk, breast-feeding may not be possible.

Pregnancy in Women with Kidney Disease

It is not always clear how the added stress of pregnancy may affect the kidneys in a woman whose kidneys are already functioning poorly. It depends on the type and extent of the kidney disease, as well as how poorly the kidneys are working. Women with mild kidney disease generally do well and are not likely to have long-term problems. Still, all women with kidney disease who become pregnant should be treated by both a nephrologist and an obstetrician specializing in high-risk pregnancies.

Most women with some degree of kidney failure have an increased risk of high blood pressure, preeclampsia, and eclampsia if they become pregnant. Women with lupus or diabetes are prone to kidney problems during pregnancy. Some moderate kidney problems can worsen if the woman becomes pregnant.

Women with severe kidney failure may find it difficult to become pregnant. If they do conceive, their pregnancies can be risky, and usually result in a premature birth. Women who are on dialysis may be able to become pregnant but require almost daily dialysis.

Commonly, the pregnancy ends in miscarriage. For these reasons, women with severe kidney conditions are usually discouraged from becoming pregnant.

On the other hand, pregnant women who have had a kidney transplant often do quite well. However, they require special care involving the transplant team and the obstetrician.

DIAGNOSTIC TECHNIQUES FOR URINARY PROBLEMS

History and Physical Exam

As with other conditions, the diagnosis of a disorder of the urinary system begins with the doctor or nurse taking your medical history and performing a physical exam. Be prepared to describe your family history, your symptoms, previous urinary tract conditions, type of diet, and so on. You may find it helpful to keep a diary of when symptoms occur and what seems to provoke them. The physical exam allows the doctor or nurse to check the strength of the pelvic floor muscles.

Usually the doctor's diagnosis is based on the results of the history, the physical exam, and specific tests. Laboratory tests, biopsies (taking samples of tissue for study), and special imaging methods for looking at the kidneys and the bladder are used.

Urinalysis

Urinalysis is the most basic test performed. It involves obtaining a clean specimen of urine and can provide much information about the function of the kidneys and bladder.

A clean specimen cannot be contaminated with blood or other substances from the vagina. Providing a clean catch urine specimen requires you to follow these four steps:

1. Wash your hands.
2. Hold your labia (lips surrounding the vagina) open and clean the area with an antiseptic towelette.
3. Void the first part of the urine stream into the toilet.
4. Catch part of the rest of the flow into a sterile cup.

If you are menstruating, you should insert a tampon into the vagina before following the steps for providing a urine specimen. Alternatively, a clean urine sample

can be obtained by catheterization. A doctor or nurse places a thin tube called a catheter through the urethra up into the bladder. A sample is obtained, and the tube is withdrawn. Catheterization is a simple but not routine way of obtaining urine.

A clean sample of urine is necessary for many tests. Laboratory tests for electrolytes and other substances normally in the urine can provide much information about how well the kidneys are working. Other tests that may be done include:

- Chemical testing for sugar, protein, blood, bacteria, and pH (acidity)
- Examination under a microscope for red blood cells (a sign of bleeding) or white blood cells and bacteria (a sign of infection)

Urine Culture

In a urine culture, a portion of the clean sample is poured on a culture plate or the plate is dipped into the sample. After allowing time for growth of the bacteria, the colonies on the plate are counted. A significant colony count denotes infection. The infecting bacteria are tested for sensitivity to a number of antibiotics, so the appropriate medication can be chosen.

Kidney Biopsy

In a biopsy, a small sample of tissue is taken from the kidney for study. With many conditions, this is the only way to make a diagnosis. In most women, a biopsy is a fairly simple procedure that can be done with local anesthesia by a nephrologist. Kidney ultrasound is used to verify the exact location of the biopsy site, and a small sample is withdrawn through a needle. The kidney tissue is looked at under several different kinds of microscopes. This provides the most accurate description of the kidney's anatomy.

The amount of tissue taken for a biopsy is so small that it does not affect the kidney's function. After a biopsy, you may have microscopic blood in your urine for a few days afterward. The risks of the procedure are low when performed by an experienced nephrologist, and biopsies are usually safe even for older women. However, complications can occur, including severe bleeding, infection, and even loss of the kidney. For safety, the nephrologist performs blood and urine tests and scans before the biopsy. After having a biopsy, you should rest for a day and avoid strenuous activity and exercise for about 2 weeks.

Imaging Techniques

There are different techniques currently available to determine the anatomy and function of the kidney. Your physician will select the imaging technique based on the information needed in your situation.

Intravenous Pyelography

Pyelography creates a picture of the kidneys and ureters. A special dye that shows up on the X-ray is injected into a vein. The dye filters through the kidneys and is excreted into the ureters and the bladder. This allows detection of kidney stones, infection, tumors, and obstructions.

This test is not done in women allergic to the dye used in these studies or in pregnant women.

Ultrasound

Ultrasound is the use of sound waves to create a picture of an organ or area of body. A small device called a transducer is rubbed over the outside of the body near the area to be studied. Sound waves bounce off the organ or area and form a picture that is displayed on a monitor. Ultrasound can be used to examine the kidney, ureters, and bladder.

Ultrasound can be used by persons who cannot tolerate the dye in pyelography. The sound waves do not harm a fetus, so ultrasound is safely used in pregnancy.

Computerized Axial Tomography

A computerized axial tomography, or CT, scan is a type of X-ray that can create a picture of the abdominal organs, including the kidneys, ureters, and bladder. It is effective in showing tumors, stones, and some problems with blood vessels.

The best pictures result when a woman having a CT scan both ingests special material that appears on the picture and has similar material injected. However, in women with kidney failure, especially those with diabetes, the injection often worsens function and is not recommended. Pregnant women should avoid CT scans because of the risk to the fetus.

Magnetic Resonance Imaging

Magnetic resonance imaging, or MRI, uses magnetic waves instead of special contrast material to create a picture. Although safe for most women, it is usually reserved for those who cannot use CT. In some kidney conditions, MRI will produce a better picture of soft tissue than CT.

Cystoscopy

During cystoscopy, the inside of the bladder is examined with a small, telescopelike instrument that is passed through the urethra into the bladder. The exam is done with local anesthesia, and most women tolerate it well. Because a woman's urethra is shorter than a man's, she is likely to find this examination more comfortable than a man would. When the inside of the urethra is examined at the same time, this is referred to as cystourethroscopy. Cystoscopy and cystourethroscopy can detect many problems in the urinary tract, including tumors, obstructions, and fistulas. Fistulas are small openings in the bladder, ureters, or urethra that allow urine to leak out.

Urodynamics

Urodynamics is the study of how the bladder functions. One type of urodynamics is cystometry, the study of how the bladder's pressure is affected by the amount of urine it contains. At its most basic, cystometry involves placing a catheter up the urethra into the bladder. Sterile saline solution (salt water) is instilled into the bladder through the catheter to mimic the effect of urine in the bladder. Special equipment measures the pressure changes in the bladder as it fills.

This test can give information about the bladder's capacity. Normal bladder capacity is about one pint. If a woman's bladder does not hold enough urine, she is at risk for urinary incontinence or infection.

The main use for this test, though, is to measure how the bladder and the urethra react to different volumes of fluid. Measurements of their ability to stretch and contract can be made. If these measurements are made while a woman coughs, jumps, or squats, it provides an idea of how well the system performs under stress. This technique is important in evaluating urinary incontinence.

WHERE TO GET MORE INFORMATION

Many conditions affecting the urinary tract can be long-term chronic problems. Fortunately, many groups can provide both information and support:

- **The Interstitial Cystitis Association,** established by women who have this condition, has been an important influence in increasing the amount of research money dedicated to discovering a cause and cure for this often-debilitating problem. For more information, contact the Interstitial Cystitis Association, PO Box 1553, Madison Square Station, New York, NY 10159; 800-422-1626.

- **Help for Incontinent People (HIP), Inc.,** and **The Simon Foundation** provide help to women who have problems with bladder control. Contact Help for Incontinent People, Inc., PO Box 544, Union, S.C. 29379; 800-BLADDER (800-252-3337). Contact the Simon Foundation, PO Box 835, Wilmette, IL. 60091; 800-23SIMON (800-237-4666).

- **National Kidney Foundation** supports kidney research and works as an advocate for people with kidney disease. It produces educational booklets, sponsors meetings, and provides support groups for patients and their families. Contact the National Kidney Foundation, 30 East 33rd Street, New York, NY 10016; 800-622-9010.

- **United Network of Organ Sharing** oversees all donations of organs and organ transplants. It also establishes and enforces regulations to ensure equality in organ transplantation and fairness in distribution of donor organs. Call 804-330-8500.

Books are another good source for information. Except as noted, many of these books can be found at a local library:

- Rebecca Chalker and Kristine E. Whitmore, *Overcoming Bladder Disorders* (New York: Harper and Row, 1990).

- Kathryn L. Burgio, K. Lynette Peace, and Angelo J. Lucio, *Staying Dry—A Guide to Bladder Control* (Baltimore, MD.: Johns Hopkins University Press, 1989).

- Katherine Jeter, Nancy Faller, and Christine Norton, *Nursing for Incontinence* (Philadelphia, PA: Harcourt Brace Jovanovich, 1990).

- Pauline E. Chiarelli, *Women's Waterworks—Curing Incontinence* is available from Help for Incontinent People.

- Lisa Delaney with Cemela Longon, *Managing Urinary Incontinence: A Patient's Guide* can be requested from the Agency for Health Care Policy and Research by calling 800-358-9295.

CHAPTER 33

The Digestive System

Susan Cobb Stewart, M.D., F.A.C.P.

The act of consuming and digesting food may appear simple, but it's actually a complex process that involves a number of finely coordinated chemical and mechanical reactions of the upper and lower gastrointestinal tract. The digestive system consists of many organs that are connected to each other, so our very survival depends on the smooth functioning of each component. It's easy to see why our entire outlook on life changes when some element of the system goes awry.

STRUCTURE AND FUNCTION

Each part of the gastrointestinal system has its own role to play in the digestion and absorption of food and the elimination of waste. (See Fig. 33.1) The major organs are the following:

- *The esophagus*, a muscular tube that connects the bottom of the throat (pharynx) with the stomach.

- *The stomach*, a pear-shaped, muscular organ situated mostly on the left-hand side below the ribs. The stomach is lined with special cells that produce acid and digestive enzymes that break down food.

- *The small intestine*, which in an adult is about 22 feet long. It consists of the *duodenum*, a short portion immediately beyond the stomach that is the place of entry for ducts coming from the liver and pancreas; the *jejunum*, the long portion of the small intestine that follows the duodenum and is lined with specialized cells that assist in diluting, digesting, and absorbing nutrients; and the *ileum*, the long portion of the small intestine that follows the jejunum and is primarily involved in absorbing nutrients and water.

- *The large intestine*, which receives all the undigested food, water, and other intestinal waste. It includes the *cecum* (where the appendix is located), which is part of the *colon*, the final 6 feet of bowel. The colon extracts much of the water from the contents of the stomach and transforms the liquid mass into solid waste, or feces. The waste material is eliminated through the *rectum*—the last 8 inches of the colon—and the *anus*, a muscular tube containing the sphincter muscles that control elimination.

- *The liver*, a large organ located in the upper right side of the abdomen, has multiple functions: it manufactures bile to digest fat, processes nutrients absorbed from the intestine, and extracts and eliminates drugs and toxins.

- *The gallbladder* is a small, pouchlike structure that is linked by ducts to both the liver and the duodenum. The main function of the gallbladder is to store bile from the liver.

- *The pancreas*, a glandular organ that branches off the intestinal tract and contains cells that

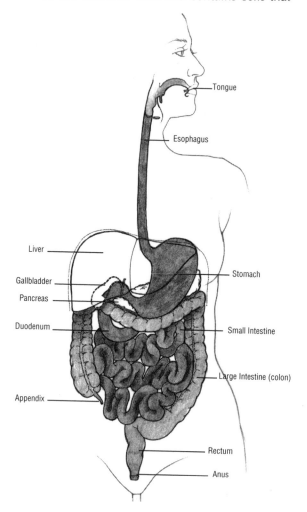

Figure 33.1 Anatomy of the Digestive System

make enzymes to digest fat, protein, and carbohydrate from consumed food. Two important hormones are produced by the pancreas, insulin and glucagon. Each is essential in the metabolism of carbohydrates.

How the Digestive System Works

Digestion begins in the mouth, where food is chewed and mixed with saliva, which contains enzymes and fluid that break down the food and make it easier to swallow. The semisolid food mass then passes down the esophagus into the stomach. The stomach responds by secreting hydrochloric acid and a protein-digesting enzyme called pepsin for a period of 3 to 4 hours. The stomach muscles mix the food with the secretions, breaking it down further. The stomach then releases small amounts of the food, now liquid containing fine particles, into the duodenum.

The presence of fat in the duodenum initiates the release of secretin, a gastrointestinal hormone that slows down the muscular activity of the stomach and causes the food to be retained in the stomach until adequate digestive enzymes are available to break down the fat. Cells in the wall of the duodenum, sensing the composition of the food, also secrete cholecystokinin, another hormone that, together with secretin,

stimulates the liver and pancreas to release digestive enzymes and bile. Complex molecules of carbohydrate, fat, and protein are then broken down into sugars, simple fats, and amino acids that are absorbed through the cells lining the jejunum.

The ileum, the last part of the small intestine, absorbs the fluids and bile acids so these chemicals can be returned to the liver and reused. By the time the food is ready to pass into the large intestine, almost all of its nutrients have been absorbed.

The role of the large intestine is to process the undigested food, fiber, and water coming from the small intestine. This liquid, called chyme, enters the colon and is dehydrated by the colon cells. Mucus from those cells and bacteria that inhabit the colon are added to the chyme. (The bacteria break down some of the dietary fiber that is not digested by the stomach or small intestine.) As the liquid mass moves across and down the colon, it becomes progressively more solid and turns into what we call *feces* or stool.

The reflex to defecate, or get rid of the feces, is initiated by the entry of stool into the rectum. Once the brain is signaled, the internal sphincter muscles relax. The brain retains control over the external sphincter, however, and ultimately makes the decision whether defecation takes place. The defecation reflex can also be signaled by the entry of food into the stomach; this is known as the gastrocolic reflex.

COMMON DIGESTIVE SYMPTOMS

We all occasionally develop minor digestive problems that are self-limiting in nature and usually clear up with time. If the symptoms persist, consult a physician.

Gastrointestinal Pain

Stomach ache is probably the single most frequent reason for consulting a doctor. But the stomach is the culprit in only a small percentage of cases. Because the gastrointestinal tract shares the abdominal cavity with organs of other systems, the pain could be originating from the spleen (left upper quadrant), the kidneys (midabdomen), the bladder (lower abdomen), or the reproductive organs—the ovaries, fallopian tubes, and uterus—(lower abdomen). (See Fig. 33.2)

Nausea and Vomiting

From time to time everyone experiences a queasy feeling in the pit of the stomach—nausea—and the forceful and uncontrolled expelling, or vomiting, of food. Centers in the brain coordinate the following events: nausea is felt in the back of the throat, the chest, or the upper abdomen; the salivary glands are stimulated to release saliva; the sphincters in the esophagus relax and the pyloric sphincter contracts; the muscles of the stomach contract violently and force the contents of the stomach up the esophagus and out the mouth.

The vomiting reflex is a complex reaction that can be initiated by a variety of causes. The stimuli from the brain may be psychological, such as a terrible sight or smell. Or there may be direct stimulation from the bal-

Figure 33.2   Sources of Abdominal Pain

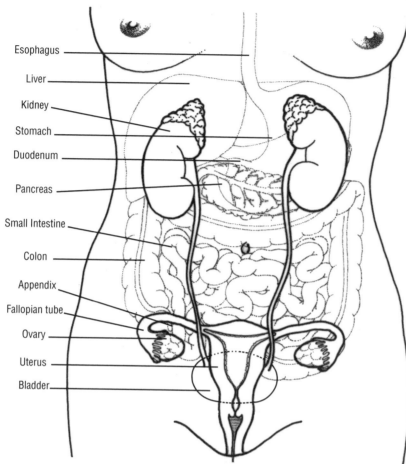

Esophagus

Liver

Kidney

Stomach

Duodenum

Pancreas

Small Intestine

Colon

Appendix

Fallopian tube

Ovary

Uterus

Bladder

Upper abdominal pain: Pain coming from the lower esophagus, the stomach, the duodenum, and the pancreas is usually felt in the mid portion of the upper abdomen. Gallbladder pain is felt on the right side and sometimes radiates around to the back. Pain from the spleen is on the left side. Kidney pain is sometimes felt in the upper abdomen but more often localizes to the back just below the lowest ribs.

Midabdominal pain: Pain from the small intestine is felt around the navel, called "periumbilical." It is often due to distention of bowel loops by gas, either from food eaten or because there is a blockage of the bowel, often caused by adhesions formed after surgery. Pain from a kidney stone in the ureter can be felt here and radiates down toward the vulva.

Lower abdominal pain: Distention and inflammation of the colon are felt in the lower abdomen, even though parts of the colon are located in the upper and mid portions of the abdomen. Appendicitis is felt in the right lower abdomen; diverticulitis on the left. In women, pain from the ovary or the fallopian tube is located on left or right; pain from the uterus or the bladder in the middle of the lower abdomen.

ance centers of the inner ear, as occurs in motion sickness. Other causes are the morning sickness of pregnancy, irritation of the stomach by an infectious agent or a chemical irritant such as alcohol, and stimulation of the back of the throat, which induces gagging and, perhaps, vomiting. More serious reasons for vomiting are an inflammation of an organ adjacent to the stomach, such as the pancreas or gallbladder, blockage of the outlet of the stomach (the pylorus), and a blockage of the intestine, usually from a tumor.

Vomiting must be distinguished from *regurgitation*, which is the sudden reflux of recently ingested food to the mouth without accompanying nausea or any particular cause. Regurgitation also can occur when there is blockage of the esophagus, usually by a stricture or

a tumor. In this situation, the food cannot enter the stomach and simply comes back up. The syndrome of reflux esophagitis, in which the sphincter between the stomach and the esophagus is incompetent, also causes regurgitation. Another type of regurgitation, called rumination, is common to the digestive processes of cattle and related animals, and has been described in some people. Rumination is the regurgitation of partially digested food, which is then chewed and reswallowed. Finally, people suffering from the eating disorders anorexia nervosa and/or bulimia often rid themselves of unwanted consumed food by inducing vomiting or learning how to periodically regurgiate food from the stomach.

Important symptoms, when medical attention

should be sought, include severe and persistent vomiting, vomiting blood, and vomiting accompanied by persistent abdominal pain.

Heartburn and Indigestion

Most people have experienced heartburn at some time in their lives, and women may experience it frequently

WHERE DOES IT HURT?

If you experience a pain in your abdominal area, it helps in the diagnosis to know the specific area of distress and the organ that may be causing it.

Upper abdomen: Lower esophagus, stomach, duodenum, liver, gallbladder, pancreas, spleen, kidney

Mid-abdomen: Small intestine

Lower abdomen: Colon, appendix (right side), ovaries (both sides), fallopian tubes, uterus, and bladder (center)

General, diffuse pain all over the abdomen usually reflects the distention of multiple organs—stomach, small intestine, large intestine—or irritation of the peritoneum, the lining of the abdominal cavity. It is also important to take note of the characteristics of the pain, which will help your doctor narrow down the diagnostic possibilities and determine which tests should be performed. Pay special attention to the following aspects of the pain:

- *Location.* Is the pain in the upper, middle, or lower abdomen? Or is it general and diffuse, over the abdominal area? Does the pain stay in the same area, or does it shoot to another location?

- *Type.* Is the pain sharp or a deep, dull ache? How severe is it?

- *Timing.* Does the pain occur at night only, or during the day? How often? Was it sudden, or did it develop gradually?

- *Relationship to meals.* Is the pain better after eating, or worse? Does it occur on an empty stomach? After eating certain foods?

- *Response to treatment.* Are there medications that seem to alleviate the pain?

- *Relationship to stress.* Does the pain occur after an emotional upset or a difficult day?

in pregnancy. Heartburn is a burning sensation that arises behind the breastbone. A component of indigestion, heartburn is caused by the reflux of stomach acid into the esophagus and usually occurs after a heavy meal.

The general discomfort that can occur after eating is called indigestion, or dyspepsia. Symptoms include a gnawing discomfort in the upper abdomen, bloating, nausea, and gas. Some people experience chronic indigestion, but in most cases it is a benign disorder and disappears on its own. The causes of indigestion include eating too fast or too heavily, and stress. You may get relief by modifying your diet, stopping smoking, eating more regular, smaller meals, and reducing the stress in your life. Avoid drinking caffeinated beverages or too much alcohol, and taking excessive amounts of aspirin, which can cause irritation of the stomach lining.

Important symptoms, when you should seek the attention of a physician, include persistent indigestion, and severe stomach pain that lasts for a few hours or wakes you up at night.

Lower Intestinal Problems: Diarrhea, Bloating, and Constipation

Diarrhea is defined as any change in bowel habit that involves an increase in frequency or a change in consistency of the stool from solid to loose. Diarrhea can be the result of an infection or irritation in the intestines, the ingestion of a nonabsorbable substance that forces the intestine to hold extra water (lactose intolerance), or a disease in the bowel itself. The characteristics most important to note are frequency of bowel movements, duration of the diarrhea, and whether it is accompanied by vomiting, fever, pain, or bleeding. If you suffer from acute diarrhea, make sure you replace the lost fluids to avoid dehydration.

Constipation refers to a change in bowel habit that results in less frequent, harder stools. It is most commonly caused by a diet inadequate in fiber or a disruption of regular diet or routine. Chronic constipation may be due to poor diet, dehydration, certain medications, stress, or the pressure of other activities that force you to ignore the urge to evacuate the bowel. Avoid excessive use of laxatives, which may lead to a dependence on the medication. Exercise, eating lots of fruits and vegetables, adequate water intake, and fiber in the diet usually improve bowel function.

Bloating is an occasional enlargement of the abdomen, usually due to excessive gas in the gastrointestinal tract. The gas can be caused by smoking, by chewing gum, by drinking carbonated beverages, or by the consumption of certain foods. More seriously, bloating can be caused by a partial blockage of the tract by adhesions (scars from prior surgery) or by a tumor or stricture in the intestines.

Important symptoms—when you should see your doctor—include severe or persistent diarrhea, constipation, or bloating, and especially the appearance of blood in the stool. Blood in the stool may indicate tears of the anus or ulcerated hemorrhoids, but also can be a symptom of inflammatory bowel disease (IBD) or cancer of the colon.

HOW TO PREVENT DIGESTIVE PROBLEMS

The maxim "We are what we eat" could be changed to "We feel what we eat" when it comes to the digestive system. The foods we eat, the liquids we drink, the drugs we take, all can affect the internal workings of the gastrointestinal tract for better or for worse. Overindulgence in food and drink can especially affect our digestive system adversely, leading to indigestion, heartburn, regurgitation, excess gas, and bloating.

The Healthy Woman's Diet

Regularity and a selectivity in food and drink pay off in a healthy gut—especially in the middle years, when many digestive problems are apt to show up. The "iron" stomach of youth—when you could eat anything—is but a memory. It's necessary to take a good, hard look at your eating habits, and change them gradually and permanently to fit a new, healthier lifestyle. A new eating program might include the following suggestions:

- *Eat regularly, but not too well.* In our society, where food is generally plentiful, the consequences of overeating are all around us. Americans have a high rate of obesity, from both eating too much and too often, from eating excessively fatty foods, and from not exercising. There are other factors, besides the availability of food, that prompt us to overeat. The sensitive neural and hormonal mechanisms that tell us we have eaten enough are constantly being disrupted by such cultural overrides as the "clean plate syndrome" (drilled into us by our parents), too large servings in restaurants, the use of food as a bribe or reward, and the urging of TV food ads to eat, eat, eat.

- Generally, however, our custom of three meals a day—breakfast, lunch, and dinner—works well with the basic physiology of the human intestinal tract. The stomach processes a meal in about 4 to 6 hours. When digestion begins, cells lining the stomach and intestines release gastrointestinal hormones that stimulate the gallbladder, the liver, the pancreas, the intestines, and the brain. These hormones keep the organs functioning and healthy.

- *Don't overload at one meal.* Eating too much at a meal causes pain from the stretching of the stomach walls, as well as the possibility of regurgitation of food into the esophagus. It may help to eat only half of what is on your plate, or wait 20 minutes before taking a second helping.

- *Avoid eating between meals.* This is often where the calories mount up and the fat collects. If you must have a snack, make it a nutritious one: fresh fruit or raw vegetables. Especially avoid eating when you are doing something else—like watching TV—because it is harder to detect the "I'm full" signals from the body when your attention is distracted.

- *Eat the right foods.* Nutrition is powerful medicine. Today, it's common knowledge that a diet including certain foods may increase the risk of disease, and a variety of other foods may reduce it. It's also important to reduce your total fat intake to 30 percent or less of your total calories. Eat 5 or more servings of vegetables and fruits every day, and keep your protein intake down. And eat lots of fiber.

- *Exercise regularly.* Just changing your diet isn't enough. It's vital to go out every day and exercise. Walk briskly, swing your arms, and breathe deeply. If you are up to it, and your doctor approves, start a jogging program or aerobic exercises. Join a health club. If you don't have the time, make the time. Once you begin to exercise, you'll feel better, look better, have an improved outlook on life (all those endorphins!), and feel more in control. The key is regularity and increasing your speed, duration, and length of exercise *gradually*, not in spurts.

- *Avoid too much alcohol.* If you want to be good to your digestive system, don't drink to excess. Alcohol can inflict serious damage on the digestive organs, including cancer of the esophagus, bleeding of the stomach wall, ulcers in the stomach and duodenum, severe inflammation and/or chronic destruction of the pancreas, and scarring of the liver (cirrhosis). If your doctor tells you that your digestive problems may be a result of too much drinking, you must seriously address the question of why you drink and whether you have lost control over your intake of alcohol. A person who has a serious medical problem caused by drinking alcohol and is unable to stop drinking is very likely to be suffering from alcoholism (dealt with in other places in this book). The successful control of alcoholism not only results in greater health for the digestive system but also leads to improved life functioning and better interpersonal relationships.

- *Don't smoke.* The list of ill effects on the body from smoking is lengthy, and the digestive system is not spared. Smokers have a higher incidence of stomach and duodenum ulcers. Cancers in the organs of the upper digestive tract—esophagus, stomach, pancreas—are more likely in smokers.

Cancer Screening of the Digestive System

Cancers of the organs of the digestive system are solid, slow-growing tumors that, once established, are very difficult to treat. Unfortunately, many are not discovered until they have invaded adjacent structures of the body. At the present time, the only gastrointestinal tumor amenable to screening is cancer of the colon. Beginning at age 50, you should have a fecal occult blood

WHY FIBER IS IMPORTANT

Your choice of food can determine whether your digestive system works well or gives you trouble. Studies have shown that the human gastrointestinal system is programmed to process foods high in undigestible fiber, such as vegetables, fruits, and the bran part of grains. Unfortunately, the diet in the United States and many European countries has eliminated fiber in favor of processed foods and the overconsumption of meat. If you habitually choose a hamburger for lunch instead of a salad, or ice cream rather than an apple, you are choosing a low-fiber diet.

The consequences of a low-fiber diet are many and long-term. Some people may not seem to suffer any immediate problems, but others may experience constipation, diarrhea, stomach upsets, indigestion, and bloating. A more serious effect is the slow transit time of low-fiber foods through the colon. This means that the contents of the intestine—food residues, products of digestive juices, bacteria—remain in contact with the cell lining of the large intestine for a longer period of time. If the diet is high in fat, as a low-fiber diet often is, the intestinal contents will be high in bile derivatives, which can break down into cancer-causing compounds. In addition, a colon receiving low amounts of fiber requires more muscular activity and pressure to push the contents through; as a result, little out-pouchings called diverticula can develop and cause a serious intestinal disease called diverticulitis.

The best diet for optimal colonic function contains about 20 grams of fiber per day, roughly the amount of fiber in three to five servings of fresh fruit and four servings of vegetables per day, and whole-grain breads and cereals. The advantages of a high-fiber diet are many. Bulkier foods take time to eat and fill the stomach, allowing time for satiety signals to reach the brain. High-fiber foods are lower in fat, so the stomach empties more easily and quickly, and there is less tendency for the formation of gas and bloating, belching, and regurgitation of food. Less fat in the diet also results in less fat and cholesterol in the blood, thus decreasing the risk of coronary disease. A smaller amount of bile is released, reducing the risk of colon polyps and cancer. Finally, because there is less abdominal straining with a high-fiber diet, there is less risk of formation of diverticula in the colon or hemorrhoids around the anal canal.

test every year and a flexible sigmoidoscopy every 5 years.

If You Have to See Your Doctor

An occasional bout of indigestion, heartburn, nausea, or diarrhea is generally self-limiting and clears up on its own, but there are instances when a digestive problem calls for prompt medical attention.

If you visit your doctor with a digestive complaint, she or he will ask for a detailed history of your problem, and question you about your digestive functions and diet. You will receive a physical evaluation including an abdominal and rectal checkup, and a spot check for hidden blood in the stool. If your symptoms or the exam suggests a particular problem, you may be asked to undergo certain diagnostic tests. Don't be afraid to ask the doctor questions. Why is the test being offered? What does the doctor suspect? What might the test show? What treatment would be recommended on the basis of the test findings? If you are offered medication, ask how the drug works and about any potential side effects.

DIGESTIVE SYSTEM SPECIALISTS

When you are suffering from a gastrointestinal ailment, the first person you should see is your primary physician. If the problem cannot be easily resolved, the primary physician will refer you to a gastroenterologist, an internist with advanced specialty training in diseases of the digestive system. She or he can do a number of procedures to diagnose and treat your illness.

Other digestive specialists are listed below:

- *Hepatologist.* A specialist in diseases of the liver. A clinical hepatologist is an internist with subspecialty training in gastroenterology, often with advanced research and clinical training in liver disease.

- *Colorectal surgeon.* A surgeon with general surgery training and advanced specialty training in diagnosis and treatment of diseases of the colon, rectum, and anus.

- *Proctologist.* A general term applied to a physician, usually a surgeon, with training and practice expertise in the conditions of the anus and rectum.

DISORDERS OF THE ESOPHAGUS

When you eat, the food passes from the back of your mouth into the esophagus, a muscular tube approximately 10 inches long that leads directly into your stomach. While the esophagus moves food along, it must also stop material from backing up and reentering the throat (regurgitation) and prevent, at the other end, the backing up of stomach acids into its interior. Two sphincter muscles—one at each end—perform this duty.

Dysphagia

Dysphagia, or difficulty in swallowing, is the most important esophageal symptom. It may indicate an active disease in the lining of the esophagus, faulty muscular action of the esophagus, or a physical obstruction that is blocking the passage of food and/or liquids.

This symptom always merits a visit to the doctor.

ESOPHAGEAL DISORDERS CAUSING DYSPHAGIA

- Peptic stricture (see Reflux, below)
- Cancer
- Motility disorders
  Spasm
  Scleroderma
  Achalasia
- Neurological disorders
  Myasthenia gravis
  Amyotrophic lateral sclerosis (ALS)

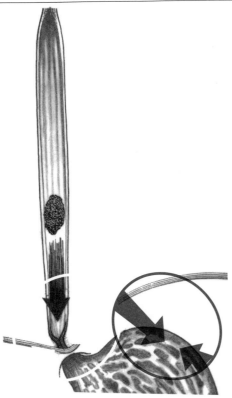

Figure 33.3A Esophageal "Peptic Stricture"
Acid and pepsin in the gastric juice can cause erosions, ulcers, and finally scar formation and thickening of the wall of the lower esophagus, leading to a narrowed area called a stricture. The first symptom is usually difficulty in swallowing solid food, like meat or bread. If the stricture becomes extremely narrow, even liquids cannot pass it. Strictures can be opened by dilators of gradually increasing size, called bougies.

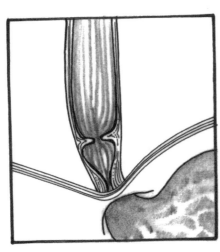

Figure 33.3B Esophageal Ring
Sometimes dysphagia (difficulty in swallowing) is caused by a thin ring of esophageal tissue called a ring or a web. Often this ring is disrupted just by passing the fiberoptic endoscope to investigate the cause of dysphagia. Sometime dilatation with bougies is required to open the ring.

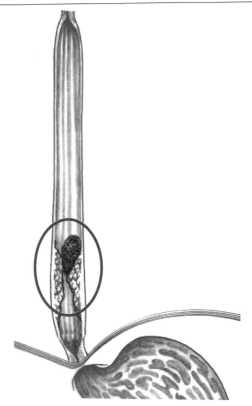

Figure 33.3C Esophageal Cancer
This tumor grows into the esophagus and obstructs the passage of food. Dysphagia to solid food occurs first. Endoscopy with biopsy will confirm the diagnosis.

Symptoms

The important characteristics of dysphagia are difficulty and pain in swallowing, regurgitation of food, and heartburn.

Aphagia, the complete inability to swallow even saliva, is a medical emergency and requires immediate medical attention.

Causes

Difficulty in swallowing may have various causes, including obstruction by stricture or tumor, or the less common motility disorders and nerve diseases. In any case, a diagnosis is always called for, and physician evaluation should be promptly sought. (See Fig. 33.3)

Reflux Esophagitis, or Gastroesophogeal Reflux Disease (GERD)

When the sphincter separating the stomach from the esophagus becomes weak or fails to function, the acid content of the stomach can wash backward, or "reflux," into the esophagus. The lining of the esophagus

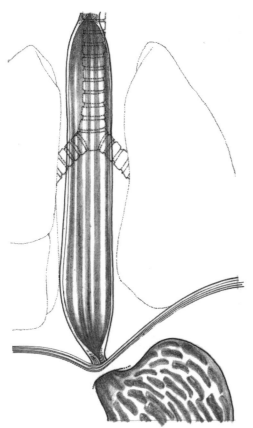

Figure 33.3D Achalasia
The lower esophageal sphincter does not relax when food is propelled down the esophagus. There is a sharply narrowed area at the end of the esophagus. Above, the esophagus is stretched and dilated.

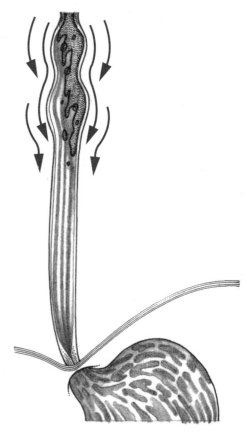

Figure 33.3E Esophageal Spasm
Uncoordinated contractions of the esophagus can result in severe chest pain, often difficult to distinguish from cardiac pain. Coronary heart disease has to be considered and eliminated in postmenopausal women or those with high risk factors. Special studies, called manometry, can detect the abnormal esophageal contractions, which can be treated by a variety of medications.

WHEN YOU HICCUP

For the most part, hiccups are a harmless annoyance. These involuntary "hics" occur when your diaphragm contracts repeatedly. As we all know, hiccups are liable to occur after a heavy meal or after drinking an excessive amount of alcohol. There are many popular remedies to get rid of an ordinary case of hiccups, including the quick downing of a glass of water while holding your breath, and breathing in and out into a paper bag. These methods may work, or the hiccups may stop on their own.

When hiccups persist for several hours or longer, see your doctor. The problem may be an irritation of the vagus nerve, which runs from the brain into your gastrointestinal system. There are also other causes of persistent hiccups, including gastritis, inflammation of the lining of the heart, and diseases of the lungs, and kidneys.

can become inflamed or irritated by this acidic fluid, sometimes to the point of ulceration. A serious long-term consequence is esophageal stricture, also called peptic stricture, in which the esophagus becomes severely narrowed and swallowing becomes difficult. Rarely the cells lining the end of the esophagus can change form, a condition called Barrett's esophagus. This condition carries a high risk for the development of cancer of the esophagus. (See Fig. 33.3A & B)

Certain conditions will cause or exacerbate reflux, including pregnancy, weight gain, the wearing of tight clothing, and straining during bowel movements. Specific chemicals or hormones can relax the gastroesophageal sphincter, such as estrogen (as in pregnancy), caffeine, and nicotine.

Symptoms

The most common symptom is heartburn, a burning sensation usually centered in the chest, although pain can occur in the upper abdomen, the back, or even the neck. Heartburn usually occurs within an hour after a meal; it can also strike at night, while you are lying in bed. Serious complications can result from night reflux if the stomach content enters the lungs, and causes nocturnal asthma or aspiration pneumonia.

Diagnosis

The doctor can make a diagnosis based on your symptoms of heartburn and prescribe accordingly. If your symptoms are particularly severe, further tests may be necessary to discover the cause of the reflux. Often heartburn is accompanied by a *hiatal hernia*, an anatomical displacement of the uppermost portion of the stomach through the diaphragm. The esophageal sphincter and the opening in the diaphragm are normally at the same level, thus producing an added pressure to keep food contents in the stomach. If you have a hiatal hernia, the reflux can occur more easily. (See Fig 33.4)

An X-ray test, called an upper gastrointestinal series (UGIS), can reveal strictures of the esophagus and the size and position of the hiatal hernia. Reflux can be demonstrated by this exam. An *endoscopy* of the esophagus and the stomach can show inflammation and ulceration of the esophageal lining as well as the presence of a hiatal hernia. Biopsies can reveal the extent of damage or the presence of Barrett's changes. *pH monitoring studies* can show if acid is in the esophagus, how often it occurs, and how long the acid re-

GI PROCEDURES

Gastroenterologists can perform a number of specialized procedures that help to diagnose and treat conditions of the gastrointestinal system. For years X-rays, using barium as a contrast agent, were the only method for getting information about the shape and condition of the structures of the gastrointestinal tract. The upper GI series examines the esophagus, the stomach, and the duodenum. The small bowel series consists of pictures taken several hours after the GI series and shows the jejunum and the ileum. The barium enema examines the colon by introducing barium, and usually air, through the rectum, filling the colon and bringing out features of its structure. Learning to do these types of X-rays was formerly part of gastroenterology training. Now these procedures are done primarily by radiologists.

Endoscopic procedures examine the inside lining of the GI tract by use of a lighted tube. Before 1970 these tubes were rigid. Some were used to perform anoscopy, examination of the anal canal, or proctoscopy (or proctosigmoidoscopy), examination of the rectum and the lowest part of the sigmoid colon. Other rigid scopes were used to examine the esophagus and the upper part of the stomach, but they took considerable skill to use and were not for routine diagnosis. Around 1970, flexible fiber-optic scopes became available. Fiber-optic technology consisted of using extremely thin glass rods bundled together. These bundles could transmit light and images, and could be bent to go around angles in the GI tract. The first scopes were made for the stomach, then scopes to examine the colon were made. Standard procedures using these scopes have been developed.

Esophagogastroduodenoscopy, or EGD, refers to the examination of the esophagus, the stomach, and the duodenum. It is also called upper GI endoscopy. Examination of the colon is called colonoscopy. In addition to examining the walls of these structures, samples of tissue (biopsies) can be taken and therapy, like cauterizing blood vessels, can be administered. The procedures are done in a specially equipped suite in a hospital or a doctor's office. For EGD, fasting is required. A local anesthetic is given to numb the back of the throat, and a sedative may be administered. For colonoscopy, a 2-day cleansing procedure is done to empty the colon. A mild sedative may be given. The time required for these procedures depends on whether biopsies are taken or therapy, like cautery of bleeding vessels, is performed.

Endoscopic retrograde cholangiopancreatography (ERCP) combines endoscopy with radiography to show the pattern of ducts coming from the liver and the pancreas. It is particularly useful in showing stones or changes in the duct systems caused by tumors or inflammations. In operative ERCP, stones can be removed, or tubes placed to bypass segments of ducts blocked by tumor.

It is beyond the scope of this chapter to describe in detail all the specialized procedures used for the GI tract. Some of them are done only in research centers and are not generally available. Reference is made to some specialized procedures in the discussions of various conditions.

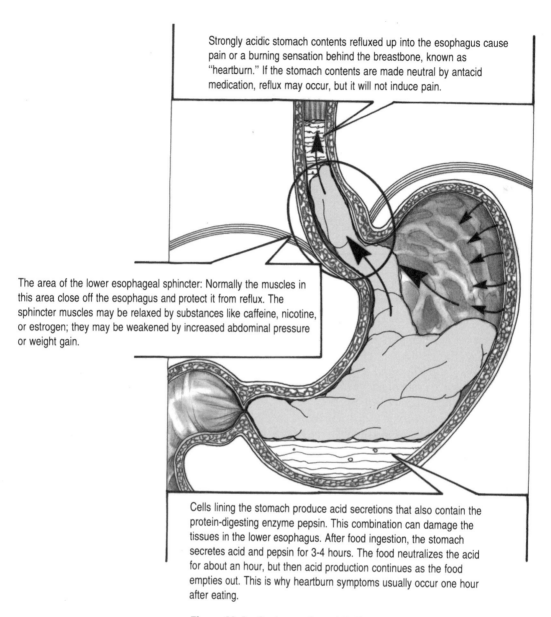

Strongly acidic stomach contents refluxed up into the esophagus cause pain or a burning sensation behind the breastbone, known as "heartburn." If the stomach contents are made neutral by antacid medication, reflux may occur, but it will not induce pain.

The area of the lower esophageal sphincter: Normally the muscles in this area close off the esophagus and protect it from reflux. The sphincter muscles may be relaxed by substances like caffeine, nicotine, or estrogen; they may be weakened by increased abdominal pressure or weight gain.

Cells lining the stomach produce acid secretions that also contain the protein-digesting enzyme pepsin. This combination can damage the tissues in the lower esophagus. After food ingestion, the stomach secretes acid and pepsin for 3-4 hours. The food neutralizes the acid for about an hour, but then acid production continues as the food empties out. This is why heartburn symptoms usually occur one hour after eating.

Figure 33.4   Gastroesophageal Reflux

mains in the esophagus. There is little to be gained from doing these ancillary diagnostic procedures unless a complication is suspected.

Sometimes there is no relationship between a person's symptoms and the findings of the diagnostic studies. You may find you have a severe peptic stricture, for example, and never recall experiencing heartburn or chest pain. Another person, suffering from severe heartburn and pain, may have a perfectly normal esophageal lining with little inflammation and no stricture.

Treatment

Pharmacological, physiological, physical, and sometimes surgical measures are used to treat reflux.

- *Pharmacological.* The first step is to neutralize the acid that is backing up into the esophagus. Antacid preparations in liquid form work better than tablets and should be taken 1/2 to 1 hour after eating, or whenever the heartburn starts. One type of tablet forms into alkaline bubbles that sit above the liquid content of the stomach and bathe the lower esophagus. It is useful for daytime treatment. The H2 blockers also inhibit acid production, and in low or high doses can alleviate symptoms. In very severe cases of reflux, acid-inhibiting drugs called sodium-potassium pump inhibitors are prescribed. Pharmacological treatment alone, however, is not enough; reflux is a chronically occurring condition, and other measures affecting diet and lifestyle must be taken.

- *Physiological*. Because the stomach reacts to food by secreting most of its acid over 3 to 4 hours, you should eat only three meals a day, with no between-meal snacks. Do not ingest any food 3 to 4 hours before retiring at night. Sharply reduce the fat in your diet, because fat delays the emptying of the stomach. Also, a large meal with a high fat content remains in the stomach a long time, accumulates acid, and gives more opportunity for reflux. A dietary regimen of low fat, moderate protein, and high carbohydrates (preferably complex and high fiber) should be your goal. Such a diet will also relieve constipation, which exacerbates reflux. Also, avoid drinking caffeinated beverages and smoking.

- *Physical*. Eliminate all factors that increase pressure on the abdomen. This means the avoidance of tight, constricting garments—girdles, long-line brassieres, belts. If your weight is above normal or you have recently gained, weight loss, as little as 5 pounds, is recommended. To avoid nocturnal reflux, elevate the head of your bed by 4 inches or so.

- *Surgical*. Anti-reflux surgery is reserved for those who, despite medical treatment, experience continued reflux leading to stricture, bleeding, or respiratory complications. The surgery corrects the hiatal hernia and creates a pressure zone at the end of the esophagus. If you decide to have this type of surgery, seek a highly skilled and experienced surgeon for this procedure.

Reflux in pregnancy

Reflux is a common problem in pregnancy—it is estimated that 25 percent of pregnant women have daily heartburn in the third trimester. There is obviously nothing that can be done about the pressure of the enlarging uterus on the upper abdomen, but there is some comfort in knowing that the symptoms will end at delivery. Some temporary measures can be taken to relieve the heartburn, including the spacing of meals, a low-fat diet, elevation of the head of the bed, and antacid medications that are approved by the obstetrician.

Stricture of the Esophagus

Narrowing of the esophagus is treated with dilation by special instruments or, in some cases, by surgical replacement with a section of bowel.

Cancer of the Esophagus

Practically all tumors of the esophagus are malignant. The most important risk factors are cigarette smoking and alcohol; the effects of these two factors are additive and increase the possibility of cancer. Malignant tumors of this type are half as likely to occur in women as in men. (See Fig. 33.3C)

Symptoms

Esophageal tumors usually do not produce symptoms until they have grown extensively and have seriously narrowed the diameter of the esophagus. The primary symptoms are difficulty in swallowing, weight loss, regurgitation of food, and vomiting of blood.

Diagnosis

A barium X-ray will reveal the form and the extent of the tumor, and endoscopy (esophagoscopy) can be done to take a biopsy and confirm the diagnosis. A CT scan may also be performed to determine the degree of the spread of the tumor.

Treatment

Unfortunately, once they are discovered, very few of these tumors are amenable to surgery. If the tumor is confined to the wall of the esophagus, and has not spread beyond that organ, surgery may be successful. In other cases, radiation and chemotherapy can shrink the tumor and relieve symptoms but do not cure the tumor.

Motility Disorders

Motility disorders of the esophagus account for some cases of difficulty in swallowing: the muscles of the esophagus propel food from top to bottom in a smooth wave. The sphincter at the bottom opens as the muscular wave reaches that point, and the food is dropped into the stomach. This normal pattern is disrupted in the case of the following disorders:

- *Achalasia*. Because of a nerve dysfunction, the lower sphincter does not open properly to allow food into the stomach and the esophageal wave becomes weak. The most common symptoms are chest pain, retention of food in the esophagus, and regurgitation of recently consumed food. Diagnosis is made by means of a chest X ray and barium esophagram, which will show the esophagus narrowing to a sharp point. Treatment consists of opening the tight sphincter either by balloon dilation or by surgery. (See Fig. 33D)

- *Scleroderma.* A collagen disease, scleroderma affects multiple organs and is more common in women. In close to 80 percent of scleroderma sufferers, the muscles in the lower two-thirds of the esophagus become thin and nonfunctional, and the lower sphincter becomes weak. As a result, these people suffer the symptoms and complications of acid reflux, esophageal stricture, and changes in the lining of the esophagus. Treatment usually consists of prescribed acid-reducing medications and other anti-reflux measures and, if necessary, dilation of the esophagus to relieve stricture.

- *Spastic disorders.* Intermittent chest pain and swallowing difficulties can be the result of diffuse esophageal spasm and other types of motility disorders. These problems are related to poorly coordinated, high-pressure esophageal contractions and a heightened sensitivity to physical and chemical stimuli within the esophagus itself. Sometimes the symptoms can be triggered by stress. It is important to eliminate any chance of the heart being the cause of the chest pain. Diagnosis can be made by barium esophagrams and manometry studies—a method of testing the motor activity of the esophagus. Treatment consists of prescribing anti-reflux measures, antidepressant medications in low doses as analgesics, smooth muscle relaxants, and, rarely, calcium channel blockers. (See Fig. 33.3E)

DISORDERS OF THE STOMACH

A pear-shaped, muscular organ, the stomach lies mostly on the left-hand side below the ribs. It receives food from the esophagus and produces the churning action that mixes the food with digestive enzymes and acid, reducing it to a thin liquid.

From time to time, the stomach fails to work properly and you may experience indigestion. The discomfort is usually self-limiting and passes quickly. If indigestion is persistent, however, it may be a sign of a more serious illness and merits consulting a doctor for a diagnosis. (See Fig. 33.5)

Gastritis

Gastritis is a term used to describe inflammation or damage to the stomach lining. (Gastritis is not to be confused with gastroenteritis, which is a short-lived illness, usually caused by a virus. Called intestinal flu, it is characterized by vomiting, diarrhea, abdominal cramps, and fever.) The two most common types of gastritis are atrophic gastritis and erosive, or hemorrhagic, gastritis. *Atrophic* gastritis is characterized by the loss of the stomach cells that are responsible for manufacturing acid, pepsin, and intrinsic factor, which is a complex protein necessary for the absorption of vitamin B12. This condition occurs in older people or those suffering from a long-term infection with Helicobacter pylori. *Erosive* gastritis occurs when shallow ulcers or sores develop on the upper layer of the stomach lining, usually because of the excessive ingestion of a stomach irritant such as aspirin or alcohol. It can occur in critically ill patients because of poor blood supply to the stomach.

Symptoms

Atrophic gastritis produces no symptoms. Bleeding is the most common symptom of hemorrhagic gastritis.

Diagnosis

Gastritis is best diagnosed by viewing the stomach interior through an endoscope. A biopsy of the gastric tissue determines the type of gastritis.

Treatment

If a B12 deficiency develops, as may occur with atrophic gastritis, you will need lifelong treatment with monthly vitamin B12 injections. In the case of erosive gastritis, you will have to discontinue the use of any substances that are irritating to the stomach, and may be prescribed medications to protect the lining of the stomach.

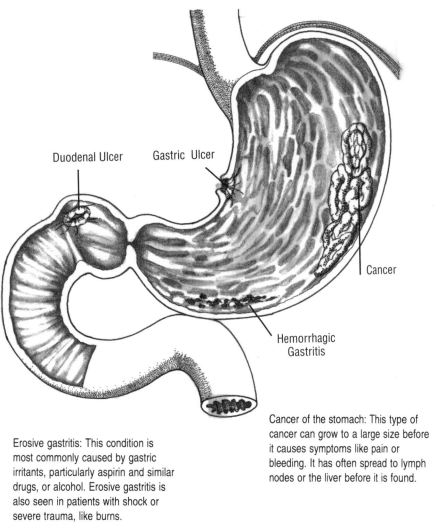

Duodenal Ulcer   Gastric Ulcer

Cancer

Hemorrhagic
Gastritis

Erosive gastritis: This condition is
most commonly caused by gastric
irritants, particularly aspirin and similar
drugs, or alcohol. Erosive gastritis is
also seen in patients with shock or
severe trauma, like burns.

Cancer of the stomach: This type of
cancer can grow to a large size before
it causes symptoms like pain or
bleeding. It has often spread to lymph
nodes or the liver before it is found.

Figure 33.5 Disorders of the Stomach

Peptic Ulcer

A peptic ulcer occurs when there is a break in the lining of the stomach or duodenum, and acid and digestive enzymes cause a sore or crater to form.

Peptic ulcers—which include duodenal and gastric ulcers—are fairly common in our society, and can occur at any time of life. The precise cause is still open to question. Contrary to popular belief, ulcers are not confined to high-powered executives or to people under a lot of stress. There is some proof, however, that the disposition to form ulcers is inherited.

The digestive enzyme pepsin and stomach acids are essential for ulcer formation. Caffeine, for example, stimulates pepsin and acid secretion. Alcohol, aspirin, and nonsteroidal anti-inflammatory drugs (NSAIDS)

can disrupt the lining of the digestive tract. Cigarette smoking is associated with ulcer formation, although the mechanism is unknown. Recent studies have discovered that a significant number of peptic ulcer patients have infection of the stomach lining with the bacterium *Helicobacter pylori*.

Symptoms

A burning, gnawing pain in the upper middle abdomen is the most common symptom of a peptic ulcer. The area surrounding the ulcer can become irritated and cause the underlying muscles to develop spasms; the nerve endings are then activated, causing pain. It usually occurs on an empty stomach, before meals, or in the middle of the night. You may also experience bloating, nausea, and vomiting.

THE SYMPTOMS OF INDIGESTION

We're all familiar with the symptoms of indigestion: discomfort or a feeling of fullness in the upper abdomen, nausea, heartburn, bloating, and a tendency to belch. Indigestion is caused by eating certain foods, too much alcohol, stress, eating too fast, or has no discernible cause.

Persistent indigestion can be a symptom of a major underlying disease, such as peptic ulcer, gastritis, gallbladder disease, or cancer. If you suffer from chronic abdominal discomfort, seek medical help. Once your doctor has established the pattern of your symptoms—when they occur, their intensity, and their duration—she or he may have to run tests to rule out any serious disorder or disease that may be causing the problem. These tests include barium X-ray studies, ultrasound, and CT scans.

It may happen that no reason is found for your abdominal discomfort. In that case, the doctor may prescribe antacids or an acid-reducing medication and advise certain modifications in your diet and lifestyle. You may be asked to stop drinking or smoking, for example, or to avoid stressful situations that may exacerbate your condition. If a specific cause for your discomfort is found—such as gastritis or an ulcer—your physician can recommend the appropriate treatment.

In some cases, a blood vessel can erode and cause bleeding. The bleeding may be detected only by a study of the stool, or massive bleeding can occur, causing the vomiting of blood. Vomited blood may appear as black particles, called coffee grounds. Alternatively, the blood may pass through the intestinal tract, resulting in a tarry stool. Weakness and dizziness may accompany the bleeding. This is an emergency, and medical help should be sought as soon as possible.

Diagnosis

Because peptic ulcer can be a chronic condition, it is most helpful to have a definitive diagnosis at the outset. If you are experiencing the typical symptoms of an ulcer, your physician will start you on a therapeutic trial of antacid therapy immediately, before any tests are performed. (A dramatic response to antacids strongly favors the presence of an ulcer.) She or he will then make arrangements for an X-ray test called an upper gastrointestinal series (GI series). The GI series will show ulcers that have penetrated the muscular wall of the stomach or duodenum, but will not detect shallow ulcers. Endoscopy detects both shallow and deep ulcers, and a culture and biopsy can detect the presence of *Helicobacter* bacterium. Evidence of *Helicobacter* infection can also be found by a blood antibody test or a breath test.

In cases of massive bleeding, the diagnosis must be made immediately. In this situation, an upper endoscopy can locate the ulcer. Active bleeding can be controlled by cautery. If this does not stop the bleeding, abdominal surgery is necessary.

Treatment

Because peptic ulcers can recur and cause serious complications, it is important to lessen any chances of a return of the condition. There is no special diet for ulcers. At one time, the typical ulcer diet consisted of bland foods, with heavy emphasis on milk and milk products, but this is no longer considered important or particularly effective. However, it *is* recommended that you eliminate alcohol and caffeine from your diet, avoid the use of aspirin and certain other drugs, and stop smoking. The mainstay of treatment is the removal of acid from the stomach. This is done by means of antacids, which neutralize stomach acid, or H2 blockers, which keep the stomach cells from making acid, or a combination of both. If the *Helicobacter* bacterium is present, antibiotics are added. Eliminating *Helicobacter* from the stomach markedly decreases the likelihood that the ulcer will recur.

Once your ulcer has healed, your doctor may advise you to continue taking a smaller dose of an H2 blocker on a regular basis, to eliminate any chance of the ulcer recurring. Duodenal ulcers are assumed to be healed in about eight weeks if the pain disappears. Healing of a gastric ulcer has to be confirmed by X-ray or endoscopy, to ensure that a gastric cancer is not responsible for the appearance of the ulcer. Surgery is seldom required, unless the ulcer does not heal with medication, or there are complications like bleeding or obstruction.

Stomach Tumors

As with tumors of the esophagus, the majority of stomach tumors are malignant. Fortunately, for unknown reasons, this type of tumor is decreasing in incidence in the United States. Diet may play a role in the formation of a gastric tumor, but there is no conclusive proof of this.

Symptoms

Because the stomach is a large and flexible organ, tumors arising from the stomach lining grow significantly and may spread to the lymph nodes and liver before they are discovered. The most frequent symptoms are upper abdominal pain, blood in the stools, weight loss, and an iron deficiency anemia resulting from slow blood loss. If the tumor blocks the esophagus or the pylorus (the outlet of the stomach), it may be found at an earlier stage, and thus have a better chance of a surgical cure.

Diagnosis

Because the symptoms of a gastric tumor are similar to those of a peptic ulcer, there is no one symptom that indicates cancer of the stomach. Again, a barium X-ray or an endoscopic examination can determine the location of the problem, and a biopsy can identify a possible cancer. CT scans may be necessary to ascertain if the disease has spread to adjoining organs.

Treatment

If the tumor is malignant, surgery is the only treatment that offers any chance of a cure, depending on the spread of the disease. Chemotherapy and radiation may shrink the tumor and provide temporary improvement, but no curative regimen has been developed to date. Even when surgery cannot cure the condition, it still may be recommended to remove blockages, arrest bleeding, or help alleviate pain.

DISORDERS OF THE INTESTINES

After food has been broken down by stomach acid and enzymes, it passes slowly into the small intestine, which consists of the duodenum, the jejunum, and the ileum. Here the nutrients are absorbed into the bloodstream through the lining of the small intestine. Undigested food, water, and other intestinal waste pass into the large intestine—consisting of the colon and the rectum—where they are solidified and prepared for excretion.

The intestines are where the major part of digestion takes place: nutrients are absorbed into the bloodstream for distribution throughout the body, water and salt are reabsorbed, and wastes are eliminated. Many of the disorders afflicting this part of the digestive system involve inflammation from infections, malabsorption, and intestinal obstructions.

Infections of the Intestinal Tract

Intestinal infections—whether viral, bacterial, or parasitic—are extremely common. Babies as well as adults get them, and travelers to other counties are especially susceptible. The infectious agents are spread mainly by food or water contaminated by human waste. *Gastroenteritis* disturbs the function of the stomach and the small intestine; *dysentery* generally refers to severe infections of the large intestine.

- *Viral gastroenteritis.* This type of infection usually begins with fever and vomiting followed by diarrhea. A number of different viruses can cause this illness, which is easily transmitted by person-to-person contact. The actual infection lasts only a few days, but symptoms, particularly diarrhea, can be prolonged by a too hasty resumption of the normal diet.

- *Bacterial gastroenteritis.* A staphylococcal intestinal infection is caused by a toxin produced by bacteria in food that is allowed to sit too long at room temperature. Vomiting begins within a few hours after eating the food, followed by diarrhea. The symptoms usually vanish by the next day. *Salmonella* is a bacterium that can be present in raw eggs or incompletely cooked chicken. *Shigella* and *Campylobacter* organisms primarily affect the colon and can cause blood to appear in the stool. (Typhoid fever, which is caused by a *Salmonella*, is rare in the United States, but travelers to developing countries who plan to spend time in rural areas are encouraged to take a course of typhoid immunization for protection.) These three organisms can be cultured from the stool and treated with antibiotics.

- *Parasitic infections.* These infections, which include giardiasis and amebiasis, are common and cause a variety of digestive illnesses. They are usually transmitted to travelers by close contact or by a contaminated water supply. Again, the agent is usually identified by testing the stool. They are treated with antiparasitic medication.

HOW TO AVOID TRAVELER'S DIARRHEA

Whether called turista or Montezuma's revenge, traveler's diarrhea (TD) can quickly put a damper on a vacation. Generally, the highest-risk destinations are the developing nations of Latin America, Africa, the Middle East, and Asia. Although the infection can be caused by a virus, bacterium, or parasite, the most common culprit is the *E. coli* bacterium, which releases a toxin that causes the intestines to pour out large amounts of secretions, especially fluids.

To prevent traveler's diarrhea, make sure to do the following:

- Drink only bottled water or beverages. Do not use ice in drinks unless it has been made from disinfected water.

- Peel raw fruits and vegetables before eating them. Do not eat raw meat or raw seafood.

- Never eat street-vendor food. Eat cooked food as soon after it is cooked as possible.

- Wash your hands even more than usual, particularly before meals and before handling food.

Traveler's diarrhea is annoying and disruptive, and every victim wants relief from cramping and the "runs." Popular remedies include a kaolin-pectin preparation (Kaopectate) and bismuth (Pepto-Bismol), which contains an anti-inflammatory agent, bismuth subsalicylate. Diphenoxylate (Lomotil) and loperamide (Imodium) slow intestinal transit. These drugs can provide temporary relief, but should not be used if the diarrhea continues for more than a few days. (It's best not to treat mild diarrhea for the first few hours; it may be the body's way of purging itself of an intestinal infection.) Severe diarrhea, which produces dehydration, fever, and blood in the stool, requires the attention of a doctor.

If you suffer from acute diarrhea, it is vital that you replace lost fluids to avoid dehydration. Drink beverages containing sugar, consomme, and bottled water.

Treatment of infectious diarrhea

When diarrhea occurs, the enterocytes, or cells lining the small intestine, replace themselves at a rapid rate. These cells are immature and are not capable of specialized digestive and absorptive functions. Eating foods that are simple to digest and then gradually adding more complex foods will provide an easier transition back to a normal diet. For example:

- *Acute phase*—plenty of fluids: tea, clear soup. Solid food should be saltine crackers, rice, dry toast.

- *Next few days*—plain meat, no fat. Other food could include banana, cooked fruits and vegetables.

As the days progress, slowly reintroduce raw fruits and vegetables, fats, and dairy products.

Malabsorption Disorders

Many different types of diseases and conditions can interfere with the normal digestive or absorptive mechanisms of the small intestine. This is called malabsorption. Vital nutrients, instead of entering the bloodstream, are eliminated in the stool. This inability to absorb vitamins can lead to anemia (loss of vitamin B12 or folate), changes in the skin (loss of vitamin A), weakening of the bones (loss of vitamin D), and disruption of normal blood clotting (loss of vitamin K).

Symptoms
The signs of malabsorption include a general feeling of weakness, weight loss, diarrhea, abdominal cramps, excess gas, bloating, and foul-smelling stools that float in the toilet bowl.

Diagnosis
The most important diagnostic test is the fecal fat test; more than 5 grams of fat eliminated in the stool over a 24-hour period indicates a significant malabsorption problem. A series of other tests, including blood tests, X-rays, and function tests, can track down the cause.

Lactose intolerance

Lactose is a sugar found in milk and other fresh dairy products. A double sugar, lactose must be split into its two components before being absorbed. Lactase, the enzyme that splits this sugar, is located on the edges of the mature small intestinal cells. Although most people are able to digest milk in infancy, those descended from populations that traditionally did not eat a dairy-based diet—African, Asian, Mediterranean, and Near

Eastern peoples—lose their ability to digest milk, usually because the amount of lactase in their intestinal cells decreases with age.

When lactose is not split and absorbed in the upper part of the small intestine, it moves on down the gastrointestinal tract and is split by the bacteria in the lower small bowel and the colon. The sugars are broken down into gases and irritating acids, which cause bloating, loose stools, cramps, and abdominal gas. The symptoms occur anywhere from 2 to 6 hours after consuming lactose. Diagnosis is confirmed by a lactose tolerance test. Treatment consists of avoiding fresh milk and foods made from milk, such as ice cream. If you want or need to drink milk, you can treat it with lactase; when you eat lactose-rich foods, you can take a lactase tablet. (Treated milk can be made into other foods.) Because the lactose in aged cheeses and yogurt has been already split by the culturing organisms, these products can be eaten without difficulty.

Celiac (nontropical) sprue

An inherited disorder, celiac disease is characterized by an intolerance to gluten, a protein found in certain grains, including wheat, oats, rye, and barley. The gluten causes an inflammatory reaction in the upper small intestine that totally changes the structure of the cells and interferes with absorption of nutrients. Common symptoms are bloated stomach, foul-smelling stools, and anemia. Celiac disease usually appears in childhood; children with the disorder lose weight and fail to grow. The main treatment is the elimination from the diet of foods containing gluten. Because gluten is a common ingredient of many processed foods, it is necessary to examine labels very carefully to make sure it is not in a particular item. People suffering from celiac disease may profit from the advice of a nutritionist, to make sure they are consuming an adequate, healthy diet.

Chronic pancreatitis

Conditions of the pancreas can lead to malabsorption. (See section on pancreas in this chapter.)

Acute Appendicitis

The appendix is a worm-shaped blind pouch of varying size that extends off the cecum, the first segment of the colon. It is located in the right lower abdomen. The appendix has some digestive function in some mammalian species, but has no known function or importance in humans except occasionally to cause trouble. Appendicitis occurs when a hard piece of stool blocks the opening of the appendix, causing swelling, inflammation, and infection. The appendix can then rupture, and a localized infection, called an abscess, can form. Or a more generalized infection can spread over the surface of adjacent organs, causing peritonitis. Both of these events are medical emergencies and require immediate surgery. (See Fig. 33.6)

Symptoms

Appendicitis usually begins with a vague pain in the middle of the abdomen. The pain becomes sharper as it localizes to the right lower abdomen. Other symptoms are loss of appetite, nausea and vomiting, and constipation.

Diagnosis

It is important, for obvious reasons, to diagnose appendicitis at the earliest possible stage. Your doctor will question you carefully about your symptoms, and

MALABSORPTION AS A RESULT OF WEIGHT-LOSS SURGERY

A few severely obese people, desperate to lose weight, choose to undergo a jejunal-ileal bypass operation, which excludes long portions of the nutrient-absorbing surfaces of the small intestine. This operation has been associated with numerous nutritional deficiencies and complications, including gallstones, kidney stones, and liver disease. One unfortunate result of the surgery is that undigested fat moves down the intestinal tract, causing the typical symptoms of malabsorption: bloating, diarrhea, and foul-smelling gas and stools.

Because of these problems, other types of weight-loss surgical procedures are now favored over the intestinal bypass operation. One such operation is a gastric bypass or gastroplasty, which drastically reduces the storage capacity of the stomach. It allows only a small amount of food to be eaten at one time but leaves the absorptive organs intact. Side effects of a gastric bypass can include deficiencies in vitamin B12, folate, and iron.

Research is also being done on a lipase inhibitor, a drug that interferes with the enzyme that is necessary for the digestion and absorption of fat.

will palpate your abdomen to elicit a "rebound tenderness" over the area where the appendix lies. The tenderness signifies that the peritoneum, the sensitive covering of the abdominal lining, is inflamed. A rectal exam will also be performed; sometimes tenderness is found above and to the right of the rectum. In women it is often difficult to distinguish appendicitis from problems affecting the right ovary and fallopian tube, so a pelvic exam is advisable. Other tests include a white blood cell count—when elevated, it can signal a bacterial infection—and a sonogram or CT scan, which will reveal the appendix and surrounding organs.

Treatment

If appendicitis is strongly suspected, surgery should be done immediately. The appendix is removed and the base tied off. Laparoscopic surgery is a recent development that can be used to treat cases of uncomplicated appendicitis.

Inflammatory Bowel Disease

Inflammatory bowel disease (IBD) is a general term that applies to two diseases of unknown cause that involve the intestines: Crohn's disease and ulcerative colitis. *Crohn's disease*—also called ileitis, regional enteritis, or Crohn's colitis—is a chronic inflammation of both small and large intestines. *Ulcerative colitis* is a chronic condition characterized by ulcers and abscesses of the large intestine only. Although these diseases can strike at any time in life, the peak time of onset is about age 20. Both conditions tend to run in some families.

Symptoms

Chronic diarrhea, abdominal cramps, rectal bleeding, fatigue, low-grade fever, and weight loss are common symptoms of both Crohn's disease and ulcerative colitis.

Diagnosis

Both Crohn's disease and ulcerative colitis are lifelong conditions that can range from mild to lifethreatening. For that reason, their management is best left in the hands of a specialist in gastroenterology. If one of these disorders is suspected, the physician will run a series of tests to establish a diagnosis. If bleeding is present, the first test is a sigmoidoscopy to examine the condition of the lining of the rectum and sigmoid colon. (See Fig. 33.7) A barium X-ray or colonoscopy, to

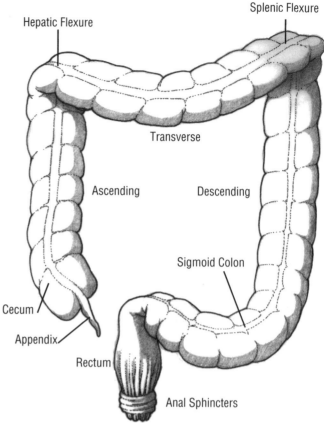

Figure 33.6 The Colon

The colon (large intestine) is distributed in a U-shape in the abdomen. Its main sections are the ascending, transverse, descending and sigmoid portions, ending in the rectum. Endoscopic diagnostic procedures on the colon are described according to how many sections of the colon are seen. Colonoscopy means that the scope was passed from the rectum all the way around to the cecum. Flexible sigmoidoscopy, the screening procedure, attempts to see the rectum, the sigmoid, and the descending colon, if possible. Cancers and polyps are more common on the left side. Proctoscopy, with a rigid instrument, covers the rectum and the beginning of the sigmoid.

see the entire interior of the colon, may be performed to determine the extent of the disease in the colon. An upper GI series with a small bowel follow-through (barium X-rays) determines whether there is involvement of the small bowel.

Treatment

A mild case of Crohn's disease may require no treatment except anti-diarrheal medication. If the problem is more acute, anti-inflammatory medications, such as sulfasalazine or prednisone, are used. Sometimes immunosuppressant drugs are prescribed to inhibit the inflammatory reaction. Surgery is done to remove obstructions. Efforts are made to avoid surgery because the condition tends to recur.

Treatment of ulcerative colitis includes medications

to control inflammation and diarrhea. A few patients may not improve and develop severe disease of the entire colon, requiring surgery to remove the diseased colon and rectum. Removing all colon tissue is curative in ulcerative colitis but results in an ileostomy—the attachment of the end of the ileum to the abdominal wall. Waste material drains into a bag attached to the abdomen. A new procedure called an ileoanal anastomosis is now being performed. This operation leaves intact the anus and its sphincter muscles, which are then attached to the small intestine, allowing waste matter to exit normally.

Active research on the causes and therapy of both these serious disorders is ongoing. To find out more about inflammatory bowel disease, get in touch with The Crohn's & Colitis Foundation of America, 386 Park Avenue South, 17th floor, New York, NY 10016-8804. This organization funds research and provides educational materials and support networks for patients and families.

Irritable Bowel Syndrome

This syndrome has several names: spastic colon, spastic colitis, mucus colitis, or functional bowel disease. *Colitis* is actually an inaccurate term, because no infection or inflammation is present. In fact, the diagnosis is based on the absence of evidence of other intestinal disorders. Because the symptoms are so variable, many people suffer with this problem for years before seeking help. Irritable bowel syndrome usually starts in the teen years or young adulthood. Women are more affected than men.

Symptoms

The symptoms seem to be the result of two disorders of intestinal function: abnormal motility (impaired contractions of the intestine) and increased sensitivity to bowel distention. Constipation, diarrhea, alternating constipation and diarrhea, cramping, gas, and bloating are all common symptoms. Typically, the symptoms occur after a meal and are often relieved by a bowel movement. Constipation is a common complaint, and many people suffering from this disorder use laxatives excessively, which exacerbates the condition. Stress and depression appear to play a role in many patients.

Diagnosis

Don't suffer in silence if you experience the chronic symptoms of irritable bowel syndrome. See your physician to make sure there is no underlying disease caus-

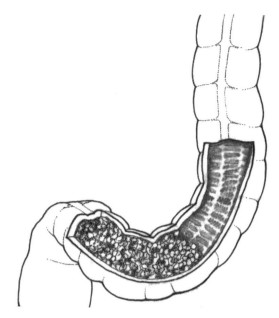

Figure 33.7 Inflammatory Bowel Disease
A segment of colon, showing colitis. The normal folds are disrupted by multiple ulcers and swollen inflamed tissue called "pseudopolyps." This tissue can bleed and secrete excessive mucus, resulting in what has been named the "currant jelly" stool.

ing the problem. A physical exam can reveal the presence of intestinal gas and variable areas of tenderness in the abdomen. Other tests, including standard blood tests, sigmoidoscopy, and possibly barium enema or colonoscopy, confirm the diagnosis by revealing no other condition. An anoscopy may find complications of constipation—hemorrhoids or fissures.

Treatment

Increasing the fiber content of the diet can improve the motor function of the bowel and result in a formed, regular stool. Adequate amounts of fiber must be consumed daily: three to five servings of fruit and four to five servings of vegetables, and whole-grain breads and cereals, for a total of 20 grams of fiber. Use bulk laxatives when there is a problem getting adequate fibrous food, as can happen when traveling. Occasionally a low dose of antidepressants, which can alter the perception of pain signals from the bowel, is helpful. Biofeedback and psychological counseling can also aid in relieving stress.

Diverticular Disease

A diverticulum is a pouch that develops in the colon and protrudes through its wall. (In an X ray, diverticula look like marbles sitting on the outside of the colon.) The pouches are caused by high-pressure pockets that occur when the colon is relatively empty—the colon lining is forced out through the weak spots where the blood vessels penetrate the intestinal muscle. *Diverticulosis* is the term used to describe the state of having diverticula in the colon. *Diverticulitis* refers to an inflammatory condition of the pouch or pouches. (See Fig 33.8)

The disease is a condition of advancing years: 10 percent of 50-year-olds have diverticulosis, and 50 percent of 90-year-olds suffer from it. The main cause seems to be our low-fiber diet, which forces the colon to generate high pressures to move the food along, leading to a collapse at certain parts of the colon wall. Once the pouches develop, they remain a lifelong threat.

Symptoms

Many people with diverticulosis have no symptoms and are not aware that they have the condition. Others suffer from various symptoms, including abdominal pain (usually on the left side), fever, nausea, and sometimes rectal bleeding.

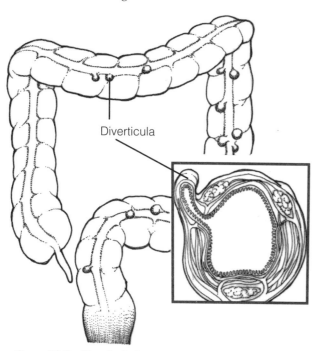

Figure 33.8 Diverticulosis

Diverticula are small pouches of colon lining that protrude through the muscular wall of the colon. They are caused by high pressure on potentially weak areas where the blood vessels penetrate the wall. They are more common on the left side of the colon than on the right. These pouches can become inflamed and infected, "diverticulitis," causing pain and fever. Occasionally they can perforate and cause a diverticular abscess.

TYPES OF LAXATIVES

There are a number of different kinds of medications that stimulate defecation:

- *Bulk laxatives*—increase the amount of insoluble fiber and stimulate more effective muscular activity of the intestines.
- *Saline laxatives*—contain unabsorbable compounds, like magnesium oxide, that keep water in the intestine and make the stool more liquid.
- *Stool softeners*—make the stool easier to pass.
- *Stimulant laxatives*—cause increased activity of the colon muscles.
- *Irritant laxatives* (castor oil)—paralyze the small intestine's absorptive mechanism, resulting in a large increase of fluid in the intestine.

Laxatives can be helpful when you have an occasional bout of constipation. However, it's rare for anyone to need laxatives on a daily basis; excessive use of laxatives can actually lead to weakness of the colon muscles, contributing to the problem they are meant to prevent: constipation. Instead of relying on laxatives, try making these changes in your lifestyle:

- Drink lots of fluids, including six to eight glasses of water a day.
- Alter your diet to include a lot more fiber. You can do this by eating more fruits and vegetables on a daily basis.
- Exercise regularly.
- When nature calls, do not suppress the urge to move your bowels. If at all possible, go to the bathroom.
- Do not use enemas on a regular basis. They interfere with the natural process of defecation.
- If you must use a laxative, use a bulk laxative.

Diagnosis

A case of diverticulosis may be noticed only incidentally, when X-rays or a colonoscopy is being performed for other reasons. If you do suffer from a severe pain in your lower left abdomen, a diverticulum may have become inflamed or infected as a result of food and bacteria lodging in it. If neglected, diverticulitis can result in infection and perforation with abscess formation, which requires immediate medical attention. The diagnosis is usually made by the clinical examination. Ultrasound or CT scanning can locate an abscess that has formed.

Treatment

Diverticulosis symptoms of pain in the lower abdomen without a sign of infection are best treated with a high-fiber diet to improve muscular function and to lower colon pressures. Severe pain with signs of infection—fever, elevated white blood cell count—usually means that the diverticulum has become obstructed and infected; in some cases there can be rupture with abscess formation. Hospitalization with intravenous feeding, antibiotics, and possibly surgery is required to control and resolve the infection. Another diverticulosis syndrome is sudden, copious, bright red rectal bleeding that is the result of erosion of the blood vessel next to the opening of the diverticulum. This usually resolves spontaneously, without treatment.

If you experience frequent attacks of diverticulitis, it may be advisable to have the involved segment of the bowel removed surgically.

Growths in the Colon: Polyps and Tumors

Polyps are small growths on the inside lining of the intestine. The muscular action of the intestine pulls on them, sometimes creating a stalk, so polyps often resemble mushrooms. (See Fig 33.9) There are several types of polyps found in the colon; the most common are hyperplastic and adenomatous. *Hyperplastic* polyps are not a health risk and are not associated with the development of colon cancer. *Adenomatous* polyps, on the other hand, have the potential to become cancerous. The discovery of an adenomatous polyp in the colon is a signal to perform a full colonoscopy, remove all polyps found, and continue to monitor the patient regularly thereafter.

Symptoms

Often there are no symptoms, and the polyps are found during a screening sigmoidoscopy or a diagnostic workup for blood in the stool. Rarely, polyps may cause visible blood in the stool or a change in bowel movements.

Diagnosis

The definitive diagnosis is made by microscopic examination of the polyp, or part of it, by a pathologist.

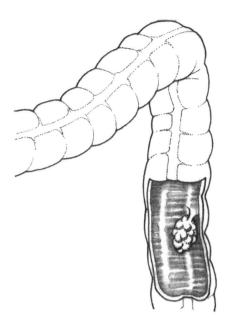

Figure 33.9 Colon Polyp
A polyp begins as a heaped-up area of tissue. As it grows, the intestinal motion pulls it, creating a stalk. Most polyps are benign (not cancerous), but some types of polyps may develop into cancer. If an adenomatous or villous polyp is discovered on screening, the entire colon should be looked at (colonoscopy) and all polyps removed.

Treatment

Most polyps are removed when detected, to eliminate any chance they will become malignant later. If an adenomatous polyp is found, you should be monitored periodically for other growths in the colon.

Colorectal Cancer

Cancer of the colon and rectum is the second most common cancer (after breast cancer) in women in the United States. Women and men are affected equally. The development of colorectal cancer is thought to be related to our high-fat, low-fiber diet as well as to specific genetic factors. The incidence of colon cancer increases sharply in those over 50, so periodic screening for this type of tumor should begin at that age. Standard screening consists of a physical examination by the physician—the digital rectal exam—plus a three-day test for occult blood in the stool, proctoscopy, or flexible sigmoidoscopy. Proctoscopy is a direct visual examination of the lower part of the colon, the rectum; a flexible sigmoidoscopy examines the rectum, the sigmoid colon, and sometimes the descending colon. (See Fig. 33.6)

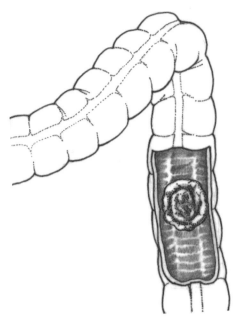

Figure 33.10   Colon Cancer
Colon cancer invades the wall of the colon and may have a flat, ulcerated appearance. Sometimes it will affect the entire circumference of the colon and produce what is called an "apple core" or "napkin ring" appearance.

Symptoms
Symptoms depend on the location of the cancer. Cancers formed in the large-diameter right side of the colon are bulky; they may break down and bleed, but the blood is not noticeable in the stool. These cancers can cause severe iron deficiency anemia, so that fatigue and weakness may be the first symptoms noticed. (One medical rule of thumb is that iron deficiency in a middle-aged person is colon cancer unless proven otherwise.) (See Fig. 33.10)

Cancers located in the narrower left side of the colon produce constipation and pain, signifying partial obstruction. Cancers in the rectum are likely to cause discomfort on defecation and visible blood in the stool. It must be remembered that these symptoms are all indicative of fairly advanced tumors. Because early colorectal cancer often causes no symptoms whatever, it is extremely important to have periodic cancer screening examinations after the age of 50.

Treatment
Surgery is the primary treatment of choice for colon cancer. The diseased colon is removed and the draining lymph nodes are checked for any sign of spreading cancer. Surgery for cancer in the rectum depends on how deeply the tumor has penetrated the wall. Radia-

tion and chemotherapy have been shown to decrease recurrence and improve the patient's chances of survival.

Anorectal Disorders

The anus is the outlet for the rectum. Anorectal disorders tend to involve inflammations, abscesses, hemorrhoids, and fissures.

Anorectal Abscess, Perianal Abscess, and Fistula

An *anorectal abscess* is usually the result of an infection of one of the anal glands. A *perianal abscess* occurs when the infection develops under the skin around the anal opening. The main complication of these infections is the development of a *fistula*, an abnormal connection or passageway between the anus or rectum and the perianal skin.

Symptoms
Anal abscesses cause dull to severe pain in or around the anal opening, accompanied by fever. If you have anal pain and fever, you should consult a physician immediately. A *fistula* will cause the skin around the anus to become itchy and irritated because of fluid and secretions draining from the hole.

Diagnosis
A physical exam is usually all that is necessary to diagnose anorectal abscess, perianal abscess, or fistula.

Treatment
Anal abscesses are a surgical emergency and must be drained.

Anal Fissure

An anal fissure is an ulcer that forms in the outer portion of the anal canal, usually in the posterior section, toward the backbone. Fissures are commonly caused by the passage of large, hard stools that cause splits in the skin in a weak area of the anal canal.

Symptoms
Anal fissures cause sharp pain during and after defecation, especially if the sphincter muscle is irritated and goes into spasm. Sometimes streaks of bright red blood appear on the stool.

Diagnosis

The fissure can usually be seen by the physician upon examination, although anoscopy may be performed to confirm the finding. Stool softeners and bulking agents can promote easier passage of the stool. A sitz bath—sitting in a tub of hot water for 20 minutes—can relax the perianal muscles and increase the blood supply to the tissue, thus promoting healing. A chronic fissure that resists healing by conservative means can be treated surgically. A colorectal surgeon or a general surgeon with extensive experience in proctology is the specialist to perform this procedure.

Hemorrhoids

Three spongy cushions, containing a rich supply of veins, lie under the lining of the anal canal. The wear and tear of elimination—and chronic constipation—can stretch these tissues and cause the veins inside them to enlarge and protrude through the canal, causing the formation of hemorrhoids, or "piles." At times, clots can form in the veins and ulcers can form, resulting in severe pain and bleeding. Pregnancy is a high-risk time for the development of hemorrhoids, especially in the third trimester. (See Fig. 33.11)

Hemorrhoids Anal Fissures

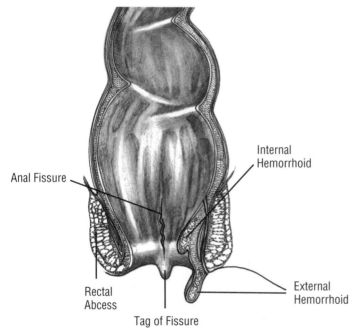

Anal Fissure

Internal Hemorrhoid

Rectal Abcess

Tag of Fissure

External Hemorrhoid

Figure 33.11 Conditions of the Anorectum
Hemorrhoids: Internal hemorrhoids originate from the upper part of the anal canal and are generally contained within it. External hemorrhoids originate from a lower plexus of vessels and may result in lumps protruding from the anus.

FECAL INCONTINENCE

In most instances, our anal sphincter mechanisms are able to control the excretion of gas and liquid or solid feces. Occasionally, even in healthy people, this mechanism can be overwhelmed, usually by a severe case of diarrhea and the absence of a readily accessible toilet. Such occurrences are embarrassing but should not be a cause for alarm. If they continue, however, consult a doctor. The most common causes are specific anal conditions, complications of anal or rectal surgery, and obstetrical injury.

Your doctor will give you a thorough physical examination, checking for normal nerve function, anatomical deformities, and the strength of the anal sphincter muscles. If necessary, you can take more sophisticated tests that measure pressure in the rectum and anus. Treatment varies according to the condition. You may profit from changes in diet and medications to make the stool solid, and exercises that increase the strength of the external anal sphincter can also be helpful. Injuries from prior surgery and obstetrical trauma can be repaired by a colorectal specialist.

Because fecal incontinence can result from previous surgery and similar trauma, it is important to remember that surgery should never be done for hemorrhoids, fissures, or fistulas unless it is patently necessary, and then only by a surgeon with extensive experience in the specialty. In childbirth, the posterolateral episiotomy incision is much safer than the direct posterior episiotomy, which can extend through the anal sphincter from the extreme pressure of the baby's head or during forceps delivery.

Symptoms

The main symptoms of hemorrhoids are feelings of pain and pressure in the anal canal, usually after a hard bowel movement, an episode of diarrhea, or lifting a heavy object. A grapelike lump may be present at the anal opening. You may also notice bright red blood on the toilet paper or on the stool itself, tenderness, and a protrusion of soft tissue at the anal opening. Rectal bleeding, whether you think it is from hemorrhoids or not, should be brought to medical attention and investigated.

Diagnosis

The hemorrhoid can usually be seen or felt during the examination by your physician. The area will be examined by an anoscope or proctoscope to confirm the finding.

Treatment

Hemorrhoids are not a disease, merely a symptom of wear and tear. The best treatment, then, is to alter the factors that lead to their formation. Treatment of acute hemorrhoids is the same as for an anal fissure—softening the stool, sitz baths, and topical anal lubricants. Most cases of hemorrhoids can be relieved by these simple measures. There are surgical procedures that can provide relief, but they are not usually necessary.

Complications of hemorrhoids

When hemorrhoids heal, they may leave a tag of redundant tissue. When numerous tags form, the anal cushions may become less competent, allowing a seepage of irritating secretions and causing a condition called pruritis ani. Rarely, hemorrhoids can be source of significant blood loss, causing anemia. Both of these conditions can benefit from surgery. As with anal fissures, only an experienced surgeon should be chosen to perform this procedure. The most important component of treatment, however, is lifelong changes in diet, weight loss, and other measures to ease the passage of stools and decrease pressure on the anal cushions.

Anal Itching

Pruritis ani, or itching around the anal opening, is a common condition that should be promptly investigated and treated. Scratching, wiping, washing, and the use of over-the-counter remedies can make this condition worse and harder to treat.

Symptoms

In rare instances, the symptom of itching can be due to pinworm, a parasite that is usually brought home by a child from school or day care and spread through the family. More commonly, the symptom is from stool left behind because of incomplete wiping, multiple hemorrhoid tags (see above), or the seepage of irritating secretions from fistulas or a weakened sphincter. Constant moisture in the area can also make the skin vulnerable to fungal infection that causes itching. In some cases, too vigorous wiping and cleaning of the anal area can lead to irritation and itching.

Diagnosis

Your physician will look for pinworm, fistula, hemorrhoids, and skin changes, and check the strength of the anal sphincter.

Treatment

Any identified problems should be treated, but often no such problems are present. If that is the case, then a concerted effort must be made to stop the scratching, which damages the skin and stimulates more itching. Other suggestions:

- Discontinue all over-the-counter anti-itch medications, since some ingredients may cause a local dermatitis.
- After using the toilet, wipe yourself with water-soaked cotton and pat gently to dry. Do not rub.
- Keep the area dry. Wear cotton panties and panty hose with a cotton crotch panel to allow moisure to evaporate.
- Eliminate certain foods from the diet—caffeinated drinks, chocolate, tomatoes, and beer. This may help.
- Most important, stop scratching. If necessary, apply a strong steroid ointment to the area to break the itch-scratch cycle.

LIVER DISORDERS

Located in the right upper abdomen, the liver is the body's largest solid organ, and one of the most complex. It has more than 500 separate functions, but its chief importance is as the center for the receipt and assimilation of food, including carbohydrates, proteins, fats, minerals, and vitamins. The liver also stores carbohydrates, regulates blood sugar levels, detoxifies drugs and substances harmful to the body, and produces important body chemicals, such as bile, blood proteins, urea, and clotting components. The liver lives up to its name—it is absolutely essential to human life.

Fortunately, the liver is protected from disease in several ways. It is capable of regeneration, meaning it can repair or replace injured tissue. Second, the liver is composed of large numbers of individual units that can take over for injured units indefinitely, or until the injury heals. However, the liver is subject to various inflammatory conditions that can injure and destroy individual cells and threaten the overall health of the organ.

Hepatitis

Hepatitis—inflammation of the liver—refers to the breakdown and dysfunction of the hepatocytes, the individual cells of the liver. One of the most common of liver diseases, hepatitis is caused primarily by viruses, although alcohol, drugs, and a variety of infections can also lead to liver inflammation. The most common hepatitis viruses are labeled A, B, and C. Other viruses, such as mononucleosis, can cause a mild hepatitis. Lupoid hepatitis is an autoimmune inflammation seen primarily in women.

Hepatitis can be acute and dramatic, or chronic and smoldering. It can clear up without a trace or leave severe scars that disrupt the functioning of the liver and block its blood flow, creating a serious condition called cirrhosis.

Viral Hepatitis—A, B, C, Delta, and E

Hepatitis A is acquired through ingesting food or water contaminated by sewage (the fecal-oral route). *Hepatitis B* is transmitted by infected blood or body fluids—the parenteral route—and is usually caused by contaminated blood products, sharing infected needles, or sexual intercourse with an infected person, particularly anal sex. *Hepatitis C* is spread primarily by the parenteral route but is less likely to be transmitted via intimate contact than hepatitis B. *Delta hepatitis* is caused by a highly specialized virus that affects liver cells only when hepatitis B is present; it increases the severity of the infection. *Hepatitis E* is acquired by the same route as hepatitis A. Rare in the United States, it is seen only in people from Asia, particularly India. It is notable for its extremely severe effects on pregnant women.

Symptoms

Viral hepatitis first shows up as a flulike illness characterized by extreme fatigue, fever, loss of appetite, and achiness. Urine may turn dark brown ("Coca-Cola" urine) and test positive for bile. This dark pigment is bilirubin, a breakdown product of the red blood cells, which is normally metabolized by the liver and excreted in the bile. When the kidneys and liver cannot remove the bilirubin, it remains in the blood and you develop jaundice, a yellow discoloration of the eyes and skin.

Diagnosis

A specific diagnosis of hepatitis is made by means of blood tests. These tests reflect the damage and destruction of the liver cells, and are the best way to monitor the progress of the disease. There are now individual tests to identify the specific type of hepatitis, although there are still a number of cases in which the cause cannot be definitely identified.

Treatment

There is no specific treatment for viral hepatitis. Rest, abstaining from alcohol, and adequate nutrition are all important in returning the liver to normal functioning. Hepatitis can vary from a mild, short-term illness to what is called fulminant hepatitis, a progressive destruction of the liver leading rapidly to coma and death. Most cases are somewhere between these two extremes, usually consisting of several weeks of symptoms, including jaundice, that reach a peak and then slowly return to normal. Some patients with hepatitis B or C never quite get over the infection and go on to develop chronic hepatitis. These people require special care and follow-up because of the danger of cirrhosis. In some cases, treatment with interferon, an antiviral substance, can enable the immune system to overcome the virus; it has worked in only about one-third of cases tested, however.

Hepatitis B carrier

In a person who is a carrier, the B virus resides in the liver cells without causing overt symptoms. The carrier is not ill, but he or she is capable of transmitting the virus to others. For example, the virus can be transmitted from a woman to her fetus in the uterus. Active and passive immunization of a baby born to a carrier mother can prevent a similar carrier state in the newborn. Some adult carriers can develop immunity by interferon treatment.

Other Types of Hepatitis

Lupoid hepatitis

Lupoid hepatitis is a chronic hepatitis associated with autoimmune phenomena. The symptoms of the disease can be improved by treatment with corticosteroid medications.

Alcoholic hepatitis.

This type of inflammation is caused by the toxic effects of alcohol. It can occur in its acute form, with symptoms of fever and jaundice, or it can be a chronic smoldering process that eventually leads to scarring and cirrhosis. Excessive alcohol consumption can also lead to fatty infiltration of the liver, which means fat is deposited in the liver cells. This condition can lead to liver swelling and discomfort in the right upper abdomen. Diabetes can also cause fatty infiltration.

Drug hepatitis

Certain medications can induce a hypersensitivity reaction in the liver. The drugs most commonly causing this condition are some blood pressure medications and medications controlling cholesterol, seizures, arthritis, and tuberculosis. Liver function tests done in the first few months after starting these drugs can identify the reaction, and alternative drugs can be substituted. Certain drugs kept past their expiration date, such as the antibiotic tetracycline, can degenerate into toxic compounds that damage the liver. Some drugs taken in large quantities are toxic to the liver—acetaminophen, for one.

Cirrhosis

Cirrhosis is a term used to indicate a condition in which the liver is progressively and irreversibly damaged by toxins or infection. In cirrhosis, normal liver tissue is replaced by scar tissue and areas of regenerating liver

---

HOW TO PROTECT YOUR LIVER

The most common serious infection of the liver is viral hepatitis. The most frequently contracted viruses are the "infectious" variety (known as hepatitis A), transmitted by the fecal-oral route, and the type of hepatitis transmitted through blood or blood products, hepatitis B or C, also known as serum hepatitis.

You can contract hepatitis A by drinking water contaminated by sewage. In the United States, the most common scenario is that campers or hikers drink water from a stream, thinking it is pure. Never drink from outdoor water sources, no matter how isolated the area. If necessary, purify the water before using. When traveling to countries where hepatitis A is common in the population, get a gamma globulin shot in advance of the trip. Gamma globulin can give you temporary immunity to hepatitis A and protect you for 3–6 months, depending on the dose. When you travel, ask your travel agent or the Department of Health whether this precaution is necessary.

Hepatitis B and C are generally more serious forms of the disease. Sensitive tests have all but eliminated hepatitis B and C from our blood supply, but posttransfusion hepatitis still occurs, caused by unidentified viruses. If you are having elective surgery, and might need a blood transfusion, ask your doctor about *autologous transfusion.* In this procedure, you donate the blood yourself, in advance of the operation.

Because some people are carriers of hepatitis B—the virus is in their bodies, even though they are not sick themselves—and because the hepatitis B virus is transmissible by intimate contact, including exchange of body fluids, always use barrier protection if you have sexual relations with anyone whose detailed medical and sexual history is unknown to you. And, obviously, never use a hypodermic needle that has been used by another person. There is now a very effective vaccine against hepatitis B. It is recommended for health care workers, patients receiving blood products (such as hemophiliacs), and spouses and intimate partners of hepatitis B carriers.

- *Medications.* A number of commonly used drugs can cause liver damage in certain individuals. Whenever you are placed on a long-term prescription medication, particularly for high blood pressure, high cholesterol, seizures, or tuberculosis, ask your doctor about the possibility of toxicity to the liver and the need for periodic tests to check for liver damage. If these tests are recommended, make sure to have them done and that you are notified of the results. Most people who are going to have an adverse reaction to the medication will have it in the first few months after starting the drug.

- *Toxins on the job.* Cleaning fluids, such as carbon tetrachloride, can induce severe liver damage if inhaled in sufficient amounts. Polyvinyl chloride, a substance produced in the manufacturing of plastics, also has been associated with liver damage. If you work in a cleaning establishment or a plastics factory, make sure that sufficient safeguards exist to prevent any chance of these toxins affecting your health. (See Chapter 6.)

cells, leading to disruption of normal liver circulation. Blood does not flow freely through the liver, and the cells are poorly nourished. High pressure builds up in the portal system, the network of veins that carries blood from the intestines to the liver. This is called portal hypertension. Reversal of blood flow may cause the spleen to enlarge. Varices (enlarged veins) may develop in the esophagus and can rupture and bleed profusely. Other circulatory disruptions cause fluid and protein to accumulate in the peritoneal cavity, a condition called ascites.

Causes

The most common causes of cirrhosis are alcohol consumption and hepatitis. Rarer causes are described at the end of this section.

Most cases of cirrhosis appear after heavy, long-term alcohol ingestion or as the end stage of a case of hepatitis that has become chronic. Occasionally an individual with no remarkable prior history presents with cirrhosis, which is called cryptogenic cirrhosis.

Symptoms

Symptoms of cirrhosis are generally related to the inability of the liver to process bodily toxins and medications, and to manufacture proteins; to the pressure of ascites on abdominal organs; and to complications from high pressure in the portal blood system. Cirrhosis symptoms include loss of appetite, weight loss, fatigue, altered mental function (from agitation to coma), jaundice, bleeding disorders, fluid accumulation, severe gastrointestinal bleeding, and the development of tiny, spiderlike blood vessels under the skin.

Diagnosis

Physical examination reveals a small liver and an enlarged spleen. Ascites and jaundice may be present. Blood tests may reveal low levels of proteins and clotting factors. A liver-spleen scan shows the size of the liver and spleen. A liver biopsy—a piece of the liver removed and studied under a microscope—can give information about the cause of the cirrhosis because of typical cellular patterns. CT scan can be helpful in defining the anatomy and size of the liver, and enlargement of blood vessels.

Treatment

All toxins (like alcohol) and mind-altering medications must be discontinued. Cleansing and acidifying the colon with a compound called lactulose can re-move nitrogenous compounds that contribute to hepatic coma. Bleeding esophageal varices can be thrombosed through endoscopic sclerotherapy. Portal hypertension can be reduced by operations that shunt the blood flow out of the portal network. These treatments can control some of the symptoms of cirrhosis, but there is no treatment to reverse the disease. The sad fact is that when the liver cell population falls below a critical mass, liver failure ensues and the patient will die. Some patients benefit from liver transplantation, but this procedure is limited by availability of organs and the complex medical care required to maintain a transplant.

Rare Conditions That Can Cause Cirrhosis

Primary biliary cirrhosis

Most commonly seen in middle-aged women, this is a rare condition in which the small bile ducts appear to be attacked and destroyed. The main symptom is severe itching, due to poor excretion of the bile acids. The cause appears to be an autoimmune phenomenon. Complications result from blockage of the bile flow and the development of scars on the liver, eventually leading to cirrhosis.

Hemochromatosis

This is an inherited (autosomal recessive) disease characterized by the accumulation of iron in the liver, pancreas, heart, skin, and other organs. The cause is the inability of the intestine to regulate the amount of iron absorbed from the diet. Premenopausal women are protected from its effects by menstrual blood loss, but postmenopausal women affected by the disease show high amounts of circulating and stored iron in the body. A liver biopsy will show the amount of iron and how much damage the liver has sustained. The condition can be controlled by removing blood from the body (phlebotomy) periodically to maintain the desired iron level.

Wilson's disease

This is a rare inherited disease caused by the accumulation of copper in the body, primarily in the brain and the liver. A young person who develops hepatitis without an obvious cause, like infection, should be checked for Wilson's disease. Symptoms may include tremors, seizures, and other neurological problems. Medications that bind and remove copper from the body can relieve symptoms; with proper treatment, the prognosis is good. Other family members, particularly siblings, should be tested for the disease.

Tumors of the Liver

Most tumors of the liver are malignant. Primary tumors, or hepatomas, arise from liver cells; secondary or metastatic tumors spread to the liver from another part of the body. In Africa and Asia, primary liver cell cancer is the leading cause of cancer death. In the United States it is an uncommon but extremely serious form of cancer that is one-third as likely to appear in women as in men. Certain factors tend to predispose a person to primary liver cancer, including chronic viral hepatitis and damage from a toxin, usually alcohol.

Benign tumors of the liver rarely occur. The most common are hepatic adenomas, which are associated with long-term use of oral contraceptives, and hemangiomas. Hemangiomas are tumors composed of abnormal collections of blood vessels. These tumors usually produce no symptoms, and may be discovered when liver scans are done for other reasons. If they do produce symptoms—pain or internal bleeding—hemangiomas can be removed surgically. Otherwise, treatment is not needed.

Metastatic liver cancer is by far the most common form of liver cancer in the United States. It is easy to see why. The liver is like a gigantic sieve, filtering the blood coming from the digestive tract through the portal system and from the lung through the hepatic artery. Tumor cells from cancers of the stomach, breast, lung, pancreas, esophagus, gallbladder, and colon can all find their way to the liver, become lodged, and start to grow.

Symptoms

Malignant tumors of the liver may produce no symptoms until the disease is far advanced. The most common signs are pain in the right upper abdomen, loss of appetite and weight, general fatigue and weakness, nausea and vomiting, and jaundice.

THE LIVER BIOPSY

If you are being diagnosed for a liver ailment, your doctor may perform a liver biopsy, in which a small piece of liver tissue is removed and examined under a microscope. A biopsy permits direct examination of the cells and structures of the liver to differentiate types of hepatitis and tumors.

You will be given a local anesthetic and instructed to lie flat on your back. Your physician will insert a special biopsy needle between your ribs on the right side and remove a small sample of liver tissue for laboratory analysis. You will then be instructed to lie on your right side and be monitored for a certain amount of time, to eliminate any risk of hemorrhage.

A liver biopsy is quite safe and carries a minimum risk of side effects or bleeding.

Diagnosis

If liver cancer is suspected, the doctor will take blood tests. A CT scan can locate the tumor. A liver biopsy of the tumor site provides the definitive diagnosis. If it does not, laparoscopy, or a small exploratory operation, a "mini lap," may be advised.

Treatment

Liver cancer is almost always fatal. In primary cancer of the liver cells, neither liver transplantation nor any chemotherapeutic regimen has been found to cure hepatoma. In rare cases when the tumor has been confined to a single site, successful surgical removal has been possible.

In metastatic liver cancer, the development of new tumors in the liver is a grave prognostic sign. Chemotherapy can shrink some tumors temporarily but will rarely destroy them completely. As with all chemotherapy decisions, the side effects of the treatment must be carefully weighed against the possible benefit.

GALLBLADDER AND BILE DUCT DISORDERS

A small, pear-shaped organ, the gallbladder stores bile, a complex substance produced by the liver. Bile contains bile acids (derived from cholesterol) and lecithin, chemicals required for the absorption of fat. It also contains cholesterol, bilirubin, and metabolized drugs and toxins that are being excreted from the body. The gallbladder removes water from the bile and concentrates it. When food containing fat is consumed, the gallbladder discharges the bile through the bile duct into the intestine.

The formation of gallstones (cholelithiasis) is the most common type of gallbladder disease.

Gallstones and Cholecystitis

Stones form in the gallbladder if the bile becomes concentrated enough to crystallize the cholesterol or the calcium bilirubinate found there. Gallstones are three times more common in women than in men, and the incidence increases with age. Not all gallstones consist of the same material. Cholesterol gallstones are the most common type; a small minority are made up of calcium salts. Often gallstones produce no symptoms. They may be detected when tests are done for abdominal symptoms, but the mere presence of the stones does not mean they are responsible for the symptoms. The most common problem caused by gallstones is cholecystitis, or inflammation of the gallbladder.

Cholecystitis commonly occurs when a stone gets stuck in the cystic duct, and the wall of the gallbladder becomes swollen and irritated. An attack of acute cholecystitis is usually precipitated by a meal containing fat, when the gallbladder, working hard, contracts vigorously and sends a stone into the cystic duct. (See Fig 33.12)

Symptoms

If a stone lodges in the cystic duct, it produces painful contractions in the upper right area of the abdomen as the gallbladder tries to empty itself of the obstructing stone. Nausea and vomiting are common. If the stone begins to travel through the duct system, it produces severe pain, called biliary colic, which is felt in the right upper abdomen and sometimes around the ribs to

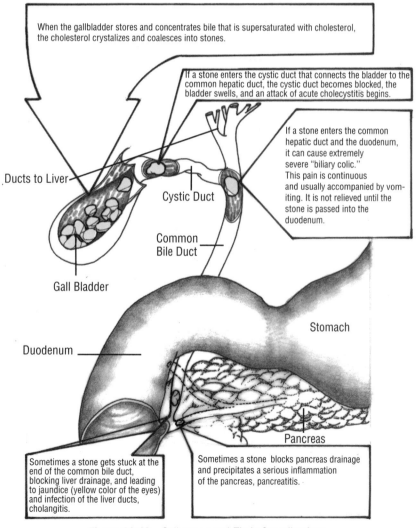

When the gallbladder stores and concentrates bile that is supersaturated with cholesterol, the cholesterol crystalizes and coalesces into stones.

If a stone enters the cystic duct that connects the bladder to the common hepatic duct, the cystic duct becomes blocked, the bladder swells, and an attack of acute cholecystitis begins.

If a stone enters the common hepatic duct and the duodenum, it can cause extremely severe "biliary colic." This pain is continuous and usually accompanied by vomiting. It is not relieved until the stone is passed into the duodenum.

Ducts to Liver

Cystic Duct

Common Bile Duct

Gall Bladder

Stomach

Duodenum

Pancreas

Sometimes a stone gets stuck at the end of the common bile duct, blocking liver drainage, and leading to jaundice (yellow color of the eyes) and infection of the liver ducts, cholangitis.

Sometimes a stone blocks pancreas drainage and precipitates a serious inflammation of the pancreas, pancreatitis.

Figure 33.12 Gallstones and Their Complications

the right side of the back. This pain is comparable in severity to renal colic (kidney stones) and labor pains. If the stone passes through the ducts to the intestine, the pain is relieved dramatically. If the stone lodges at the end of the common bile duct, it can block the passage of bile from the liver, causing obstructive jaundice. It can also precipitate an infection in the bile duct system (cholangitis), or bring on an attack of acute pancreatitis. The possibility of these serious complications makes it imperative to remove the stone from the common bile duct (see treatment).

Chronic cholecystitis may develop in women who experience many episodes of gallbladder inflammation. The wall of the gallbladder thickens, affecting the cellular lining. The gallbladder no longer functions effectively, nor is it able to concentrate the bile.

Diagnosis

If your symptoms fit the clinical picture of cholecystitis, your physician will give you tests that are most helpful in confirming the diagnosis. These tests include an ultrasound of the abdomen, which can show stones in the gallbladder, and an HIDA scan, which reveals blockages in the flow of bile.

Treatment

The good news about gallstone disease is that it can be completely cured by removal of the gallbladder. This operation is called a *cholecystectomy*. A standard cholecystectomy is a major surgical procedure with a 6-to-8-week recovery time. It usually leaves a slanting scar in the right upper abdomen, under the rib cage.

In the late 1980's, a new procedure called *laparoscopic cholecystectomy* became available. This procedure uses multiple instruments introduced through several small incisions in the abdomen. The recovery time is much shorter than with the standard operation. Laparoscopic surgery is most useful for uncomplicated acute cases with little or no scarring around the gallbladder. Since a laparoscopic procedure may have to be converted at any time during surgery to a standard operation, it should be done by a surgeon who has had extensive experience in standard cholecystectomies and specific training and experience in the laparoscopic technique.

If a stone becomes lodged in one of the ducts, it is extremely important to remove the obstructing object before severe complications ensue. In a standard cholecystectomy, the surgeon will explore the common bile duct to make sure that all the stones in the duct system are removed. If you have complications or you are too ill to withstand major surgery, you can be treated by sphincterotomy, a procedure using an instrument called an endoscope, which opens the muscles at the end of the common bile duct, releasing the stone.

Some cases of gallstone disease can be treated without surgery. Medication derived from bile acids can change the balance of chemicals in the bile and dissolve the crystallizing cholesterol. This treatment works best when there are many small stones and the gallbladder cells are functioning well in removing water from the bile. A good candidate for this treatment does not have severe symptoms or complications. It is also beneficial for those patients unwilling or unable to undergo surgery because of other medical problems. After the gallstones are dissolved, a maintenance dose of medication must be taken to keep the cholesterol from forming new stones.

Other Bile Duct Disorders

Sclerosing cholangitis is a rare disorder affecting the bile duct system. The walls of the duct become thickened and irregular, causing jaundice and infection. Sclerosing cholangitis sometimes is found in patients suffering from ulcerative colitis, one of the inflammatory bowel diseases.

Cancer of the biliary tract is very rare, but it can occur in the gallbladder, the large bile ducts, or the duct system in the liver. *Cancer of the gallbladder* occurs only in association with chronic gallbladder inflammation and may be found only when the gallbladder is removed in a cholecystectomy. As with many other intestinal cancers, these tumors do not cause symptoms, such as pain or jaundice, until they are well advanced, and cannot be removed successfully with surgery. At that point, treatment is usually palliative, directed at relieving symptoms.

DISORDERS OF THE PANCREAS

A large, complex gland located in the upper abdomen, behind the lower part of the stomach, the pancreas has two distinct functions. Scattered small groups of cells within the pancreas, called the islets of Langerhans, manufacture insulin and other essential hormones that regulate the body's sugar metabolism. Its second function is to produce enzymes required for the digestion of starch, fat, and protein. These enzymes are secreted in response to hormones signaled by the presence of food in the intestine. The enzymes flow into the duct system that joins the common bile duct as it empties into the duodenum. Because the drainage system of the liver is adjacent to the pancreas, conditions in the pancreas can affect the liver, causing jaundice and giving the first clue that something is wrong with the pancreas. Conversely, because the drainage ducts of the liver and the pancreas are connected, gallstones from the biliary ducts can interfere with pancreatic drainage and lead to pancreatic inflammation.

Acute Pancreatitis

Pancreatitis occurs when a chemical, toxin, pressure, or infection causes the enzyme-manufacturing cells of the pancreas to rupture, leading to irritation and swelling of the pancreatic tissue. The most common causes of acute pancreatitis are gallstone disease and excessive alcohol ingestion. Rarer instigators are the viral illness of mumps and high blood levels of certain fats, the triglycerides.

Symptoms
The main symptoms of acute pancreatitis are severe upper abdominal pain that often begins 12 to 24 hours after a large meal or a bout of heavy drinking, followed by vomiting, fever, and chills.

Diagnosis
The physical exam reveals severe tenderness in the upper abdomen. The diagnosis is confirmed by the finding of elevated levels of the enzymes amylase and lipase in the blood.

Treatment
The course of pancreatitis can range from mild pain to massive destruction of the pancreas and death. If you are suffering from acute pancreatitis, you will be hospitalized and all food intake will be stopped. The aim is to quiet the gland, stopping the flow of enzymes as much as possible. Food is given intravenously, and the stomach is drained with a tube to remove all stimuli to the pancreas. Severe cases will require complex care in the intensive care unit. The most important element of long-term treatment is to eliminate the cause of the

pancreatitis by removing the gallstones, or stopping alcohol ingestion, or controlling blood lipids.

Cancer of the Pancreas

Pancreatic cancer is one of the more common cancers, ranking just behind cancers of the lung, colon, and breast. It is perhaps more frequent in people who smoke, drink heavily, or have chronic pancreatitis or diabetes, but it can and does occur in individuals with none of those factors. It is less common in women than in men.

Symptoms
The signs of pancreatic cancer depend on the location of the tumor. Most of these cancers produce no symptoms until the cancer has spread outside the gland. One exception is when the tumor is located near the common bile duct or the main pancreatic duct. When the liver ducts are blocked, the liver malfunctions and jaundice can develop; when the pancreatic duct is blocked, malabsorption with diarrhea can occur. In most cases, however, the common symptoms of lack of appetite, weight loss, nausea and vomiting, and abdominal pain occur after the cancer has spread elsewhere in the body.

Diagnosis
A physical exam may reveal an upper abdominal mass. Liver tests may show signs of bile duct obstruction. A course of pancreatic enzyme medication may stop the diarrhea, pointing to the pancreas as the cause. Ultrasound or a CT scan can locate the tumor and determine whether the duct systems are dilated, and if there are enlarged nodes or metastatic tumors in the liver.

Treatment
The survival rate for those with pancreatic cancer is poor. In rare cases, surgery on the pancreas is successful in removing the tumor. More commonly, because the tumor is far advanced, treatment consists of reestablishing the flow of bile and pancreatic secretion into the intestine by placing drains through the tumor via an endoscope or by a surgical bypass operation. There is no chemotherapeutic regimen developed to date that eradicates pancreatic cancer.

CHAPTER 34

The Musculoskeletal System

Laura L. Tosi, M.D., F.A.A.O.S., and Patience White, M.D., F.A.A.P., & Judith Petry, M.D., F.A.C.S., and Francesca Thompson, M.D., F.A.A.O.S.

The bones that make up the skeleton, along with the muscles and connective tissues that bind them together, form the musculoskeletal system. This system provides a framework that allows the body to move. When the system is working properly, motion is full range and painless. Problems in the musculoskeletal system can restrict movement and affect daily living activities. Certain aspects of your lifestyle can affect the health of your musculoskeletal system. Seek medical advice if warning signs of problems occur, because some disorders can progress, becoming disabling and chronic if not treated.

STRUCTURE AND FUNCTION

Bones provide support for the body and anchor and protect the internal organs. The 206 bones come together at joints, which allow the skeleton to be flexible. The bones are connected at the joints by ligaments. Muscles, which are responsible for all movement, are attached to the bones by tendons. All the parts of the system work together to perform the thousands of acts that make up your capacity to move within your environment.

In addition to supporting the body and its organs, bones encase and protect certain organs. The skull protects the brain, and the rib cage shields the lungs and heart. Bones also serve as a storehouse for fat and minerals, the most important of which are calcium and phosphorus. Other minerals stored in the bones include potassium, sodium, sulfur, magnesium, and copper. These stored minerals are released into the bloodstream and are carried to all parts of the body as they are needed. Inside the bones is a cavity filled with soft, fatty, vascular tissue called marrow, which produces the oxygen-providing red blood cells, an important component of blood.

Each bone in the skeleton contains different proportions of two basic types of bone tissue called cortical bone and cancellous bone. Cortical bone is hard and dense, whereas cancellous bone has a honeycombed appearance similar to a sponge. Most bones in the female skeleton are the same shape as the bones in the male skeleton, but a little smaller. One exception is the pelvis. A woman's pelvis is usually broader than a man's and has a larger space in the middle. The shape allows for the head of a baby to pass from the uterus through the pelvis during childbirth.

The location where two bones meet is called a joint. The ends of the bones are covered with cartilage, which serves as a cushion between the bones. The joints are connected by fibrous tissue called ligaments and the joints are lined with a thin membrane called synovium. The synovial membrane produces fluid which provides nutrition for the cartilage and lubricates the joint, reducing friction and wear and tear (see box).

The joints are also cushioned by bursae. These sacs contain synovial fluid that helps prevent friction during activity. Bursae are located in areas of the body where ligaments, muscles, skin, or tendons rub against bone or against each other.

Ligaments attach bones together, and provide support for joints. The more ligaments located at a joint, the stronger it is. Joints are further strengthened by tendons that attach muscles to bone. The better the muscle tone, the stronger the joint.

Muscles are bundles of fibers or cells bound together by connective tissue. They are responsible for the movement of the body itself as well as the organs within the body. Muscles can translate messages from

TYPES OF SYNOVIAL JOINTS

Synovial joints can be classified by how they function:

- Plane joints (hand and foot) allow slipping or gliding movements in all directions.

- Hinge joints (elbow, knee) move in only one direction.

- Pivot joints (forearm, head, and neck) allow rotation of one bone against another.

- Knuckle and saddle joints in the fingers and thumb, respectively, fit together to permit a wide range of movement.

- Ball and socket joints (shoulder, hip) are the most freely moving of joints.

various parts of the body into mechanical energy to exert force. They also maintain posture and generate heat in the body to maintain normal temperature.

Muscle has the ability to contract or shorten when tensed, to extend or lengthen when relaxed, and to resume its original length after being contracted. Some muscles are voluntary (under conscious control) and others are involuntary (cannot be consciously controlled). There are three types of muscle:

- **Skeletal muscle** controls body movements on voluntary command.
- **Cardiac muscle** controls the involuntary beating of the heart.
- **Smooth muscle** controls the involuntary function of organs such as the stomach, urinary tract, and lungs.

Each skeletal muscle fiber has a nerve ending that controls its activity. To meet its energy needs, each muscle is served by an artery and one or more veins that circulate oxygen-rich blood to the muscle and remove byproducts (see Chapter 26). Each skeletal muscle is attached to bone or other connective tissue, such as cartilage or fibrous membranes, at a minimum of two points. Body movement occurs when muscles contract across joints, resulting in activity of the joint such as bending or stretching.

The skeleton—including bones, cartilage, joints, and ligaments—makes up about 20 percent of the body by weight. (See Fig. 34.1) Nearly 50 percent of the body's mass is muscle. These structures are made up of living, growing cells that renew damaged areas and change with age. Bone especially is subject to constant change as it is removed and replaced in a process called remodeling (see ''Bone Remodeling'').

During adolescence, a growth spurt changes the skeletal structure. The legs become longer, the hips and chest become wider, and the trunk lengthens. Skeletal growth stops around age 25. Around age 40, bone mass begins to decrease. The rate of bone loss is faster in females than in males.

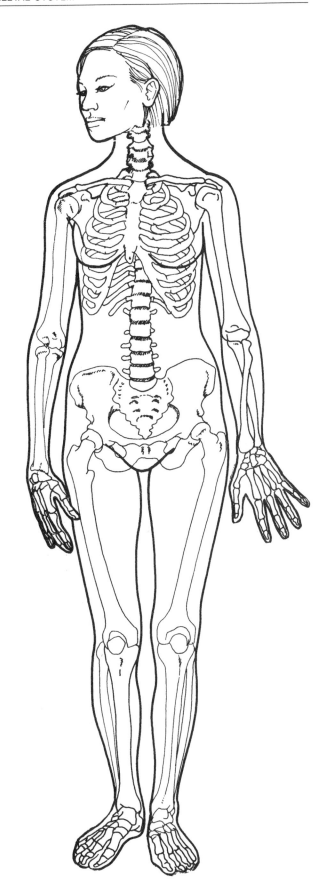

Figure 34.1 The Skeletal System
The skeletal system is made up of 206 bones. The hardest living tissue, bones provide a supportive framework, make movement possible, and are a source of calcium and red blood cells.

BONE REMODELING

Bone is renewed through remodeling, a continual process of breaking down old bone and depositing new bone. In healthy young adults, bone mass stays the same, in other words the amount of bone deposited and the amount of bone broken down is about equal. As a person ages or experiences certain hormonal changes, more bone is broken down than deposited, resulting in a loss of bone mass.

Bone deposition occurs at sites of bone injury or where added bone strength is required. Bone is broken down by cells called osteoclasts. As the minerals in the bones are dissolved, calcium is released into the blood, serving a number of important functions in the body. Most of the calcium in the body comes from the bones. The body draws calcium stored in the bones as needed. If levels of calcium in the blood are low, it will be removed from the bones and the bones become weakened by being broken down faster than new bone is laid down.

Bone remodeling is regulated by hormones in a cycle that controls the level of calcium in the blood:

1. When levels of calcium in the blood are low, a hormone from the parathyroid gland triggers release of calcium from the bones, causing the breakdown of bone.
2. As bones are broken down, the level of calcium in the blood increases. The thyroid gland then releases a hormone that halts the breakdown of bone and causes calcium to be removed from the blood and deposited in the bones.
3. As calcium is deposited in the bone, the level of calcium in the blood decreases. The parathyroid gland then signals an increase in the breakdown of bone so calcium can be added to the blood.

Bone remodeling is also affected by the amount of stress placed on bones. Stress can occur in the form of exercise, which strengthens bones. It is also exerted in the legs, ankles, and feet by the pull of gravity. Heavy use of bones results in increased bone deposits and heavier, stronger bones.

HEALTH CARE PROFESSIONALS

Health care professionals who treat disorders relating to the musculoskeletal system include the following physicians and therapists:

- *Orthopedic Surgeon*—a physician with advanced surgical training who specializes in the diagnosis and treatment of musculoskeletal disorders.
- *Physiatrist*—a physician who specializes in the evaluation and treatment of musculoskeletal and neurological diseases and conditions to effect rehabilitation of neuromuscular functioning (also called a specialist in Physical Medicine and Rehabilitation [PM&R]).
- *Rheumatologist*—a physician who specializes in internal medicine and has advanced training in rheumatology, which is devoted to diseases of the immune system and the musculoskeletal system, including the joints, muscles, and bones.
- *Physical Therapist*—a professional who helps patients return to normal musculoskeletal functioning following illness or injury.
- *Occupational Therapist*—a professional who helps patients achieve maximal independence in tasks of daily living after injury or illness.

Other specialists in related fields may be involved depending on the type of disorder:

- *Oncologist*—a physician who specializes in cancer, which can occur in bone primarily or spread there from other parts of the body.
- *Neurologist*—a physician who specializes in diseases relating to the nervous system, which can affect the musculoskeletal system.

KEEPING THE SYSTEM HEALTHY

The development of a strong skeleton begins early in life and can be affected by several factors, including exercise, diet (particularly calcium intake), and hormones.

The health of bones is affected by the amount of stress placed on them. The pull of muscles and gravity on bones makes then stronger and heavier. Good muscle tone also helps stabilize joints. Bones and mus-

OSTEOPOROSIS: PREVENTION AND TREATMENT

A gradual loss of bone mass, generally beginning about age 35, is a normal occurrence for both men and women. After growth is complete, women usually lose 30 to 50 percent of their bone density, while men lose 20 to 30 percent. If bone is no longer replaced as quickly as it is removed, a condition called osteoporosis develops, in which the bones become thin and brittle. This condition particularly afflicts postmenopausal women, who are often unaware that they have osteoporosis until a fracture occurs.

The exact medical cause of osteoporosis is not known, but a number of factors are known to heighten the risk, including a calcium-poor diet, physical inactivity, reduced levels of estrogen, heredity, excessive cortisone or thyroid hormone, being underweight, smoking, and excessive alcohol use. The disease can be prevented if your diet contains the necessary calcium and vitamin D during childhood, adolescence, and adulthood. (See Chapter 3, Diet and Nutrition) The National Institutes of Health (NIH) recommends the following daily calcium intake:

11–24 years: 1,200–1,500 mg.
Pregnant or nursing women 19 or older: 1,400–2,000 mg
Before menopause: 1,000 mg
Menopausal, postmenopausal women not taking estrogen: 1,500 mg
Premenopausal, postmenopausal women taking estrogen: 1,000 mg

Vitamin D plays a major role in calcium absorption, so you should also increase your intake of this vitamin after menopause. Other recommendations to prevent osteoporosis:

- Exercise. You should engage in regular weight-bearing exercises, such as walking—one of the best methods of maintaining bone strength—jogging, hiking, tennis, bicycling, dancing, aquatic exercises, and weight training. The emphasis should be on an activity that combines movement with stress on the limbs. Start exercising slowly, especially if you have been inactive. Consult your doctor before beginning any exercise program.

- Maintain a healthy lifestyle. Eliminate smoking and excessive alcohol use; these cause bone loss and increase your risk of a fracture.

- Take medications to prevent further bone loss. Ask your physician about hormone replacement therapy, calcitonin, or other medications that will help to slow down the rate of calcium absorption in the body.

- Get medical help as soon as possible. If you think you are at risk of developing osteoporosis, consult your medical advisor. Treatment plans should be initiated as early as possible, because once bone is lost it is difficult to replace.

cles lose their bulk when they are not used, so it is important to exercise these vital parts of the musculoskeletal system to maintain its overall health. This is especially true for women, who have less bone density than men to begin with, and who are even more susceptible to bone loss in later life.

Bone mass, and the rate of bone formation and loss, can also be affected by diet. Calcium and vitamin D intake are needed throughout life in order to makes bones strong enough to carry weight and resist breaking under stress. Both men and women gain fifty percent of their bone mass between the ages of 10 and 20. Adequate calcium intake of at least 1,200–1,500 mg of calcium each day in adolescence, combined with regular exercise, will promote a strong peak bone mass. Between the ages of 20 and 30 years, the bone mass increases only slightly. After age 30, bone loss begins to occur. Therefore, taking care to build strong bones

in adolescence and young adulthood goes a long way to preventing osteoporosis later.

These dietary points are particularly important for women, because of their unique biological functions. Pregnancy and breast feeding require extra calcium. If a woman does not have adequate calcium in her blood, it is removed from the supply in her bones, thus weakening them. Smoking tobacco and drinking alcohol also promote bone loss. The hormone estrogen is responsible for regulating the woman's use of calcium from bone, promoting long bone growth, and helping to protect bone. However, the ovaries stop producing estrogen at menopause, hastening the loss of bone. This can lead to a condition called osteoporosis, or brittle bones that can break easily.

Osteoporosis in postmenopausal women can be slowed through exercise and increasing calcium intake to 1,500 mg/day. This can be accomplished by eating

PREVENTING HIP FRACTURES

A broken hip, especially after menopause, is a serious injury. Although modern orthopedic surgical techniques and care can assist in healing of the bone, most hip fracture patients require extended periods of rehabilitation. They may need assistance from their family or home care, or may be transferred from hospitals to long-term care facilities. Walking aids may be necessary for several months after the injury, and many patients will permanently require canes or walkers to move around the house or outdoors.

Who is at risk for hip fractures? For one, women over 65. Slender women with small bones may be more prone to such fractures than large, heavy-boned women, and a family history of fractures in later life is another important indication of vulnerability. Women who have a low dietary intake of calcium, smoke, or drink alcohol excessively are also in the higher risk category, as are those with arthritis, poor balance, coordination, and eyesight.

Obviously, prevention of hip fractures is far better, and far less costly, than treatment after the bone is broken. A diet high in calcium, regular exercise, and the correct medications can all help to prevent weak bones and the possibility of a hip fracture in the future. Remember, too, that most of these injuries occur as a result of a fall, usually in the home. There are steps that you can take to minimize your chances of such an accident:

- *Stairways.* Provide enough light to see each step clearly. Repair loose stairway rugs. Do not leave objects on the stairs. Install handrails on both sides of the stairway.

- *Bathrooms.* Install grab bars on the walls around the tub. Place a skid-resistant rug next to the bathtub for safe exit and entry. Use a nonskid rubber mat or textured adhesive strips on the tub and shower floor. Install a night light.

- *Bedrooms.* Place a lamp and flashlight near your bed. Keep the floor clear of clutter, and make sure the route between the bedroom and bathroom is clear of objects and illuminated by a night light.

- *Living areas.* Keep pathways clear of furniture, plants, lamps, and electrical cords and wires. Secure loose area rugs and runners with tape, tacks, or slip-resistant backing. Avoid standing on unsteady stools, chairs, or ladders to clean or to reach distant objects.

IF THE SHOE FITS

Many common foot problems are caused or made worse by improper size and fit of shoes. According to the Council on Women's Shoewear of the Orthopedic Foot and Ankle Society, most women wear shoes approximately $1/2$ inch narrower than their foot, resulting in foot pain and deformities such as bunions, hammer toes, and calluses.

Many women wear shoes that are too small because the shoe must be snug in the front to stay on the back. The foot has only one bone in the heel, which stays narrow throughout life. The front of the foot, in contrast, is made up of many bones connected by ligaments. Over the years, these ligaments stretch, and the front part of the foot widens; in addition, the arch may sag, and the foot becomes longer. This can increase the shoe size.

Here are some guidelines for selecting shoes:

- Your feet may vary in size, so ask the salesperson to measure the length and width of each foot.

- The shoes you buy should be fitted to your longer and wider foot.

- Feet expand when bearing weight, so stand while your feet are being measured.

- Feet tend to swell during the course of a day, so shop for shoes at the end of the day.

- Never select a shoe by size alone. A size 8 in one brand or style may be smaller or larger than the same size in another brand or style. Buy the shoe that fits well.

- Don't assume that you will always have the same size feet. As you grow older, the size may change, so have your feet measured regularly.

- If shoes feel too tight, don't buy them. Remember, there's no such thing as "breaking in" a shoe. You can sustain considerable foot pain and damage while you wait for a shoe to stretch and fit properly.

- Shoes are not always sized correctly. To make sure, take a 6-inch ruler to the store with you to measure the shoes.

Women often have problems finding shoes that are sized correctly and are appropriate for their work and social functions. Sometimes compromises are necessary. Because of the long-term consequences, however, women should avoid wearing shoes that don't fit properly or that can cause deformities in their feet.

foods high in calcium, or by taking supplements. Hormone replacement therapy, or estrogen taken after menopause to replace that which is no longer being made by the ovaries, can also help prevent osteoporosis.

Osteoporosis can lead to hip fractures. A hip fracture is a break in the femur bone, just below the hip joint or in the upper thigh bone. Over 280,000 hip fractures occur in the United States each year, and most of these fractures occur in women. Women over the age of 65 have a 1 in 5 chance of suffering from hip fracture during their lifetime. Most hip fractures require extensive care, and many result in long-term disability and even death as a result of complications. In addition to taking steps to avoid osteoporosis, a woman should also try to make her home as safe as possible to prevent falls and accidents (See Preventing Hip Fractures).

Exercise strengthens bones and decreases the rate of bone loss. To be most effective, the exercise should be weight bearing. Weight can be applied to the bones by the weight of the body, such as with walking, or by lifting or holding weights. Exercise also strengthens muscles and joints and helps make connective tissues more flexible.

Careful weight management is important to the health of the musculoskeletal system. Although heavier women have stronger bones, and thus are less at risk of osteoporosis, being overweight causes stress and strain on certain joints, especially the knees and hips. Women who have been overweight most of their lives are more likely to have a kind of arthritis called osteoarthritis, the gradual wearing away of cartilage and bone in the joints. Extra weight can also increase the pain involved with this condition.

The feet are the foundation upon which your whole body rests. They play an important role in the musculoskeletal system as well as in your overall health, comfort, and ease of activity. Proper foot care, including the selecting and fitting of shoes, can help prevent foot problems that plague many women (see ''If the Shoe Fits'').

Cancer can occur in bones just as it does in other parts of the body (see Chapter 36). It can begin in the bone or spread there from other areas. Because breast cancer often spreads to the bone, it's important to perform monthly breast self-examination (see Chapter 25) and get regular checkups to detect breast cancer early, before it has spread.

As with many health problems, the first sign of a problem in the musculoskeletal system is usually pain. Any symptoms should be evaluated by a doctor, who may consult with a variety of health professionals, depending on the problem (see ''Health Care Professionals'').

SIGNS AND SYMPTOMS

Problems in the musculoskeletal system usually appear first as pain. Pain can occur in the affected area or be felt elsewhere. This is called referred pain. Pain in smaller joints is usually more sharply localized, whereas pain in larger joints can be felt in a general area. Certain characteristics about pain aid in the diagnosis:

- Is the pain located in one spot, or does it occur all over the body?
- Does the pain involve one joint, or are several joints affected?
- Does the pain move from one joint to another, or has it steadily progressed to include several joints?
- Did the pain occur suddenly or develop over time?
- Has the pain become steadily worse, or does it come and go?

- How long has the pain lasted, and does it occur, worsen, or improve at certain times of the day?
- What factors make the pain better or worse?
- In what setting did the pain develop, and was it related to injury or excessive use of the body part affected?

In addition to assessing the nature of the pain and how it arose, related factors are considered in the diagnosis:

- Limitation in the normal range of motion of joints.
- Signs of inflammation, including swelling, tenderness in or around a joint, increased heat, or redness.
- Stiffness.
- Skin conditions or other symptoms occurring elsewhere in the body.

These signs and symptoms can help pinpoint the diagnosis. Their significance depends on the part of the body affected and the pattern of the symptoms. Treatment is based on the cause and can range from medication to surgery. Anti-inflammatory medications are often used in the treatment of musculoskeletal disorders (see box).

Back Pain

The S-shaped curve of the spine makes it prone to problems. The backbone includes 24 individual vertebrae, as well as the sacrum and the coccyx at the end of the spine. (see Fig. 34.2) It is divided into three regions:

- Lumbar (lower back)
- Thoracic (chest)
- Cervical (neck)

The spinal cord runs through the middle of the spinal column. Nerves branch out from the spinal cord to the rest of the body. Thus, problems in the back can affect other parts of the body and cause pain.

Pain in the back is a frequent complaint. Fortunately, most back pain is the result of mild injuries or strains that are not serious and go away within a short time. In many cases, the cause of back pain is not known. Conditions which may cause chronic back pain include:

- **Disc herniation:** This occurs when the fibrous cushion between vertebra bulges out and causes pressure on one or more spinal nerves.
- **Spinal stenosis:** This occurs when the canal containing the spinal cord becomes narrowed, and thus the nerves traveling in the canal are squeezed and pinched.
- **Tumors:** Destruction of normal bone by tumors can cause chronic pain.

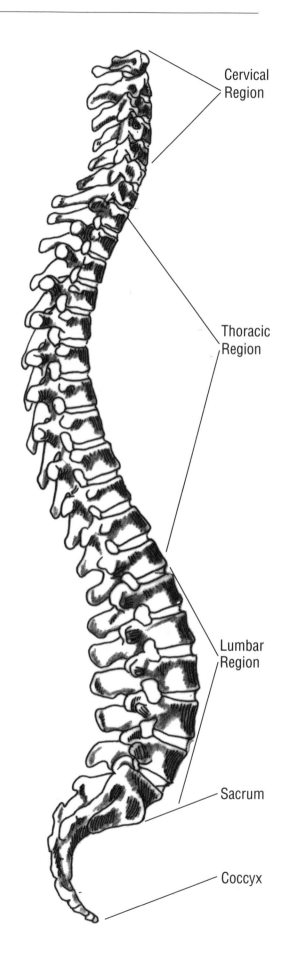

Figure 34.2 The Spine
The spine, or vertebral column, is made up of interlocking bones called *vertebrae*. The 26 bones of the spine include the 7 *cervical*, the 12 *thoracic*, and the 5 *lumbar* vertebrae. Five fused vertebrae form the single bone called the *sacrum*. The *coccyx* consists of two to four fused vertebrae that represent the tail of our prehuman ancestors.

- **Arthritis:** This can result in joint surfaces being worn away and the development of bone spurs. Both can result in back pain.
- **Fibromyalgia:** The condition is characterized by aching and pain in muscles, tendons, and joints all over the body and especially along the spine.
- **Trauma:** This can cause fractures, injuries to the ligaments, or muscle tears. It may result in compression fractures of the vertebrae.
- **Referred pain:** This is pain which originates in other organs, such as the pancreas or kidney, but is felt in the back.

Lower back pain is centered in the small of the back and is often caused by unusual exertion or physical strain. It can also be caused by muscle spasms. Other causes of lower back pain include disc problems, arthritis, and spinal stenosis. Pain in the middle or thoracic part of the spine in women can be caused by muscle strain due to poor posture, fibromyalgia, or compression fractures that result from osteoporosis. Pain in the neck region is often related to disc problems and arthritis.

Back pain is cause for concern when pain or numbness travels down the legs, when bladder or bowel function is disrupted, or when the pain continues without improvement. The buttocks and legs may be affected. In some cases, pain may become more severe with coughing, sneezing, or bending.

Back pain is diagnosed by obtaining a history of symptoms, mapping the location and pattern of the pain, and physical examination. Additional studies may include X-rays, a computed tomography (CT) scan, magnetic resonance imaging (MRI), or bone scans.

Lower back pain may be treated with rest, moist heat, massage, and medication. Other treatments include weight reduction, exercise, and in some cases physical therapy and psychological counseling. Surgery is reserved for those patients in whom a treatable cause has been identified, such as disc herniation, or spinal stenosis.

Foot and Ankle Pain

Pain in the foot is often related to wearing improperly fitting shoes. Ill-fitting shoes can result in corns, calluses, and bunions, which are thickening and hardening of the skin over bony protrusions caused by friction. Wearing high heels can contribute to a condition called metatarsalgia, an inflammation of the metatarsal bones of the foot that causes pain in the ball of the foot. Another cause of foot pain is neuroma, in which swelling from a nerve causes pain between the toes.

Heel pain is caused by inflammation of the plantar fascia, a ligament-like structure that begins at the heel and ends in the forefoot. In this condition, pain begins at the heel and extends along the arch of the foot. Problems relating to the Achilles tendon, which connects the calf muscle to the heel, can also cause pain. This tendon can become inflamed or torn, usually as the result of an injury. Pain in the ankle is often due to sprains. The ligaments that support the ankle joint can become stretched or torn, usually as the result of a twisting injury. Severe pain, swelling, and bruising may occur.

The diagnosis of heel and foot problems depends on the location of the pain, whether it occurred in relation to an injury, and the nature of the pain. Usually the diagnosis is based on the results of an examination. An x-ray exam may be used to detect bone spurs or rule out fractures.

Hip Pain

Pain in the hip is a frequent complaint that can be hard to pinpoint. Pain from the hip can be felt in the groin area or the top of the thigh or the knee. Osteoporosis can lead to weakening of the bones and fractures, especially in elderly women. Pain along the outside of the hip can be caused by inflammation of the bursae located around the hip. If a disc in the spine presses on a nerve, it can cause sciatica, which can result in pain in the buttocks or pain radiating down the back of a leg. The location of the pain helps determine the diagnosis. In elderly women, hip fracture should be suspected, especially after a fall, even if they have only minor pain. If the fracture is unrecognized, it may become displaced (the bones may move out of place) and require more extensive surgery than might otherwise be required.

Joint Pain

Pain in a joint that is not swollen or inflamed is called arthralgia. Joint pain with inflammation and swelling is called arthritis. Certain disorders that result from infections, such as rheumatic fever, rubella, or Lyme disease, can cause joints to ache and become swollen. The autoimmune diseases, like lupus, can affect multiple joints. The pain can occur in a single joint, multiple joints, or move from one joint to another. Arthritis can be diagnosed by physical examination, blood tests, examination of the fluid from the joint, and imaging tests such as X-rays or MRI, and arthroscopy (direct viewing into the joint).

Leg and Knee Pain

Leg pain can be related to an injury or to muscle cramps. It can also be caused by problems in circulation, which are serious and should receive immediate medical attention (see Chapter 26). Shin splints are injuries that occur as a result of repeated pounding on hard surfaces, such as with jogging or tennis. The fibers that tie the muscle to the bone become inflamed and cause pain in the shin. They can be relieved through rest, applying cold, and elevating the injured area.

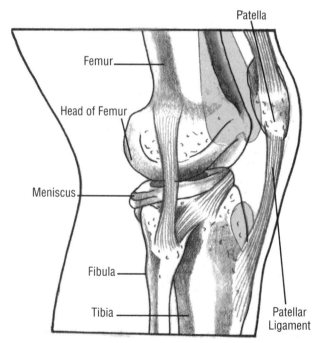

Figure 34.3 The Knee
The knee joint is one of the most complicated joints in the human body; it helps balance the entire weight of the body. It is surrounded by cartilage and ligaments that support it and allow movement. A crescent-shaped pad of cartilage, the *meniscus*, cushions the *femur*, or thigh bone, where it meets the *tibia*, the larger of the two bones in the calf and the stoutest bone in the body. (The *fibula*, the smaller of the two calf bones, forms part of the ankle joint.) The *patella*, or kneecap, is attached to the femur and tibia by the *patellar ligament*.

A muscle cramp is a spasm of the muscle that produces sudden and intense pain. It can occur as a result of muscle strain or as a result of overexertion, especially in warm weather when there is a risk of dehydration. Calf muscle cramps can also occur at night. Muscle cramps are not serious and usually can be relieved by gently stretching the affected limb. Massaging the muscle and applying heat, either in the form of a hot bath or heating pad, may also relieve the pain.

Pain in the knee is often the result of an injury, either new or old. Injuries commonly occur in athletic younger women. In older women, particularly those who are overweight, knee pain can be caused by osteoarthritis. Pain felt at the front of the knee, which can become worse when climbing stairs or exercising, can be caused by problems with the kneecap fitting into its groove and moving smoothly, a condition called chondromalacia patellae. It can also be caused by disorders in the cartilage and bone supporting the kneecap. Inflammation of the bursae, tendon, or synovial space in the joint between the thigh and calf bones can cause knee pain, as can a tear in the meniscus, the cartilage "washer" between the knee bones that cushions the joint. (See Fig. 34.3) The diagnosis depends on how the pain arose and other symptoms present. Severe pain and fever could be a sign of an infection and should receive medical attention right away.

Shoulder and Elbow Pain

Pain felt in the shoulder is often referred from another area, such as the neck. A heart or lung problem can also cause shoulder pain. One of the most common musculoskeletal causes of shoulder pain is a condition called subacromial impingement, also known as rotator cuff tendinitis. The rotator cuff, the muscles and tendons that make up the shoulder joint, can become inflamed, usually as the result of an injury or repeated motion. Injury or continued motion also can cause the rotator cuff to tear. The tendon that attaches the biceps muscle to the shoulder also can become inflamed as a result of repeated movement. If movement is constricted because of the pain, a "frozen" or severely limited, shoulder may result. Although arthritis is not as common in the shoulder as it is in other areas, it can occur.

Pain along the outside of the elbow can be caused by small tears where the muscles are attached. This condition is called tennis elbow (or lateral epicondylitis), but it can occur for reasons other than playing tennis, mostly related to overuse or stress of muscles at the point of attachment to the bone. Grip strength is usually reduced and shaking hands with someone can be painful. The diagnosis is based on a physical examination, and treatment begins with rest and avoiding overuse. Exercises may be done to strengthen and stretch the forearm muscles, and wearing a forearm band or wrist splint may be helpful.

Hand and Wrist Pain

The hand is an intricate structure that is in constant use. The activities of everyday living subject the structures of the hand to repeated trauma. Pain in the hands can be caused by arthritis, infection, inflammation of the muscles and tendons, injuries, problems with circulation, or tumors. The complex and delicate anatomy of the hands complicates treatment of hand injuries.

Arthritis can affect any of the many joints in the hand, resulting in limited use. Inflammatory arthritis, such as rheumatoid arthritis, can affect all of the hand joints while osteoarthritis may affect only some of them.

A relatively minor injury to the hand can result in an infection that limits function. In addition to pain, other signs of infection include redness (especially a red streak on the arm), swelling, fever, and heat. If these signs occur, seek medical attention immediately to prevent permanent damage to the skin, soft tissue, and bone. Infection of the hand can be caused by bacteria or a virus, such as the herpes simplex virus. Bacterial infections can arise as a result of a bite, either from a human or an animal. Treatment may involve surgical drainage of the wound and antibiotics.

Some of the most frequent complaints related to hands are the result of the inflammation of these constantly used structures. Tendons and their lining, muscles, and joints of the hand can become inflamed through repeated use, causing pain and swelling. Tendinitis can occur with an unusual activity, such as painting, or as the result of an arthritic condition. Although it can occur anywhere in the hand, tendinitis most often occurs around the wrist. Muscles of the hand, particularly those in the fleshy part of the thumb, are subject to stress and can become swollen and painful. Severe swelling may rupture muscle fibers.

Pain in the wrist or hand can be caused by repeated use. Carpal Tunnel syndrome, which causes pain, tingling, and weakness in the hand and wrist, results from compression of the median nerve. (see Fig. 34.4) Pain that occurs with movement of the thumb is often caused by a condition called DeQuervain's tenosynovitis, a condition in which the thumb tendons become inflamed.

Tendons and nerves of the hand are very close to the skin of the top of the hand, so a cut that appears to be minor can cause major damage. A cut on the finger or hand that results in the inability to bend or straighten the finger suggests that a tendon has been severed. Seek medical attention if any numbness, loss of motion, or severe pain on motion occurs after a laceration or cut. If a wound is dirty, it must be cleaned by a qualified health care professional. If a tendon or nerve has been injured, surgery may be required. Tendon injuries must be protected with a splint during healing. Physical therapy may be required to restore full function.

A fingertip may be crushed, such as when a car door is slammed on it; if the fingernail becomes discolored and there is swelling and pain, the nailbed may be injured. This may cause the nail to be mal-

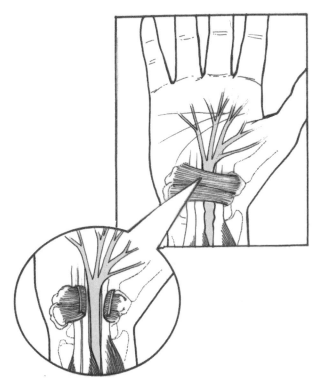

Figure 34.4 Carpal Tunnel Syndrome
Carpal tunnel syndrome is caused by compression of the *median nerve*, which runs through a sheath of muscle, the *retinaculum* ("carpal tunnel") at the wrist. The syndrome is common in pregnant women and in people who engage in repetitive hand and wrist movements.

formed when it regrows. An injured nailbed may require surgical repair.

Certain problems can cause tightening of the skin that pulls the finger or wrist into an abnormal position and restricts motion. Scarring, either from injury or from burns, also can interfere with hand motion. In some cases the skin can be released with surgery and a skin graft applied. Other conditions that result in tight-

ening of the skin include scleroderma, a connective tissue disease, and Dupuytren's contracture, a disorder in the connective tissue of the palm.

Some disorders that affect the hands are caused by problems in the blood vessels or nerves that supply them. A tumor called a ganglion can also arise from tendons and disrupt hand function. Treatment of these conditions varies based on any underlying disorder.

DISORDERS

Problems affecting the musculoskeletal system can either be limited to a specific area (usually due to an injury to that area) or can affect multiple areas. Such problems include infections, trauma, tumors, osteoporosis, certain medical disorders, and inflammatory conditions such as arthritis. Treatment is directed to the cause.

Achilles Tendon Injuries

The Achilles tendon links the leg muscles in the calf to the bone at the back of the heel. With exercise or strain, such as that which occurs with jogging or aerobic exercise, the tendon can become inflamed and even tear. Wearing high heels also may cause the tendon to become shortened, causing strain when the foot is flat. Symptoms include a dull ache or pain in the heel, especially with exercise. Swelling and tenderness may be noted as well. Since injury is usually the cause, the diagnosis is based on the patient's history and examination.

Treatment involves rest, applying ice to the ankle (when the injury is acute), and taking nonsteroidal anti-inflammatory drugs to provide relief. Occasionally a splint may be used. Heel lifts also may be used to raise the heel. Running or jumping is prohibited until the tendon has healed, then stretching and strengthening exercises can be done. If the tendon has ruptured or torn, it may have to be reattached with surgery.

Arthritis

Arthritis causes pain, swelling, and stiffness in joints. There are various types of arthritis based on the cause and the disease process involved. Some types of arthri-

tis result from mechanical wear on the parts, whereas others occur for no known reason. Arthritis can also be caused by infections.

Osteoarthritis

Also known as degenerative arthritis, this condition is a chronic wearing away of the cartilage that protects the joint. With normal use, the cartilage in joints becomes worn, so many people develop osteoarthritis with age; osteoarthritis affects women more than men and usually occurs after age 40. Rarely, an injury, a birth defect, or overuse of a joint such as from being overweight may cause osteoarthritis at an earlier age.

Osteoarthritis may affect any joint in the body if there is a prior injury but is mostly found in the knees, big toes, and small joints at the ends of the fingers. Pain often occurs after using the joint and improves with rest. There is little or no morning stiffness and the joint may be swollen but is rarely hot or red. The disease is confined to the joints, so other symptoms usually are not present. The diagnosis is based on the history and physical examination. X-rays may help assess any damage to the joint. Treatment consists of applying heat to the joint, and weight reduction, particularly for arthritis in the knee and hip. (See Fig. 34.5) Exercises to keep joints mobile and to strengthen the muscles surrounding them may be helpful, and medications can be used for pain relief. Surgery to replace the hip or knee joint is occasionally required.

Rheumatoid Arthritis

This form of arthritis is a chronic inflammatory process that affects the lining of a joint, the synovium. It results in swelling and destruction of cartilage and bone over time. Women between the ages of 30 and 50 are most often affected. The cause of rheumatoid arthritis is not known. It could be related to a combination of inher-

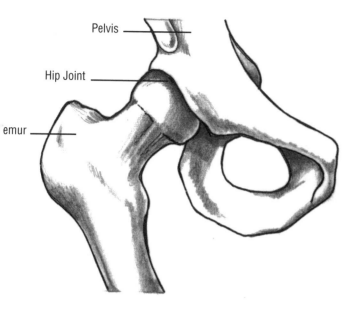

Pelvis

Hip Joint

emur

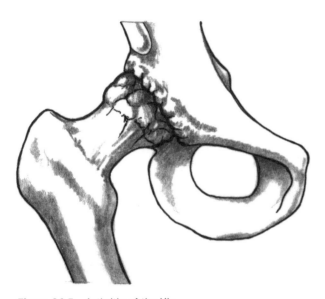

Figure 34.5 Arthritis of the Hip
Arthritis of the hip joint can cause a once healthy joint (top) to become painful as the cartilage is worn away and becomes scaly (bottom).

ited and environmental factors. It could also be an autoimmune disorder, by which the immune system mistakenly begins to attack specific tissues in the body.

Like other forms of inflammatory arthritis, rheumatoid arthritis causes joints to become stiff, painful, swollen, and warm. It usually affects the hands, feet, wrists, knees, elbows, and ankles, and it can begin in one joint and progress to others. Stiffness occurs after rest. Unlike osteoarthritis, people with rheumatoid arthritis can also have flu-like symptoms of fatigue, low-grade fever, and muscle aches. The diagnosis is based on the pat-

tern and the progression of disease. Blood tests and X-rays can be used to provide further information. Treatment depends on the severity of the condition and can include nonsteroidal anti-inflammatory drugs, steroids, and drugs that suppress the immune system. Exercise can strengthen muscles and bones so they can continue to support the joints.

Infectious Arthritis

Infections with bacteria can cause arthritis. These are acute forms of arthritis, coming on suddenly, whereas osteoarthritis and rheumatoid arthritis are chronic, with slow but steady progression. One such acute infection is Lyme disease (discussed later). Another is gonococcal infection, which is transmitted sexually. It is reported 10 times more often in women than in men, and about one-third of women who contract the disease have pain in several joints. Symptoms of gonococcal arthritis are joint pain and swelling that come on suddenly, especially if they are accompanied by red sores on the skin of the extremities. Seek medical treatment immediately to avoid long-term complications from the disorder. It is treated with antibiotics. Both sexual partners must also be treated and should abstain from sex until treatment is completed.

Bursitis

A bursa is a sac-like structure near areas of the joints that are subject to heavy movement. Bursae cushion the tendons moving near joints and help reduce the amount of friction. Bursitis occurs when the bursae become inflamed because of strain or injury. Repeated physical activity, such as swinging motions involved in tennis, golf, or baseball, can lead to bursitis. Most commonly, it can affect the shoulder, knee, elbow, or hip. Pain and swelling can occur at the affected area or near a joint as fluid accumulates in the bursa. The diagnosis is based on a physical examination and assessment of recent activities. During the examination the doctor can locate the area of tenderness and swelling and check the range of motion of the joint. Diagnostic X-rays may be taken to detect any other causes or to show old injuries.

Drugs such as a nonsteroidal anti-inflammatory will ease the pain, and often bursitis disappears on its own within a few weeks. If it persists, however, some of the fluid may be removed from the bursa with a syringe to relieve the pressure. Corticosteroids may be injected directly into the bursa in the area of the affected joint or, rarely, it may need to be removed by surgery.

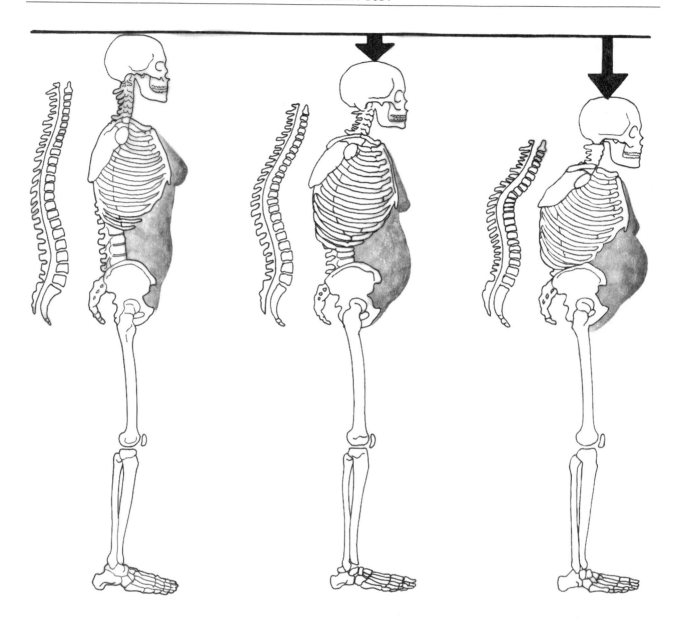

Figure 34.6 Osteoporosis
Osteoporosis causes bone mass to be lost, which can result in compression fractures in the spine. As normal vertebrae (left) begin to lose bone mass and weaken under the body's weight (middle), the spinal column collapses and shortens (right), causing the characteristic "dowager's hump" seen in individuals with this condition.

Compression Fractures

These fractures can occur with minimal injury, often because bones are weakened by osteoporosis. The most common cause of back pain in the thoracic region is compression fracture due to osteoporosis. About one in every four women has a vertebral fracture by the time she reaches age 60. (See Fig. 34.6)

A woman may lose height as a result of compression fractures of the spine. She may feel pain in the middle of the back, but often there are no symptoms, however. The condition is diagnosed by x-rays. There is no treatment for osteoporosis, but its progress can be slowed through diet high in calcium, exercise that strengthens the bones and helps prevents bone loss, and hormone replacement therapy.

Disc Problems

Discs are pieces of cartilage between the spinal vertebrae that separate and cushion the vertebrae as you move. A disc can be ruptured when injury, compression fractures, or wear and tear cause the gel-like center to squeeze against the spinal cord or one of the nerves. When this occurs, the disc is said to be herniated, prolapsed, or "slipped." This is most likely to happen in discs in the lower back and neck, although it can occur in any of the vertebrae in the spine.

A prolapsed disc in the lower back may arise acutely from an injury such as lifting. A woman often reports she felt a sudden "snap" in her low back while performing a task. In other cases, the symptoms may come on gradually. Pain may be felt in the lower back only or in the buttock and travel down the thigh and leg. This type of pain is called sciatica because it is felt along the course of the sciatic nerve. A prolapsed disc in the neck may cause sudden, extreme pain in the neck that is made worse by moving the neck, coughing or straining.

As a woman ages, her discs gradually dry out and lose elasticity. The bones of the neck may respond to this by forming spurs known as osteophytes. This combination is called cervical spondylosis. It can cause the spinal cord, as well as spinal nerves, to be compressed. This can result in pain with movement of the head, which can radiate to the shoulders, upper extremities, and chest area. Reflexes and sensations may also be affected.

Spinal stenosis occurs in the lumbar spine when the channel that hold the spinal cord becomes narrowed by thickened ligaments, breakdown of the vertebrae, and protruding discs. This can cause pressure on multiple nerves and result in pain in the legs and back after prolonged standing or walking. The pain can be on one or both sides and can go deep into the thigh. Other symptoms, such as weakness, loss of feeling in the legs, or urinary problems, also may occur.

A prolapsed or herniated disc is diagnosed based on symptoms and clinical findings on examination. The nature of the symptoms depends on the disc and nerves affected. If a prolapsed disc is suspected, a CT scan or MRI of the neck or spine can locate the area where the disc is out of place. Treatment depends on the disc affected and whether there are signs of nerve damage. A prolapsed disc in the neck is treated by immobilizing it with traction, or resting on a collar and giving medication for pain and muscle spasms. A prolapsed disc in the lumbar region is treated with bed rest and pain medication. Surgery may be required if the con-

dition does not improve or there are signs of neurologic impairment.

Dupuytren's Contracture

This disease of the palm causes the fingers, especially the ring and small finger, to be gradually pulled into the palm. The disease causes a shortening, thickening, and hardening of the connective tissue just under the skin of the palm. There is a tender lump in the palm, which may progress to becoming a cord that extends to the fingers. The cause of the disease is unknown, but it runs in families and seems to be associated with epilepsy, diabetes, injuries, and alcoholism.

If a finger is left in the bent position, the joint stiffens. Surgery is indicated when one or more fingers cannot be straightened completely. It involves removal of the diseased tissue to release the fingers. Although surgery has a high success rate, the disease may progress to other fingers.

Fibromyalgia

This condition affects more women, especially those over middle age, than men. The cause of the disorder is unknown, but those women who don't get enough deep or rapid eye movement (REM) sleep seem to be at higher risk.

Aching and pain occur in the muscles, tendons, and joints all over the body. The condition often affects the back and can cause muscle tenderness. The pain may take the form of a tingling sensation. The joints don't swell but may feel stiff. Multiple tender spots are located along the spine and the extremities. The condition is associated with extreme fatigue and sleep disturbance, which may be severe.

The diagnosis is based on the history, excluding other causes of these symptoms, and treatment is with sleep-promoting drugs, nonsteroidal anti-inflammatory drugs, and lifestyle changes involving a reduction of stress, exercises, and relaxation techniques.

Foot Problems

Many foot problems in women are caused by ill-fitting shoes. The most common problems are bunions, corns, and calluses. In some women, arthritis can occur in the joint of the big toe, causing extra bone to pile up at the joint and produce pain. Most of these problems can be prevented or helped by proper footwear.

Bunions

A bony protrusion on the outside of the joint at the base of the big toe occurs when pressure is concentrated on the big toe, changing the normal profile of the foot. Over time, the big toe may turn sideways so you are walking on the bony inner side of the toe instead of the bottom, where the padding is. (See Fig. 34.7) The bun-

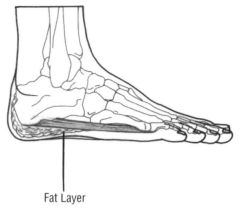

Fat Layer

Figure 34.8 Foot Padding
The foot is padded at the heel with a layer of fat that helps cushion the impact of movement.

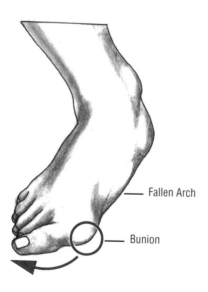

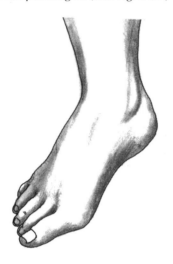

— Fallen Arch

— Bunion

Figure 34.7 Bunions
Bunions are bony protrusions that form on the joint at the base of the big toe. A normal-appearing foot (top) can become bent (bottom), so that weight is placed on the inner part of the foot, causing the arch to collapse.

ion is often subjected to constant rubbing, which results in a thickening of the skin (callus) and pain. The cause of bunions is usually wearing shoes that are too narrow. The best therapy is wearing shoes that have ample room for toes and that do not put pressure on them. (Fig. 34.8) When shoe changes do not relieve the bunion pain, surgery may be considered.

Corns and Calluses

Constant pressure or repeated friction on the skin produces a thickening and hardening of the skin. This often occurs on and between the toes, causing discomfort. Some women get hard calluses, called corns, on the top of their toes or soft calluses between their toes. Corns are often associated with hammer toes and claw toes, when the toe becomes permanently bent from being in that position. Corns and calluses on the feet are usually caused by poorly fitting shoes and high heels, and can be relieved by wearing soft shoes of the proper shape. The thickened skin of corns can be gradually removed with a towel or mild abrasive (such as a pumice stone or file) after it has been softened by a shower or bath. If the problem persists, the tissue may need to be removed surgically.

Neuroma

This condition involves a painful swelling of a nerve located between two toes, usually between the second and third or third and fourth toes. It arises from excessive pressure inside the foot. Symptoms include intermittent burning pain between the toes, particularly while bearing weight. Pain can become worse with running or walking, and may be eased by sitting down, removing the shoe, and rubbing the foot. The diagnosis is based on a physical examination. Treatment may involve pads under the ball of the foot to cushion it, nonsteroidal anti-inflammatory drugs, and steroid injections. Relief is usually obtained by widening the shoe, lowering the heel, and softening the insole. Rarely, surgery may be required to remove the growth if the pain is disabling.

Metatarsalgia

This is aching pain felt directly under the bones of the forefoot, especially when weight is placed on the foot. It is usually related to too much pressure being placed on the metatarsal part of the foot, often the result of wearing thin soled or very high-heeled shoes. The diagnosis is based on an examination. Therapy is oriented toward unloading the pressure on the metatarsals by wearing a cushioning pad or a custom-molded shoe with a pad. Shoes with ample room for the toes allow weight to be evenly distributed over all the metatarsals so they can share the weight. This condition can also be caused by arthritis in the metatarsal area.

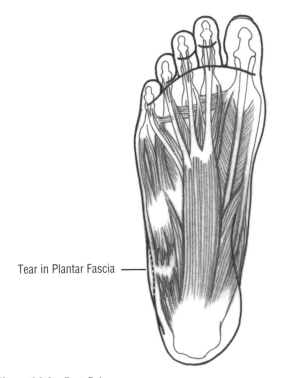

Tear in Plantar Fascia ————

Figure 34.9 Foot Pain
A tear in the *plantar fascia*, the wide ligament that stretches from the heel to the front of the foot, can cause inflammation, pain, and swelling.

Plantar Fasciitis

The plantar fascia are multiple bundles of connective tissue arranged in sheets underneath the foot. Chronic strain on these structures can cause them to become inflamed. Bone spurs of the heel may occur as a by-product of the inflammation. (See Fig. 34.9) Pain is localized to the heel and does not radiate to the rest of the foot. It is usually most severe on awakening or at the end of a long day of standing or walking. The heel is tender to the touch, especially if the first toe is extended.

The diagnosis is usually established by an examination. An X-ray may reveal a bone spur. Treatment is usually nonoperative and includes nonsteroidal anti-inflammatory drugs, heel stretching, rest, decreased weight bearing, and cups to cushion the heel. Steroids may be used, but multiple injections may cause atrophy of the heel pad. Surgery to remove a bone spur or release the plantar fascia may be required.

Ganglion

A benign (noncancerous) tumor that occurs on a tendon or at a joint, a ganglion is a thin fibrous capsule enclosing clear fluid. It ranges in size from a pea to a golfball and often appears in the hands and wrist, although it can occur in other places as well. It may occur as a result of an injury or repetitive strenuous wrist activity, but often there is no apparent cause. Discomfort may be caused by pressure on adjacent structures. A ganglion may go away on its own. A large painful ganglion can be treated by removing fluid from its center with a needle, or removing it with surgery. It may recur, however.

Gout

This condition occurs when uric acid, one of the body's waste products that is normally passed out of the body through the urine, builds up in the blood and is deposited in the joints. It is inherited, and it can be worsened by high-protein diet and overconsumption of alcohol. It can also be caused by some medications. Uric acid crystals cause inflammation in the joints and can accumulate in the kidneys and urine, causing kidney stones. Symptoms include sudden onset of pain, swelling of a single joint (usually the joint between the big toe and the foot), and redness of the overlying skin.

There can be a fever. If the disease is not treated, the soft tissue may become inflamed around the joint and the joint may become deformed because of uric acid deposits.

The condition is diagnosed by detecting high levels of uric acid in the blood and finding uric acid crystals in a sample of joint fluid. Treatment consists of NSAIDs (not aspirin) or a drug called colchicine. Those who experience recurrent attacks can be given a drug that lowers the levels of uric acid in the blood. Another option is to take a drug that increases the excretion of uric acid by the kidneys.

Infections

Infections of the bone—called osteomyelitis—have become increasingly rare because of the widespread availability of antibiotics. Before antibiotics were available, chronic infection of the bone (often as a result of trauma) or of the joints (as a result of tuberculosis) were crippling and sometimes fatal. Today chronic infection of bone usually occurs after a compound fracture, when a broken bone punctures the skin. When this occurs, the ends of the bone can die and lose their blood supply. Bacteria can live here easily and multiply quickly. Because of the poor blood supply to the bone ends, antibiotics cannot reach the bone easily. For this reason, open fractures are treated with thorough cleansing in the operating room to prevent infection. Similarly, an orthopedic operation can interfere with the blood supply of bones. Antibiotics are used to prevent infection after surgery.

Other types of infection can also cause problems in the musculoskeletal system. Certain types of bacterial infection cause arthritis. These include gonococcal infections, which are sexually transmitted, and Lyme disease, which is carried by ticks (see "Arthritis" and "Lyme disease").

Gangrene

This infection of the muscle usually occurs from an open wound. It spread rapidly and produces toxic effects throughout the body that, if untreated, can cause severe illness. Symptoms usually occur 2-4 days after the wound, and the first symptom is sudden and severe pain at the site. The diagnosis is based on clinical findings and identification of the infecting organism. Treatment involves giving antibiotics and removing the infected tissue with surgery.

Lyme Disease

This disease is named after the location in Lyme, Connecticut, where it was first discovered in 1976. Since then it has spread rapidly and is now most prevalent in New England, New York, New Jersey, and areas of the Mid-Atlantic and the Mid-West. Lyme disease is caused by a spirochete (a type of bacteria) infection of the blood that spreads to the connective tissues and causes symptoms of arthritis. The bacteria is carried by a deer tick, which lives on a variety of animals, including deer, mice, and dogs and cats that are outside. The tick is smaller than a regular tick and thus can be hard to detect.

Lyme disease can have three phases:

- Early localized infection: A red mark can form at the site of the bite. The rash can then spread to cover the entire back or leg. The rash is present in about one quarter of those affected and often disappears within a few days. General flu-like symptoms of fatigue and nausea often are present.

- Early disseminated infection: A rash may occur. The heart muscle may become inflamed and cause an irregular heartbeat. Nerves, especially the facial nerve, may be affected, resulting in paralysis or a condition called Bell's palsy.

- Persistent infection: Sixteen weeks or more after the initial infection, arthritis can occur. Areas most affected include knees, shoulders, elbows, ankles, and wrists, in that order. The joint of the jaw also may be affected. Up to 10 percent of patients can develop chronic arthritis in one or both knees, even after treatment.

However, someone with Lyme disease may proceed from the early stage to the persistent phase of the illness and be completely asymptomatic. Similarly, individuals with Lyme disease may first develop symptoms at the early localized, early disseminated, or persistent phase.

Most patients develop antibodies to the infection within 6 weeks after they are exposed to it. Although antibodies are usually produced by the body to prevent it from further infection, these antibodies do not seem to offer future protection against this disease.

The best way to protect against Lyme disease is to prevent tick bites. Use insect repellents containing DEET and wear long pants, preferably white ones that will show the ticks, when hiking through grass. The ticks are often brushed off deer and stay on tall grass. Check yourself and your children regularly for ticks and remove them promptly, making sure to remove both the head and the body. Use tweezers.

If symptoms develop, consult a doctor as soon as possible. Tests can be performed to detect the antibody to the infection. Unfortunately, current laboratory tests are not perfect in diagnosing the disease. Also, since it takes 6 weeks for antibodies to develop, the test will not be positive until that time.

Lyme disease is treated with antibiotics. In early localized infection with a rash, a 2–3 week course of treatment is usual and will prevent progression of the disease. In persistent infection, longer courses of oral or intravenous antibiotics may be required.

Medial Meniscus Tear

The medial and lateral menisci of the knee are half-moon shaped wedges of cartilage that act as a buffer or bumper in the joint between the thigh and the shin bones to soften the force of weight on that joint. The meniscus can tear from trauma or a sudden twisting injury of the knee. When this occurs, there is severe pain over the inside of the knee and swelling that does not go away quickly. The condition is diagnosed by physical examination and MRI. Surgery may be required to repair or remove the meniscus. Arthroscopic surgery has had a major impact in improving the management of this problem.

Osteoporosis

Osteoporosis is a condition that results in bone loss with aging. (See Fig. 34.10) As a woman's bones become weakened, she is susceptible to fractures, which can occur with only minor injury. Osteoporosis can lead to compression fractures of the vertebrae and back pain, particularly in the thoracic region of the back. It can also increase the risk of hip fractures, which should be suspected if hip pain is present, even if a woman cannot recall an injury. If the hip fracture is not displaced, that is, if the bones are still in place and have not moved—the fracture is relatively easy to treat. If not treated, however, a hip fracture can become displaced and require major surgery to repair. Treatment can involve placing a pin in the hip to hold it in place or replacing part or all of the hip joint.

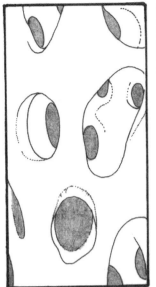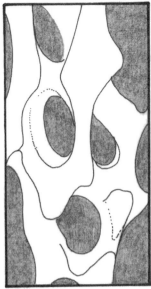

Figure 34.10 Osteoporosis
Osteoporosis is a condition in which normal bone (left) begins to lose the cells that produce new bone. This results in decreased bone mass, giving the bone a spongy appearance (right). Osteoporosis is more common in women than in men because of the natural decline in the hormone estrogen, which plays a role in bone cell production, that occurs with menopause.

Osteoporosis can be slowed through exercise, a diet high in calcium, and hormone replacement therapy. Back pain related to osteoporosis can be improved through the use of nonsteroidal anti-inflammatory drugs and exercises that strengthen the back muscles. With any pain, particularly in the wrist, collar bone, or hip, a fracture should be suspected, especially in older women.

Paget's Disease

In this disease, new bone is produced faster than old bone is broken down. The new bone is more spongy than compact, which leads to weakening of the bones. As new bone continues to be produced and old bone is not broken down, the bones may become thickened and the bone marrow cavity filled. The cause of this disorder is unknown, but it may be linked to a viral infection. It may affect many parts of the skeleton but is usually localized to the spine, pelvis, femur, and skull, which can become deformed and painful. The condition can be diagnosed with blood tests and X-rays. Treatment focuses on medications that strengthen the bones and relieve pain.

Polymyalgia Rheumatica

This disease of unknown origin affects people over 50, especially women. It causes pain in the hip and the shoulder regions and may be associated with a general sensation of not feeling well, weight loss, and fever. Symptoms of aching and stiffness may come on suddenly.

This condition may be related to another called giant-cell arteritis, or temporal arteritis. The temporal artery, which passes just in front of the ear and across the temple, becomes inflamed and interferes with the blood supply to the optic nerve. Blindness can result if the condition is not treated promptly. The first sign of this arthritis is a headache that recurs and is usually more severe on one side. Scalp tenderness also may be noted, and the artery may be enlarged.

Polymyalgia rheumatica is diagnosed by history, physical examination, and blood tests. If giant-cell arteritis is suspected, a biopsy of the artery may be performed. Complications can be avoided by early diagnosis and treatment with nonsteroidal antiinflammatory drugs (NSAIDS) and/or corticosteroids.

Polymyositis

These disorders of unknown cause affect the muscles and connective tissue, and some types are much more common in women. The disorder may have an autoimmune or genetic cause or be related to a viral infection. Symptoms can begin slowly and include weakness in the hip or shoulder muscles. In some cases, symptoms can come on suddenly and include fever or skin rash, rapidly progressing muscle weakness, and pain and tenderness. This disorder is diagnosed based on the physical findings, laboratory tests to detect muscle enzymes in the blood, electromyography to measure electrical responses of muscle contraction, and muscle biopsy to look for changes in the cells. The goals of treatment are to suppress the inflammatory response and reduce the loss of muscle and its strength. Results are best when treatment is given in the early stages. Treatment consists of corticosteroids or drugs that suppress the immune response. Physical therapy can teach patients exercises that reduce weakness and shrinking of muscles.

Raynaud's Disease

A disorder of the blood vessels, Raynaud's disease affects 3-4 times as many women as men. The symptoms are related to exposure to the cold and emotional stress, which cause pain, numbness, and a bluish or white color to the fingers and toes. Once the area is rewarmed, it is very pink for a time until normal color and sensation return. The spasmodic narrowing of the blood vessels that occurs with this disorder decreases blood flow and can lead to the development of ulcers or infection of the skin. Raynaud's disease can occur along with other disorders, such as scleroderma, lupus erythematosus, and arthritis.

Drugs that increase blood flow to the fingers and prevent the abnormal narrowing brought on by cold and emotional stress can be very effective in limiting attacks. The condition also can be treated with surgery of the nerves, but it is not always effective and complications are common. When Raynaud's disease is associated with other diseases, both problems must be treated.

Reflex Sympathetic Dystrophy

This is a poorly understood, disabling condition that can occur after what appears to be minor injury or surgery. It can occur in any extremity, and may be associated with overactivity of nerves that control the opening and closing of blood vessels and regulation of skin temperature. Symptoms include burning pain, swelling of the extremity, sweating, bluish discoloration, and stiffness. Treatment consists of nerve blocks or biofeedback to regulate the nervous system, physical therapy, and medication.

Scleroderma

A connective tissue disease that affects many organ systems, scleroderma involves the progressive replacement of normal tissues by dense, thick, scar-like tissue. The cause is unknown. It occurs most often in women between the ages of 30 and 40. In early stages, scleroderma can appear in the hands as tight skin limiting mobility. In later stages, the skin becomes increasingly thick and tight, hair and the ability to sweat are lost, and the skin may have the consistency of wood. Years after this stage has been reached, the skin may soften again. The treatment for scleroderma of the skin includes daily exercise of all joints, keeping the skin moisturized, and some specialized medications. Without proper treatment, the disease can affect interior organs, often fatally.

Spinal Curvature

The normal spine curves gently backward (kyphosis) in the upper back and gently inward in the low back (lordosis). However, there are several conditions that cause exaggeration of the normal curvature. Some are present at birth and some result from disease, poor posture, and the effects of aging. If very severe, abnormal spine curvature can interfere with movement and with body functions such as breathing. Mild cases are common, however, and may not require treatment.

Lordosis

When exaggerated, this condition is also called "swayback." It can be caused by disease, but more commonly results from abnormal weight distribution, such as with pregnancy or obesity.

Kyphosis

Also known as "roundback," kyphosis is an exaggerated rounding of the normal part of the spine. It can worsen during adolescence or it can result from compression of vertebrae that occurs with aging, particularly with women who have osteoporosis. It can also occur as the result of disease.

Scoliosis

An abnormal curving of the spine to the side, most often in the thoracic or thorocolumbar region. It commonly appears during adolescence, especially in girls. Although most progression of the curve occurs prior to the end of growth, severe curves can continue to progress during adulthood. (See Fig. 34.11) In severe

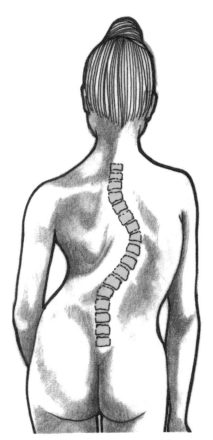

Figure 34.11   Scoliosis
Scoliosis, or curvature of the spine, has a number of possible causes, including abnormalities of the vertebrae, weakness of the muscles that support the spinal column, and inherited birth defects.

cases, body braces or surgery are needed before growth ends to prevent deformity or breathing problems.

Systemic Lupus Erythematosus

An autoimmune disorder in which the body's immune system attacks healthy cells, lupus can cause inflammation throughout the body. It can affect the skin, kidneys, lungs, heart, and nervous system, as well as the musculoskeletal system. The condition is much more common in women than in men, and usually occurs between the ages of 15 and 40, although it can occur at any time. Those who have a family history of the disorder are more at risk, and it may be linked to hormonal or environmental factors.

Systemic lupus erythematosus causes aching and swelling in the joints, often accompanied by fever, weight loss, and morning stiffness. Other symptoms include a butterfly-shaped rash on the face, chest pain, hair loss, swelling of the legs, high blood pressure, and depression.

People who have lupus have certain antibodies circulating in their blood. The diagnosis is based on the history, the symptoms, and the presence of these antibodies. The condition can get better or worse over a period of years. Therapy is directed toward suppressing inflammation and relieving symptoms. Treatment varies depending on the organ system involved and may include NSAIDs, corticosteroids, and drugs that suppress the immune system.

Tendinitis

Tendinitis is an inflammation of the tendons, the fibrous cords that attach the muscles to bones, usually caused by injury or overuse. It causes painful tenderness over the affected area, and the tendon is usually slow to heal because the muscle is in constant use. The area can become stiff because of the natural tendency to favor a painful area by not exercising it. Tendinitis often occurs in the shoulder in the form of rotator cuff tendinitis. It can also occur in the elbow (tennis elbow), and in the wrist.

Physical examination confirms the diagnosis of tendinitis. Sometimes X-rays are needed to rule out a bone injury. Treatment includes several days of rest and splinting of the affected area. Ice can be applied to reduce discomfort and swelling right after injury, and pain can be relieved with nonsteroidal anti-inflammatory drugs. After a few days of rest, gentle exercises can be done to increase the range of motion and flexibility of the joint. Often heat works better than ice at this point. Ultrasound or massage therapy may be recommended by your doctor. A recurrence can be avoided by warming up before exercise and cooling down afterward. In severe cases, an injection of corticosteroids may be recommended.

Trauma

Many problems in the musculoskeletal system are caused by injuries. They can result from sports activities or accidents and can affect most of the bones and joints in the body, although some are more susceptible than others. Examples of such injuries are fractures, sprains, and dislocations (see chapter 21, Trauma and Emergencies).

Fractures

A break in a bone is called a fracture. The break occurs as a result of the bone being stressed by physical forces greater than it can withstand. In a young person, the fracture usually occurs with a major injury, such as a motor vehicle accident or a sports-related injury. In older adults, fractures commonly occur with a fall. Adult bone gets weaker with age and will break with less force. Older women may suffer compression fractures of the vertebrae or fractures of the hip as a result of osteoporosis.

There are different types of fractures, classified according to the way the bone is broken:

- **Simple fractures** occur when the bone snaps but does not break the skin. (See Fig. 34.12A)
- **Open fractures** occur when the bone snaps and breaks through the skin. (See Fig. 34.12B)
- **Incomplete fractures** occur when the bone is cracked but not broken. (See Fig. 34.12C)

With all fractures, the first symptom is intense pain and swelling. A bruise may appear over a bone, and there may be numbness in the area. Pain becomes more severe when the affected area is moved or when pressure is applied. Fractures are diagnosed by physical examination and by X-ray. First aid involves giving support to the injured area and keeping it from moving with a splint (see Chapter 21). There is a risk of bone infection with an open fracture, so precautions should be taken to keep the injured area clean and to get prompt medical attention.

Fractures are treated with a process called reduction, in which the ends of the bones are aligned. They can be manipulated back together by a physician's hands, or surgery can be performed and the bone ends can be secured with wires, pins, and metal plates. The broken bone is then immobilized by a cast or traction to allow healing. It takes about 6–8 weeks for a broken bone to mend, and the healing time is longer with large bones and with elderly patients.

Sprains

An injury to a ligament, the tough bands of fibrous tissue that connect bones to each other and hold joints

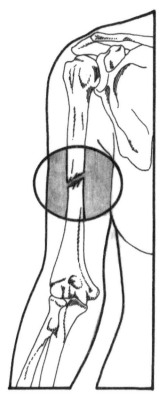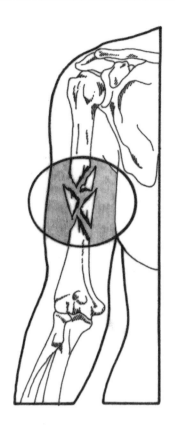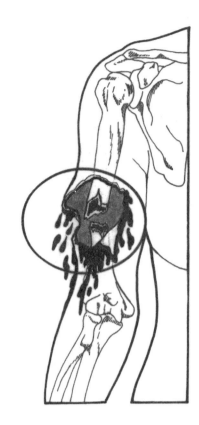

Figure 34.12 Fractures
Types of bone fractures include *simple* (or closed), in which the bone breaks in one place and the skin remains intact (left); *comminuted*, in which the bone breaks into several pieces (middle); and *compound* (or open), in which the skin is broken and there is an open wound down to the level of the bone itself.

in place, is a sprain. If excessive demands are made on a joint, the ligaments that hold the bones together may be stretched or torn. Any joint can be sprained, but the joints at the ankles, knees, wrists, and fingers are particularly susceptible to this type of injury. There are various types of sprains, depending on the degree of injury:

■ **A first-degree sprain** is a minor stretching injury, but the joint is still stable and able to function.

■ **A second-degree sprain** is a partial tear in the ligament, but the joint is still stable.

■ **A third-degree sprain** is a complete tear in the ligament, and the joint is no longer stable.

Symptoms include pain and tenderness, swelling, and sometimes bruising. The amount of pain depends on the amount of injury. If the pain is severe or if weight cannot be borne on the joint, medical attention should be sought. An X-ray may be required to distinguish a sprain from a fracture. These problems are best treated with a basic approach known as RICE:

Rest;
Immobilization, such as using a splint;
Cold to reduce pain and swelling; and,
Elevation. If pain is severe, if it persists, or if there are other symptoms present, immediate medical attention is required. A mild sprain can be supported with an elastic bandage on the joint. A second- or third-degree sprain may require a cast.

Dislocations

When two bones that make up a joint are no longer in contact, it is called a dislocation. This usually results from a major force great enough to tear the ligaments that support the joint. It can cause damage to the soft tissues that normally hold the joint in place. The main symptom is intense pain. The joint may look misshapen and become swollen, bruised, and immovable. Any joint can become dislocated, but this injury is most common in the shoulder, knee, hip, and fingers.

X-rays are done to show whether the bones are out of their normal position. The bones are repositioned in their normal place, possibly with the aid of an anesthetic to reduce pain. Sometimes surgery may be needed to reposition the bones and to repair damaged structures. Afterward, the joint will be immobilized for two or three weeks so the damaged tissues can heal. Sometimes dislocations can recur. It may be possible for the bones to be repositioned by the patient. This should be done under the guidance of a physician and evaluated afterward to ensure it was done properly.

Tumors

As with any cells of the body, bone cells are constantly reproducing so new cells can replace old ones. As with other parts of the body, bone cells can multiply and divide more than normal and result in tumors. These tumors may be benign (not cancerous) or cancerous, and they may arise in the bone or spread there from another source.

Benign Tumors

A benign tumor is one that stays localized to its original site and does not spread throughout the body.

Malignant Tumors

Malignant tumors invade and infiltrate local healthy tissue and damage or destroy that tissue. A primary malignancy refers to a tumor whose cells arise from the local area. Cancer cells that spread from another site are called metastatic or secondary tumors. Malignant tumors that begin in the bone are rare in adults. Secondary cancers in adults are most commonly from breast, kidney, lung, and thyroid cancer.

Soft tissue tumors are often first discovered as a lump or mass, while bone tumors frequently are discovered because a woman complains of a deep "boring" pain that interferes with sleep or activity. About 10 percent of bone cancer patients have fractures due to the weakening of bones by cancer cells. Diagnosis is based on a careful history, physical examination, and imaging studies, which may include X-ray, bone scans, CT, or MRI. A biopsy may be done so the cells can be examined under a microscope. The biopsy is usually performed by an orthopedic surgeon who specializes in oncology (tumors).

Treatment varies depending on whether the lesion is primary or metastatic. For a primary cancer, treatment often involves removing the cancer to prevent its spread. This can be done by a combination of surgery,

LIMB SALVAGE

Amputation was the standard treatment for primary bone cancer for many years. Today new techniques in limb salvage have allowed many limbs to be saved. In this technique, the patient often receives chemotherapy to first shrink the tumor. The tumor is then removed along with some normal tissue to be sure no cancer cells are left behind. This leaves a large gap in the bone, which can be filled by a bone from a human body, by shortening of the limb, or by replacement with a custom-made metal joint. The type of reconstruction takes into consideration a number of factors, including the patient's needs, age, and lifestyle. Long-term studies have shown that this technique is as safe as amputation in most cases. It adds to the quality of a woman's life because her limb is spared and thus function is maintained.

radiation, and chemotherapy. Sometimes, artificial bone can be put in place of the bone that is removed. One of the major advances in the management of primary bone cancer has been the development of limb salvage techniques (See box).

Treatment of bone cancers that have arisen from cancer in other parts of the body is mostly geared to relieving pain, supporting the structure of the diseased bone, and maintaining the function of the limb. Depending on the type of cancer, it may first be treated with chemotherapy or hormonal agents. If there is a risk of fracture or if fracture has occurred, the bone may be repaired with metal implants.

Wrist Problems

The wrist is susceptible to damage from repetitive tasks, overuse, and injuries. Some of these problems are work-related and are thus hard to prevent. All wrist problems should receive prompt medical attention, however, so further injury can be prevented.

Carpal Tunnel Syndrome

This condition is caused by compression of the median nerve at the wrist, usually because of overuse. Extra fluid in the tissues around the joints and bone narrow the space between the joints and joint capsule, causing pressure. The condition is fairly common in women, especially those who are pregnant or are of middle age or older. It may occur in women with diabetes, thyroid disease, or rheumatoid arthritis. Workers who engage in repetitive tasks that involve movement of the wrist, strong grip, or exposure to vibration (typists, for instance) are especially at risk. Symptoms include hand and wrist pain, tingling, and thumb weakness. Numbness may occur in the thumb, and index, middle, and part of the ring fingers. Many women find the symptoms are worse at night. They may have a burning sensation that improves with shaking the hand. Many women note difficulty holding objects.

The history is critical to the diagnosis. Tests such as electromyography may be done to reproduce the symptoms and to measure responses of the muscles and nerves. Treatment is directed to treating any underlying medical problem, if present. Efforts should be made to eliminate any stress that may come from repetitive use. A splint may be used on the wrist, particularly at night.

Medications such as NSAIDs and steroid injections may provide relief. In severe cases, a surgical procedure to release the constricting tunnel of fibers through which the nerve passes may be required.

deQuervain's Tenosynovitis

This condition is an inflammation of the tendon sheaths that contain the muscles that lift the thumb. It is often seen in the last three months of pregnancy and immediately after pregnancy. Usually the patient has a history of chronic, repetitive movements of the wrist and thumb. Women often complain of a "triggering" sensation when they move their thumb. The diagnosis is based on the history and examination. Treatment involves keeping the thumb immobile with splints, nonsteroidal anti-inflammatory drugs, and occasionally injections of steroids. In severe cases, surgery may be required to release the tendon sheath.

SPECIAL CONCERNS DURING PREGNANCY

Musculoskeletal complaints are common during pregnancy. The three most frequent areas of concern are the lower back, the wrist, and the leg. The problems usually go away after pregnancy.

Lower Back Pain

Lower back pain occurs in more than two-thirds of pregnant women. Pregnant women notice dull pain and stiffness in the middle and lower back. The pain is usually mild and occurs mostly in the last three months of pregnancy. Fortunately, back pain in pregnant women rarely develops because of disc problems or nerve irritation and the pain usually goes away after pregnancy.

The pain can have a mechanical or a hormonal cause. First, as the uterus enlarges, it causes the body's center of gravity to move forward, and there is an increase in the normal curve of the lower back (lordosis). This puts added stress on the joints and ligaments of the lower back. Second, hormones produced during pregnancy cause the ligaments around the pelvis to loosen and the joints in the pelvic region to open up so that the baby's head can exit the birth canal safely during

delivery. Sometimes the ligaments stretch out so much that women will complain of "popping" or "catching" in these joints. These symptoms usually improve with rest.

In general, pregnant women can minimize their lower back pain by following a regular exercise program beginning early in pregnancy. In addition, women should take care in lifting heavy objects, including children, while pregnant. Back pain in the early months of pregnancy, particularly if it is accompanied by vaginal bleeding or stomach cramps, should be evaluated by the woman's obstetrician or family physician. This may indicate problems in the pregnancy such as an impending miscarriage. Finally, the beginning of labor can be felt as persistent back pain, particularly if the pain differs from previous occurrences of back pain. It could signal the beginning of labor and the woman's physician should be consulted immediately (see chapter 4, Exercise).

Wrist Pain

Both carpal tunnel syndrome and DeQuervain's tenosynovitis occur frequently in pregnancy. Carpal tunnel syndrome has been reported in 20 percent of pregnant women. Both conditions usually respond to splinting during the pregnancy and go away after pregnancy. Steroid injections or surgery are rarely required.

Leg Cramps

Leg cramps occur in 15–30 percent of pregnant women. The cause is not well understood, but many women find that calcium supplementation can result in a decrease in the frequency and severity of these cramps.

TESTS AND PROCEDURES

Tests and procedures used to diagnose and treat the musculoskeletal system include imaging tests, tests to measure the responses of nerves and muscles, and surgical procedures. Imaging studies such as X-ray, CT scans, and MRI scans are often used, as well as specialized tests to study bone.

Bone Scans

This test uses radioisotopes to create images of areas inside the body. A small amount of radioactive material is injected into the blood stream and gathers in specific parts of the body, depending on the element used. The element then breaks down in the body and produces gamma rays. These rays are reflected back into a special camera that creates an image of the area. Because gamma rays have good penetration through hard surfaces, they are useful in the study of bone. This test is often used to look for problems such as occult fractures, bone infection, and cancer.

Electromyography

This test is used to record the electrical properties of skeletal muscle. Electrodes are placed on the skin to measure whether the muscle is contracting. A small needle may be placed into muscle to assess normal or abnormal muscle responses while a muscle is at rest and while it is contracting. The results are shown on a video screen and audible signals are given to show the nature and location of any problem in the muscle. The response of the muscle also can be measured by electrical stimulation of the nerve to the muscle.

Arthroscopic Surgery

Fiberoptic technology has led to the development of the arthroscope, an instrument that allows a physician to look directly into a joint, diagnose problems, and

MEDICATIONS

Nonsteroidal anti-inflammatory drugs, NSAIDs, and corticosteroids are often used in treating disorders that cause swelling of joints and pain. In most cases, they relieve the pain but do not cure the problems. These drugs can bring relief, but they do have side effects and should be used with caution, especially long-term.

- NSAIDs include drugs such as aspirin, ibuprofen, and naproxen sodium that can be obtained without a prescription and are taken by mouth. They relieve pain and reduce inflammation. These drugs also may cause stomach upset or internal bleeding, so they should not be used by anyone who is anemic or has ulcers or kidney problems. Long-term use should be avoided.

- Corticosteroids are synthetic versions of hormones made in the adrenal gland that must be used under a doctor's direction. They reduce swelling, pain, redness, and heat. They can be taken by mouth, applied to the skin, dropped into the eye, or injected into an affected area. There is a risk of side effects with the long-term use of corticosteroids. These include weight gain, bone loss, muscle weakness, water retention, hypertension, and skin changes. Long-term use should not be stopped suddenly but rather slowly tapered off so the body can readjust.

often repair or relieve many of these problems at the same time.

The arthroscope is a long thin metal tube that contains coated glass fibers and a series of magnifying lenses. The fibers carry light into the joint and relay a magnified image back to the operator. After anesthetic is administered (either local or general), a small cut is made into the joint. The arthroscope is then inserted through the incision, allowing the physician to view the joint either through an eye piece or on a video monitor. Once inside the joint a biopsy specimen also can be obtained and surgery performed.

Prior to arthroscopic surgery, surgeons opened joints to inspect and repair them. The joints were opened through long incisions, and wound healing and recovery of function required a great deal of time. Unlike traditional procedures, arthroscopy rarely takes more than an hour, and the patient can usually return home the same day. Most normal activities can be resumed in a week.

Joint Replacement Surgery

In a healthy joint, smooth, glistening cartilage covers the ends of bones and allows the bone ends to move smoothly and painlessly through a wide arc of motion. However, osteoarthritis, characterized by the breakdown of joint cartilage, occurs in many joints, particularly with aging. Although this can involve many joints, the hip, knee, and shoulder are usually affected.

Joint replacement surgery allows the surgeon to remove the diseased joint and replace it with a synthetic one. Like a healthy joint, the artificial one also has smooth gliding surfaces that allow painless joint motion.

Most joint replacements require replacement of both sides of the joint. For example, both the ball and the socket of the hip joint are often replaced in surgery for osteoarthritis. Sometimes after fracture only the ball portion of this ball and socket joint will be replaced. The decision of when to replace a diseased joint is based on a number of factors, including the degree of disability, lifestyle, age, and the patient's ability to withstand the risks of surgery.-

CHAPTER 35

Skin, Hair, and Nails

June K. Robinson, M.D., F.A.A.D., & Elizabeth A. Abel, M.D., F.A.A.D, Zoe Diana Draelos, M.D., F.A.A.D, Patricia Engasser, M.D., F.A.A.D., Judith Petry, M.D., F.A.C.S., and Frances J. Storrs, M.D., F.A.A.D.

Y ou live inside a paper-thin, tough, flexible envelope—your skin. It forms a protective barrier around the delicate internal workings of your body. Totaling about 2 square yards on average and constituting approximately 12 percent of your body weight, the skin is a unique and complex organ. One square inch of skin contains millions of cells, thousands of nerve endings, and numerous oil glands, sweat glands, blood vessels, hair follicles, and muscles.

This remarkable organ also performs multiple functions. It protects the rest of your body from physical and environmental trauma, such as sunburn, frostbite, chemical burn, and friction. It controls your internal temperature, transmits sensations, and regulates water transportation into and out of your body. By its texture, color, and temperature, your skin can relay information about your general health. Constantly in contact with the world, your skin is an early-warning system for your body, signaling the brain of impending hazards.

There are a vast array of regional differences in the skin surface topography: the thickest skin is on the palms of the hands and the soles of the feet, and the thinnest on the eyelids. The skin also varies in color—the amount and concentration of a black pigment, melanin, determines the coloring of your skin and helps protect it from ultraviolet light. Keratin, a specialized component of skin, creates fingernails, toenails, and hair.

Our skin is the part of the physical self that we show the world. Not surprisingly, people of all ages are concerned about the appearance of their skin; unsightly pimples, lesions, rashes, and other skin disorders can affect us psychologically as well as physically.

To take care of our skin properly, we first have to understand how the skin is structured and how it functions.

THE STRUCTURE OF THE SKIN

The skin is composed of two layers: the epidermis, or surface layer, and the dermis, the deeper layer that contains blood vessels and nerve fibers. Between the skin and musculoskeletal structures lies the subcutaneous tissue, which acts for the body much as insulation acts in the walls of a house. (See Fig. 35.1)

The Epidermis

The top layer of the epidermis consists mostly of dead skin cells, and the bottom layer is composed of living basal cells. The basal cells divide every day to create new skin. Every four weeks, the new cells move up through the epidermis, gradually changing from soft, rounded cells to the hard, flat, lifeless cells that cover the outer surface of the skin. This surface layer of dead cells protects the body from the harmful elements of the external environment. The protein of the dead epidermal cells, called keratin, prevents tissue injury, and the dry surface inhibits the growth of microorganisms. After a short period of time, the dead cells flake off as new ones take their place.

The flexibility of the outer layer of skin depends on its water content. Generally, the skin remains flexible by reacting to fluctuations of humidity in the air and drawing water from the underlying skin tissues. In an area of low humidity, a pint of water may move through the skin in a 24-hour period, evaporating as invisible perspiration.

The Dermis

Dense and rich in nerves and blood vessels, the dermis lies under the epidermis. Like the epidermis, it is thickest on the palms and soles. It is composed mostly of a strong protein called *collagen* and elastic fibers called *elastin.* Collagen, along with other structural features of the skin, enhances the strength of the skin and helps build scar tissue when it is damaged. Elastin gives strength and flexibility to the skin. Also embedded in the dermis are nerve endings, blood vessels, muscle cells, hair follicles, and glands.

As we age, our skin loses the suppleness and elasticity supplied by collagen and elastin. There is a gradual reduction in the number and thickness of the connective tissue fibers, which is perceived externally as a decrease in texture and firmness.

The Subcutaneous Layer

Lying directly under the dermis is subcutaneous tissue, which is attached to the underlying musculoskeletal structure of the body by bands of connective tissue. In

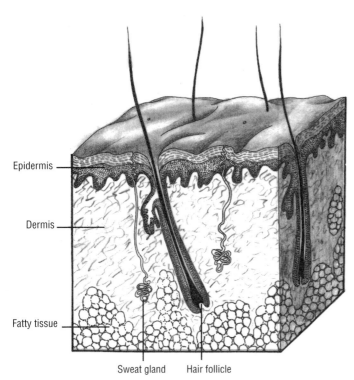

Figure 35.1. Structure of the Skin
The top layer of skin, the epidermis, covers the dermis, which contains hair follicles, sweat glands, and blood vessels.

Labels: Epidermis, Dermis, Fatty tissue, Sweat gland, Hair follicle

WHY SKIN PATCHES WORK

Your skin has a unique ability to absorb certain substances. It does this by

- Absorbing the substance on the surface of the skin
- Diffusing the substance through the skin surface
- Diffusing the substance into the upper layers of the epidermis and upper dermis to reach the capillaries
- Diffusing the substance through the capillary walls into the bloodstream to circulate throughout the body.

The skin acts as a reservoir, building up and releasing chemicals. This ability makes it an ideal transmitter of medications such as nitroglycerine, estrogen, and nicotine. Substances that can be dissolved in oils penetrate the skin best; penetration is enhanced when the skin surface is wet and free of hair. This ability of the skin to absorb medications over a period of time forms the basis for the success of patch-delivery systems. (See Fig. 35.2)

some parts of the body the subcutaneous layer is amplified by fat accumulations—breast and buttocks—and in others by tough fibrous bands—palms, soles, scalp. As we age, this layer thins out and disappears.

Sweat Glands

The body has two kinds of sweat glands: the eccrine glands and the apocrine glands.

Eccrine glands are a highly developed and extensive part of the thermoregulatory system of the body. They manufacture and pump a solution of salt, chemicals, and water to the surface of the skin for evaporation and cooling in times of heat stress. If you are particularly affected by the heat, or emotionally stressed, 2 or 3 quarts of sweat may be produced in a very short period of time, or about a gallon a day. The eccrine glands are distributed throughout the body, but your palms, soles, forehead, and underarms have the most abundant supply.

Apocrine glands are specialized sweat glands that are found in the armpits, ear canals (there they form a portion of what we know as ear wax), and around the

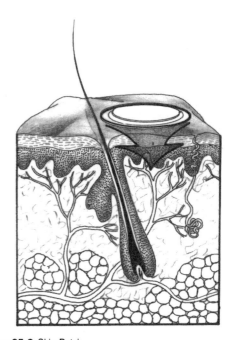

Figure 35.2 Skin Patch
Medications can be absorbed slowly in the bloodstream through a patch applied to the skin.

nipples and genitals. Apocrine glands become active during adolescence and are influenced by sex hormones. These glands respond to strong emotions, not heat, and contribute to the production of adult body odor.

Melanin

All skin color comes from the same substance, the pigment melanin. Melanin is produced by specialized cells called *melanocytes* that are found in the epidermis, the dermis, and hair follicles. Octopus-shaped, with long, irregular "arms" that reach out from the cell body, melanocytes transfer the melanin to adjacent cells in the epidermis. Regardless of skin color, all human beings have about the same number of melanocytes; differences in skin color are a result of the amount and concentration of melanin produced by the cells, which are inherited.

Melanin absorbs ultraviolet (UV) rays and converts them into harmless infrared rays. People who tan have more melanin in their bodies than fair-skinned people who burn. A tan is the body's attempt to defend itself against the damaging rays of the sun. Several factors control melanin production, including genetic influences, hormones, and environmental hazards.

Blood Vessels

The dermis contains an extensive network of blood vessels that, in concert with the sweat glands, helps in controlling the temperature of the body. When the environmental temperature is high, or you have generated heat through exertion, the small blood vessels dilate and bring blood closer to the surface of the skin. In this way, the interior body heat is transferred outside the body. When the body is cold because of falling outside temperatures, the blood vessels contract, decreasing the blood supply at the surface and conserving body heat.

The superficial blood vessels of the face and upper chest are sensitive to emotions and stress, which makes possible the common and sometimes embarrassing phenomena of flushes and blushes.

The Hair

Human beings are as hairy as other mammals, but the hair that covers most of our bodies is fine and cannot

be seen. The only thick growths of hair are in the pubic area, under the arms, on the scalp, and on the faces of men.

Hair protects us from the sun and, in the case of hair on the scalp, from external trauma. Each hair grows from a single live follicle that has its roots in the subcutaneous layer under the dermis. (See Fig. 35.1) Hair follicles are distributed over the entire body, except the lips, palms, and soles of the feet. Adjacent to the hair follicles, and connected to them by short ducts, are the sebaceous glands. These glands produce sebum, a waxy, oily material that naturally moisturizes the skin and hair, and acts as a shield against toxic substances. Sebum also carries dead cells and debris from the inner skin to the surface of the skin. Sebum contains chemicals that, when triggered by the ultraviolet rays of the sun, become vitamin D.

Hair is similar to skin cells, in that it grows and is shed regularly. The average rate of growth is about 1/2+ inch a month.

The Nails

Your fingernails and toenails are made of keratin, the same tough protein that makes up the epidermis and constitutes the greater portion of the hair. The nail plate grows outward from the nail root, or matrix. (See Fig. 35.3) Fingernails grow at the rate of 1/8 inch a month, although this rate slows in old age. As with the skin and hair, the appearance of the nails can signal an illness or a dysfunction in some part of the body.

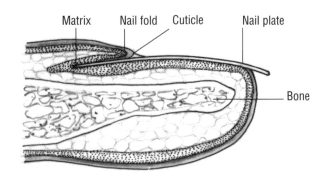

Figure 35.3. Cross-section of a Fingertip
The nails are made in the matrix from the protein keratin and protect the tips of the fingers and toes.

THE HEALTHY WOMAN'S GUIDE TO SKIN, HAIR, AND NAIL CARE

Looking great and feeling good are important to most women. Your appearance and your sense of well-being are linked, and are products of conscious decisions affecting habits and lifestyle. Proper diet, adequate sleep, and regular exercise are the components of good health, which includes a smooth, glowing skin; thick, shiny hair; and smooth, flexible nails.

Good grooming and the commonsense use of cosmetics and beauty preparations can promote both a healthy skin and an attractive appearance.

Care of the Skin

Sensible skin care is important throughout your life. A good skin care regimen doesn't need to be expensive, elaborate, or time-consuming. In fact, the three rules of skin care are very simple indeed.

Rule #1. Protect the skin from the sun. The soft, unlined skin you were born with can be maintained for many years if you follow the first rule of skin care: Protect the skin at all times from the ultraviolet light of the sun. Whether it is dark or light, skin exposed for long periods of time to the sun becomes wrinkled, dried out (leathery), and prematurely aged. You can see this for yourself if you compare an area of your skin that rarely sees the sun—your buttocks, for example—with your face, hands, or arms.

Of course, it is impossible to avoid the sun completely. Sunscreens can provide chemical and physical protection during the day, and their use should become part of your daily routine. Sunscreens are now an ingredient of many cosmetic products, including foundations, lipsticks, and moisturizers. There are other ways to avoid the sun (see Skin Cancer).

Rule #2. Keep the skin clean. The use of soap and water on the face discourages bacteria and possible infections. The type and amount of cleaning necessary for your face depends on the amount of natural oil (sebum) that your skin produces. There are three basic skin (and hair) types: normal, oily, and dry. Normal skin is well-balanced, neither too oily nor too dry, but probably will become dry with advancing years. Oily skin is caused by overactivity of the sebaceous glands. This type of skin tends to be thick, with large pores, and acne may be a problem. Dry skin is caused by underactivity of the sebaceous glands, by environmental con-

ditions, or by the normal aging process. The skin is thinner, has smaller pores, and is easily irritated. Some people have combination skins, consisting of oily regions—usually around the nose or forehead—and drier regions.

Whatever your skin type, you probably should wash your face both morning and evening.

- Normal skin requires a mild cleansing bar. In the drier winter months, use a superfatted soap.

- Oily skin may require more than two washings. Use a deodorant or antibacterial soap that will help prevent the formation of blackheads and pimples (see Acne).

- Dry skin does best with a superfatted soap. Many specialty cleansers other than soap are available commercially, but these products do not have any advantage over soap and water. Soap and water washing does not promote the development of wrinkles.

Proper cleansing is an important strategy in protecting your skin and enhancing its appearance. Here are some cleansing tips:

- Before washing your face in the evening, remove all facial and eye makeup. Apply a gentle cleansing cream and wipe it off with tissue. To remove eye makeup, use cotton balls and a hypoallergenic eye makeup remover solution.

- Use tepid water—never hot water—to wash your face. Occasionally, use a washcloth to remove dead cells. When bathing, never use hot water or strong soap. Frequent bathing has the tendency to dry out the skin.

Rule #3. Use a moisturizer. Moisturizers are designed to replace natural skin oils that normally form a barrier to prevent water evaporation from the skin. If you have oily skin, you probably don't need a moisturizer. If you have dry skin, combination skin, or even a normal skin, you will need to use a moisturizer after washing your face and before applying makeup. Moisturizers are especially beneficial if the humidity is low, as happens when cold weather and central heating create dry environmental conditions, and if excessive bathing strips away too much of your natural sebum, creating dry, cracked skin.

There are basically two types of ingredients used in moisturizers: occlusives and humectants. *Occlusives* are oily substances, such as petroleum jelly, mineral oil, and lanolin. (A recent study demonstrated that petroleum jelly is the most effective moisturizer. Unfortunately, it tends to be sticky, greasy, and staining.) *Humectants* are substances that attract water and include glycol, glycerin, sorbitol, and gelatin. Many of the moisturizers on the market today contain urea, a chemical that effectively binds water to the skin but may be irritating to some women.

What is the best moisturizer for your skin? The answer depends on how the product seems to you—what feels ''greasy'' to some may appeal to others. It's not necessary to spend a lot of money. Most of the money spent on expensive moisturizers is more for their packaging and their aesthetic values—smoothness, pleasant feel, fragrance—than for their innate moisturizing properties. And it is unproven and questionable whether certain ingredients, such as vitamins and collagen, penetrate the skin to work their ''magic.'' The only exception is tretinoin (retinoic acid, a form of vitamin A), which is of value in the treatment of severe acne and may reverse some sun damage to the skin. In the final analysis, your skin is best maintained by a nutritious diet, commonsense hygiene, and basic skin care.

Care of the Hair

From the medical point of view, hair is superfluous. It provides insignificant protection from the sun and does not insulate us against heat and cold. It is merely a cosmetic appendage to the body. But abundant hair that is becomingly arranged is important to women. Beautiful hair enhances the appearance, and the way it is styled is an expression of the personality. Good hair care, then, is a priority for most women. Millions of dollars are spent each year for hair care products, in the hope that a particular shampoo, conditioner, or styling gel can beautify and tame wayward hair. There are differences in hair care products but, despite advertising to the contrary, none are miracle workers.

Shampoos

Basic hair care starts with clean hair. Too much cleansing, however, can be damaging to hair. The scalp makes a valuable oily substance called sebum, which coats each hair and keeps it looking shiny and soft. This natural scalp oil also protects the hair shaft from developing the static electricity that contributes to frizzy, unmanageable hair. Shampoos are designed to remove sebum from the hair shaft, because too much oil makes the hair greasy and dirty. Removing excess oil is desirable, but overly aggressive cleansing contributes to dry, harsh-feeling hair that looks dull and is difficult to manage. It is important, then, to handle your hair gently and to choose a shampoo that removes just the right amount of oil. Fortunately, there are a great many shampoos on the market, and trial and error can help you find the right one for you.

- *Detergent shampoos.* These hair cleansers are beneficial for women with oily scalps but are too drying for those with dry or normal scalps.

- *Low ph shampoos.* Women with especially dry hair, or hair that is dyed, permanently waved, or straightened, should use a shampoo designed for dry or damaged hair. These shampoos are milder than detergent products and do not completely strip the hair of sebum.

- *Dandruff shampoos.* These products help control scalp flaking. They tend to be harsher than other shampoos, however, so use a conditioner afterward.

- *Protein shampoos.* Contrary to some advertising claims, these shampoos do not penetrate the hair shaft, but they do coat it, giving your hair more bulk. Some protein shampoos include conditioners.

If you regularly use hair spray, styling mousse, or sculpturing gel, be aware that these water-resistant products are somewhat difficult to wash away with only a mild shampoo. In fact, a buildup of styling products can make your hair look lifeless and dull and contribute to scalp problems. One solution is to shampoo more often—frequent shampooing should not damage the hair as long as it is done gently. Make sure you rinse thoroughly.

Hair conditioners

Conditioners are designed to replace the sebum that is removed from the hair shaft by shampooing. Too much conditioner will leave your hair limp; too little may leave your hair unmanageable and subject to static electricity during cold weather. There are many different types of conditioners on the market, including in-

THE PROBLEM OF LIMP, FINE HAIR

In general, fine hair tends to be poor at holding a style. Too much conditioner increases limpness and makes the hair even more difficult to manage. If you have this type of hair, avoid using deep conditioners unless absolutely necessary, and then not more than once a month. Leave-in conditioners, with the exception of mousse, may not work well either. Instant conditioners are your best bet, especially if you choose one formulated for extra body or limp hair. These products generally contain less conditioner and tend to prevent that limp look; and because they contain protein, they may thicken the hair temporarily.

stant, deep, and leave-in. (Before you spend a lot of money on fancy conditioners, remember that the hair does not "eat," so vitamin and protein deficiences that contribute to poor hair formation and growth cannot be treated by applying various exotic substances to the hair. Vitamins and proteins must be part of a balanced diet to have any effect on hair growth.)

- *Instant conditioners.* These quickie conditioners come premixed in a bottle and are applied to the hair immediately following shampooing and rinsing. Instant conditioners contain conditioning additives including herbal extracts, aloe, vitamins, balsam, and lanolin. These products counteract static electricity and give a sheen to the hair, but are only mildly conditioning.

- *Protein conditioners.* These products, like other conditioners, lubricate your hair between washings. Although the protein does not penetrate the hair shaft, it may thicken your hair temporarily.

- *Deep conditioners.* These products, although they contain all of the agents found in instant conditioners, are more concentrated and are meant to remain on the hair for a longer period of time. Sold as hot-oil treatments or protein packs, deep conditioners are applied to the hair and left on for about 20 minutes. Instructions for use may include the application of heat, because warmth causes the small breaks or holes in the hair shaft to enlarge. If you

have damaged hair, use a deep conditioner containing protein at least once a month.

- *Leave-in conditioners.* These products include blow-drying lotions, hair glazes, and hair thickeners. They are applied to shampooed, towel-dried hair and are not removed until the next washing. These products increase shine in dull hair but do not mend split ends or eliminate frizziness.

After shampooing, gently towel-dry your hair. Never comb or brush wet hair, because it is more susceptible to stretching and breakage when it is wet. Wait until it is damp before styling. If possible, let your hair dry naturally. If you use a blow-dryer, use a moderate heat setting and never overdry.

Be cautious about dyeing your hair. Regular stripping and dyeing can cause cumulative damage, although it may take years before there are obvious signs of hair breakage. Instead of using a permanent dye, try a rinse or a temporary dye.

Permanent waving is generally safe for healthy hair, although you may find that the process results in drier hair and split ends.

Care of the Nails

Nature gave you nails to protect the tender tissue of the fingertips, but nails can also be an attractive asset. Good nail grooming takes both these functions into consideration. First, never bite, pick, or injure your nails. Always wear rubber gloves when handling detergents, chemicals, or abrasive cleansers. Trim your nails every few weeks to keep them smooth and looking good. Common sense is the key to nail care: don't abuse your nails. Since nails grow at the rate of about 1/8 inch a month, you can improve your nails with care and patience.

Manicuring

Manicuring your nails is a safe practice, but don't overdo it—your nails do best when they are just left alone. When you style your nails, leave a rounded tip and square corners to maximize nail strength and minimize breakage. To do this, use a sharp nail clipper, then file with an emery board to remove any rough edges that could snag and tear. As with your skin, it is important to moisturize your nails and the adjacent skin to prevent splitting and cracking, especially during

TAKING CARE OF YOUR TOENAILS

Toenails profit from regular care and grooming. To trim your toenails, clip them straight across. Don't cut them too short. Toenails tend to be thicker than fingernails, so the best time for a trim is after a bath or shower.

If you cut your nail improperly, especially on the big toe, you risk an ingrown toenail. Ingrown toenails occur when improper cutting or pressure—often caused by ill-fitting shoes—forces the side of the nail into the skin. The area then becomes swollen, red, and infected. If you have a mild ingrown toenail, place a wisp of sterile cotton under the corner of the nail plate to elevate it from the painful area. Apply an antibiotic ointment to the inflamed area two or three times daily. Wear loose-fitting shoes and discard tight, pointed-toe shoes. If the nail is painful and you notice a discharge, see your doctor.

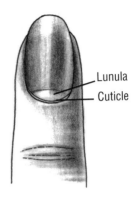

Figure 35.4. Fingernail
The lunula is a crescent or moon-shaped area at the base of the nail. The cuticle seals the skin around the nail and protects the matrix from damage.

the winter months. Use moisturizers containing lactic acid, glycolic acid, or malic acid.

The cuticle is vital to nail maintenance and health. It functions as a type of gasket, preventing water and other substances from damaging the cells that produce the nail. (See Fig. 35.4) Injury to this cluster of cells, called the nail matrix, can result in a deformed nail or, if the damage is severe, in the failure of the nail to grow. Never cut, clip, or remove a cuticle. A mutilated cuticle could be a point of entry for bacteria or a fungus. Apply moisturizers to the cuticle to keep it soft and supple; if necessary, you can occasionally push it back gently with an orange stick.

Nail Cosmetics

Many products on the market today promise sparkling, hard, long, and long-lasting nails. They include enamels, polishes, buffers, undercoats, overcoats, strengtheners, cuticle removers, and artificial nails. Use them only occasionally, because most of these products damage the nails if used in excess.

Nail polishes or enamels add color to the nail but provide no other benefit. Their regular use can cause dryness of the nail plate, leading to brittle, breaking nails, because the polish must be removed with a harsh chemical. Polish removers tend to weaken and dry the nails. However, there is little harm in occasionally applying nail polish or using nail polish remover.

Nail strengtheners reinforce the nail plate by adding nylon or rayon fibers to nail polish. If you use strengtheners regularly, you may find that your nails are discolored and break more easily. Sculptured nails or nail tips use synthetic polymers (plastic) shaped like fingernails. Of all the nail products on the market, sculptured nails account for the majority of nail problems—abnormally shaped nails, fungus infections, bacterially infected nails, and nails that detach from the nail bed.

DISEASES OF THE SKIN

Your skin is a complicated organ that is constantly exposed to the environment. It is no wonder that occasionally you may suffer from some type of skin disorder, including dermatitis, acne, sunburn, and other mild skin conditions. Some of these problems are amenable to home treatment, while others may require care by a dermatologist. Some skin diseases are more serious and more difficult to treat, such as psoriasis and cancer of the skin.

Dermatitis

Dermatitis is an itching inflammation of the skin. It includes a number of conditions, among them atopic dermatitis (eczema), irritant and allergic contact dermatitis, stasis dermatitis, and seborrheic dermatitis (dandruff).

Atopic Dermatitis

An inherited disorder, atopic dermatitis or eczema first appears in infancy. It usually continues into adult life, although attacks may occur far less frequently then. Stress can cause the symptoms, as can environmental allergens, medications, and extreme temperatures.

Symptoms

In the mildest form, people with atopic dermatitis have very dry skin. More severe cases show itchy, thickened, cracked skin, usually in the folds of the body, including the neck, bends of the arms, and the skin behind the knees.

Treatment

The treatment for atopic dermatitis has changed radically with the advent of corticosteroids. These medications are safe if used properly. Hydrocortisone lotions, used in conjunction with other topical emollients, are especially valuable. Wet dressings are sometimes used, and antihistamines can relieve the itching.

There are no cures for this disorder, but the symptoms can be relieved by keeping the skin well lubricated, by avoiding irritating fabrics and substances, by treating any infection of the skin promptly, and by striving to maintain a less stressful and more emotionally balanced life. (See Fig. 35.5)

Irritant and Allergic Contact Dermatitis

Irritant contact dermatitis occurs when the skin is exposed to a mild irritant, usually a detergent, harsh soap, or other powerful cleaning substance. Commonly called "housewife's eczema," irritant contact dermatitis is an occupational hazard that commonly affects, besides homemakers, people working with irritating chemicals and solvents, such as hairdressers, health care workers, machinists, and restaurant workers.

Allergic contact dermatitis occurs when a specific substance comes into contact with a person who is allergic to that substance. The most common examples of allergic contact dermatitis are reactions to poison ivy and poison oak. Not everyone reacts to these common allergens in the environment; the tendency seems to be

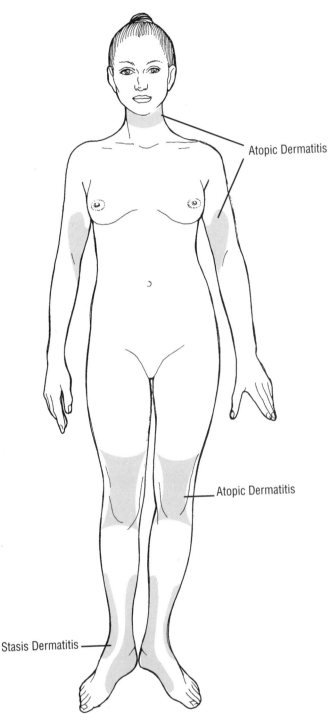

Figure 35.5. Dermatitis
Atopic dermatitis affects the folds of the body, including the neck, bends of the arms, and the skin behind the knees. Stasis dermatitis occurs on the lower legs as a result of poor circulation.

inherited. Other materials that commonly cause allergic reactions are listed below.

- *Nickel.* After poison oak and poison ivy, nickel is the most common cause of allergic contact dermatitis. Women are particularly prone to develop a nickel allergy because of exposure to nickel-alloy jewelry. For example, about 15 percent of women who pierce their ears will become sensitive to the metal. To avoid an allergic reaction, wear stainless steel, sterling silver, or gold earrings. Nickel is also found in metal buttons, belt buckles, watches, and some coins. A nickel allergy usually shows up as an itching plaque at the contact site.

■ *Cosmetics and perfumes.* Various makeup products have a tendency to cause problems if you are already suffering from irritant dermatitis, atopic dermatitis, or seborrheic dermatitis (dandruff). A cosmetic allergy usually develops in patches, and is most often seen on the eyelids and sides of the neck. Perfumes are notorious for causing this type of allergic reaction. If you are prone to other types of dermatitis, buy cosmetics that contain no perfumes nor dyes. Another common cause of cosmetic contact dermatitis is the preservatives used to extend their shelf life. Buy cosmetics that are free of preservatives such as formaldehyde. The preservatives that cause the fewest problems are the parabens—methyl paraben, ethyl paraben, and propyl paraben. The ingredients are listed on the labels of all cosmetic products, so check before you buy.

■ *Hair products.* "Acid" or "3-part" permanent waves can cause allergic reactions in both the hairdresser and the customer. If an allergic reaction appears on the face, it may take months

COSMETIC CHEMICALS TO AVOID

The preservatives and other chemicals in cosmetics can cause allergic contact dermatitis. The ones to avoid are the following:

Quaternium-15
2-bromo-2-nitropropane-1
Diazolidinyl urea*
Imidazolidinyl urea
Formaldehyde
3-diol
* Most likely to cause problems

to cure because the permanent wave chemical has saturated the hair shaft. Cutting the hair short and frequent shampooing may help. The offending chemical is glycerol thioglycolate, found in the wave solution. To prevent any problems, ask for an "alkaline" or "cold wave" perm.

Hair dyes that contain the chemical paraphenylen diamine are another source of allergies. Reactions to hair dyes can be severe, and occasionally require hospitalization. To prevent these problems, many hairdressers pretest their customers before beginning the procedure.

Shampoos are rarely the cause of allergic dermatitis. If it occurs, it will usually appear behind the ears.

■ *Nail products.* Toluene sulfonamide formaldehyde resin in nail polish is a possible cause of allergic contact dermatitis. It often appears first on the eyelids and the sides of the neck, seldom on the fingers or nails themselves. Acrylic artificial nails cause a dermatitis similar to the nail polish variety. This kind of allergy can be severe, resulting in the loss of a fingernail. At the first sign of irritation, remove and discard the artificial nails, and do not attempt to wear them again.

■ *Chemicals in fabrics.* Certain dyes in clothing can cause a severe and acute allergic contact dermatitis. Formaldehyde-releasing chemicals used in many fabrics also cause these reactions, which appear at the point of contact on the body. Natural fabrics, such as linen, silk, wool, and wrinkling cotton are unlikely to be treated with formaldehyde-releasing finishes. Nonwrinkle cotton, however, may contain these chemicals, as do combination fabrics and rayon. Nylon and polyester are usually safe.

■ *Medications.* Almost any substance that is applied to the skin can cause an allergy. Medications used for irritated skin, minor cuts, and abrasions, including neomycin, bacitracin, and benzocaine, are most likely to cause problems. if your dermatitis worsens, stop using all medications and consult your dermatologist. Substances containing iodine and lidocaine are usually safe to use.

Symptoms
The most common symptoms of allergic dermatitis are redness, swelling, and itching at the site of the

affected area. In severe cases, there may be blisters and sores that "weep" fluid. The skin may become tight, stiff, and dry, causing painful cracks and fissures.

Irritant dermatitis often begins in the web spaces of the fingers, since this is an area that is prone to damage by water. It takes about three months to develop after a first exposure to a "wet" work environment. Although it does not usually spread, the affected area can extend to include the tops and palms of the hands.

Diagnosis

There are no tests that ascertain the causes of irritant and allergic contact dermatitis. You and the dermatologist may have to do a little detective work before the source of the irritation is found. Clues may be found by looking at your medical history, doing a patch test to determine if you are allergic to a given substance, and by the process of elimination. Often people with a history of atopic dermatitis are particularly vulnerable to these other types of dermatitis. The association is so strong that individuals who suffered eczema as children should avoid employment that involves water and irritating substances.

Treatment

To speed the improvement of contact dermatitis, minimize your exposure to water and eliminate all topical chemicals that may be causing or aggravating the problem. To identify the cause of the allergic contact dermatitis, your physician may have to use a patch test, in which small quantities of the suspected chemical are applied and covered by a dressing for about 2 days. If a rash develops, you have an allergy to that substance. Patch tests are scientifically sound, but they are not foolproof. The actual offending material may not be tested, other allergies may show up and be misleading, and your skin may not react to a substance in the patch test in the same way that it does in real life.

Severe cases of dermatitis that involve the skin around the eyes, mouth, or genitalia may be treated with corticosteroids, such as prednisone, which is taken orally. Prednisone is used for short periods and is very effective. (This medication cannot be used if you suffer from diabetes, a bleeding ulcer, or an acute infection.) Cortisone ointment or cream can be used on the hands and elsewhere on the body. For milder cases, you can purchase a 1 percent hydrocortisone ointment in the drugstore, without a prescription. (Unfortunately, many creams are prepared with formaldehyde releasers. Use a hydrocortisone ointment in plain petroleum jelly, if available.) There can be side effects. Using a strong cortisone ointment on the face or in the folds of the body may result in the formation of blood vessels on the face, or atrophy or thinning of the skin. Some people even develop a contact dermatitis from cortisone. Consult your physician about the proper application of these powerful drugs and follow all instructions on their use.

In the case of severe dermatitis on the hands, removing the hands from the wet–dry cycle and decreasing exposure to water is important. Rubber gloves provide protection from water and from strong chemicals found in cleansers and other products. When you use the gloves, avoid getting water in them. Turn them inside out after use, to drain any water left in them, or wear cotton gloves inside the rubber gloves. On removing the rubber gloves, apply a simple grease (petroleum jelly) to the hands. Always apply any lubricants when the skin is still moist, so any water is trapped in the skin.

Stasis Dermatitis

This kind of skin irritation occurs on the lower part of the legs, usually in older women who have varicose veins or suffer from thrombophlebitis (an inflammation of the lining of the veins) of the legs. Poor circulation of the blood causes the skin to become inflamed. The constant irritation leaves the skin thickened, scarred, and discolored. In severe cases, open ulcers may form that are slow to heal and can recur.

Preventive measures include the wearing of elastic bandages or support stockings. Another option is rest and elevation of the legs while sitting or lying down. Wet astringent dressings can give some relief and prevent infection. (See Fig. 35.5)

Seborrheic Dermatitis (Dandruff)

One of the more common skin problems, seborrheic dermatitis is an inflammation of the scalp that results in stubborn, itchy dandruff and red, scaly patches at the sides of your nose, eyebrows, and face, behind your ears, and on your chest. Sometimes a reddening and scaling of the eyelids and a mild conjunctivitis accompany the disorder. The cause is unknown.

In mild seborrheic dermatitis, you can control the flaking and itching by using over-the-counter shampoos that contain zinc pyrithione, sulfur, salicylic acid, selenium sulfide, or tar derivatives. More severe cases require a dermatologist's intervention. The doctor can prescribe stronger shampoos and ointments containing corticosteroids, sulfur, and antibiotics. (See Fig. 35.6)

located on the lower face and neck. Because acne is expected to disappear after adolescence, you may find this type of adult-onset acne to be particularly frustrating and embarrassing.

Acne is a disorder of the pilosebaceous unit of the skin, which consists of a hair follicle and the sebaceous gland attached to it. The cells lining the tiny well of the hair follicle become sticky, clump together, and form plugs. If the cells adhere near the surface of the pore, blackheads or whiteheads form. Blockage deeper in the follicles creates inflamed pimples or pustules, or acne's most scarring form of lesion, the cystic nodules. Once the plug has formed, oil (sebum) from the sebaceous glands and bacteria build up behind the attached keratin-producing cells. The pressure builds up, forming a bump or pimple. If the follicle is stretched too far or the pimple is squeezed, the contents spill out into the surrounding skin, causing further inflammation. More red, tender, deep pimples form, which may ultimately result in permanent scarring. (See Fig. 35.7)

Some substances and situations seem to trigger the overproduction of sebum and the formation of pimples and lesions.

- *Hormones.* The sebaceous glands become activated in puberty in response to androgenic (male) hormones. Women naturally produce small amounts of these hormones in their adrenals and ovaries. The rate of production varies over the menstrual cycle; some women note that their acne flares up in the premenstrual period.

- *Stress.* Many women report outbreaks of acne in times of stress and emotional upset. To add to the problem, some women develop a habit of squeezing and picking at the acne blemishes, which often results in deeper and longer-lasting lesions and scarring. In these cases, you may want to consider a stress-reduction program that includes sufficient rest and regular exercise.

- *Diet.* Years ago, youngsters suffering from acne were admonished to avoid chocolate, sugar, and greasy foods. Diet restrictions are no longer part of acne therapy because there is no evidence that food plays any role in its development.

- *Cosmetics.* Many women use facial cosmetics, and many wonder if these products cause or aggravate their acne. It is true that some ingredients in cosmetics may cause follicular plug-

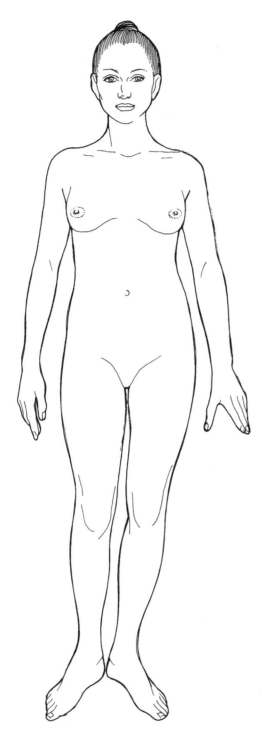

Figure 35.6. Dandruff
Seborrheic dermatitis, or dandruff, produces red, scaly patches on the scalp.

Acne

Acne is not limited to teenagers. In fact, acne is quite common in women in their twenties, thirties, and beyond. In adult women, the lesions and pimples are

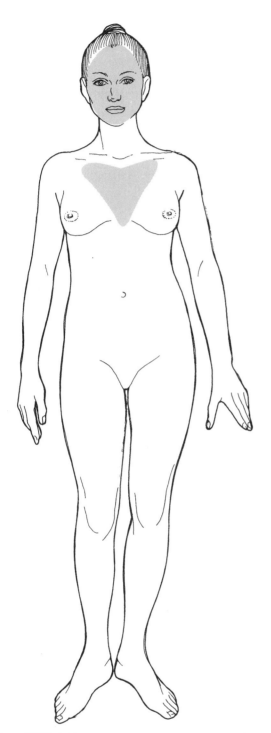

Figure 35.7. Acne
Acne usually appears on the face, neck, chest, and back.

ging, although most manufacturers test their beauty products carefully to avoid this kind of problem. The cosmetics that have passed this testing are labeled noncomedogenic. If you suffer from acne flare-ups, select your cosmetics from this screened group.

Symptoms

Acne usually appears on the face, neck, chest, and back. It can be an occasional blemish, a continual smattering of red bumps, or a mixture of noninflamed lesions called blackheads (open comedones), whiteheads (closed comedones) papules, pustules, nodules, and pimples. At its worst, the acne lesions are tender and painful.

Diagnosis

Acne is easy to diagnose, although sometimes the pimples and pustules may be confused with a disease like rosacea (see below).

Treatment

There is no one single treatment or medication that can cure acne. Rather, a long-term and consistent combination of self-help therapies and medications offers the best chance of relieving the acne and clearing the skin.

Self-help treatments. Acne involves plugged pores caused by bacteria breaking down the oils in the follicles, so it is extremely important to cleanse the skin regularly and *gently*. *Gently* is emphasized because you cannot scrub acne away, and irritating the skin only worsens the condition. Furthermore, skin products such as scrubs, abrasives, and masks do not release the deep oil plugs inside the follicles. Use a mild medicated soap or detergent to remove surface oils and bacteria. Wash your face gently several times each day.

Benzoyl peroxide is the most commonly used medication in the treatment of acne. It has a mild loosening effect on follicular plugs, it dries the skin and promotes peeling, and it is a potent antibacterial. Benzoyl peroxide lotions, soaps, and gels are available over the counter. Do not use these medications to excess, however, because they can cause severe dryness and a red, scaly rash.

If you use cosmetics, choose products that are water-based. There are many such products, made especially for women with oily skin or acne, on the market.

Some women believe that the sun helps their acne, although studies have not supported their claims. Tanning certainly may bring a much-needed cosmetic improvement, but caution must be observed when deciding to undergo sun therapy or to use a commercial sunlamp. Because of the long-term harmful effects of sun on the skin, this treatment is definitely not recommended.

In the past it was noticed that women on birth control pills had dryer skins and less acne. When these

are significantly helpful in acne treatment. Nevertheless, it is not uncommon to see a flareup of acne when a women stops taking birth control pills.

Medical treatments

Women with varying skin types develop acne, so careful planning is needed to tailor a complete and effective regimen of care. Medications should not be simply dotted on pimples; the entire area of skin involved must be treated according to the severity of the acne. Often the most important elements for successful care are patience and persistence.

For many decades, topical preparations containing salicylic acid, sulfur, and resorcinol have been used to peel the skin and produce some mild improvement in acne. These preparations are still included in the formulas for many topical acne treatments, available over the counter and by prescription. Benzoyl peroxide, the most popular substance now on the market, can be purchased over the counter and by prescription. Several other acne treatments are effective, if used with caution.

- *Antibiotics.* Antibacterial preparations of erythromycin, clindamycin, tetracycline, and meclocycline are available by prescription in topical forms. Because it is important to reduce bacterial counts deep in the follicle in order to eliminate redness and inflammation, topical applications of antibiotics are often useful.

- *Tretinoin (Retin-A).* Topical tretinoin, a vitamin A derivative, loosens and releases acne plugs. It is available in varying concentrations, by prescription, as a cream, gel, or solution. Tretinoin can cause a good deal of dryness, peeling, and irritation of the skin, and its use requires care and patience. It should be introduced gradually, never applied to the skin immediately after cleansing, and never used in conjunction with other potentially irritating skin products. Sun protection is required when using tretinoin, because the skin becomes abnormally sensitive to ultraviolet light. Despite great care, some patients are unable to tolerate this medication.

  Oral vitamin A derivatives such as 13-cis-retinoic acid (Accutane) are potent drugs that have been linked with serious birth defects. At present, however, there is no evidence that any topical application of tretinoin can be absorbed sufficiently into the body to cause serious con-

ACNE MEDICATIONS ALERT

Many oral drugs used for acne treatment are generally safe as long as they are used properly and with care. There are several precautions that must be followed.

- None of the oral medications in "Systemic Treatments" should be taken during pregnancy.

- Although it is not proven, these antibiotics may diminish the blood concentration of birth control pills.

- Taking oral antibiotics always increases the risk of developing a vaginal infection caused by a fungus—a yeast vaginitis. Indeed, there are a few women who cannot use oral antibiotics for acne treatment because of recurring candida vaginitis, despite therapy for this condition.

- Accutane, or 13-cis-retinoic acid, is an oral vitamin A derivative. It is especially effective for cases of nodulocystic, scarring acne that does not respond to oral antibiotics. Taking an adequate dosage of Accutane for approximately four months usually results in a long-term or permanent remission of the acne. This potent drug suppresses sebum production and reduces the formation of comedones in the follicles. Unfortunately, Accutane also has potent side effects, which means that only reliable patients who cooperate fully can be considered for this treatment.

The most important side effect involves unborn children. Women who are considering Accutane therapy should be aware that this drug can cause severe birth defects in the developing fetus, including serious deformities of the brain and nervous system. For that reason, noncelibate women should be counseled by their doctor to take oral contraceptives as well as use a backup means of birth control for at least a month before initiating Accutane therapy. Routine serum pregnancy testing is done throughout the course of treatment.

Other side effects may include changes in liver function and elevation of serum lipids (fat levels) in the blood. Again, monitoring with blood tests is necessary during Accutane therapy. Everyone who takes the drug experiences some dryness of the skin and lips.

The benefits of Accutane for informed patients with severe acne are impressive, but they can be realized only by close collaboration between physician and patient.

sequences. Nevertheless, physicians prefer to be cautious in this area, and most counsel women against using tretinoin before becoming pregnant or during pregnancy.

Systemic (oral) medical treatments

When topical preparations are not sufficient to subdue acne, oral medications are used. Oral antibiotics, used judiciously, have a 40-year record of safety and efficacy.

- Tetracycline, the first antibiotic used for acne, is highly effective. Take it 1 hour before or 2 hours after meals. Milk, milk products, and medications containing calcium or iron can reduce its absorption and compromise its effectiveness. Tetracycline is not without potential side effects, but most are mild. Among them are intestinal upsets (including constipation and diarrhea), yeast infections, and sensitivity to sunburn. Pregnant women cannot take tetracycline because it affects the normal bone and tooth development of the fetus.

- Doxycycline and minocycline are related to tetracycline but are absorbed more readily. Some patients find them to be more effective than tetracycline. Potential side effects include sensitivity to the sun (doxycycline) and headaches and dizziness (minocycline). After long-term use of minocycline, the drug may be deposited in the skin, causing the appearance of dark blotches. These blotches usually disappear once the medication is stopped.

- Erythromycin is another safe and effective antibiotic used orally for the treatment of acne. It is less likely to interact with oral contraceptives than tetracycline, and for this reason is used more often. All antibiotics may cause gastrointestinal upset, but this symptom appears to be more frequent with erythromycin. However, this problem occurs less with certain forms of the drug. Erythromycin can also cause serious side effects if it interacts with Seldane, Hismanal, or theophylline. Any long-term antibiotics program, especially one that uses erythromycin, requires a detailed discussion with your physician and a complete list of any other medications you are currently taking.

Acne Rosacea

As the name implies, acne rosacea is a chronic inflammation of the cheeks, nose, mid-forehead, and chin. In a few individuals, this persistent flushing of the face becomes permanent, and acnelike blemishes erupt on the red skin. Rosacea usually begins between the ages of 30 and 50, and women are affected more than men. The causes of this condition are unknown, although it seems to be a disorder of blood vessels that are extremely sensitive to emotional and physical stimulation.

Symptoms

The face becomes inflamed, especially around the cheeks, nose, forehead, and chin. In some cases, pustules and pimples form on the reddened areas. The nose may become red and bulbous, especially in men.

Treatment

Diet is an important part of the treatment for rosacea. You will want to avoid hot or spicy foods, and alcohol, which may aggravate the condition. It also helps to avoid emotional upset and stress. Other treatments may be similar to treatments for acne, including tetracycline, other antibiotics, and topical medications.

Psoriasis

A noncontagious, chronic skin disorder that can appear on many areas of the body, psoriasis affects over 3 million Americans. It can appear at any age when both the genetic predisposition and certain triggering factors are present. Psoriasis is a particularly distressing affliction because of its visibility. Women suffering from psoriasis often have psychological and social concerns that can inhibit their interpersonal and sexual relationships.

In psoriasis, the skin cells multiply more rapidly than normal cells as they move toward the surface of the skin. These cells shed as scales before they develop normally. The cause of psoriasis is unknown, although there seems to be a genetic predisposition to the disease. Current theories focus on immune system abnormalities as well as cellular, biochemical, and metabolic defects. Diet does not appear to affect the disease, but other triggers can precipitate an attack. (See Fig. 35.8)

- Bacterial or viral infections, particularly streptoccal, can lead to the development of psoriasis or a flare-up of the condition.

- Extremely dry skin—common in winter and associated with low humidity—can make the

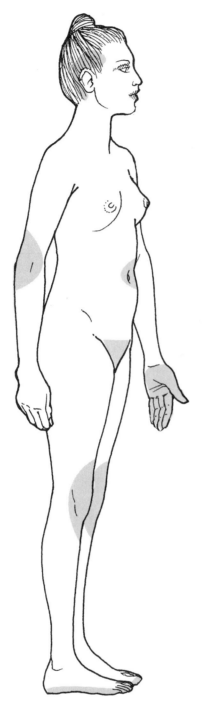

Figure 35.8. Psoriasis
Psoriasis produces red, scaling patches over the body, particularly the knees and elbows, under the breasts, and in the genital area.

skin more vulnerable to itching, scratching, and attacks of psoriasis.

■ Certain medications, such as lithium (used for manic-depressive disorders), beta blockers (used as antihypertensives and antimalarials),

and even certain nonsteroidal anti-inflammatory agents can cause psoriasis.

■ Irritation or trauma to the skin, such as cuts, burns, and insect bites, can aggravate existing lesions or cause new lesions at a particular site.

■ Emotional and physical stress is associated with flare-ups of the disease.

Symptoms

Psoriasis first appears as red patches on the skin that thicken into plaques with silvery scales. Occasionally the disease begins as a group of little pimples following a streptococcal infection. The disease ranges from a few localized plaques of varying sizes to large areas of involvement or redness and scaling over the entire body. The progress of the disease also varies. It may be chronic, stable, or progressive with periods of remission and exacerbation. Common sites of involvement are pressure points such as the knees and elbows, as well as the scalp, trunk, palms, soles, and genitalia.

When the face is affected, psoriasis may be accompanied by seborrheic dermatitis. Psoriasis often appears in skin fold areas, such as under the breasts, in the armpits, and in the genital area. At times it may appear as white, spongy skin that can be mistaken for a fungal infection. The disease can also attack the nails of the fingers and toes, causing a thickening of the nails, a yellow-brown discoloration, or scaling under the nails. In mild cases, there may be pits or small depressions on the nails; in severe cases, the nails may separate from the nail beds. Between 10 and 40 percent of patients have problems with their finger joints as well as other joints, as part of a severe nail involvement.

About 5 percent of psoriasis patients suffer from a form of arthritis that is similar but not identical to rheumatoid arthritis. The severity of the arthritis varies from person to person, but it commonly affects the hands and, at times, the large joints and spine.

Treatment

There is no cure for psoriasis, but there are many effective treatments that can result in periods of remission ranging from months to years. Treatment varies according to the extent and severity of the disease, as well as the location of the plaques. For localized plaques, the use of various topical medications is a first-line approach, although there are advantages and disadvantages to each. All of the following preparations and therapies can be particularly effective when used in combination with other treatments.

■ Corticosteroid creams and ointments can reduce the inflammation, ease itching, and slow the rapid turnover of skin cells. Prolonged use of high-potency topical steroids, however, can lead to tolerance and relative resistance, as well as to thinning of the skin.

■ Crude coal tar ointment is often prescribed, but the thick black substance is messy and aesthetically unappealing. Commercial refined tar products are more cosmetically acceptable, but these, too, have a strong tar odor.

■ A synthetic drug that is similar to tar, called anthralin, acts to normalize skin cell growth. It must be carefully applied to localized skin areas, because it can cause irritation and temporary discoloration of the skin.

■ For those with widespread psoriasis, a course of sunlamp (UVB) therapy is sometimes administered three to five times weekly over a long period. This treatment is called the Goeckerman regimen when combined with the use of topical tar preparations. Some people are sensitive to ultraviolet light, however, and care must be taken not to cause burns.

■ PUVA therapy combines the use of an oral medication followed by exposure to ultraviolet light (photochemotherapy). The dose of UV light is carefully regulated and increased in increments to avoid a sunburn-like reaction. The eyes are shielded with wraparound UV-blocking goggles during treatment, and the patient is carefully monitored afterward to avoid any increased risk of lens opacities or cataracts. PUVA therapy can produce a significant clearing of the skin within an average of 25 treatments, administered two to three times a week. It does carry an increased risk of the common sun-related type of skin cancers, particularly squamous cell carcinoma.

Certain systemic, or internal, medications can be used only in cases of severe and disabling psoriasis. These drugs include the following:

■ Methotrexate, a type of drug used in treating cancer. In the treatment of psoriasis, it interferes with the rapid proliferation of cells. The patient must be monitored carefully, because this drug can affect liver function and increase blood lipids.

HELP FOR PSORIASIS SUFFERERS

Psoriasis is a subject of active interest and investigation. Research scientists throughout the world are attempting to find a cure for this distressing and sometimes disabling skin disease. An increasing number of topical and systemic drugs are under study, including calcipotriol, vitamin D, new retinoids, and immunological agents.

In addition to the traditional approaches, you may want to try alternative treatments, including stress-reduction techniques, group therapy, and preventive methods to avoid attacks in the future. For additional information, contact the National Psoriasis Foundation. A patient advocacy group, this organization supports research in psoriasis and helps to educate the public about this important skin disorder.

■ Etretinate, a type of vitamin A derivative that is similar to Accutane. It is often administered in combination with PUVA therapy in severe cases of psoriasis. It has potent side affects, however, including liver damage and an increase in blood cholesterol and triglycerides. Of particular concern is the potential of this drug for causing birth defects. Because etretinate has a long half-life and can persist in the body for years, the drug cannot be used in women of childbearing age.

■ Cyclosporine can be used in transplant patients to prevent organ rejection. It has been found to be very effective for severe psoriasis, perhaps because of its effects on the immune system. The psoriasis dramatically clears after a course of therapy with the drug but tends to recur when the cyclosporine is stopped. Because of the potential for serious side effects, particularly on kidney function, the drug cannot be given indefinitely.

Hives

A hive is an itchy, red swelling that comes and goes in a matter of hours. A single hive is usually an allergic reaction to an insect bite or some other external irritant. Multiple hives, or urticaria, are usually caused by

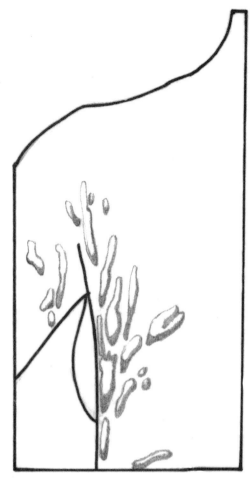

Figure 35.9. Hives
Urticaria are multiple itchy, red hives usually caused by
an allergic reaction to medication or food.

an internal allergic reaction and can last for a longer
period of time. (See Fig. 35.9) Internal irritants can be
medications or foods. The chief medical offenders are
aspirin and penicillin; chocolate, strawberries, shellfish, nuts, and eggs are typical foods that cause this
type of reaction.

The first step is to find and eliminate the substance
causing the hives. In the case of foods, you may have
to keep a diet diary, listing all the foods you eat and
whether the hives appear after a particular food is ingested. In the case of medications, the source is much
easier to find and eliminate. To alleviate the immediate
symptoms, your doctor may recommend lotions and
soothing baths to relieve the itching. Antihistamines
are the drug of choice; if one does not work, another
will probably do the job. If the hives are particularly
severe, or if the allergic reaction is acute, you may get
an injection of adrenalin or corticosteroids. See Chapter 31)

Skin Cancers

Skin cancer is as common as all other types of cancer
combined. More than 500,000 Americans develop skin
cancer each year. More than 90 percent occur on skin
that is exposed to the elements, and exposure to ultraviolet radiation from the sun is considered to be the
cause. Exposure to artificial sources of UV radiation,
such as sunlamps and indoor tanning booths, poses
similar hazards.

Although anyone can get skin cancer, those at
greatest risk have fair skin and blue eyes, freckle easily,
and sunburn readily.

Other risk factors include where you live now and
where you lived as a child; this is especially true in the
case of malignant melanoma (see below). If you live in
an area that receives high levels of UV radiation from
the sun, the risk is greater than if you live in an area that
is often overcast. For example, although many blue-
eyed blondes live in Minnesota, skin cancer is more
common in Texas, where the UV rays of the sun are
more intense, than in Minnesota. Because skin cancer
risk is a cumulative product of a lifetime of exposure to
the sun, sun protection should be started as soon as
possible—in early childhood—in order to lower the
risk of skin cancer later in life.

Types of Skin Cancer

A cancer occurs when normal cells lose their ability to
limit and direct their growth. The affected cells divide
rapidly and grow without any order. Some of these
deviant skin cancer cells also metastasize, or spread, to
other parts of the body and form new tumors. There are
three types of skin cancer.

ARE YOU AT RISK OF SKIN CANCER?

High risk: Your skin and hair are light, and you
usually burn and freckle easily. Your eyes are blue,
green, gray, or hazel.

Moderate risk: Your skin and hair may be light or
dark. You tan, but can burn if you stay in the sun too
long. Your eyes may be light or brown.

Less risk: Your skin is beige or brown, and it takes a
great deal of sun to make you burn. Your eyes are
brown or black.

- *Basal cell carcinoma.* This is the most common skin cancer. It is slow-growing, remains local, and rarely spreads to other parts of the body. If left untreated, however, it can invade nearby tissue and bone.

- *Squamous cell carcinoma.* Found mainly on the head, face, and hands—areas exposed to sunlight—this type of cancer can spread to other parts of the body. Early detection and treatment can minimize the invasion and the destruction of adjacent tissue.

- *Malignant melanoma.* This form of cancer has a high risk of spreading to other parts of the body, and is responsible for most of the deaths from skin cancer. It begins as a growth that develops in the pigment cells (melanocytes) of the skin.

Symptoms

The most reliable warning sign of skin cancer is any noticeable change on the surface of your skin. A new growth or a sore that fails to heal after two or three weeks should not be lightly dismissed. Although basal and squamous cell cancers are found mainly on sun-exposed areas of the skin—face, neck, scalp, ears, hands, arms—they can occur anywhere on the body. Malignant melanoma especially is not always found on frequently exposed areas. A regular checking of all of your skin should be an essential part of your self-care program.

Examine yourself in a room that has adequate lighting. The best time to do this is after a shower or bath. Use a full-length mirror and a hand-held mirror, so you can view all areas of your body. Check between the buttocks and in the genital area. Section your hair to see any growths that may be on the scalp. Especially check for a new mole or a change in an old mole or mark on the skin. If you find something that disturbs you, and the growth persists for three weeks, have your doctor evaluate the area. Here are signs to look for.

- A small (¼ inch or less in diameter), smooth, shiny, waxy, or pale bump

- A red bump or sore that develops a crust and bleeds.

- A flat, red spot that is rough, dry, or scaly.

- A mole or dark spot that has the ABCD characteristics:

    Asymmetry (irregular in shape)

    Border notching or jaggedness

Color in variations of shades of brown or, especially, blue-black

Diameter greater than 5 millimeters (the size, of an eraser on a #2 graphite pencil)

In additions to the ABCDs, other warning signs for malignant melanoma are moles or growths that change in size and in elevation, itch, are tender and painful, bleed, or develop scaliness or crusting.

Diagnosis

Your dermatologist will inspect the area in question. If he or she thinks it is suspicious, a biopsy can be performed in which a small section of your skin is removed for examination under a microscope. If it appears that you have a skin cancer, your dermatologist can weigh the options for the treatment that is best for you.

Treatment

The goal of skin cancer treatment is to remove all the cancer while affecting as small an area and leaving as small a scar as possible. Your physician must consider the type and size of the cancer, its location, and the risk of scarring. Your medical history and general health also may influence the treatment. There are several options.

- *Surgical excision.* The tumor is cut out with a scalpel and the wound is closed with sutures. This is the most common treatment for skin cancer, and it is often performed under a local anesthetic.

- *Curettage and electrodesiccation.* Curettage uses a sharp, spoon-shaped instrument to scoop out the cancerous area. An electric current (electrodesiccation) controls bleeding and kills any remaining cancer cells around the edges of the wound. This procedure often leaves a flat, white scar.

- *Mohs micrographic surgery.* This surgical technique removes and examines one thin layer of skin at a time. The amount of tissue removed depends upon the extent of the tumor growth. Mohs surgery is especially helpful in difficult-to-see places, such as the borders of a tumor, and on hard-to-treat areas, such as the eyelid. A variety of surgical repairs may be done to restore the removed tissue.

- *Cryosurgery.* An extremely cold chemical, liquid nitrogen, is used to treat precancerous conditions and some small skin cancers. The cold application kills the visible abnormal cells and a small surrounding border of normal skin. A few days later, a scab forms over the wound; it falls off after about two weeks. In stubborn cases, more than one treatment may be needed to remove the growth completely. Side effects include swelling, some discomfort, and some scarring.

- *Topical chemotherapy.* This treatment, usually reserved for precancerous conditions, uses anticancer creams or lotions. These topical medications are applied to the affected area over a 3-week period. Sometimes, in a series of treatment sessions, anticancer medications are injected directly into the tumor. Side effects include inflammation; scars do not usually occur.

- *Laser therapy.* Lasers are instruments that produce high-energy light of a very specific wavelength. Generally reserved for precancerous conditions, laser therapy uses this light to remove suspicious cells from the uppermost layers of the skin. Scarring can occur.

- *Radiation therapy (radiotherapy).* Radiation treatment is the use of high-energy rays to damage cancer cells and stop their growth. This method is used for areas hard to treat with

MINOR GROWTHS AND BENIGN TUMORS

As we age, our skin is subject to various bumps, lumps, and spots. These benign tumors are usually quite harmless, although at times they may become irritated and should be removed. The most common of these minor growths are listed below.

- *Keratoses.* There are two types of keratoses—seborrheic and solar. *Seborrheic* keratoses are flat, slightly elevated, brown, rough-surfaced spots that can appear in large numbers on the back, chest, face, and arms. They are not caused by a virus or the sun, and can easily be removed by cryosurgery or a simple surgical procedure. *Solar* keratoses are more dangerous. Caused by exposure to the sun, more than 20 percent of these flat, raised, red, scaly spots become cancerous. Methods of removal include curettage, topical chemotherapy, and cryosurgery.

- *Cherry angiomas.* "Cherry spots"—small, red bumps on the skin—become increasingly common with age. You can safely ignore these generally harmless benign growths unless they become unsightly or start to bleed. Angiomas are easily removed with cryosurgery or electrosurgery.

- *Liver spots.* These flat, light-brown or black spots are extremely common after age 50. They almost always occur in fair-skinned people, usually on the face and the backs of the hands. Liver spots are associated with exposure to the sun, but they are harmless. You can have them removed by cryosurgery, acid peeling, or electrosurgery.

- *Moles.* By adulthood, most people have a quantity of moles scattered over their bodies. These flesh-colored, brown, or black growths are made up of collections of melanocytes, pigment-manufacturing cells. African-Americans tend to develop fewer moles than the white population, but they are subject to the development of multiple, small, black growths on their face that may be cosmetically unsightly. These "moles" are really a type of keratosis and can be removed electrosurgically by a dermatologist.

    Most moles are harmless, but they can become cancerous. If you notice any changes in existing moles on your skin—scaliness, change of color, increase in size—see your dermatologist.

- *Warts.* Common warts, small, hard, flesh-colored growths, are caused by a viral infection. They can occur anywhere on the body, but usually pop up on hands and feet (plantar warts). Appearing more commonly in children and younger people, warts are contagious, but usually only to the person who has them. They are harmless growths, and usually disappear on their own. Over-the-counter medications can remove some warts, or they can be eliminated by a dermatologist using cryotherapy, electrosurgery, or strong acids or other chemicals.

surgery, including the eyelid, nose, and ear. A rash may develop on the treated skin, and changes in skin color and texture may become apparent over the years.

Although most skin cancers are cured by using one of these methods of treatment, there are situations when a combination of radiation therapy, local chemotherapy, and systemic chemotherapy is advisable. A small number of cancers may also recur. If you have one episode of skin cancer, you are at increased risk for developing another. If you are in a high-risk group, examine your skin thoroughly once a month, and have a skin checkup from your dermatologist annually. Early detection can improve the cure rate, and there is less scarring.

Infections of the Skin

Most skin infections are noncontagious, minor annoyances, but some can develop into more serious conditions if they are neglected or improperly treated. Disease-producing bacteria and viruses, for example, may infect hair follicles or a wound in the skin and cause a number of skin conditions, including boils, impetigo, erysipelas (cellulitis), cold sores and canker sores, and shingles. Fungal infections can result in ringworm and yeast infections.

Boils

Staphylococcus bacteria can infect one or more hair follicles and cause an inflammation that quickly spreads into the surrounding skin. Boils can occur anywhere on your skin, but commonly appear on the upper back and the nape of your neck. Physical conditions such as diabetes, acne, and severe dermatitis can cause boils, or they may be the result of poor hygiene, low immunity, or irritations.

Symptoms

Boils are painful, red, swollen nodules that may be accompanied by fever or a feeling of fatigue. Solitary boils are common, and many people treat them themselves. The boil usually comes to a head and bursts, discharging a pus-filled core.

Diagnosis

If the boil persists or recurs, or you have a series of boils, see your dermatologist for an evaluation. The strain of *Staphylococcus* bacteria may be especially virulent, or there may be an underlying disorder that needs to be attended to.

Treatment

For a single boil, apply hot compresses to the area for about 30 minutes every few hours. It will usually burst, drain, and disappear on its own. Keep the area clean—use an antiseptic soap—and avoid contaminating other areas of the skin with the drained matter. Never squeeze or try to lance a boil yourself; you may spread the infection and make it worse. If the boil recurs, or you are suffering from a cluster of boils, your doctor can surgically drain them and prescribe antibiotics to prevent their recurrence.

Impetigo

Impetigo, a superficial bacterial skin infection, is common in babies and young children, but can also occur in adults. The infection starts when *Streptococcus* bacteria enter through a small opening in the skin surface, usually caused by an abrasion, minor cut, fever blister, or insect bite.

Symptoms

Impetigo causes the infected skin to become covered with blisters that break and form red, itchy sores. Yellow or gray crusts then form on the sores, which fail to heal normally.

Diagnosis

Impetigo is often diagnosed only when the disease spreads to other parts of the body. Your doctor can confirm the diagnosis by taking a tissue culture.

Treatment

The therapy for impetigo depends on the severity of the infection. Antibiotic ointments and lotions are effective for minor and limited infections; oral antibiotics are usually prescribed for more severe cases. Care must be taken to avoid spreading this contagious infection.

Erysipelas (Cellulitis)

Erysipelas, once called St. Anthony's fire, is a severe inflammation of the skin caused by *Streptococcus* bacteria. In most cases, a small crack in the skin provides entry to the bacteria, which then spread rapidly.

Symptoms

Erysipelas generally begins with a fever, headache, chills, and muscle pains. The ensuing rash consists of patches of hot, red, swollen skin. This infection can be fatal if left untreated.

Diagnosis

Because of confusing symptoms, erysipelas is sometimes dismissed as a viral infection or as a common rash. Your doctor will examine you thoroughly for the shiny, sharply defined borders of the characteristic erysipelas rash.

Treatment

Antibiotics usually stop the infection quickly. Within a matter of hours, the fever drops and other symptoms quickly subside. The rash may take longer to disappear.

Cold Sores, Fever Blisters, and Canker Sores

Among the most common of virus infections, cold sores (also known as fever blisters) affect over 70 percent of the U.S. population. These recurrent skin infections are caused by the *Herpes simplex* I virus, which is contagious. The virus may remain dormant in the body for long periods of time, but sooner or later the infection recurs. Certain factors trigger a *Herpes* episode, including sun exposure, illness, emotional stress, even menstruation. Facial *Herpes* outbreaks commonly occur on the lips, around the mouth, and on the nose or cheeks. (See Fig. 35.10)

One of the more annoying and painful of the trivial ailments, canker sores form inside the mouth and can make eating difficult. The cause of canker sores is unknown, although it is thought that an immune reaction is involved. Women tend to suffer from canker sores more than men.

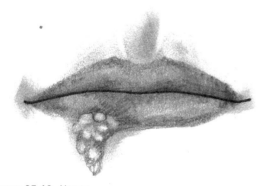

Figure 35.10. Herpes
Herpes is an infection with a virus that causes cold sores on the lips and around the mouth.

Symptoms

The initial *Herpes* infection is the most severe. There may be local tenderness, fever, and then small blisters that form, break, and ooze. Crusts will form and then slough off. Recurrent attacks are much milder: you may feel a tingling or burning sensation for a few hours before blisters start to form.

Canker sores begin as a sore spot in the mouth, then develop into painful lumps. Some people experience fever, fatigue, and swollen glands.

Diagnosis

Both of these infections can be readily diagnosed upon examination by a physician.

Treatment

An antiviral compound, acyclovir, is the drug that is used most often to treat the first attack of *Herpes* and to prevent recurrent eruptions. There are also over-the-counter ointments and lotions that may be helpful in relieving the discomfort. Unfortunately, there is little you can do for canker sores. Your doctor can prescribe anesthetic solutions or antihistamine mouthwashes that can provide some relief; avoid eating spicy or acidic foods until the sores have healed.

Shingles

Shingles is caused by the same virus (*Herpes zoster*) that is responsible for chicken pox. The virus remains dormant in the body until something triggers its reappearance, which takes the form of a localized rash. Shingles can occur at any age but is most common after 60. Recurrence is possible but rare.

Symptoms

Shingles is often preceded by tingling or pain in the affected area. The skin reddens, and blisters appear on one side of the body or on the face. These blistering areas follow the path of a spinal nerve. (See Fig. 35.11) In some cases the pain persists throughout the attack, which lasts for about 2 to 3 weeks, and even long after the rash has healed. This postherpetic neuralgia seems to occur more often in chronically ill or elderly people.

Diagnosis

The characteristic blistering rash, along with your other symptoms and medical history, can help your doctor reach a diagnosis.

Treatment

If caught in the early stages, your doctor may prescribe the antiviral agent acyclovir to lessen the sever-

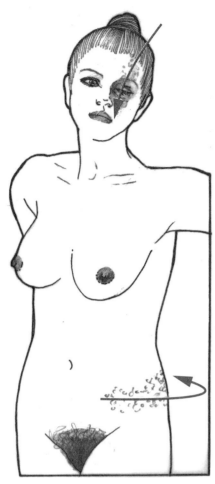

Figure 35.11. Shingles
Shingles are caused by a virus that produces patterns of painful redness and blisters that follow the paths of nerves in the body. The rash can circle the waist, cross the shoulder, or affect the face and eyes.

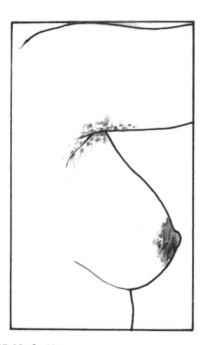

Figure 35.12. Scabies
Scabies is caused by parasitic mites that burrow under the skin in areas such as the armpit and under the breast, producing an extremely itchy rash.

ity of the attack and to minimize any danger to your eyes, if the virus is on the face. Oral corticosteroids, if given early enough, can also prevent the prolonged postherpetic pain that occurs in some people. You may also get some relief from wet compresses, soothing lotions, and analgesics.

Fungus Infections

A form of plant life, fungi can cause a number of skin infections, including ringworm and *Candida albicans,* a yeast infection. Ringworm—there is no worm involved—actually refers to several different forms of the same fungus that infect different parts of the body. For example, athlete's foot and jock itch are similar fungal infections. (See Fig. 35.13) Symptoms include a red, scaly rash and intense itching. The central area of the

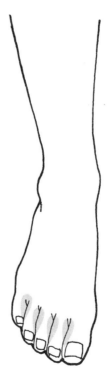

Figure 35.13. Athlete's Foot
Athlete's foot is a fungus infection that produces a red, scaly rash and intense itching.

BUGS, TICKS, AND INFESTATIONS

Your skin is vulnerable to small insects that attach themselves and feed off your blood. Many of these parasitical problems are merely annoying and embarrassing, but sometimes these insects transmit viruses or bacteria that cause serious illnesses in humans.

- *Fleas.* The ordinary flea is perfectly happy to live on domestic pets but, given the right circumstances, will settle for a diet of human blood. Fleas are able to jump great distances, so bites often appear on a pet owner's ankles or legs. The bites appear as an itching, localized rash. Soothing lotions will help relieve the irritation, but the problem will continue until the fleas are eliminated. This can be done using sprays and aerosol bombs, or a professional exterminator. Obviously, the source of the fleas must be treated by a veterinarian at the same time the patient is treated.

- *Scabies.* Scabies is an intensely itching rash that can affect people of all ages, races, and classes. It is caused by tiny mites that burrow into certain areas of the skin, such as between the fingers, in the armpits, on the breasts and genitals, and on the buttocks. (See Fig. 35.12) Highly contagious, scabies is spread by intimate personal contact, as well as by using the linens, towels, and clothing of affected persons. It is most often treated with strong creams and lotions that are applied all over the body and left on all night. One application should be enough to kill all the adult mites, although some physicians recommend a second application some days later.

- *Head and pubic lice.* Lice are tiny parasitic insects that can infest the hair, the body, and the pubic region. They cause intense itching and allergic reactions. Body lice are usually associated with poor hygiene, extreme poverty, or wartime deprivations. Head lice are very common among schoolchildren. Both can be eradicated using pesticide shampoos or a preparation for body lice. With body lice, all clothing and linens must be washed in very hot water, and mattresses must be dusted with an appropriate powder.

- Pubic lice, or crabs, come from intimate contact with an infected person. They can be eliminated by using the appropriate medication. The sexual partner should be examined and treated if infected.

- *Ticks.* Ticks, small, flat insects that feed on blood, are found in wooded areas in all parts of the United States. They may be carriers of Rocky Mountain spotted fever or, more commonly, Lyme disease. A typical skin rash—a red mark that spreads out to form a large ring 2 to 3 inches in diameter—is often the first symptom of Lyme disease. Other signs of infection—such as fever, headache, muscle aches, sore throat, swollen glands—usually develop later. Early treatment with antibiotics is essential, or complications may ensue. Since the results of a blood test may take several weeks, your physician may decide to start treatment immediately if there is any chance that you do have Lyme disease.

pills were first introduced, the formulas had a high estrogen component, which suppressed sebum production and often resulted in dramatic improvement in acne. In modern oral contraceptives, the estrogen content has been markedly reduced, and few of these drugs sore eventually heals, leaving a ring on the skin. Ringworm is highly contagious. Pets also can transmit the disease. *Candida* yeast infections include diaper rash and oral thrush in babies, and genital infections. You may be more susceptible to yeast infections if you have diabetes, are pregnant or obese, or are taking certain medications.

There are many excellent medications available to treat fungus infections, including over-the-counter products. Your physician may prescribe an oral anti-fungal medication if your case is particularly severe.

Hair and Nail Disorders

Hair Problems

Hair loss

Obviously, the worst disorder affecting your hair is its loss. We all lose hair on a regular basis, as a part of normal hair growth and regeneration. It is also normal, as we age, for our hair to thin out gradually. Called female-pattern hair loss, this means you might have, besides thinning, moderate loss of hair on the crown and at the hairline.

In younger women, there are other reasons for a heavier-than-normal loss of hair. Childbirth is one of the most frequent causes of a temporary type of hair loss, and is probably hormone-induced. Women who discontinue the use of birth control pills may experience a similar pattern of temporary hair loss. Certain diseases and stress can also affect your hair cycle, including a too-rapid loss of weight (crash dieting) and severe emotional shock, although this is harder to prove.

Temporary hair loss is nothing to worry about. It is when hair falls out in patches, as in the disorder *alopecia areata,* that you should consult your dermatologist. Unfortunately, there is not much that can be done for this type of severe hair loss. Corticosteroids may arrest or decelerate hair loss, but there are no medications that can restore hair.

Hirsutism

Sometimes women believe they have excessive hair, especially on the legs, arms, cheeks, and upper lip. The amount of hair in these regions of the body varies with genetic background and age. Too much or too little hair is a matter of personal perception and social norms. Luckily, it is easier to get rid of hair than to grow more. There is no completely satisfactory method of eliminating unwanted hair, but the following options are available:

- *Plucking.* This is a popular and easy way to get rid of a few stray hairs. Use good tweezers, and pull out the hair in the direction in which it is growing.

- *Shaving.* This is a generally safe and simple method of hair removal, although some women find it unattractive because it leaves a stubble. Contrary to popular belief, shaving does not make the hair grow faster or more coarsely.

- *Bleaching.* Using inexpensive hydrogen peroxide, or the more expensive bleaching creams, is a relatively simple way to make arm and leg hair less conspicuous. Follow the instructions, and do a patch test to avoid an irritation or allergic reaction to the product.

- *Waxing.* This technique—hot wax is applied to the area and then quickly peeled off—is gener-

ally done by a trained cosmetician in a beauty salon. Waxing can be painful, but the hair does take longer to grow back.

- *Depilatories.* These products are chemical agents that dissolve hair protein and leave a smooth, hairless skin surface. They can be irritating to the skin, so test the product first on a small patch of skin.

- *Electrolysis.* This is the only method that removes hair permanently. A fine needle is inserted into the hair follicle, and an electrical impulse is delivered to the sensitive hair bulb. This procedure should be done by a trained technician, because damage to the tissue around the hair follicle can cause scarring. The procedure is also long, tedious, and expensive.

Nail Problems

Nails are subject to a number of ailments, including chronic breaking, superficial infections, and fungus infections.

Brittle and splitting nails may be a result of drying out of the nails, particularly if you are exposing them to household irritants and chemicals, as well as a low-humidity environment. Brittle, breaking, and splitting nails have nothing to do with nutritional deficiencies. Try wearing rubber gloves when you do housework or handle chemicals, and use a lubricating ointment when you manicure your nails.

Infection of the nail, or *paronychia,* is caused by minute breaks in the skin around the nails that allow bacteria and fungal agents to enter. The injuries are usually due to the biting off of hangnails or injury to the cuticle. When paronychial infections are caused by the *Staphylococcus* bacteria, you will experience redness, swelling, and extreme pain. Your doctor can prescribe hot soaks and antibiotics, and sometimes will perform a surgical incision to release the pus.

A fungal infection of the nails causes a more low-grade infection, with minimal pain and tenderness. However, the nail may become thickened, loosened, and shed, or it may be destroyed. Contrary to the treatment accorded paronychial infections, the nail affected by a fungus must be kept absolutely dry. Although your physician can prescribe the appropriate oral antifungal medications, there is no guarantee that the fungus can be eradicated.

CHAPTER 36

Reconstructive and Plastic Surgery

Jane A. Petro, M.D., F.A.C.S., and
Linda G. Phillips, M.D., F.A.C.S.

The term "plastic" comes from the Greek word *plasticos,* which means "to shape or mold." Plastic and reconstructive surgery is a medical specialty whose practitioners are concerned with improving appearance or restoring form and function of a part of the body affected by injury or deformity. The specialty is usually divided into cosmetic surgery and reconstructive surgery, although the distinction is not always clear. The goal is to achieve the best possible result, in terms of both aesthetics and function.

Plastic surgery may be done to correct a birth defect, reconstruct a breast after mastectomy, restore the use of a hand after injury, or repair tissue after burns or disease such as skin cancer. It can also be performed to provide a more pleasing appearance, counteract effects of aging, and boost the self-confidence of those who are troubled with some aspects of the way they look.

Plastic surgery is often elective surgery—that is, the woman chooses whether she wishes to have it. Before deciding on plastic surgery, she should carefully consider a number of factors. Those who are well prepared in advance usually have more realistic expectations and are more likely to be pleased with the results.

GENERAL CONSIDERATIONS

Some of the things to think about before having plastic surgery are the qualifications of the surgeon, the reasons for having the surgery, what the procedure will entail both preoperatively and postoperatively, and what, in general, can be expected. Because plastic surgery is elective, it often is not covered by insurance, and many plastic surgeons require payment in advance. Plastic surgery may be performed in a physician's office or in a hospital.

Selecting a Surgeon

As with any medical specialist, it is important when selecting a plastic surgeon to find a doctor who not only is qualified to render care but is also accessible (see box). The selection process should begin by seeking a referral. In an emergency situation, the plastic surgeon on call for the hospital usually provides care. When selecting a plastic surgeon for an elective procedure, referrals can be obtained from a primary care practitioner, friends, local hospitals, the county medical society, or the American Society of Plastic and Reconstructive Surgeons (see "Resources" at the end of this chapter.)

A board-certified plastic and reconstructive surgeon has completed a residency of specialized training after medical school and passed an examination to be certified by the American Board of Plastic Surgery. Specialists from a variety of fields—dermatology (skin), otolaryngology (ears, nose, throat), ophthalmology (eyes)—can have advanced training in plastic surgery.

A physician who has had training in a specific procedure is qualified to perform that procedure.

Plastic surgeons are frequently thought of as cosmetic surgeons, but the training for plastic surgeons includes extensive training in general surgery and more specifically in reconstructive and cosmetic surgery. The specialty of plastic and reconstructive surgery is becoming increasingly subspecialized. Some physicians perform pediatric plastic surgery, whereas others may do only hand surgery, head surgery, cancer surgery, breast surgery, or cosmetic plastic surgery. It is still most common, however, for a physician to do a mix of these types of procedures, perhaps with an emphasis on a particular area.

Preoperative and Recovery Preparations

There are things a woman can do to prepare for surgery. With some minor changes in lifestyle and advance preparations, she can ease discomfort, speed healing, and help ensure that she is ready for surgery.

Exercise
Being physically fit helps the lungs and heart deliver oxygen throughout the body. Fitness improves lung capacity during surgery, increases blood flow for fast healing, and encourages joint flexibility, which helps keep joints from stiffening after lying on the operating table for several hours. A woman who exercises should continue to do so. A woman who does not exercise should begin a program 3 weeks before sur-

EVALUATING A SURGEON

Any doctor can identify herself or himself as a cosmetic and/or plastic surgeon after completing medical school and obtaining a license to practice medicine. Although this is legal, it does not necessarily mean that such a physician is qualified or certified to perform cosmetic surgery. There are a number of ways to evaluate the qualifications of a surgeon:

- Check for certification by the American Board of Plastic Surgery or consult *The Official ABMS Directory of Board Certified Medical Specialists*, published by the American Board of Medical Specialists and Marquis Who's Who. It is available in most public libraries.

- Check for membership in the American Society of Plastic and Reconstructive Surgeons (ASPRS) and the American Society for Aesthetic Plastic Surgery (ASAPS). These professional societies have members who are certified by the American Board of Plastic Surgery.

- Check the surgeon's hospital affiliation. An appointment to the surgical staff of a hospital means that a surgeon has been reviewed and judged acceptable by medical colleagues.

- It is appropriate to ask the physician about board certification, training and qualifications, and hospitals where the surgeon has privileges. It is also appropriate to ask about the physician's experience in the area.

Talk candidly with the surgeon. During an initial consultation the surgeon will examine you and discuss preoperative considerations and postoperative care. You should feel comfortable discussing your expectations and the procedure with your surgeon. Discuss fees and insurance. Costs vary widely and depend on the complexity of the surgery, where the surgery is done, and the anesthetic that is administered.

gery. At least 10 minutes every other day should be spent bending, stretching, and deep breathing. Brisk walking can be done on alternate days.

Nutrition

Both dieting and bingeing should be avoided before surgery. Dieting adds stress to the trauma of any surgery. The body burns extra protein during and after surgery, so extra protein should be eaten beginning about 2 weeks in advance. A multivitamin should be taken daily 2 weeks before surgery. The recommended daily dosage should not be exceeded because high levels of vitamins can be dangerous. Vitamin E and fish oil, for example, slow blood clotting.

Drugs

Most drugs—legal and certainly illegal—should be stopped two weeks before surgery. Consult your physician if you are taking any prescription or nonprescription drugs on a regular basis. You should also avoid tobacco during this time. Tobacco slows healing, increases the risk of complications, and reduces the body's ability to fight infection. Illegal drugs such as marijuana and cocaine can cause life-threatening complications during surgery. The physician should be informed of all prescription drugs being taken so any risks can be determined. Aspirin and nonsteroidal anti-inflammatory drugs such as ibuprofen should not be taken because they may cause bleeding. The only pain reliever that can be taken before surgery is acetaminophen; it is helpful to have a supply available afterward as well.

Blood Flow

Blow flow in the legs can slow during and after surgery, causing them to ache. This can be relieved by doing stretching exercises (point toes down, then bend ankles back) 10 times per day before surgery. The exercises can be continued after surgery to keep the blood moving. Elastic stockings also help prevent swelling and aching.

Planning for Recovery

Preparations should be made for taking time off—from work outside or at home—for 2 weeks, and all activities should be limited during that time. It is helpful to have family or friends available to help with household duties. Food and medicines (including bandages and tape) for that period should be stocked in advance. It is good to have a supply of prepared foods, juices, and dried fruit. Pain medication can cause constipation that juices and fruit can help relieve. Last-minute preparations include arranging the bedding so it will be ready after the surgery, removing nail polish so the color of the nails shows (reflecting the amount of oxygen in the blood), and making an appointment for a postoperative visit. The healing process can be helped by special care during recovery (see box).

HEALING

The healing process starts during surgery when blood, flowing through a wound, dries into a scab, forming an airtight, moisture-resistant, temporary bandage. Beneath the surface, skin replacement goes into high gear. After about 6 weeks, gentle massage, combined with a lubricating cream or vitamin E oil to help reduce inflammation, and antihistamines can help relieve itching during the healing process. Scratching should be avoided; it can cause scar buildup.

Infections slow the healing process. Signs of infection are redness, heat, or tenderness that persists more than a few days or any signs of pus. Immediate treatment is needed to allow natural healing to resume.

Good nutrition is vital for rapid healing. Ample protein is needed for building new tissues. Vitamins play a key role, both in healthy cell growth and in preventing infection. Vitamin A (in fish oils) and vitamin C (in green vegetables and citrus fruits) are linked with skin repair.

Anesthesia

Most people have heard the terms "general anesthesia" and "local anesthesia." With local anesthesia, a specific area of the body is made numb by an injection of medication at the site. An example is the kind of anesthesia given in a dental office for a filling. Sometimes a sedative is given with a local anesthetic to help the patient relax. General anesthesia puts the patient to sleep, leaving no memory of the procedure. It can be given through an injection or a mask. It must be given by an anesthesiologist.

The choice of anesthetic depends on the type of procedure and whether it is performed in a hospital or a doctor's office. General anesthesia is usually given in a hospital and often has a higher risk of complications.

Complications

No surgery is riskfree. The patient's health and whether she smokes can affect the success of some procedures. Many procedures should not be done on patients who continue to smoke (such as facelifts). Surgery cannot stop aging; it can diminish some effects of aging, but the results are not permanent. Serious complications

SCAR REMOVAL TECHNIQUES

Biochemical changes continue to take place for months after surgery or a traumatic injury to the skin. It may be months before a doctor can begin to deal with new scars. Most scars are raised, red, and firmer than other skin. Others are deep, pitlike areas lying below the surface. To erase or "revise" scars, marks higher than the skin are lowered, and scars that are depressed are raised to the skin's normal surface level. Scars from surgery can be removed or disguised with several procedures. The cause, size, and location of a scar influence which revision technique is used.

- **W and Z incisions.** The simplest technique is to cut away the scar and repair the wound with fine stitches; this works best when the wound was not stitched in the first place. W and Z incisions are small cuts made to camouflage the scar by making it irregular or reorienting its direction to fit into natural creases. "Z-plasty" lengthens the scar at an angle and is best for knees and elbows.

- **Sanding.** Dermabrasion is one of the most common procedures performed to decrease scarring caused by surgery, trauma, fine wrinkling, or acne. In the past, dermabrasion was done several months or a year after the injury, to allow a scar to heal properly and mature. Today, dermabrasion is performed before healing is complete. This produces collagen fibers and results in flatter, better-healing wounds.

- **Collagen.** This type of protein, derived from animal sources, is similar to the one that appears naturally in skin. Collagen can be injected beneath a deep scar to raise the area to the normal level, eliminating or minimizing pitting. Collagen also can lift some birthmarks and plump out wrinkles. Several injections about 4 weeks apart can lift most pitted scars or small depressions.

- **Freezing and Melting.** Cryosurgery freezes the skin by spraying or painting it with liquid nitrogen (−195.8° C). The cold slows or stops scar-producing collagen formation, making scars less dense. It is also possible to shrink a scar with cortisone injections, which "melt" the tough collagen tissue.

are rare, but they can occur and include infection, bleeding, and nerve damage. In most cases these complications are apparent soon after surgery and may require further surgery.

Scars are a result of almost any kind of surgery, since all surgical incisions cause scarring. Placement of the incision, surgical technique, and suturing can minimize scarring, however. The degree of scarring depends on a number of factors, including the type of surgery and its extent as well as the individual woman's ability to heal. Certain procedures can be performed after the initial surgery to correct scars.

BREAST SURGERY

Breast surgery may be cosmetic or reconstructive or both. It can be done to reduce or enlarge the breasts or to reconstruct them after mastectomy.

Breast Reduction

Breast reduction is designed to decrease the size of a woman's breasts. The procedure does not affect the woman's chest size. Breast reduction is often done for medical reasons and is not performed for cosmetic purposes alone. Thus, it is covered by most medical insurance policies, depending on the amount of breast tissue to be removed. It may be wise to obtain authorization from the insurance company in advance.

Women with very large breasts often complain of neck, back, or shoulder pain caused by the weight of their breasts. They have difficulty finding bras that fit; without this support, breasts tend to sag. Although manufacturers use thicker straps in large size bras, the straps may cause grooves to form in the shoulder from the weight of the breasts. Sweat accumulates where the breasts rest on the upper abdominal skin, leading to irritating rashes. Large breasts often prevent active participation in sports, cause ready-made clothing to fit poorly, and can be a source of embarrassment.

Breasts enlarge at puberty and during pregnancy. The use of birth control pills or a substantial weight gain also can cause breasts to enlarge. In these situations, however, the breasts will usually decrease in size when the conditions are no longer present. Large breasts may also be a family tendency.

Reduction surgery is performed under general anesthesia. Most women are hospitalized for 1 or 2 days after surgery and must avoid strenuous exercise or heavy lifting for a while. Wearing a well-fitted bra night and day for 2 to 3 weeks after surgery will support breasts and relieve pain.

Before surgery the physician measures the patient's breasts and marks where incisions are to be made and where the nipples are finally to be placed. Ideally, the nipples will be placed symmetrically, at a position on the chest level with the middle of the upper arm. If a woman's skin is stretched or a complication develops, a breast mound and nipple may shift position.

Most breast reductions are designed to give the breast a conical shape. The skin is cut around the nipple and to the crease of the lower breast. The nipple and areola (pink or brown skin surrounding the nipple), and the blood and nerve supply, are left intact. Wedges of skin and breast are cut out on either side of the lower breast. The skin flaps are then brought together, and the nipple is repositioned. Breast reduction may also be done by a modified liposuction technique.

Breast reduction produces scars that surround the areola, running from the base of the areola to the breast fold and in the crease below the breast. If the breasts were very large, the scar may extend toward the back and even cross the midline. These scars may widen if a woman gains weight after surgery or a wound complication arises. Internal scarring can develop after surgery, changing the appearance of the breast on a mammogram (a procedure done to detect breast cancer). For this reason, women over 30 or with a strong family history of breast cancer should have mammography before surgery.

A woman may be unable to breast-feed after the surgery. Most women will experience a loss of nipple sensation. The two most common complications are bleeding and infection. They can lead to further surgery and hospitalization to stop the bleeding or drain an abscess. Infection can lead to death of tissue resulting in the loss of a nipple, some of the skin, and even some of the breast tissue. These complications may require later surgical revisions.

Breast Enlargement

Breast augmentation is performed for women who want larger breasts. Occasionally one breast is enlarged if it is much smaller than the other. However, because there is usually not a medical reason for the surgery, breast enlargement is considered a cosmetic procedure and is not covered by medical insurance. An increasing number of companies are also refusing to cover the complications of this type of surgery. Breast enlargement makes it more difficult to perform mammography, although extra views may be taken to compensate.

Women considering breast enlargement should thoroughly explore the question of size with their physician before any surgery is performed. Many women envision larger breasts than the build of their bodies will permit.

Breast enlargement is usually performed under a local anesthetic, perhaps with the addition of injections to block the nerves connecting to the chest wall. Sedation is usually given to keep the woman comfortable. Most physicians make an incision in the fold beneath the breast to form a pocket. An implant is then placed either under the breast, resting on the muscle, or under the muscle, resting on the ribs. (See Fig. 36.1)

Until recently, most breast enlargements were done with silicone gel implants. The Food and Drug Administration (FDA) has ordered that silicone gel implants cannot be used for cosmetic procedures. There is some evidence that some women may develop a reaction to the silicone that can lead to an autoimmune disease like scleroderma. Currently the only implant that can be used for breast enlargement consists of a silicone shell filled with saline solution.

Saline implants are firmer than silicone gel implants. The rate of saline implant rupture is higher. The rupture of an implant results in a sudden change in shape and loss of size in a breast. Implants can rupture spontaneously, presumably due to age of the silicone sheeting. They also may rupture as the result of trauma—for example, hitting the steering wheel in an automobile accident.

The most frequent complications after breast enlargement surgery include loss of nipple sensation and bleeding. Numbness of the nipple may recede with time, but often the condition is permanent. Bleeding can lead to a buildup of blood that needs to be drained to avoid infection. Infection often requires temporary removal of the implant and its replacement weeks or even months later. Infections can occur well after sur-

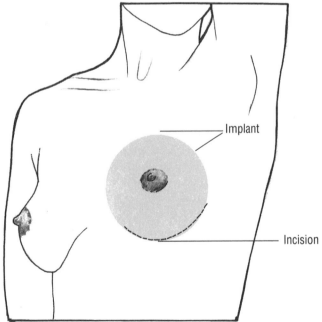

Figure 36.1A Breast Enlargement
The incision used for breast enlargement is usually made in the fold of skin underneath the breast, where it is least noticeable.

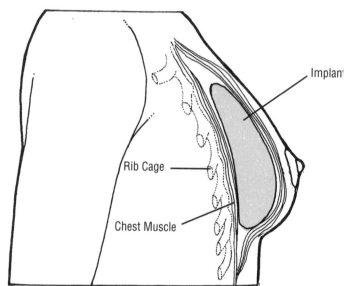

Figure 36.1B Breast Implants
Breast implants may be placed under the breast and on top of the chest muscle (shown here) or underneath the chest muscle and on top of the rib cage.

gery has been completed, perhaps triggered by an infection elsewhere in the body or even dental work. Many physicians caution their patients that they require antibiotic treatment if they undergo extensive dental work.

All women form some degree of scar tissue around implants. Scars can become firm and may make the breast appear more globular or higher. Tight, firm scars resulting from scar shrinkage, called capsules, can be painful and may need to be released externally by applying pressure or internally by surgically cutting the capsule. Some physicians believe that oral administration of vitamin E may decrease the risk of this firm scar. Capsules are less likely when implants are placed under the breast muscle. However, implants placed this way often are high in the breast. With vigorous arm motion, these implants move toward the shoulder, which troubles some women.

Augmented breasts are more difficult to study with mammography. Excessive compression during a mammogram may cause implant rupture.

Breast Reconstruction

Breast reconstruction is undertaken to help women who have lost breast tissue primarily through the surgical removal of tumors. Only 30% of the women who require mastectomy for breast cancer choose breast reconstruction. (See Fig. 36.2) Although breast reconstruction should not be done if it will interfere with treatment, in most women there is no medical reason that it should not be done. There are so many types of breast reconstruction available that a type can usually be found to suit a woman and give a fair match to her remaining breast.

Many women experience a profound improvement in their mental attitude after breast reconstruction. They feel free to be more active without the worry of displacing an external prosthesis. Even if a woman chooses not to undergo breast reconstruction, simply being aware that this option is available may be reassuring. Some women feel that reconstruction can put an end to the psychological trauma that often results from the removal of a breast.

A woman considering the procedure should think about several choices, the first being whether to select reconstruction. The decision should represent an agreement among the patient, oncologic surgeon, chemotherapist, and reconstructive surgeon. It should reflect the woman's desires, the need for additional therapy, and the woman's health.

After the removal of a breast, the size and shape of the surviving breast determine how symmetric the woman will appear. A woman's physical activities influence how comfortable she will be with an external

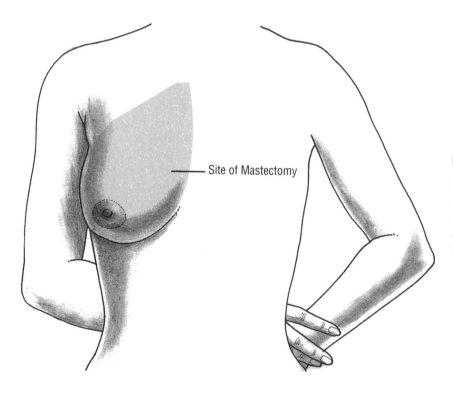

Site of Mastectomy

Figure 36.2 Mastectomy
In a modified radical mastectomy, all breast tissue is removed. Many women undergo breast reconstruction after a mastectomy to produce a more natural and symmetrical appearance than that afforded by an external prosthesis.

prosthesis designed to correct the appearance of asymmetry. If a woman decides to undergo breast reconstruction, there are several types of procedures from which to choose. They include insertion of an implant or tissue expander under existing skin, creation of a muscle flap under which an implant is inserted, moving body tissue from other areas to reconstruct a breast, and nipple reconstruction.

Implants

The simplest type of breast reconstruction involves the insertion of an implant filled with either silicone gel or saline solution. This procedure is similar to breast enlargement. Silicone gel implants, avoided in purely cosmetic operations pending proof that they do not increase a woman's risk of autoimmune disease, are still frequently chosen for breast reconstruction. Saline-filled implants result in a firmer-feeling breast and have a higher rate of deflation. All implants increase the risk of infection following surgery because they represent a foreign substance introduced into the body. All of them can cause a scar to form within the body to wall off the foreign body. As with breast enlargement, this scar can shrink and form a capsule, which may be uncomfortable and require release.

Skin Expanders

The placement of an implant alone is relatively easy but results in a fairly small breast in a high position. Depending on the size and shape of the other breast, this may not make a good match. After a modified radical mastectomy, in which the entire breast is removed, the remaining skin envelope may not be large enough to accept an implant of sufficient size. The skin envelope must then be enlarged, usually by stretching it with a tissue expander.

Tissue expanders are like water balloons; they are placed under the skin and connected to a tube that can be felt through the skin. At weekly intervals, additional saline solution is injected into the balloon to fill it and expand the overlying skin. Most physicians expand the skin envelope slightly more than the minimum needed. When a smaller implant is placed in this skin envelope, a more natural appearance results.

Muscle Flaps

Some women are unable or unwilling to return on a weekly basis for tissue expansion. If a woman has had radiation therapy for breast cancer, she is not a good candidate for tissue expansion. Such women will need additional skin brought to the area by a flap trans-

fer procedure. Tissue from the upper abdomen or from the back can be moved into position on the chest to admit a larger implant or to achieve a greater droop to match the opposite breast. This is a much more complex procedure. The woman usually remains in the hospital for up to a week after this procedure.

More and more patients now choose procedures that use their own body tissue instead of foreign implants. Muscle, fat, and skin can be taken from the lower abdomen and repositioned on the chest. This tissue, or "flap," as it is called, can retain its original blood supply or be attached to blood vessels of the chest by microsurgery. This tissue can be trimmed and draped to match the other breast quite closely. To produce a large breast, a large amount of tissue can be relocated, depending on the size of the woman's abdomen.

Completely separating the flap and reconnecting it to the blood vessels somewhat increases the risk of thrombosis (clotting) of the artery and the vein, which could lead to the loss of the entire flap tissue. Less of a bulge in the woman's upper abdomen results when a free flap is used, than when the muscle is left attached.

Other options for reconstruction of the breast include use of the upper or lower buttock or the upper outer thigh. These are not very good options for very slender women; they are more suitable if a fairly large amount of fat is present. Use of buttock fat results in a very long scar and flattening of the buttock. The lower buttock flap especially results in an irregular contour that can be visible when the patient wears a bathing suit or tight clothing. The lower buttock flap yields only a very short segment of artery and vein to be attached to vessels in the chest wall. This may require the removal of a portion of rib to attach the blood vessels.

Nipple Reconstruction

Not every women who opts for breast reconstruction desires reconstruction of her nipple and areola. Even for those who do choose it, this reconstruction is commonly delayed a month and a half or longer after formation of the breast mound to ensure that there are no complications or loss of the flap. If the nipple-areola is positioned at the same time the mound is formed, and a complication resulting in loss of some of the breast mound follows, the placement of the nipple and areola is distorted and obvious asymmetry will result. Reconstruction of the nipple and areola consists of composite skin grafts, which are raised at specific locations to achieve projection of the nipple. Tattoo pigments may be used to match the color.

COSMETIC SURGERY

Cosmetic surgery is performed on women of all ages to improve their appearance. The most common procedures sought by women include liposuction, breast augmentation, and fat or collagen injections. The most common procedures sought by patients under age 20 are rhinoplasty, ear pinning, and breast reduction. The most common procedures for individuals over age 50 include facelifts and other skin rejuvenation procedures, such as collagen injections and eyelid surgery.

Brow Lift

Horizontal wrinkles on the forehead often appear on an otherwise youthful face. A sagging in the skin of the forehead may cause sagging of the eyebrows, resulting in a tired or sad expression. Deep vertical frown lines can appear between the eyebrows. The brow lift is designed to correct or improve these problems.

The procedure is usually performed under local anesthetic. An incision is made on the top border of the eyebrow, and an elliptical piece of skin is then removed. When sutured, the eyebrow is returned to its former, higher position. Another procedure, usually done with a general anesthetic, involves incisions made behind the hairline, above the ear, and passing over the crown of the head. In some cases, incisions may be placed in front of the hairline to make improvements beneath the skin and on the deep muscles. The skin and muscle are then tightened to give a fresher, more youthful appearance. The brow lift may be done in conjunction with other procedures.

After surgery, temporary swelling and discoloration may involve the eyelids and lower portions of the face. There will also be temporary numbness of the scalp. The stitches or skin clips will be removed a week or so after the operation. Temporary hair loss may result from the shock to the hair follicles. The most common complication is bleeding. Other complications include infection and nerve damage.

Cheek Augmentation

In some cases cheekbones may be built up to give a sculptured appearance to the face. This is done by placing an implant over the cheekbones. Augmentation of the cheekbones also lifts the tissue of the face, resulting in a more youthful look.

Cheek augmentation is usually performed through an incision within the mouth, at the junction of the inside of the upper lip with the gum. Tunnels are made leading to the tissues of the cheek, and a pocket for the implant is created. Some surgeons like to suture the implant in position.

Side effects include numbness. On rare occasions, infection can occur and require that the implant be removed. After a chin or cheek augmentation, most women are able to return to their normal activities in 1 or 2 weeks.

Chemical Peels

Chemical peels are effective for removing fine lines and smoothing out the skin. They are based on the theory that removing the upper surface of the skin will expose newer, clearer, and more attractive skin. After removal of the upper layers of the skin, a crust forms and a new layer of skin develops beneath the crust. Chemical peels can be used in areas, such as eyelids and areas about the mouth, that cannot be reached with a face lift.

Deep chemical peels applied by a physician use phenol or other strong chemicals. Chemical peels are confined to the face because facial skin regenerates more quickly than skin elsewhere. Application of the caustic peeling solution burns away the upper layers of the skin. The chemical solution is applied with a cotton swab and the area is then taped. Approximately 3 days after surgery, the tape is removed. Antiseptic powder is then applied, and a crust forms. Pain medication may be taken if needed. The crust will drop away when new skin covers the treated area.

Swelling of the treated skin will be noticeable for about 7 days. After peeling, the skin loses its ability to tan, so sunblocks should always be used. Phenol can be dangerous if it reaches toxic levels or if it is given to someone with a heart condition. Chemical peels by milder agents like trichloroacetic acid or glycolic acid may be appropriate for many people, giving the skin a fresh, youthful look. The recovery time from this is short, depending on how deeply the peel affects the skin.

Chin Augmentation

Chin augmentation (genioplasty) can enhance the appearance of a receding chin by increasing the projection of the chin. It also can create a better proportion and balance between the chin and other facial features, particularly the nose in profile. Chin augmentation sometimes is suggested in place of rhinoplasty (nose surgery). It does not affect the mouth or teeth structure, the bite, or the jaw.

There are two techniques for enhancing chin prominence and recontouring the chin. One is performed through an incision inside the mouth, at the bottom of the inside of the lower lip. An implant is inserted beneath the skin, fatty tissue, and muscle. It fits against the jaw. The other technique is performed through an incision under the chin. If genioplasty is done under the chin, a small scar will result. Occasionally a more major procedure, advancing the mandible may be necessary, improving both the appearance and dental occlusion.

There may be swelling and numbness around the jaw for a few weeks after the operation. To permit proper healing following chin augmentation, a liquid diet is suggested for several days and a soft diet for about a week. The area may be taped or bandaged.

Dermabrasion

Dermabrasion is done to remove lines and some scarring, such as scars that result from acne. It will not remove deep scars, however. Deep dermabrasion is done with a high-speed rotary wheel similar to fine-grained abrasive paper. A bandage is placed on the treated area until healing takes place, in approximately 7–14 days. The skin remains pink and susceptible to sunburn for 6 months. Dermabrasion may be replaced by chemical peels for some conditions.

Eyelid Surgery

Bags beneath the eyes, wrinkled, drooping layers of skin on the upper eyelids (hooded eyes), and sagging eyebrows detract from a youthful appearance. Eyelid surgery can brighten the face and restore a more youthful appearance by reducing the fat and extra skin that cause these conditions. Eyelid surgery, or blepharoplasty, can be performed alone but is often performed along with a facelift.

Before the surgery the amount of skin that will be removed is marked with indelible ink. During the surgery this skin is removed, along with any sagging muscle and protruding fat. The edges of skin on the upper lids are sutured together so the line of incision falls in the natural fold of the eyelid, where it will not be seen. The outside corners of the eyelid can be elevated and the shape of the eye can be changed for a more flattering look. Because eyelid skin is thin, there may be some black-and-blue discoloration after surgery.

Bags beneath the eyes are removed through an incision made just below the lashes, along the length of the lower eyelid. The skin is pulled in an upward and slightly outward direction, excess skin and muscle are removed, and the edges are sutured. Surgical scars around the eyes will be almost invisible in about 2 months. There may be some tearing or dryness. Wearing dark glasses for several weeks will protect the eyes outdoors, and it is best to avoid eyestrain. Puffiness of the eye may be approached through the conjunctiva removing fatty tissue from below the eye without making an incision in the eyelid skin. Each person's eyes are different, and the approach chosen should be individualized.

Facelift (Rhytidectomy)

A facelift can reduce sagging skin of the face and neck. Bone structure, heredity, and skin texture are all important elements in estimating how successful the operation may be. The same elements determine how long the effects of the facelift will be apparent. The goal is to give the face a firm appearance.

The operation is performed one side at a time, with incisions that are placed in the hairline and then pass in front of and behind the ears. The incisions are designed to keep the scars as inconspicuous as possible. When necessary, fatty deposits beneath the skin are removed and sagging muscles are tightened. The slack in the skin is then taken up, and excess skin is removed. If there is loose skin beneath the neck, a small additional incision is made in the natural fold beneath the chin. Incision lines and sutures are located within the hair (it is not shaved). Most scars will be hidden within the hairline or within crease lines in front or back of the ear.

After surgery there will be bruising, swelling, and a tightness or numbness in the face and neck. Healing is gradual, and it often takes several weeks or months before the total effect can be seen. Major complications that can occur include bleeding, nerve damage, and poor healing. The procedure is best avoided if it is impossible to stop smoking.

Liposuction (Suction Lipectomy)

A procedure introduced from France to the United States, liposuction has become one of the most popular cosmetic procedures. It is a technique used to suction away fat deposits under the skin and resculpt the body's contours.

Using a high-vacuum device, the surgeon can suction fat from the legs, buttocks, abdomen, back, arms, face, and neck. It leaves only a small scar, often as small as 1/2 inch or less. Fat removal leaves the body firm and slender. However, liposuction does not remove skin, and thus cannot correct sagging. It is important to have healthy, elastic skin that has the capacity to shrink evenly after surgery.

After making a small incision, the surgeon inserts a hollow tube into the fatty tissue. A back-and-forth motion is used to loosen and vacuum fat cells from the body. The fat comes first, then blood from the torn small blood vessels. Nerve endings also are removed, resulting in some numbness. During and after the surgery the patient is given fluids to replace those lost by the body. Blood transfusions also are given if necessary.

If the suctioning has been confined to a small area, the procedure can be done in the surgeon's office and the patient can go home the same day. There may be some discomfort, and brown blotches may appear on the area suctioned. There is an increased risk of blood clots and phlebitis (inflammation of the veins in the legs, causing swelling and aching) with this procedure. Snug elastic bandages or underwear should be worn for at least a week after the procedure. Skin may shrink irregularly, leaving a pebbled appearance. This may improve with time—3–6 months—or require additional liposuction to give a more even appearance.

Nose Surgery (Rhinoplasty)

Rhinoplasty can reshape a nose to improve appearance in several ways. The size and shape of the bridge and tip of the nose can be changed, as can the shape of the nostrils. This procedure is often performed on teenagers when the nose is near full development. It can

change appearance dramatically, and many enjoy improved self-esteem. Rhinoplasty also can improve breathing.

The nose is supported by two bones that are attached to other bones of the face. Further down the length of the nose, the tissue of the nose is cartilage rather than bone. The nose is reduced or built up by adjusting the supporting structures—either removing or adding bone and cartilage. The skin and soft tissues are then reshaped around the new bone. The tip of the nose is tilted at an angle, and the nostrils are adjusted. In some cases, an internal deformity can affect breathing. This may be due to an irregularity in the central structure of the nose, called a deviated septum.

Reshaping is generally done through incisions inside the nose, but there may also be an incision passing across the central portion of the nose, between the nostrils. This is sometimes necessary to narrow the base of the nose or reduce the size of the nostrils. A small piece of skin is removed at the base of the nostrils. The resulting scars usually fade very well, and ultimately should not be noticeable.

After surgery there may be some pain, swelling, and bruising, but these side effects will gradually subside. A splint is worn for about 10 days after the procedure, and sports or other strenuous activities are restricted for another week. The final shape of the nose will not be seen until it has healed completely, in about 6 months. Complications include bleeding and infection, or an unsatisfactory appearance. There may occasionally be a temporary or prolonged decrease in the sense of smell.

Tummy Tuck (Abdominoplasty)

A major weight loss, multiple pregnancies, or weakened abdominal muscles can leave the skin flaccid and without elasticity. Surgery can tighten abdominal muscles and remove stretch marks (stretch marks are removed along with the excess, sagging skin). Women who have fat that is concentrated in the abdomen but are otherwise of normal weight can benefit. The procedure will remove excess skin and fat and tighten the skin.

The operation requires hospitalization for a short time. To smooth the abdomen, the surgeon works through a low abdominal incision that spans the hips. Because sagging skin will be pulled down and out over the abdomen before fat is removed, it is necessary to release the skin from the navel. Resulting scars across the pubic area and around the navel are permanent, but they will flatten and lighten within months of the procedure. To remove extra skin, an abdominoplasty is often performed in combination with liposuction.

When skin laxity and muscle weakness are confined to the lower part of the abdomen, a modified abdominoplasty, which limits tissue removal and muscle repair to the area below the navel, can be performed.

Surgery will provide a firmer, flatter stomach area and a smaller waist. After the surgery patients are advised to wear a light support garment for 2 to 3 months and to restrict strenuous activity for a few weeks.

CHAPTER 37

Cancer in Women

Claudia R. Baquet, M.D., M.P.H.

Cancer is characterized by an uncontrolled growth and spread of abnormal cells in the body. If not caught early, this proliferation of abnormal cells—called a tumor—can result in death. You should be aware, however, that cancer is not a hopeless disease, but one that can be cured with prompt treatment. Recent advances in cancer therapy have led to nearly 50% of cancer patients remaining alive and free of disease some 5 years after the initial diagnosis.

Cancer occurs in larger numbers among the elderly. It is much more common in people over 65; about 73 million Americans are eventually expected to develop cancer in their later lives. Lung cancer is the leading cause of cancer-related deaths in both men and women, followed by breast cancer in women. The incidence rates and the death rates vary in men and women and in different ethnic groups, based on the type of cancer.

CAUSES OF CANCER

Why does cancer occur? What triggers an occurrence? The reasons are still largely unknown, although the mechanisms of the disease have long been recognized.

The body renews and replaces it cells through a constant process of cell division and growth. Cells exist, repair themselves, die, and are reborn. Old tissues are replaced with new, injuries are repaired, and the body grows and develops. Normally, the body has control mechanisms that limit abnormal cell growth. Cancer cells, however, continue to grow without restraint, dividing many more times than do normal cells. The abnormal cells form tumors, which compete with normal, healthy tissue for nutrients.

Tumors can be benign (harmless) or malignant. Benign tumors can be removed with surgery and usually do not recur. Malignant tumors, on the other hand, can grow, invade, and destroy nearby areas of the body. They can spread, or metastasize, to distant organs and form new tumors. If malignant tumors aren't removed or killed early in their development, they can spread to other parts of the body.

Some cancers spread quickly, whereas others develop slowly. Because cancers can be most successfully treated before they spread (metastasize), it is important to be aware of cancer warning signs and steps that can be taken for early detection of the disease.

METHODS OF EARLY DETECTION

The American Cancer Society has identified certain warning signs that should alert you to see your doctor promptly (see "Warning Signs of Cancer"). None of these signs necessarily means that you have cancer, but each one is important and warrants immediate medical attention. Pain is seldom a symptom of early types of cancer, so don't wait until it hurts if the other symptoms don't disappear on their own.

Certain tests can also help detect cancer in early stages. These screening tests are often done routinely for people who may have symptoms of a disease and for those who have risk factors, such as age and family history. Every woman should have a physical examination annually and undergo the following routine screening tests as needed.

- Pelvic exam and Pap test (annually after age 18 or once sexual activity has begun) to detect cancer of the cerix, ovary, or uterus.

- Mammography (every 1–2 years age 40–49; yearly thereafter) to detect cancer of the breast. High-risk women may benefit from earlier screening.

- Fecal occult blood test (annually after age 50) to detect hidden blood in the stool, which may be a sign of cancer of the colon and rectum

- Sigmoidoscopy (every 3 to 5 years after age 50) to detect changes in the colon or rectum that could be a sign of colon and rectal cancer

THE SEVEN WARNING SIGNS OF CANCER

1. Change in bowel or bladder habits
2. A sore that does not heal
3. Unusual bleeding or discharge
4. Thickening or lump in the breast or elsewhere
5. Indigestion or difficulty swallowing
6. Obvious change in a wart or mole
7. Nagging cough or hoarseness

These tests may be done earlier in women who have special risks. For instance, if you have a family history of cancer of the breast or colon, you will benefit from having tests to detect these diseases more than women who have no family history of disease. Colonoscopy, a test used to view the inside of the entire colon, is rec-ommended in women age 40 and older who have had inflammatory bowel disease or who have a family member who had cancer of the colon or rectum at an early age.

Be alert to any changes in your body. Besides scheduling a yearly pelvic exam, you should regularly examine you breasts. Many breast lumps have been found through self-examination. It is best to do the breast examination at the same point in your menstrual cycle each month (or on the same day of the month if you're postmenopausal), because breast tissue changes with your cycle. It will be easier for you to detect anything unusual if you follow this suggestion. Check out other areas of your body, including your skin, for any suspicious signs.

Have your mouth checked periodically by a dentist. In addition, use a mirror to examine your mouth. Changes in the color of the gums, lips, or cheeks as well as sores, swelling, bleeding, or thickening of any tissue should be reviewed by your doctor.

RISK FACTORS OF CANCER

About 80 percent of all cancers may be related to the things we eat, drink, and smoke and to the quality of our environment and workplace. Repeated and long-term contact with cancer-causing agents (carcinogens) can damage cells or change cells that are already damaged and lead to cancer. For example, tobacco smoke is one of the most potent carcinogens, and it acts with other elements, such as alcohol, to increase the risk of certain cancers.

Tobacco

Smoking is a major risk factor for cancer. The risk of dying from lung cancer is 12 times greater in a smoker than in a nonsmoker. Overall, smoking causes 30 percent of all deaths from cancer. In addition to contributing to lung cancer, it also increases the risk of cancers of the cervix, mouth, throat, esophagus, pancreas, bladder, and possibly the stomach. Smokers also have a higher rate of cardiovascular and respiratory disease. Household members of smokers are also at risk for cancer.

If you smoke, quit. As soon as you stop smoking, your risk of cancer decreases.

Diet

A high-fat diet has been linked to certain types of cancer, including cancer of the breast, colon, rectum, and ovaries. Obesity has been linked to increased cancer death rates. The exact link between diet and cancer is not clear, but most health practitioners agree that it is best to eat a variety of foods, to limit saturated fats and cholesterol, and to eat foods high in fiber. Eating fresh fruits and vegetables daily may decrease your risk of cancer by as much as 50 percent. An increased daily intake of vitamins A, C, and E may also boost your protection against lung cancer.

Sunlight

One of the most common forms of cancer in the United States is skin cancer, which is caused by exposure to ultraviolet (UV) radiation from the sun. Repeated exposure to the sun may be especially harmful for people who have fair skin or who burn or freckle easily. Take steps now to avoid the sun, especially during the hours of 10:00 A.M. and 2:00 P.M., when the sun's rays are strongest. If you are out during those times, wear protective clothing, including a hat. Use sunscreen to block the UV light. Remember, a tan is really the body's attempt to protect itself against the sun.

Alcohol

Cancers of the mouth, throat, esophagus, and liver occur more often among heavy drinkers, especially those who smoke as well. Alcohol also poses a number of other health problems. If you regularly drink more than two drinks a day, you should probably consider cutting back or stopping drinking altogether.

Chemicals

Exposure to certain industrial agents or chemicals increases the risk of various types of cancer. Exposure to these chemicals may occur in the workplace, outdoors, or at home. They include

- Asbestos fibers
- Nickel, chromate, and vinylchloride
- Solvent cleaners, cleaning fluids, and paint thinners
- Lawn and garden chemicals (pesticides and fungicides)

Avoid inhaling any of these chemicals, especially in areas that are not well ventilated. Read labels carefully and avoid having these agents come in contact with your skin or household items (see also Chapters 5 and 6).

Hormones

Certain cancers are stimulated by an excess of the female hormone estrogen. Estrogen occurs naturally in reproductive-age women. It is also the main component of birth control pills and hormone-replacement therapy after menopause. Birth control pills have not been linked to cancer in most women, however, and they may even protect against some types of cancer. Replacement of estrogen alone can increase the risk of endometrial cancer in postmenopausal women, but when it is combined with the hormone progesterone, the risk is lowered. Before taking estrogen, discuss the risks with your physician.

Genetics

Some cancers may be inherited. The risk of breast, colon, and skin cancer, for instance, is higher in some families than in others. Your risk for these cancers is high if you have a first-degree relative (mother, father, sister or brother) who developed one of these cancers. If you have close relatives who have had cancer, tell your doctor. He or she may advise that you receive regular checkups and tests.

TYPES OF CANCER

Cancer in women can be nongynecologic or gynecologic. *Nongynecologic* cancers occur in both men and women. *Gynecologic* cancers, however, are unique to women; they occur in the female reproductive and genital organs. (Although breast cancer can occur in both men and women, it is considered here as a gynecologic cancer, because it is much more common in women than in men.) For more details about all of these cancers, see the chapters where the specific body parts are discussed. (See Fig. 37.1)

Nongynecologic Cancers

Lung

Today, lung cancer is the most common cause of cancer death in American women, resulting in the death of 59,000 women in 1994. The rate of occurrence as well as the death rate from lung cancer is on the rise in both white and African-American women.

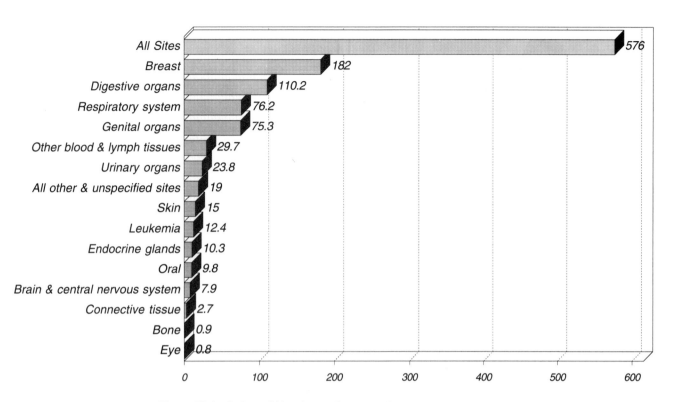

Figure 37.1 Estimated New Cancer Cases and Deaths in Women, 1994.

The main cause of lung cancer is cigarette smoking. Other less common causes are exposure to radon gas, asbestos, and radiation.

The specific warning signs of lung cancer are as follows:

- A cough that won't go away
- Sputum streaked with blood
- Chest pain
- Repeated attacks of pneumonia or bronchitis

There are no screening tests for lung cancer, and it can be difficult to diagnose. Nearly 90 percent of patients diagnosed with lung cancer receive care too late to be cured. Diagnosis is based on chest X-rays, examination of the cells in the sputum, biopsy of the suspicious area, and imaging tests of the bronchial tubes. Survival rates are low and based on the stage of disease. Surgery is the main form of treatment, followed by chemotherapy. Some cancers will be treated by radiation therapy. The best way to combat lung cancer is prevention by stopping smoking.

Colon and Rectum

Cancer of the colon (the large bowel) and rectum (the last 8 to 10 inches of the large bowel, which leads to the anus) is the second most common cancer in women. Although the death rate from colon and rectum cancer is decreasing in white women, it is remaining steady for African-American women. This form of cancer occurs more often in older women, in those who have a history of inflammatory bowel disease, and in women who have a family history of cancer of the colon or rectum. A diet high in saturated fat and low in fiber appears to increase the risk of this disease, and increased daily intake of fiber, fruits, and vegetables seems to protect against it.

Cancer of the colon and rectum can be detected early. The following persistent symptoms are warning signs of a possible problem:

- Diarrhea or constipation (recurring or alternating)
- Blood in or on the stool
- Stools that are narrower than usual, indicating obstruction

- General abdominal discomfort (bloating, fullness, or cramps)
- Frequent gas pains
- A feeling that the bowel doesn't empty completely

These symptoms could be a sign of a number of things, so it's important to ascertain the cause without delay. The diagnosis is based on a physical examination and tests that detect blood in the stool or growths in the colon or rectum. Sometimes a piece of a growth can be removed for further study (biopsy). The most common treatment for bowel cancer includes surgical removal of the diseased area, and follow-up chemotherapy may be recommended.

Bladder

Each year, more than 13,000 American women will be diagnosed with bladder cancer. If the disease is treated early, the cure rate is good. Cancer of the bladder is twice as likely to occur in women who smoke as in women who don't smoke. The main symptom is blood in the urine and the need to urinate more often than normal. Pain rarely occurs in the early stages, and there may be no symptoms at all.

Diagnosis is based on physical examination, laboratory tests, and imaging studies. A urine sample may reveal cancer cells. Since the cancer usually occurs inside the bladder, a test may be done using a thin lighted tube that is inserted inside the bladder. A sample of any growth may be removed for further study. Bladder cancer is usually treated surgically.

Skin

Skin cancer is the most common form of cancer in the United States, with about 700,000 new cases annually. It is estimated that 40 to 50 percent of Americans who live to age 65 will have skin cancer at least once. Caused by exposure to ultraviolet light, skin cancer occurs more often in regions that traditionally have more sunlight. Basal cell carcinoma, a slow-growing cancer that usually does not spread to other parts of the body, accounts for more than 90 percent of all skin cancers. It usually appears as pale bumps or red scaly patches. Squamous cell skin cancer can spread to other areas and must be removed surgically. Multiple melanoma is invasive and life threatening. It first appears as a molelike growth that gets bigger, darker, and more inflamed. (See Fig. 37.2)

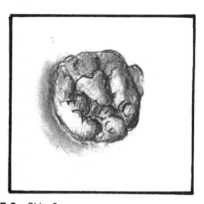

Figure 37.2 Skin Cancer
Basal cell cancer is the most common type of cancer and looks like pale bumps or red scaly patches.

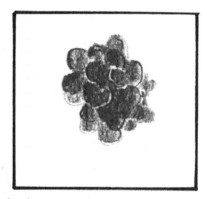

Melanoma is a less common but more severe type of skin cancer that looks like a mole but grows bigger and darker.

Warning signs of skin cancer include

- A change in the size or color of a mole or wart
- Scaliness, oozing, or bleeding
- Itchiness, tenderness, or pain in a bump or a mole
- A sore that does not heal

Regular self-examination is the best way to detect skin cancers. Inspect all moles carefully and look for any changes. Examine all parts of the body, because melanoma can appear in places that have not been exposed to sunlight. The cure rate is nearly 100 percent if skin cancers are treated before they spread.

Pancreas

The pancreas, a large gland located behind the stomach and in front of the spine, makes enzymes that digest food as well as insulin, which controls the amount of sugar in the blood.

Cancer of the pancreas is a common cause of death in women. It is known as a *silent* disease, because there are no symptoms in the early stages. As a result, the cancer has often spread by the time it is diagnosed, which makes for low survival rates. Symptoms are pain in the upper abdomen and sometimes the back, nausea, loss of appetite, weight loss, and weakness.

Oral

Cancers of the mouth, lips, gums, cheeks, teeth, jaw, and tongue are usually found in people over age 45. The best way to detect oral cancer is through self-examination. Look for the following warning signs:

- A sore that bleeds easily and doesn't heal
- A lump or thickening
- A red or white patch that doesn't go away
- Difficulty chewing, swallowing, or moving tongue or jaws

Women who smoke, especially if they also drink alcohol, are at an increased risk for oral cancer.

Diagnosis is established by taking a biopsy of any lump or abnormal area and examining it under a microscope. Imaging tests also may be done to see if the disease has spread to other parts of the body. If caught early, many of these cancers can be cured.

Gynecologic Cancers

Breast

Breast cancer is occurring in epidemic proportions in the United States. About one of every nine women will develop breast cancer during her lifetime. African-American women, who are less likely than white women to develop breast cancer, are more likely than white women to die from it. Formerly, it had been thought that African-American women postponed seeing a doctor or did not have access to care, resulting in the disease being diagnosed in later stages. Recent research, however, indicates that a more aggressive form of the disease may afflict African-American women, particularly younger ones.

Women who have a mother or a sister who has had breast cancer are at increased risk of getting the dis-

ease. The risk is also higher in women who have not had children or who had children later in life. Breast cancer has also been linked with alcohol use and a high-fat diet.

The best way to detect breast cancer is by doing a monthly self-examination, seeing a doctor annually for an examination, and by having periodic mammograms. The warning signs of breast cancer are

- Changes in the breast that don't disappear—a lump, thickening, swelling, or dimpling
- Irritation of breast skin
- Nipple distortion, retraction, or scaliness
- Discharge from the nipple

The earlier breast cancer can be found and treated, the better the chance of cure. Breast cancer can spread to the bones, liver, lungs, or brain, making it very difficult to treat in later stages.

The first stage in diagnosis is feeling for any breast lumps. Your doctor may use a needle to withdraw fluid or a piece of the lump so that it can be studied in a laboratory. Treatment of breast cancer depends on how advanced the cancer is at the time of diagnosis. (See Chapter 25).

Cervix

The cervix, the narrow neck of a woman's uterus, can go through a series of changes that eventually can lead to cancer. Cervical cancer is the third most common form of cancer of the female genital tract and accounts for 19 percent of these cancers. Cervical cancer occurs almost twice as often in younger African-American than in age-matched white women; over the age of 65, African-American women develop cervical cancer about three times more often than white women. Death rates follow similar patterns, with African-American women dying more often from the disease.

Risk factors for cancer of the cervix include having sex at an early age, having multiple sexual partners, and smoking. Women without any of these risk factors can also develop cervical cancer, however.

A precancerous or localized condition of the cervix can develop over time into invasive cancer. There may be no warning signs with early cervical cancer. More advanced cervical cancer can be signaled by abnormal bleeding or vaginal discharge. Changes in the cervix can be detected through regular Pap tests. Precancerous changes in the cervix can be treated before they become cancerous.

To confirm the diagnosis, a biopsy is done. A sample of tissue from the cervix is removed and studied under a microscope. If detected early, the cancer can be removed surgically. For prevention, always have a Pap smear test done at least once a year after the age of 18.

Endometrium (Uterus)

Cancer of the uterus accounts for 5 percent of all cancers in women and is the most common gynecological cancer. Most cancers of the uterus occur in the endometrium, the lining of the uterus.

Endometrial cancer occurs most often in older women; it is rare before age 40. Cancer of the endometrium is more likely to affect women who are infertile, began menstruating at an early age, don't have children, have menstrual problems, and go through menopause at a later age. Other risk factors include obesity, diabetes mellitus, hypertension, and use of estrogen. Gallbladder disease and thyroid disease may also be associated with increased risk.

The most common symptom of cancer of the endometrium is abnormal bleeding or discharge from the vagina. Because this disease often occurs in women around the age of menopause, they may mistake this symptom for a menstrual period. Any bleeding or discharge that appears after menopause should be checked by a doctor.

Cancer of the endometrium is diagnosed by removing a piece of the lining of the uterus for further study. A hysterectomy (removal of the uterus) is the usual treatment.

Ovary

The ovaries are located on either side of the uterus; each month during ovulation one of the ovaries re-

leases an egg. These glands also produce estrogen. Cancer of the ovary is the second most common gynecologic cancer and the fourth leading cause of death from cancer among women.

Risk factors for cancer of the ovary include a family history of the disease. It generally develops after menopause and is seen more often in women who have had no children or who had trouble conceiving. It is often hard to detect until it is in the advanced stages, when the following warning signs occur.

- Discomfort in the pelvic region
- Indigestion, gas, or bloating
- Pain during intercourse
- Abnormal vaginal bleeding
- Pain and swelling in the abdomen

There is no good method of screening for cancer of the ovary, although the use of two tests, ultrasound and a blood test for a protein called CA125, show promise. Any abnormality should be checked by a doctor. Imaging tests may be done to get a better idea of the size of a growth. Surgery to remove the ovary, and any other affected organs, is an important part of treatment.

Vulva and Vagina

Cancer of the vulva and vagina are rare and occur most often in older women. Warning signs include a lump or sore on the vulva (external genitals) or in the vagina.

Risk of vaginal cancer is increased after radiation of the cervix, chronic irritation, and uterine exposure to the hormone DES. Diagnosis is determined by removing a sample of tissue for further study. If detected in the early stages, cancers of the vulva and the vagina can be treated successfully.

TYPES OF CANCER TREATMENT

Although a diagnosis of cancer is serious, it no longer carries the dire consequences it once did. Nearly 50% of all patients diagnosed with cancer can now be cured because of advances in early detection and treatment. The type of treatment is based on the stage of disease. It can involve surgery, radiation therapy, chemotherapy, or a combination of these. Emotional support is invaluable in helping patients with cancer deal with the physical and psychological aspects of their disease.

At the time of diagnosis, the extent of the disease is determined. Called *staging*, this is a useful way to determine whether cancer is localized or has spread to other areas. Additional staging is used to determine types of treatment and possible outcomes. One method of classification is *historical stage*, which relates the extent of cancer at the time of diagnosis to the natural history of the disease. The *localized stage* refers to a cancer that is confined to its place of origin. The *re-*

THE AFTERMATH OF CANCER: WHAT YOU CAN DO

Cancer changes the life of the person who has it as well as the lives of the family and friends of that person. If you suffer from cancer, you may have initially reacted to the disease with anger and denial and now feel a range of emotions from hope to despair. More important, you may feel that you have suffered physical and emotional losses that you find hard to deal with and that prevent you from moving ahead to continue on with your life.

Support groups, psychologists and psychiatrists, and families and friends are important recovery resources.

---

gional stage refers to disease that has spread beyond its place of origin to surrounding areas. The *distant stage* is cancer that has spread extensively to distant tissues or organs.

For localized cancer, surgery is often used to remove the affected tissues. During the surgery, a lymph node or nodes may be removed for examination to see if cancer has spread to the lymphatic system, where it can be spread to other parts of the body.

Radiation therapy is another form of local therapy. Treatment can be directed to particular areas of the body, or radioactive units can be implanted at the site of the cancer. For other cancers, the whole body may receive radiotherapy. Radiation can be used occasionally before surgery to shrink tumors or after surgery to destroy any remaining cancer cells.

Drug therapy, known as chemotherapy, uses drugs to destroy cancer cells. These chemicals interfere with the cells' ability to grow and multiply. The drugs may be administered orally or intravenously. Chemotherapy can destroy healthy cells as well as cancer cells. Side effects of chemotherapy vary and are strongly related to the specific drug or drugs given as well as the type and extent of disease.

Antihormonals block the body's production of specific hormones. The growth of some cancers is stimulated by hormones, and antihormonal drugs limit that stimulation. One such drug is tamoxifen, which is used to treat some breast cancer. Because this drug interferes with the actions of estrogen, women who take it may develop symptoms of menopause.

Some types of cancer therapy have side effects, some more severe than others. Many side effects are temporary, and many can be successfully managed so that the patient is as comfortable as possible.

THE FUTURE OF CANCER RESEARCH AND CANCER CARE

Research in new areas of cancer prevention and treatment is ongoing. One area of research is directed toward examining cancer at the molecular level. By identifying genes that may cause cancer or may make one more susceptible to cancer, scientists hope to be able to target people who are at risk so they can receive early treatment and may even be able to avoid getting cancer at all.

Other research efforts are being directed toward antioxidants, chemicals that consume free radicals, which are waste products produced by our bodies. Some evidence suggests that free radicals may cause cell damage and degeneration. Other research is trying to find ways to boost the body's natural immune response, so it can fight cancer wherever it appears in the body.

CHAPTER 38

Pain Evaluation and Management

Kathleen M. Foley, M.D.

The term *pain* is pervasive throughout our society, as shown in our common expressions, such as "a pain in the neck" or "no pain, no gain," both of which imply our negative feeling toward pain. Actually, pain can be positive or negative. On one hand, pain warns a person that there is something wrong with part of her body. On the other hand, chronic pain often serves no useful purpose, giving only lifelong trouble to the person dealing with it.

Long ago, pain was thought to be the body saying something was wrong with one of its physical parts. Now we know pain is not only physical, pain also has mental components. The unique pain felt by a specific woman with an injury or disease depends on the situation, on the woman, and on her genetic makeup. No matter how individual each person's pain is, however, pain is a reality that causes many people discomfort, disturbance of sleep and appetite, and even depression.

WHAT IS PAIN?

Physical pain is a physiological response of the body to a stimulus. It occurs when any of the body's pain receptors has an internal or external physical reaction to a stimulus that activates the nerves. Pain is defined as an unpleasant sensory and emotional experience associated with the actual physical or potential tissue damage. This subjective experience cannot be measured in any quantifiable way. Psychological pain usually has no apparent injury or physiological explanation, even though the patient describes the symptoms in terms of physical hurt (see Table 38.1).

How We Feel Pain

The feeling of pain occurs when nerve endings detect damage to the body. These free nerve endings, or pain receptors (nociceptors) sense the changes in the body that are translated in the brain as pain. Pain receptors respond to three conditions: pressure, such as hammering a finger; heat, such as burning an arm; and chemical changes around the nerve endings, such as prostaglandins, chemicals released by damaged cells.

Pain-generating nerve endings are in the skin, organs, muscles, joints, and tendons; they can be external or internal. External pain is caused by outside influences, such as cutting a finger or stubbing a toe; internal pain may be more disturbing, as the stimulus—and often the hurting internal organ, muscle, or bone—cannot be seen. Headaches and migraines are examples. Pain originating in visceral or internal organs is not well understood, as they can be cut, burned, or crushed without any pain to the patient; yet chemical burns, spasms, and ischemia (tissue anemia) can provoke intense pain in certain organs. Not all pain

TABLE 38.1 COMMON SOURCES OF PAIN

Imbalances in the Body

Digestive (gastroenteritis, ulcers, irritable bowel syndrome, hemorrhoids, diverticulitis, gas, inflammatory bowel disease, appendicitis)

Urinary (bladder infection, kidney or ureteral stones)

Reproductive system (menstrual symptoms, menopause, pregnancy, fibroid tumors, ovarian cysts, endometriosis, cervical polyps)

Upper respiratory system (pneumonia, colds, flu)

Brain and nerves (aneurysm, thrombophlebitis, neuralgia)

Physical Injuries

Back (aches and disk)

Eyes (eyestrain, infections, pink eye)

Ears (altitude related ear pain, infection)

Face (TMD, neuralgia)

Hand and arm (carpal tunnel syndrome, bursitis, tendonitis, Raynaud's syndrome)

Leg and foot (bone spurs, corns and bunions, varicose veins, muscle cramps, thrombosis, ingrown toenails)

Nose and throat (sore throat, strep throat, sinusitis)

Teeth and gums (gingivitis, periodontitis, toothache, mouth sores)

Skin (frostbite and sunburn, fire burns)

Pain from Disease

Contagious diseases (mumps, chicken pox, shingles, measles)

Degenerative diseases (bones and joints—arthritis, osteoporosis, gout)

Sexually transmitted diseases (herpes, AIDS, pelvic inflammatory disease)

Other disease (diabetes, cancer, heart disease, sickle cell anemia)

comes as the result of a direct stimulus—indirect problems from pain are also possible. For example, an arthritis victim may walk in a different way because of pain, thus causing another type of pain unlike the change in walking patterns.

When you feel pain, certain reactions take place in less than a second. Nerve fibers carry chemical signals from the pain receptors to a specific area of the spinal cord: C nerve fibers signal slow, burning, aching, and long-term pain, such as the residual ache from a burned finger, or the chronic pain from cancer. Thick, A-delta nerve fibers signal faster, more localized or acute pain; these are responsible for our faster pain-induced reactions, such as instantly removing a hand from a hot stove.

Fibers from other sections of the body join at certain sites along the spinal cord, and from there, fiber bundles, or tracts, carry the pain messages to the brain stem cortex. Even as the pain signal is sent to the cortex, other information is sent from the spinal cord to various parts of the brain controlling specific parts of the body. The heart rate and blood pressure may increase, breathing increases, and the pupils dilate; adrenaline and sugar may rush into the bloodstream to increase energy to prepare the body for the possible stress of pain. When the nerve signals reach the thalamus, deep in the middle of the brain, they are translated to indicate where the pain is and what type of pain it is. At the same time, signals are sent back down to the spinal cord to modulate the sensation of pain, thus raising our threshold of pain.

The overall nervous system has many overlapping and redundant features, such as densely packed pain receptors that deliver information to the brain and other parts of the body when pain is felt. This is an indication that pain is a primitive sense, built into our systems to allow us to better survive. Too much pain would disable us. Conversely, having no nerves to detect and deliver pain information would threaten our survival as we would not be aware of trauma or infections.

NATURAL HIGHS

The opiate peptides called endorphins are present throughout the brain and appear to control pain principally at the brain stem. Enkephalins act mainly within the spinal cord where this natural painkiller blocks the transmission of pain signals. Researchers studying why the synthetic painkiller morphine effects the body eventually discovered the body's endorphins in 1975. *Endorphin* is a contraction of "endogenously manufactured morphinelike substance," or a morphinelike chemical manufactured by the body.

Researchers have connected the release of endorphins to many other body functions and responses; they believe endorphins significantly alter the body's blood cholesterol levels (in reaction to stress), memory, learning, sexual activity, depression, and schizophrenia. A well-known effect of endorphins (in particular, beta-endorphins) occurs after vigorous aerobic exercise. Also known as a runner's high, the release of endorphins occurs after about 12 minutes of strenuous workout. This may be the body's way of coping with the pain of exercise—by raising its resistance to pain.

Beta-endorphins are uniquely different than the other opiate peptides found in several regions of the brain. Beta-endorphins occur only in cells around the brain's highest levels and in the pituitary gland, which releases beta-endorphins at the same time it releases ACTH, a stress hormone. During World War II, wounded soldiers required fewer painkillers than civilians undergoing elective surgery; even though the soldiers were subjected to terrible battle wounds, the stress of combat increased the amount of endorphins, and thus ACTH, altering the soldiers' perception of pain.

NATURAL PAIN RELIEF

The delicate balance between our perception of too much or not much pain is controlled by chemicals produced naturally within our body. This special system helps the body to deal with stress and pain. A chemical called substance P is thought to be important in transmitting the pain signals from the skin to the spinal cord. Thus, people who are insensitive to pain are thought to be deficit in substance P. The body also produces at least eight naturally occurring opiates, including endorphins and enkephalins. All are more powerful than any opiates derived from plants such as opium.

Natural opiates are molecules of pain-suppressing chemicals also called neurotransmitters; they transmit information among and between the roughly 100 billion cells (neurons) in the brain. The neurons fire electrical chemical impulses at varying rates, triggering the release of the neurotransmitters and causing other nerve cells to fire. In the nervous systems of most vertebrate animals, the natural painkillers (also called neurochemicals or opiate peptides) endorphin and enkephalin interact with some nerve cells on sites called opiate receptors (as do opiate drugs such as morphine). When the painkillers bind with the opiate receptors, usually at an area of gray matter surrounding a fluid-filled canal in the brain, they modulate the nerve impulses across the nerve synapses, reducing or relieving pain.

HOW TO COMMUNICATE WITH YOUR PHYSICIAN ABOUT YOUR PAIN

The most common way to describe pain to your health care provider is by using her terminology:

- *Generalized pain* is a hurt felt all over the body with no real specific central location, such as certain pains from cancer.

- *Local pain* is a hurt in one specific region, such as a broken finger.

- *Referred pain* is a hurt felt at a site that is at a distance from the injury or diseased part. For example, a toothache may be referred to the ear, because they share the same sensory nerves; angina, a chest pain caused by a reduction in blood supply to the heart, often is felt in the left arm or shoulder. Even an injury in the knee can be felt in the hip area.

- *Acute pain* is a response to some physical ailment or stimulus of sudden onset. It usually occurs as an injury, such as the hammering of a finger, or as the result of a previous and continual exposure to a pain-causing stimulus, such as a sunburn or postoperative pain. An attack of appendicitis or kidney stones can cause acute pain. Most acute pain can be a warning signal that something is wrong and that to avoid further damage your should seek medical attention. Some injuries cause a delayed or subacute pain, such as whiplash that is felt hours or days after an accident.

- *Chronic pain* occurs as a symptom to an underlying disease or problem. It usually lasts more than 3 months. Chronic pain often develops gradually, such as a back or shoulder ache, or arthritis. After an injury or disease is cured, chronic pain can still persist, often due to permanent nerve damage or scar tissue buildup. Chronic pain can be barely noticeable to debilitating; it can vary as to the times it strikes—ranging from constant, or minute to minute, to every other day. *Chronic pain syndrome* causes changes in a person, including physical problems (sleep and appetite disturbance, fatigue), psychlogical problems (irritability, depression), family problems, and social withdrawal.

There are several additional ways to talk with a doctor about your pain: If you know the source of your pain, such as a bee sting, or recurrent sinus infection, explain to your doctor what happened or prior occurrences of a certain pain. This helps the doctor pinpoint how to treat your pain. Be specific about your pain: describe its timing, nature, location, severity, or if it radiates from one spot.

Note if the pain occurs at certain times during the day (such as after you eat or when you exercise), if any foods trigger the pain (such as shellfish or milk products), or if you have had the same pain in the past.

Pain is the most common symptom causing patients to seek medical attention. Not everyone responds in the same way to pain, making it a highly individual experience. Even two people feeling pain from the exact same stimulus and under similar conditions feel their pain in different ways. Commonly, these two people would define their pain differently, even though they are experiencing the same disease or stimuli. This is why methods to relieve pain may work for one person but not work for the next.

Realize that there may not be a cure for your pain. Some types of pain go on indefinitely and it is necessary to live with such pain. When you need relief from chronic pain, ask your doctor to help you manage your pain or to refer you to a pain clinic or specialty group that can help you to understand and better cope with the pain.

ANXIETY AND PAIN

There is a direct connection between pain and anxiety, an emotion that accompanies most feelings of pain. Most of the time, we experience little anxiety with familiar types of pain, especially a hurt that can be easily explained such as sunburn or banging the head on a open cabinet door. We feel more anxiety when we do not understand the pain or when it is excessive, such as sudden excessive painful aches in the head or abdomen.

Such pain leads to worries about dreaded diseases or incurable pain; and these thoughts cause the body to react: the pulse quickens; breathing, heart rate, and sweating increase; and muscles become tense. Often such a reaction worsens the feeling of pain, causing the person to perceive that she is experiencing even more pain. Studies have shown that such excessive anxiety also can affect the recovery of a patient undergoing surgery for a painful physical ailment. A patient with less anxiety going into surgery recovers faster and has less pain associated with the surgery than one who is anxiety-ridden before surgery.

CHEST PAINS

Contrary to popular belief, chest pains have a variety of causes. Anxiety causes some chest pains, most often from the quicker intake of breaths during times of such stress. We normally breathe about 14 to 16 times per minute; when anxiety strikes, our breaths become shallow and almost double in number. Thus, less oxygen can reach our chest muscles and help them work. This results in a tenderness around the cartilage connecting the ribs and the breastbone. Colds (upper respiratory infections) or pneumonia can cause chest discomfort, especially from excessive coughing.

Also, chest pain may originate from angina pectoris, or a pressure in the chest that comes and goes, usually during physical activity or emotional stress when the heart needs more oxygen-rich blood than it receives. The lack of oxygen—most often caused by a plaque partially blocking the walls of arteries leading to the heart—can cause a constricting chest pain that can spread to the jaw, neck, and arms. It usually lasts less than 10 minutes. Most angina patients have prescriptions, including nitroglycerin tablets that open up constricted blood vessels, to alleviate the pain of angina.

The chest pain associated with a heart attack feels like a pressure in the chest that can range from mild to unbearable. The signs and symptoms of a heart attack include breathing difficulty and sweating. The pulse may be fast, slow, or irregular, while the victim is pale or bluish in color. The overall symptoms that indicate a heart attack are usually associated with pains in the shoulder and down the left arm or to the jaw.

CHOICES IN THE MANAGEMENT OF PAIN

Patients have numerous choices to eliminate or reduce acute or chronic pain under certain conditions. The most common approaches include (1) pain relievers that alter the body chemistry, and (2) physical, psychological, cognitive, anesthetic, and neurosurgical methods. No one can tell you the best method to relieve pain from your body; you must weigh the risks and benefits of various approaches. With your physician's help, you can tailor a treatment approach for your body and circumstances.

Drug Therapy

The most frequently used approach—mainly because it is fast and most in demand—is drug therapy. Even so, drug therapy is not always the safest way to eliminate pain; certain drugs can have side effects. Consult your physician before taking any medication; when a physician prescribes a medication for pain, ask about the possible side effects. Drug therapy utilizes anti-inflammatory drugs, narcotics, and antidepressants.

Anti-Inflammatory Drugs

The three types of anti-inflammatory drugs are corticosteroids, nonsteroidal anti-inflammatory drugs, and analgesics (although not all analgesics block pain). All three drugs also are used for other purposes. Most anti-inflammatory drugs are pain relievers to take care of the redness and burning associated with inflammation and help relieve general pain.

Corticosteroids

Corticosteroids are made from synthetic hormones and are used as anti-inflammatories, bronchodilators for asthma, and immunosuppressives.

Nonsteroidal Anti-Inflammatory Drugs

Nonsteroidal anti-inflammatory drugs (NSAID) include more than 20 substances and work by blocking the production of prostaglandins. These drugs are effective against slow, prolonged tissue damage and the associated pain, such as in the socket of an extracted tooth or arthritic joint, and general or localized pains, such as back pain, menstrual cramps, and headaches. NSAIDs are not effective against pain triggered by events that do not produce inflammatory reactions.

Analgesics

Analgesics include simple analgesics, such as aspirin and acetaminophen, for mild pain and narcotic analgesics, such as codeine and morphine, for severe pain. Analgesics such as aspirin work by reducing inflammation. They also prevent the production of prostaglandins, chemicals that the body produces when tissue is damaged (these chemicals combine with the opiate receptors on the surface of cells in the brain and spinal cord). Acetaminophens are the only analgesics that work by blocking pain impulses in the brain and preventing the perception of pain.

For patients with moderate to severe pain, doctors often combine narcotic analgesics with non-narcotic drugs. These include drugs such as hydrocodone, codeine, and propoxyphene that are useful for moderate pain often associated with mild trauma, headache, toothache, or backache. For patients suffering severe pain, the strong narcotic analgesics are useful; these include morphine, hydromorphine, and methadone. Doctors use this class of drugs most commonly to help patients manage acute postoperative pain and the severe chronic pain of cancer. Narcotic analgesics work by binding to the opiate receptors on the peripheral nerve as well as the central nervous system. Patients need to be aware that all of these analgesic drugs have side effects.

Local anesthetics are locally applied analgesics used for reducing pain; they include bupivaocaine and lidocaine, which can be injected to deaden the nerve so pain is not felt during a dental procedure. Doctors use local anesthetics to facilitate treatment of skin wounds and to numb areas of the body before surgery.

Narcotics

Narcotics are opiate drugs that block pain signals and inhibit the patient's perception of pain. Doctors use narcotics when pain is short-term and intense, such as with kidney stones, severe burns or injury, heart attacks, or after surgery. Narcotics are prescribed for chronic pain, only if other drug or nondrug therapies do not relieve the pain. In most cases, the dosage is such that the pain is brought to a bearable level so the patient can still mentally function.

Antidepressants

People who suffer from pain, especially chronic pain, often become depressed and are prescribed antidepressants. Low doses of such drugs can have an effect on pain. For example, low doses of mood-elevating drugs called tricyclic antidepressants seem to block pain messages traveling to the spinal cord or may change the way the nerve acts at the injury site. These antidepressants work best for nerve damage pain (such as diabetes, injuries, amputation, or viral infections that attack the nerves like shingles); they include doxepin, amitriptyline, imipramine, and desipramine.

Regardless of the drug approach you and your doctor choose, it must be individualized for your pain problem. This includes the choice of drug, the way it is administered, and the time frame for its use.

Nondrug Techniques

Some nondrug techniques are just as good for certain pain reduction problems as drug therapy; often they carry less risk to the patients than medications. The success rate of such ministrations varies; it is up to the patient, with the help of the doctor and other experts, to determine the best treatment. They must consider the nature, site, and intensity of the pain. Most commonly, doctors combine drug and nondrug approaches to provide patients with comprehensive treatment.

Heat

One of the most ancient ways to decrease pain is to use heating techniques; no one knows why heat makes pain decrease. It is doubtful that heat speeds up repair of an injury. However, locally applied heat using simple methods such as heating pads, moist heat, and hot water bottles does reduce low to moderate levels of pain due to such injuries as bruises, torn muscles, and arthritis, and such pains as menstrual cramps or backaches. Ultrasound raises the temperature in deep structures under the skin to treat pain in joints or bones.

Cold

Another ancient technique to decrease pain is to use cold that constricts local blood vessels and makes the area feel numb. Researchers believe that the cold acts similar to acupuncture by producing a burning pain that may block pain signals. Ice has been used to decrease dental pain by massaging an ice cube on the back of the hand between the thumb and index finger. Ice also relieves the pain and swelling from sprains, bumps, and subsequent bruises.

TENS

The transcutaneous (across the skin) electrical nerve stimulation units (TENS) are available only through prescription. TENS units send a small electrical current pulse—less than 10 percent of a 60-watt lightbulb—that stimulates the nerve fibers just under the skin, blocking pain signals along the nerves. TENS units are used for just about every type of pain: wound pain; nerve injuries; face, mouth, and tooth pain; diametric nerve damage; cancer pain, itching; postoperative pain; labor pain; arthritis; headaches; and so on. The unit, about the size of a television remote control, is worn on the belt; the patient places the electrodes carrying the current at the site of the pain or over the acupuncture point near the pain. The pain is relieved while the unit is turned on or a short time after it is turned off. Many patients report that after over a year of use, the TENS unit loses its therapeutic abilities; apparently the nerve system begins to ignore the electrical stimulation and allows pain signals to break through.

Behavioral Techniques

Behavioral techniques that relieve pain use the mind to modify or eliminate pain, especially chronic pain. Although not for everyone, behavioral pain relief methods can replace medication; they should be taught in a professional facility by therapists who can provide advice and assistance.

Biofeedback

Feedback is a word taken from electronics that means information in a loop that is recorded and fed back into the system to adjust the operation. Biofeedback is similar, using the mind to control the body when tension is the cause of pain, rather than arthritis, cancer, or nerve damage. After being attached to sensors that monitor body readings, patients are able to see or hear muscle tension, temperature, and other body processes. With practice, patients eventually gain enough control over the process to change what they see or hear on the monitors. For example, temperature biofeedback is used for the treatment of migraine headaches; the temperature sensors show that as blood vessels narrow, body temperatures decrease. Patients learn to increase the blood flow to these areas with biofeedback; thus, by controlling their thinking they can decrease the occurrence of painful migraines.

Visualization

Visualization is a mental technique similar to biofeedback. Athletes use visualization to enhance their performance; over and over they see in their minds the perfect pitch, or precise pole jump. Visualization does not necessarily have to be in the mind; patients also can draw their illnesses, using the images to get rid of their pain or illness on paper. One type of visualization called guided imagery gives the patient a visual goal to accomplish, such as picturing being free of pain, or visualizing an image of a shrinking tumor. The patient is trained to ignore the pain by evoking imagery that is incompatible with the pain. Researchers believe that such visualization techniques cause the body to become less stressed.

Relaxation

Relaxation is the release of stress, anxiety, and often pain. Relaxation techniques include deep breathing, muscle relaxation techniques, and meditation. One of the best ways to relax is to meditate: Sit or lie down in a comfortable position, deeply relaxing all your muscles. Breathe at a relaxed rate through the nose, releasing all thoughts from your brain. Some people repeat one word over and over, focusing their attention on that word. This is usually done for about 20 minutes; however, there is no real set time to use relaxation techniques. Each individual develops her own rhythm of relaxation.

Hypnosis

Pain patients often turn to hypnosis; by using this form of relaxation they can shut out distraction and focus intensely on one particular subject, such as getting rid of pain. Not everyone is a candidate for hypnosis because patients must be receptive to suggestion. After the diagnosis of a pain problem, hypnosis can be used as a potential alternative to treat the pain. It is used mainly for chronic pains, such as recurring headaches; or for relaxation, such as helping a woman to relax and thus experience less pain during labor.

Physical Techniques and Specialists

Exercise

Exercise is thought to relieve pain by forcing a patient to concentrate on something other than the pain; in addition, vigorous exercise causes the body to release natural painkillers into the bloodstream, thus decreasing pain. Exercise such as running, walking, skiing, biking, and hiking increase cardiovascular and overall endurance. Weight training increases muscular strength and decreases the chance of painful injuries because the body is in shape. Exercise can include some of the more gentle motions that benefit organs and internal body structure. Some yoga instructors also include deep breathing and meditation with more traditional yoga exercises.

Massage

At one time or another, we have all rubbed a sore shoulder, or stretched an aching hamstring muscle to relieve pain. For deeper pains such as backaches, highly trained professionals use techniques that apply mechanical pressure to relieve the pain. There are many massage techniques; some massage the area of pain, while others use pressure on various parts of the body to relieve the pain.

Physical Therapy

Physical therapists are trained professionals who treat the musculoskeletal system; they cannot diagnose medical problems or prescribe medication. They use their hands and technology to treat a wide variety of pain problems, including cancer, strained or sprained muscles, and lower back pain. They customize each treatment, using techniques such as exercise programs, ultrasound, massage and heat and cold applications.

Physiatry

Physiatrists are medical doctors who use physical methods and agents to treat patients, including those suffering pain. They can evaluate and prescribe treatment regimens for disabilities due to pain. Physical medicine emphasizes rehabilitation and uses other health care professionals in a team approach to diagnose and relieve pain.

Alternative Health Techniques

Alternative health methods provide an alternative to drugs and drug therapy; they use numerous healing techniques to relieve pain.

Acupuncture

Acupuncture, the ancient Chinese healing art, uses various therapeutic techniques including the insertion of various size needles at specific points on the body called meridians. Classic texts describe 365 acupuncture points, each associated with specific organs. According to acupuncturists, the needles allow the body to flow; they are used to maintain health or eliminate imbalances in the body, including the relief of pain. Researchers believe that acupuncture may work because the stimulating needles cause the release of endorphins, thus lessening pain or giving the patient a feeling of well-being.

Acupressure

Very similar to acupuncture, acupressure is a method of using pressure to work on the meridians of the body to treat specific pain symptoms or disorders.

Hydrotherapy

Hydrotherapy uses water to relieve the constant pressures on certain parts of the body and reduce pain. The most common types of treatment are swimming and water exercises, usually for chronic back problems.

Surgery

Surgery to relieve pain often is a last resort. It may seem as if just cutting a nerve will cause the feeling of pain to disappear. In reality, cutting nerves to cut pain usually leads to other complications such as numbness. Nerve blocks to temporarily deaden neural pathways that conduct pain also have been used to control pain; they leave the area insensitive to a pinprick. Chronic pain patients report the pain still persists even though the area is numb.

CHILDBIRTH AND PAIN

Most women experience pain with contractions during childbirth, with the peak intensity of pain between the time when the cervix opening is fully dilated and contractions in the uterus push the baby into the vagina and out of the body. During labor, there are several ways to reduce the pain:

Change your position by adopting an upright position, kneeling on all fours, or squatting. Breathe slowly and rhythmically to help you relax. Narcotics, usually used to help the mother relax, are commonly administered in the middle of labor but not at the last part of labor, as they may cause the baby to have difficulty breathing. Local anesthesia is used for a forceps delivery or episiotomy. General anesthesia usually is used if a Cesarean section is warranted.

Epidural anesthesia, an anesthetic drug injected in the spine, numbs the mother from the waist down when other pain-relieving measures during labor pain do not work. This anesthesia generally wears off when the baby is being delivered, so the mother can still push the baby effectively. The issue of using drugs during childbirth to reduce pain is highly debated. Several issues are involved, including the rights of the mother to experience the birth without clouding her thinking; the ease of delivery with or without drugs; and the effects the drugs will have on the baby. And, there are tradeoffs to all the aspects of drugs and childbirth. For example, early in labor drugs to control vomiting are administered in case narcotics or anesthesia must be given later due to an emergency; these may alter the mother's awareness. Local anesthetics are frequently used, which leave the mother's mind clear, but partially paralyze the lumbar area; this weakens the contractions and slows down the labor.

What are the best alternatives to using drugs to ease the pain of childbirth? Although it does not appeal to everyone, many women choose to use prepared childbirth training. Such training includes the Lamaze training that prepares the mother so she knows what to expect and decreases the anxiety that can increase her pain. It features relaxation training to help the mother calm herself when the contractions increase in number and intensity; using techniques to distract attention from the pain; and breathing exercises to help relax and aid in the birthing process.

The following neurosurgical approaches have been tried to relieve pain, but there have been very few successes. Pain often returns in a different place or is more intense than before surgery.

- The patient's sympathetic system can be surgically or chemically destroyed; the sympathetic system supplies the blood vessels and glands, and affects blood flow and pressure. This operation is difficult and usually does not relieve pain.

- A cordotomy involves cutting the tracts in the spinal cord. This usually cuts the paths to the spinal cord, and disrupts signals to the thalamus; there are so many nerve fibers destined for the thalamus that it is a difficult operation. The major problem is that the effect fades as months go by.

- Cerebral (brain) operations have been used in the past, directly targeting the pain centers even though the true sites of pain are still not known; these operations have very few successes.

Psychological Help

Pain does not always follow physiological paths—the patient's mental state also has a direct effect on her perception of pain. In many cases, part of an injured patient's stress is emotional distress as well as the awareness of physical injury. During childbirth, or after surgery, emotional distress may be a major aspect of the patient's pain. Research has shown that the intensity and duration of pain for postoperative patients has a direct relationship to the patient's psychological preparation before the operation by counselors and the physician's explanation of the operation.

Because of this direct link between pain and emotion, doctors realize that some patients' pain, especially chronic pain, may be helped using psychological approaches. In fact, psychological pain usually cannot be treated physiologically. The psychologists try to understand how much of the patient's pain is due to psychological factors, such a depression, or job or family difficulties. They work with patients' families to increase their awareness of the patients' pain and to decrease factors in the home that may contribute to their pain. For patients who are thinking too much about the pain—concentrating so hard on the pain that it is more overwhelming than reality—psychologists help them overcome such feelings.

Psychologists also look at patients' pain in terms of behavior: Are they getting out of a stressful situation by using their pain as an excuse? Are they getting attention because of pain? Another situation often occurs: Even if they have had the pain for months or years, patients are in a constant state of alarm, believing there is really something else wrong. As such anxiety continues, patients become worse; their fears are confirmed by a self-fulfilling prophecy.

Most psychological situations involving pain can be helped by psychological techniques. Psychologists use such techniques as having patients make goals for themselves; positive thinking; tuning out the pain; and helping patients answer hard questions about their pain. Another way patients can cope with pain is by attending group therapy sessions; often these include patients who are trying to cope with the same types of pain.

IS IT ALL IN MY HEAD?

One of the main questions for those suffering from chronic pain is whether the pain is all in their heads. This question usually is asked about long-term pain or when no real diagnosis for the pain has been made. Pain almost always has a real physical basis; only about 5 percent of chronic pain is psychological rather than physical.

Patients who experience psychogenic or psychological pain do so for two major reasons: They have hallucinations (or a false perception of reality) or delusions (usually depressed patients have a false belief relating to their bodies). Less frequent reasons include conversion reactions in which sensations (such as the complaint of a pain) are compensating for some intense emotion; and hypochondriasis, in which the patient has a fascination with the experience of illness.

GETTING HELP

Patients who experience pain—either chronic or acute—are not alone. Pain clinics and organizations can help them understand their options, including how to talk about, understand, and cope with the pain. For a person in chronic pain, this can be the difference between living a fulfilling life or existing in a debilitating situation.

Often pain patients are advised to set goals for themselves; working toward their goals gives them a feeling of accomplishment. The goals should be the antitheses of pain, such as setting goals at work (even if it means changing careers), taking classes for enjoyment, or actively working so many hours or minutes a day in the garden (even with adaptations to make it easier).

The pain patient should be realistic about her pain. For example, a patient with degenerative joint problems must be realistic about the chronic pain, and understand that when all the alternative cures or treatments are exhausted she must live with the pain. This is probably the most difficult step of all, but it is most important in coping with chronic pain.

Pain patients are encouraged to become as active as they can in their work, recreation, and social activities. It does no good to ignore the mental and physical health benefits of being active in all aspects of their lives. Pain patients are encouraged to talk with others about their hurt—especially other pain patients—and continue optimistically with life.

There are numerous pain clinics across the country. When looking for a pain clinic, keep the following points in mind:

- Make sure the program is legitimate; pain centers that are part of hospitals or rehabilitation centers usually offer a more comprehensive treatment than stand alone clinics.

- The program should have several types of professionals on staff, including physicians (neurologist, psychiatrist, physiatrist, or anesthesiologist with expertise in pain management), registered nurse, physical therapist, biofeedback therapist, vocational counselor, family counselor, personnel trained in pain management intervention, and occupational therapist.

- Patients should look for a program that is convenient for them and their families to attend; they should make sure that their families can be included in their pain care. The facility should be close enough to enable patients to comfortably commute every day or as often as their programs demand.

- Patients should examine the clinic to see if it has the following features: biofeedback, relaxation, and stress management training, counseling (individual and family), TENS unit, physical therapy, educational program (explaining medications and pain management), group and occupational therapy, assertiveness training, and aftercare.

Other patient concerns when selecting a clinic include: what your insurance company covers; whether the program is part of a hospital; what will be required of you during your stay (including what you should bring with you); does the clinic have all your previous medical records, including allergies; can you interview past and present patients at the clinic to learn about their experience at the clinic.

Pain Organizations

To discover which pain clinics are closest or best for you, contact one of the following organizations. You may also want to join some of the groups, as they often offer newsletters or booklets on coping with pain.

1. Commission on Accreditation of Rehabilitation Facilities (800-444-8991)
2. The American Chronic Pain Association (916-632-0922)
3. American Pain Society (708-966-5595)
4. The American Academy of Physical Medicine and Rehabilitation (312-922-9366)
5. The Chronic Pain Support Group (216-657-2948)
6. National Committee on the Treatment of Intractable Pain (301-983-1710)

CHAPTER 39

Managing Medication

Jean A. Hamilton, M.D., and
Kimberly A. Yonkers, M.D.

More than half of all visits to a doctor result in at least one prescription, and over a lifetime women make more visits than men. Women will likely be prescribed more drugs than the average man. Yet, until recently many new medications were tested and studied more extensively in men. Doctors know much less about how medication use affects their prime recipients, women.

It is known, however, that the sexes respond differently to certain kinds of medicines. Their bodies may process the medication differently, and they may experience beneficial or negative side effects. Some of these variations are related to the differences in body type between men and women. But women experience many physiological and psychological changes in their lives; the way women respond to medicines may alter as they go through menstruation, pregnancy, menopause, and aging.

Many doctors prescribing medications today were educated before all this new information was understood and accepted. Some still have a paternalistic attitude toward women and their health concerns. Thus, many doctors are playing catch up, prescribing medications with an imagined male model patient in mind, whether or not the real patient is a woman or a man. When you realize the special sex-related issues of medication, both you and your doctor benefit from a better knowledge of how a particular medication is likely to affect you, the real patient. But first you have to understand how medications work in the body.

A QUICK COURSE IN PHARMACOLOGY

Pharmacology is the study of medications. *Pharmacotherapy* refers to the practice of using medications for therapeutic or preventive purposes. Because some groups of people respond differently to a given medication than do others, the goal of research is increasingly to make drug treatments work for members of various groups. Optimizing medication use for women is part of a larger, positive trend.

How Medications Work

How well medications work in the body depends on many factors. These factors can be simplified to the following four main steps needed for safe, effective medication use:

1. The medication must be *absorbed* into the body.
2. The medication must be *distributed* to the place in the body where it's needed.
3. The medication must be *metabolized* (broken down into parts) so that dangerously high levels do not build up.
4. Unabsorbed medication and broken-down medication must be *eliminated* from the body.

Any factor that affects how a medication is absorbed, distributed, metabolized, or eliminated affects the safety and effectiveness of the medication.

Absorption

The absorption of a medication into the body is determined by the health of the body, the type of medication, and the route by which the medication is taken. Many medications taken by mouth are digested in the intestines, where they are passed into the bloodstream. For these medications to be properly absorbed, the intestines need to be functioning normally. If not, much of the medication may pass uselessly out of the body.

The type of medication plays a role, too. Some types are more readily absorbed in an empty stomach; others enter the body faster when taken with food. Pills with coatings to protect the stomach from irritation have to be broken down in the intestines, so they are absorbed more slowly than pills without such a coating. Some medications can enter the body more readily through the membranes of the mouth, and get into the bloodstream quickly. This method is particularly useful for medications like nitroglycerin, which is used to relieve the chest pains of angina, a condition of decreased blood supply to the heart.

Distribution

Once medications have been absorbed into the bloodstream, they must be distributed to the place in the body where they're most needed. The size and composition of the body—the amount of blood and fluids and the percentage of muscle versus fatty tissue—affect distribution. Some medications are more likely to be stored in fatty tissue than others.

Metabolism

To prevent toxic, or dangerous, levels of medications from building up, the body has to find a way to break down the medication. This happens through a process called *metabolism*. Generally the metabolic process is done by enzymes, special types of proteins that act to break down or bind drugs to other substances. The metabolites, products that result from metabolism, may be "active," have a drug effect, or they may be inert.

Medications that pass from the stomach and intestines into the bloodstream first stop off in the liver. There, the liver gets a chance to metabolize the medicine before it gets into the general bloodstream and spreads throughout the body. With repeated circulation more and more of the drug is broken down by the liver. So, a healthy liver is a must for the proper metabolism of medications.

You need the right enzymes to break down the medication, too. Your genes and chromosomes, the body's blueprint, control the production of enzymes. Some women may inherit a blueprint in which an enzyme is absent or present in subnormal amounts. If this happens, the rate at which the body can break down certain medications slows.

Sometimes, one medication will speed up metabolic activity in the liver. This may cause other medications to be broken down faster, leading to lower levels of the drug in the body. These lower levels are less effective and so higher doses are needed. In this way, *tolerance* to medications occurs. Tolerance is particularly a problem with medications that can be abused, such as narcotics (heroin, morphine), sleeping pills (barbiturates), depressants (alcohol), and stimulants (amphetamines, caffeine, nicotine).

Elimination

Medications that have not been absorbed by the body and the elements resulting from the process of metabolism need a way to exit the body. As might be expected, most medications are mainly eliminated either through the liver into the bile to the feces or into the urine. Disturbances in the digestive system or urinary tract can affect how this occurs, however. If you have diarrhea, for example, food and medications rush through your digestive tract without getting a chance to be absorbed. The amount of medication you eliminate might be higher than normal and not enough of the medication would be available for use by your body. If there is a blockage to the biliary system in the liver, medications would not be eliminated by this route. In the urinary tract, kidney function can affect whether drugs and their metabolites are eliminated rapidly or slowly. If kidney function is significantly decreased, the dosage of drugs eliminated by this route must be decreased.

There are other routes out of the body, though, and some amounts of many medications can be found in tears, sweat, and saliva. Women who are breast-feeding can excrete some medications in their breast milk. Breast-feeding women should always consult their obstetrician or pediatrician before taking such medication.

Measures of Effectiveness in Medication

Pharmacologists and doctors often summarize the activity of medications in terms such as:

- *Bioavailability.* The amount of medication that the body can actually use.
- *Blood levels.* The amount of medication in the blood, which is related to the effectiveness (or efficacy) of the drug and its side effects.
- *Clearance.* The removal of a medication from the body.
- *Half-life.* The amount of time it takes for half of the medication to be eliminated from the body.

Bioavailability

One of the ways doctors compare the effectiveness of a medication is bioavailability. Not all of an ingested medication reaches its target. Some is eliminated without being used. When a medication has good bioavailability, it means that more of the medication is available for use. If the bioavailability is poor, less of the medication can be used, so more must be taken.

A similar measure of medication effectiveness is potency. Potency refers to the effectiveness in relation to the amount of drugs used. Less medication is needed if it has high potency, while more is needed if it is low.

Blood Levels

Once medication is absorbed into the bloodstream, its concentration in the blood can be measured. This is very helpful to doctors in determining how well the medication is working. If the blood levels are too low—which is known as low efficacy—the medication will not produce an adequate effect. If the blood levels of medication are too high, the risks for toxicity and side effects increase. Some side effects are just a nuisance, but others can be serious or even life threatening. Toxicity refers to a situation in which high levels of a drug can become dangerous, like a poison rather than a helpful medication.

Clearance

Clearance, or the removal of a medication from the body, can also be measured. If clearance is slower than normal, the medication can build up to dangerous lev-

els. If clearance is faster than normal, the medication may be eliminated from the body before it has had a chance to act.

Half-Life

A medication's half-life refers to the amount of time it takes for one-half of the medication to be broken down in the body or eliminated. Medications with short half-lives are only active for hours; those with a long half-life are active for days. Half-life dictates dosing schedules—whether a drug is taken several times daily or once daily. Some medicines are specially treated with coatings that make them "slow releasing (SR)," so that they can be taken only once daily.

HOW SEX DIFFERENCES AFFECT MEDICATIONS

Many medications are processed differently by men and women, although a greater number *do not* show sex differences. (See Table 39.1.)

When sex differences are noted, women tend to

Table 39.1. SAMPLE OF MEDICATIONS THAT DO NOT SHOW SEX DIFFERENCES

Medication	Reason Used
Acebutolol	Lowers high blood pressure
Bupropion*	An antidepressant
Caffeine†	A stimulant found in coffee, tea, and some pain-killing medications
Cimetidine	Suppresses stomach acid production; used in treating ulcers
Clonazepam	Prevents and treats seizures
Metoprolol	Treats high blood pressure
Phenytoin†	Prevents or treats seizures
Theophylline	Opens the blood vessels; used to treat asthma and other breathing problems, also stimulates the heart
Triazolam	A tranquilizer

* Although buprorion does not show sex differences, a person with the eating disorder bulimia is more likely to have seizures when taking this medication. Bulimia is much more common in girls and women than in men.

† This medication may be affected by hormones, either those naturally found in the body or those taken as medication (for example, birth control pills).

Table 39.2. SAMPLE OF MEDICATIONS THAT SHOW SEX DIFFERENCES

Medication	Reason Used
Acetaminophen	A pain killer
Alcohol	A sedative
Amitriptyline	An antidepressant
Chlordiazepoxide	An antianxiety medicine
Clozapine†	Treats severe schizophrenia
Diazepam†	Antianxiety medicine, tranquilizer
Flurazepam	A sleeping pill
Fluphenazine decanoate†	Treats schizophrenia
Imipramine	An antidepressant
Lidocaine	An anesthetic
Lorazepam†	Antianxiety medicine, tranquilizer
Oxazepam	Antianxiety medicine, tranquilizer
Piroxicam‡	Fights inflammation, used in treating arthritis
Propranolol§	Treats high blood pressure
Temazepam	A sleeping pill
Thiothixene†	Treats psychotic disorders
Trazodone	An antidepressant

With the exception of trazodone, all these medications tend to be cleared faster from a man's body than from a woman's. Older men seem to have a slower clearance for trazodone than do women.

† This medication probably has sex differences.

‡ This medication may have a sex difference in older persons.

§ This medication may have a sex difference in younger persons.

show *greater bioavailability*—that is, more of the medication is available for use. They also display *slower apparent clearance*—the slower elimination of the medication from the body—compared with men. These sex-related differences suggest that the standard dose for a medication (probably based on studies of men) may be fairly high for women. Unless your doctor adjusts the dosage of a medication, your risk of having side effects or building up dangerous levels of the medication is higher. In fact, women tend to have side effects from medications about twice as often as men. (See Table 39.2 for some examples of sex differences in medications.) Researchers believe that mediations that affect the brain and behavior (the psychotropic drugs) are more likely to show sex differences.

What causes these variations? Some of the important factors in men and women that are known to affect medications include

- Body size and weight
- Stomach emptying
- Secretion of stomach acids

- Lean body mass
- Body fat
- Total body water
- Blood flow to the brain
- Activity of enzymes in the liver
- Function of the kidneys

In some cases, the difference may be due to only one factor, such as weight. Many other times, however, sex differences are due to a combination of factors. This happens, for example, even when dosages are modified to reflect a woman's weight. Taken together, then, men and women may differ on average in many of the factors that affect medication absorption, distribution, metabolism, and elimination.

Sometimes sex differences exist but have no real effect. The medication may have a large margin of safety, which means there is a wide safety zone between the amount that is effective and the amount that is dangerous. Thus, even if a woman has higher blood levels of the drug than a man, she does not have much of an increase in risk.

LIFE CHANGES AND DRUG EFFICACY

Over the years, the way a woman responds to medication changes according to the stage of her life cycle. Many of these changes are coordinated by hormones. Female hormones, such as estrogen, change throughout a woman's monthly menstrual period and provide a woman with the ability to have a child. They also affect her response to medication. When female hormones are prescribed for a woman—for example, for birth control or hormone replacement after menopause—they also can play a role in at least some women.

During the years that a woman is sexually active, medication can affect this part of her life (see "Medications and Sex"). As a woman ages, her response to medication changes again.

The Menstrual Cycle

The menstrual cycle probably does not affect how most women respond to medication. However, a small group of women—maybe 5–10 percent—do show menstrual effects.

In some cases, the blood level of a medication drops a few days before a woman has her period. Sometimes the blood level is so low that the medication isn't effective any more. Women who have these premenstrual drops in medication effectiveness may need to take higher doses of a medication before their periods, but this should be discussed first with the doctor. Once the period is over, they can go back to their regular doses. Other women find that their medications reach higher levels in the blood in the time before their periods. These women may have a higher risk of side effects.

If you find that your period seems to affect how you respond to medicine, talk with your doctors. They can study your blood levels and help decide whether changing doses would help increase the medication's effectiveness or reduce the risk of side effects.

Pregnancy

Pregnancy affects how a woman responds to medication, and it may affect the fetus. Because of fears of harming the fetus, few studies have been done on the effects of medications in pregnant women. For obvious reasons, medication should be carefully chosen in pregnancy. Because so little is known, it is best to avoid medicines at this time, even those available without a prescription.

When a woman is pregnant, her body must produce not only enough blood for her needs but also enough to circulate through the fetus. A pregnant woman's blood volume may increase by about 20–30 percent. As a result, she retains fluid and her total body water increases. Because this extra fluid tends to water down, or dilute, any medicine she takes, higher doses may be needed during pregnancy. In some medicines, though, the effective level in the blood may be very close to the hazardous level (a narrow therapeutic index). During pregnancy, this can be risky. Pregnant women who must take these kinds of medicines should have their blood levels checked often.

Medication can affect the fetus if it can cross the placenta, the organ where nutrients and oxygen are delivered to the fetus from the mother's blood.

The 9 months of a normal pregnancy can be divided into three trimesters of 3 months each. Medications taken in the first trimester have the greatest risk of causing birth defects. While medicines taken later in pregnancy are less likely to cause birth defects, they can cause other problems like low birth weight or delayed development.

Tell your doctor as soon as you know you are pregnant. The doctor can explain what medicines are safe to use during pregnancy. If you have a serious medical condition that requires medication, often you can be switched to one that is safer for the fetus. For example, warfarin, an anticoagulant used to prevent blood clots, can cause birth defects if used in pregnancy. Pregnant women who need to use an anticoagulant can choose heparin instead, which poses less risk to the unborn child. In some cases, it is believed that certain drugs (e.g., tricyclic antidepressants, but not lithium) are relatively safe during pregnancy. Even when such medications in pregnancy have not been formally tested, some women have taken the drug before they knew they were pregnant. Such information helps establish whether to take certain drugs in pregnancy. Work with your doctor to weigh the risks *and* benefits of medication use during pregnancy, for both mother and child.

Women who choose to breast-feed should be aware that medications can be excreted in breast milk and passed on to the baby. If you are breast-feeding, have any medication cleared by your physician (obstetrician or pediatrician) before taking it.

Menopause

The possible effects of menopause on various medications is largely unknown. What *is* known is that at menopause, a woman's blood levels of estrogen drop dramatically. This development can contribute to annoying symptoms such as hot flashes and can increase the risk of weak bones (osteoporosis) or heart disease. To replace the estrogen their bodies once made naturally, some women choose to take synthetic hormones. These hormones are sometimes similar to the ones in birth control pills, so their effects may resemble those of pills.

BIRTH CONTROL AND MEDICATION

Certain birth control methods contain synthetic hormones similar to the ones a woman's body makes naturally, including:

- Birth control pills
- Hormone injections
- Hormone implants

Contraceptives like these can affect other medications or results on lab tests. If you use one of these methods, be sure to tell any doctor who prescribes medicine for you.

About 25 percent of U.S. women 15–45 years of age use birth control pills. The estrogen and progestin (a synthetic version of progesterone, a natural female hormone) in the pills can affect how the liver functions. When a woman who uses the pill takes other medications that are metabolized through the liver, she may have higher blood levels and more toxic side effects than a woman who uses other methods of birth control or no birth control at all. In this case, the pills exaggerate the differences that already exist because of the difference in sex. The effect may be greatest for pills with high amounts of progestin.

A birth control pill that contains only progestin (the minipill) is available. Hormone injections and implants also contain only progestin. Inform your doctor if you are taking birth control pills.

See Table 39.4 for more information.

MEDICATIONS AFFECTING SEXUAL FUNCTION

Medication	Reason Used	Effect on Sexuality
Alprazolam	Treatment of anxiety	Changes in sex drive, sexual problems
Amiodarone	Corrects irregular heart beat	Decreased sex drive
Atenolol	Lowers high blood pressure	Decreased sex drive
Amitriptyline	Antidepressant	Increased or decreased sex drive
Clofibrate	Lowers fat levels like cholesterol in the blood	Decreased sex drive
Clonidine	Lowers high blood pressure	Decreased sexual activity decreased sex drive
Danazol	Treatment of endometriosis or fibrocystic breast disease	Vaginal dryness, increased or decreased sex drive
Diazepam	Treatment of anxiety	Changes in sex drive, sexual problems
Fenfluramine	Used in weight loss programs	Increased or decreased sex drive
Fluoxetine	Antidepressant	Decreased sex drive, painful intercourse
Guanabenz	Lowers high blood pressure	Decreased sex drive
Methodone	Detox treatment for heroin abuse	Decreased sex drive
Methyldopa	Lowers high blood pressure	Decreased sex drive
Mexiletine	Corrects irregular heart beat	Decreased sex drive
Nafarelin	Treatment of endometriosis	Vaginal dryness, decreased sex drive
Nifedipine	Relieves the chest pain of angina	Can cause sexual difficulties
Phentermine	Used in weight loss programs	Changes in sex drive
Protriptyline	Antidepressant	Increased or decreased sex drive

Sources: S. M. Wolfe and R. E. Hope, Public Citizen Health Research Group. *Worst Pills Best Pills II* (Washington, DC: Public Citizen's Health Research Group, 1993) (for drug names); *Physicians' Desk Reference,* 48th ed. (Montvale, N.J.: Medical Economics Data Production Company, 1994) (for description of effect and confirmation of interaction)

Older Women

Medication is a particularly important issue for women over 65. In general, both metabolism and elimination of medications are slower in older people. The elderly tend to weigh less, too, so they may need less of a drug. Their livers and kidneys may not work as well, and they may have problems clearing medicines out of their systems. And even healthy older women are more sensitive to the effects of medicine.

The effects of age seem to be greater in men than in women, however, which means that older women may not need as low a dose after all. Generally, doctors should choose the right dose to use on the basis of each woman's needs, rather than use a standard dose for everyone.

Another problem is multiple medications. Older women tend to have more health problems than younger women, and they may be on a variety of drugs. For example, an older woman may suffer from diabetes, heart trouble, and arthritis. She could easily be taking a different medicine for each problem. These medications may have side effects, and they may interact with each other.

These interactions are more likely if a woman sees several different doctors, all of whom are prescribing medication for her. None of them may know what the others have prescribed. If you take a number of medicines, note all of them on a card that you keep with you. Better yet, make sure that a copy of your list is presented to any and all doctors at each visit. This precaution will help doctors to prescribe the right medicines for you.

It is also wise to talk periodically with your doctor about whether all of the drugs you are using are really needed. Some may even result in tolerance and addiction if they are used too long. If medication is stopped, sometimes annoying and debilitating symptoms will disappear on their own. Others, like insomnia, may be relieved by lifestyle changes such as getting more exer-

Table 39.3.   SAMPLE MEDICATION INTERACTIONS WITH FOOD

Medication	Reason Used	Foods That Interact	Effect of Interaction
Isoniazid	Treatment of tuberculosis	Cheese or fish	In some people causes sweating, chills, headache, faintness and palpitations, and red, itchy skin
Lithium	Treatment of manic depression	Sodium; coffee, tea	Lithium levels can be affected by rapid changes in amount of salt in diet; large amounts of tea or coffee can cause lithium to build up
Methoxsalen	Treatment of severe psoriasis (skin condition)	Limes, figs, parsley, parsnips, mustard, carrots, celery	May increase sensitivity of skin to light
Monoamine-oxidase inhibitors (e.g., isocarboxazide, phenelzine)*	Treatment of depression	Foods high in tyramine (red wine, beer, some cheeses, fava beans, herring, and chocolate)	Can cause a serious rise in blood pressure
Potassium-sparing diuretics (for example, amiloride, spironolactone)	Increases the excretion of urine	Foods high in potassium (dried fruit and salt substitutes)	Potassium could rise to dangerous levels in the body
Tetracycline	Antibiotic	Milk products	Milk reduces absorption of tetracycline

Source: C. B. Clayman, *The American Medical Association Guide to Prescription and Over-the-Counter Drugs* (New York: Random House, 1988).

* Procarbazine, a medication used in cancer treatment, can have similar effects.

cise and limiting beverages containing caffeine. Don't be afraid to question your doctor. You have a right to ask questions about the treatment you are receiving. If your physician is not responsive, find another one who is.

Taking medicines as prescribed is often a problem for the elderly who may have poor and declining sight. Plus, the more medicines she has to remember, the more likely she is to forget to take one or mix up her instructions. Making a list each night of all the medicines to be taken the next day and noting when to take them can help. Another alternative is to use a daily or weekly pill box dispenser. In some cases a family member can help to fill the pill box properly.

Sadly, some families actually encourage an old person to take more medications. Rather than spending time with a woman who complains about her aches and pains, her family and doctors may suggest that she take tranquilizers, sleeping pills, or antidepressants to make her feel better. Actually these only make her easier to handle. That's not a good reason to take medications, nor is it good medicine.

GETTING THE MOST FROM YOUR MEDICATIONS

When you buy an over-the-counter medication at a drugstore or a grocery, you frequently have the option of buying the less expensive store brand or the brand name. Often, you have the same choice with prescription medicines: you can buy the generic version or the brand name. It costs a lot to develop and advertise a new drug, so the price of a new, brand name medication may be high. Initially only the company that developed the medicine is allowed to make it, so it can set the price as high as the market will bear.

After a medicine has been available for some time, other companies are allowed to produce their own ver-

Table 39.4. SOME MEDICATION-MEDICATION INTERACTIONS

Medication (Reason Used)	Interacts with (Reason Used)	Type of Interaction
Amantadine (treatment of Parkinson's disease)	Anticholinergics (treatment of urinary incontinence and irritable bowel syndrome)	Increased effect of anticholinergics
Antacids (relieve stomach upset)	Digitalis (treatment of heart failure)	Reduced absorption of digitalis
	Iron (treatment of anemia, also found in multivitamins)	Reduced absorption of iron
	Isoniazid (treatment of tuberculosis)	Antacids containing aluminum can reduce absorption of isoniazid\
	Quinine (treatment of malaria)	Antacids containing aluminum can reduce absorption of quinine
	Tetracycline (antibiotic)	Reduced absorption of tetracycline
Anticoagulants (prevent blood clotting)	Aspirin (pain killer)	Increased anticoagulant activity
	Barbiturates (sleeping pills)	Decreased anticoagulant activity
	Carbamazepine (prevents and controls seizures)	Decreased anticoagulant activity
	Chloramphenicol (antibiotic)	Increased anticoagulant activity
	Clofibrate (lowers fat levels like cholesterol in the blood)	Increased anticoagulant activity
	Griseofulvin (antifungal)	Decreased anticoagulant activity
	Thyroid hormones (adjust activity of thyroid gland)	Increased anticoagulant activity
Antidepressants, tricyclic (treatment of depression)	Barbiturates (sleeping pills)	May increase metabolism of antidepressants
	Guanethidine (lowers high blood pressure)	Decreased effectiveness of guanethidine
	Monoamine oxidase inhibitors (antidepressants)	Serious effects on nervous system, including seizures and death
Antihistamines (treatment of colds and allergies)	Anticholinergics (treatment of urinary incontinence and irritable bowel syndrome)	Increased anticholinergic effects of antihistamine (dry mouth, etc.)
	Monoamine oxidase inhibitors (antidepressants)	Dangerous rise in blood pressure
Birth control pills (prevention of pregnancy)	Barbiturates (sleeping pills)	Decreased effectiveness of birth control
	Phenytoin (prevents and controls seizures)	Decreased effectiveness of birth control
	Rifampin (antibacterial used in treatment of tuberculosis)	Decreased effectiveness of birth control
	Tricyclic antidepressants	Increased blood levels of the antidepressant may occur and dosage may need to be decreased.
Cephalosporins (antibiotics)	Aminoglycosides (antibiotics)	Possibly increased risk of kidney damage
	Probenecid (treatment of gout)	Increased level of cephalosporin in blood
Digoxin	Indomethacin	Rise in digoxin level (could be toxic)
Propranolol (treatment of high blood pressure, angina, and irregular heart beat)	Cimetidine (treatment of ulcers)	Increased levels of propranolol in blood
	Indomethacin (relieves pain and inflammation)	Reduced effectiveness of propranolol
Pseudoephedrine (nasal decongestant)	Antihypertensives (reduce blood pressure)	Decreased effectiveness of antihypertensive
	Monoamine oxidase inhibitors (antidepressants)	Dangerous rise in blood pressure

Source: C. B. Clayman, *The American Medical Association Guide to Prescription and Over-the-Counter Drugs* (New York: Random House, 1988); J. E. Knoben and P. O. Anderson, *Handbook of Clinical Drug Data*, 5th ed. (Hamilton, Ill.: Drug Intelligence Publications, 1983).

sions. These generic versions must have the same basic effects as the brand name variety but, by law, generic medicines are allowed to vary a little bit in the bioavailability of their active ingredients. The bioavailability may be a bit higher or lower. This small difference does not matter for many medications, and generics are often far less expensive than name-brand drugs. Some medications, however, such as some birth con-

Table 39.5   MEDICATION INTERACTIONS WITH ALCOHOL

Drug Name	Reason Used	Interaction with Alcohol
Aspirin	Headaches and other body pain, blood thinner	Increased risk of bleeding in the stomach or intestines
Disulfiram	In alcohol treatment programs to develop aversion to alcohol	Dilation (expansion) of veins, low blood pressure, headache, breathing problems, nausea, vomiting, chest pain, weakness, and confusion
Methotrexate	Cancer treatment, rheumatoid arthritis, psoriasis	Increases methotrexate's risk of liver damage
Metronidazole	Fungal infections, such as vaginal infections	Reactions similar to those with disulfiram
Nitroglycerin	To treat pain of angina	Both drugs dilate (expand) the veins, so low blood pressure may occur
Phenytoin	To prevent seizures	Phenytoin more rapidly metabolized with long-term use of large amounts of alcohol

Source: Condensed from J. E. Knoben and P. O. Anderson, *Handbook of Clinical Drug Data,* 5th ed. (Hamilton, Ill.: Drug Intelligence Publications, 1983).

SIGNS OF MEDICATION TAMPERING

Before buying or using any medication, whether an over-the-counter product or a prescription medication, check the following:

- Are the inner and outer wrappings tight and secure?

- Does the container appear to be too full or not full enough?

- Are the expiration date, lot number, and other information the same on the container and its outer wrapping or box?

- Is a liquid medicine the normal color and thickness?

- Do tablets look different than they usually do (unusual spots, dull and rough instead of shiny and smooth)?

- Do tablets all have the same imprint?

- Do capsules look cracked or dented?

- Does the medicine smell or taste different than usual?

SOURCE: Adapted from United States Pharmacopeial Convention, *United States Pharmacopeia,* DI vol. II, *Advice for the Patient: Drug Information in Lay Language* (Rockville, Md.: USPC, 1993).

trol pills and heart medications, require very specific blood levels of the medicine for safe use. If you must take these kinds of drugs, think carefully before you request a generic version. Also, certain psychoactive drugs may differ in bioavailability.

The active ingredient is only a small portion of each pill. The rest is made up of various fillers. Generic medicines are allowed to have different fillers than the brand-name product. If you are intolerant of any of the common medication fillers, such as lactose (milk sugar) or to certain dyes, or you need to watch your intake of salt, sugar, or alcohol, ask your doctor or pharmacist about the fillers used in the generic version.

Generics are a good choice, especially if cost is a concern. In many states and many health plans, a pharmacy will fill a prescription with a generic version unless the doctor specifically requests the brand name.

When selecting an over-the-counter drug or picking up a prescription medicine from the pharmacy, be alert to signs that the medicine has been tampered with (see "Signs of Medication Tampering"). If a box, container, or medicine shows signs of tampering, do not buy it. If you only discover the problem at home, do not use the medicine. Take it back immediately to the store or pharmacy and ask for a replacement.

Safe Medication Use

The most important things you can do when taking medications is to take them as directed. Doing so increases the chance that the medication works as it's supposed to, and decreases the risk of side effects. Taking extra medicine because "it doesn't seem to be working" can be very risky. Stopping medication early because symptoms have cleared up can cause problems, too. For example, if you are being treated for an infection, it is very important that you take *all* the medication prescribed for you. If antibiotics (the common treatment for infections) are stopped early, the infection may come back. The bacteria causing the infection may then build up resistance, so that the same antibiotic doesn't work as well later, if you need it (see

WHAT A WOMAN NEEDS TO KNOW ABOUT HER MEDICINES

To the extent possible, there are a number of things you should know about each medicine you are taking, including

- The medicine's generic and brand names. This can be overwhelming.
- How it will help you and the expected results. How it makes you feel. How long it takes to begin working.
- How much to take at one time.
- How often to take the medicine.
- How long it will be necessary to take the medicine.
- When to take it. Before, during, after meals? At bedtime? At any other special times?
- How to take it. With water? With fruit juice? How much?
- What to do about a missed dose.
- Foods, drinks, or other medicines not to be taken while taking a medicine.
- Restrictions on activities while taking a medicine. May you drive or operate other motor vehicles?
- Side effects to be expected. What to do if they appear. How to minimize them. How soon should they go away? Insist that the physician give you side effects *in writing* (AMA sells these to doctors).
- When to seek help, if there are problems.
- How long to wait before reporting no change in symptoms.
- How to store the medicine. Should the unused portion be saved for future use?
- The expiration date.
- The cost of the medicine.
- How to have the prescription refilled, if necessary.

SOURCE: Adapted from United States Pharmacopeial Convention, *United States Pharmacopeia*, DI vol. II, *Advice for the Patient: Drug Information in Lay Language* (Rockville, Md.: USPC, 1993).

READING A PRESCRIPTION

It's only natural to want to know what you're putting in your body, so it may be important for you to be able to read prescriptions your doctors hand you.

Unfortunately, reading a prescription isn't quite as simple as reading a label. A prescription may look like it's written in a foreign language because it is. Prescriptions have their own set of abbreviations and codes, many of which are based on Latin. Being able to read a prescription can help you double-check that you're being given the instructions the doctor intended.

This list includes some of the terms that show up most often on prescriptions:

ac	Before meals (ante cibum)
ad	Right ear (auris dextra)
ad	Up to (ad)
ad lib	As desired (ad libitum)
as	Left ear (auris sinistra)
bid	Twice a day (bis in die)
c	With (cum)
et	And (et)
gtt(s)	Drop(s) (gutta)
h *or* **hr**	Hour (hora)
hs	At bedtime (hora somni)
M	Mix (misce)
nr	Do not repeat (non repetatur)
od	Right eye (oculus dexter)
os	Left eye (oculus sinister)
pc	After meals (post cibum)
po	By mouth (per os)
prn	As needed (pro re nata)
q	Each (quaque)
qd	Each day (quaque die)
qh *or* **q hr**	Each hour (quaque hora)
qid	Four times a day (quarter in die)
s	Without (sine)
ss	One-half (semis)
Sig	Mark, write (signa)
stat	At once (statim)
tid	Three times a day (ter in die)
ud *or* **ut dict**	As directed (ut dictum)

"What a Woman Needs to Know About Her Medicines").

Be prepared to tell a doctor about all other medicines you are taking, including those that can be bought without a prescription. As suggested earlier you can jot this information down on a small card that you carry in your wallet. The card should also include any medical conditions you may have, along with any allergies to medicine.

Many medicines can interact with each other, or with food or alcohol. Be aware of any possible interactions with the medicine you've been prescribed. If medications that have the same type of effect are taken together, the effect can be greater than desired. For example, both alcohol and sleeping pills slow down the nervous system. If these products are taken together, the system can falter dangerously. Many deaths have resulted from this lethal combination.

On the other hand, products that have opposite effects reduce each other's effectiveness. For example, if a barbiturate is taken with a stimulant, such as a diet pill, these two types of medication may cancel each other out (see Tables 39.3–5). This type of up-down treatment is hard on the body too.

SAFE STORAGE OF MEDICATIONS

The bathroom cabinet may be a convenient place to store medicines, but the hot, steamy environment of a bathroom can make them break down into other products that can be useless or even dangerous. Store most medicines at room temperature in a dry, dark place. Don't store a medicine in the refrigerator unless the label says to do so.

All medications should be thrown away once you have taken the prescribed amount. Self-treating with old medications or with drugs prescribed for someone else is dangerous. Over-the-counter products like pain killers should be thrown out once their expiration date is passed.

Store medications away from children and pets. Today, many medications come in child-proof containers. If you find that the container is adult-proof as well, and there are no children in the house, your pharmacy can usually provide you with a regular container instead. It may be best to flush old or extra medicine down the toilet rather than leaving it in the trash for a child or pet to find.

Diagnostic Tests

Claudia I. Henschke, M.D., PH.D.

Laboratory Procedures

Imaging Tests

    Radiographic Imaging
    Angiography

Nuclear Medicine
Ultrasonography
Computed Tomography
Magnetic Resonance Imaging

There arenumerous techniques available to help physicians look inside a patient's body to see if there is a problem. Some tests tell the story through the analysis of substances that naturally circulate through the body, whereas others show an image of the organs and their function. Still other techniques enable physicians actually to view inside parts of the body. There have been major advances in diagnostic techniques used to assess symptoms and diagnose disorders. These techniques have allowed diseases to be diagnosed more quickly and have virtually eliminated the need for diagnostic surgery. Each technique has advantages and limitations. The benefits must be weighed against the costs, risks, and overall value to the patient.

There is increasing emphasis on patient involvement in the approach to treating a disease once it is diagnosed. Similar emphasis needs to be given to the diagnostic workup. Patients should ask about all the available tests, their accuracy in making the diagnosis, and the agents that will be used and their side effects. Women should also ask about the sequence of the tests to find out what the next test will be if the answer is not found or if further information is required. Any examination that has even a slight chance of serious side effects will require a consent form to be signed by both the patient and physician. The patient should be given a full explanation about the potential risks and benefits prior to giving informed consent.

LABORATORY PROCEDURES

Used along with a patient's medical history and physical examination, laboratory tests can extend the physician's power of observation. They can provide information relating to the cause of a problem that can be obtained through no other means. The results of laboratory tests are considered along with other findings to determine a diagnosis. Laboratory tests are performed on any body fluid, including samples of blood, urine, or even feces. Tests may be used to assess the makeup of these substances or to detect factors that could be a sign of a disorder.

Laboratory tests may be used to detect disease when there are no symptoms present. They are part of a routine check-up. Other routine tests are a complete blood count (to measure white blood cells, red blood cells, hemoglobin in red blood cells, and the shape of blood cells) and urinalysis (to check the urine for its appearance, acidity level, protein, and abnormal cells). The results can be helpful in detecting early signs of disorders such as anemia or diabetes.

The results of these tests may be used to establish a diagnosis or to exclude the presence of disease. For instance, special blood tests can detect thyroid disease or heart damage. Normal values can rule out the presence of disease. This can be helpful when there are several diagnostic possibilities. Tests may also be useful to measure the severity of disease or to assess whether the present treatment has been effective.

Laboratory tests can aid in the regulation of therapy. They can be used to measure the level of a drug or medication in the blood to see if its concentration it is too high or too low so that adjustments can be made. For some drugs, it is important to maintain a certain blood level in the body, so that it can be effective without doing harm or becoming toxic.

Laboratory tests have a wide variety of uses in all levels of patient care. In addition to diagnosing disorders, they are used to check blood types and test compatibility before transfusion or transplants, to detect genetic disorders, and to protect the blood supply from infections.

It is important to remember, however, that these tests can produce false results. The results can vary from one laboratory to another, and the interpretation of the results may vary from one region to another. In some cases, it may be necessary to repeat a test or perform additional tests.

IMAGING TESTS

The technology that allows physicians to create an image of the body has become increasingly advanced. Imaging tests are often not only complex but also costly. There are five basic ways of creating an image of the inside of the body: radiography, computed tomography (CT), ultrasonography, nuclear imaging, and magnetic resonance imaging (MRI). In addition to showing an image of a part of the body, some of these tests also show body function and movement.

All imaging tests involve sending some form of energy into the body, detecting the energy that comes out, and converting the detected signal into an image. Radiography and CT scanning use X-rays, nuclear medicine uses gamma rays, MRI uses radio waves, and ultrasonography uses sound waves.

X-ray penetration of the body tissues depends on their composition, since different parts of the body register differently on the X-ray film. The thicker or more dense the tissue, the lighter the image, and conversely the less dense or thinner the tissue the darker the image. For this reason, radiography can easily identify calcium, fat, and air, but cannot as easily differentiate between soft tissues of similar densities. CT scanning is 10 to 20 times more sensitive than radiography in showing differences in tissue densities, and MRI is even more sensitive than CT scanning.

Certain parts of the body, such as bones and lungs, are easily studied on radiographic images because they contrast naturally with surrounding tissues. Other parts of the body—such as the brain, gastrointestinal tract, genitourinary system, liver, and spleen—cannot be easily viewed via X-rays. Contrast agents—swallowed or injected into the veins—are used to help make these body parts stand out more clearly on X-rays.

Barium is one such contrast agent. If barium is swallowed, the upper gastrointestinal tract (esophagus, stomach, and small bowel) can be studied on X-ray film. If it is introduced in an enema, the lower gastrointestinal tract (large bowel) can be viewed. A technique called fluoroscopy allows an X-ray image to appear on a television monitor which shows live action and can show movement during the X-ray exam. The combination of regular X-ray and fluoroscopy allows the entire gastrointestinal tract to be examined. Barium coats the bowel and allows the inside of the bowel to be seen during fluoroscopy; this also shows the movement of the barium through the bowel.

Other contrast agents can be injected into the veins and arteries. The contrast agents contain iodine compound and mix with the blood to give it increased density. By injecting a contrast agent into the veins and using both fluoroscopy and rapid filming techniques, blood vessels in many parts of the body, including the heart and the brain, can be evaluated. This is called angiography. Once contrast is diluted in the blood it is eventually removed by the kidneys; this also allows us to view the kidneys and bladder.

Nuclear medicine studies use radioisotopes that emit gamma rays. Gamma rays are identical to plain X-rays except that they originate from radioactive material that can be placed inside the patient. These materials only last inside the patient for short periods of time and expose her to an amount of radiation similar to that of a regular X-ray. The radioisotopes are injected into the veins to assess organs such as the brain, liver, bones, heart, kidneys, and gallbladder. Specific isotopes are concentrated in the different organs and emit gamma rays; they are captured by a device (gamma camera) that creates an image by detecting the radiation in the body. Another technique, called positron emission tomography (PET) scanning uses radioisotopes, which are very sensitive in measuring the functional activity of different organs, including the brain and heart. The equipment also produces cross-sectional images.

Advances in computer technology have created new methods to acquire and display images. Ultrasonography, computed tomography, and magnetic resonance imaging use various forms of energy to create a signal that is then computerized into a cross-sectional image. Whereas an X-ray is a photograph that shows structures along their length and width, these cross-sectional images obtain multiple views at different levels in the patient, allowing the viewer to see the patient in three dimensions.

Advances in radiologic imaging have allowed physicians to view the body in more detail while using lower doses of radiation. Both X-rays and gamma rays are ionizing radiation, however, and can harm cells at high levels with prolonged exposure. Ultrasound causes no known damage and is the preferred imaging technique for pregnant women for that reason. MRI is also safe at the strengths currently used.

Side effects can be caused by contrast agents, particularly those which are injected. Some side effects, such as skin rashes, hives, and itching, are temporary. More serious side effects, such as swelling of the larynx (voice box) and high or low blood pressure, require immediate treatment. If you've had any previous reactions to contrast agents, you should tell your doctor before a procedure is performed. Medication can be given in advance to prevent some reactions or another agent or study can be used instead.

New techniques, combined with the use of contrast agents, have dramatically improved the ability of physicians to diagnose problems. This technology has reduced the number of surgical procedures required for diagnosis and provides detailed information on the anatomy and function of the organs before a procedure is performed. Before undergoing any imaging study, patients should ask about the latest developments, the options available, and the contrast agents that will be used.

Radiographic Imaging

Plain X-Rays

X-rays can be used to evaluate all parts of the body. Either a single film or a set of films taken in different views can be performed to gain additional information. These films are obtained by positioning the patient in front of a tube that generates the X-rays. The X-rays penetrate the tissues and expose the X-ray film, which is placed inside a plastic holder on the side of the patient opposite the tube. The X-ray film is later developed in a developer similar to a developer for photographic film.

The GI Tract: Upper GI Series

Radiographic imaging of the upper gastrointestinal system includes studies of the esophagus, stomach, and small bowel. A contrast agent (barium) is swallowed by the patient and its progress through the body is followed using fluoroscopy. Additional films may also be taken of specific problem areas. Delayed films, sometimes even an hour later show the progress of the contrast agent as it moves beyond the stomach, and through the small bowel to the colon.

Barium Enema

The large bowel is studied by introducing the contrast agent through an enema. Fluoroscopy is used to follow the agent's progression from the rectum (the 8 to 10 inches of the large bowel that connect to the anus) to the opposite end of the colon near its junction with the small bowel. Air may be introduced to bring out the fine structure of the bowel lining.

Intravenous Pyelogram (IVP)

The urinary tract can be studied by injecting a contrast agent, containing iodine, into a vein which mixes with the blood. As the agent is extracted by the kidneys, images are obtained to assess the kidneys themselves as well as the tube connecting the kidney to the bladder (ureter), which carries the urine to the bladder. From the bladder, the agent is voided through the

urethra. Images are obtained at regular intervals after the contrast agent is injected to allow the physician to view the different structures of the urinary tract as the contrast passes through them.

Mammography

Mammography is a radiographic examination of the breast that uses specialized equipment designed specifically to evaluate features of soft tissue (See Fig. A.1). A device is used to compress the breast and to hold it in place during the examination. Compression makes the breast thinner during the exam, which allows for both better images and the ability to see fine details as well as better distribution of the various tissues within the breast. Although this part of the procedure may be somewhat uncomfortable, it does not last long or cause any harm to the breast. Two images of each breast are routinely taken, one from the top to the bottom and

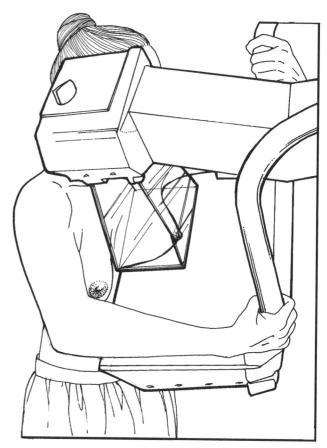

Figure A1.   Mammography
Mammography uses X-rays to examine the breast tissue. The breast is compressed between two flat plates for the procedure. Multiple views of each breast from different angles allow all of the breast tissue to be examined for any lumps or masses. The level of radiation delivered during mammography is very low, making the risks of the procedure minimal.

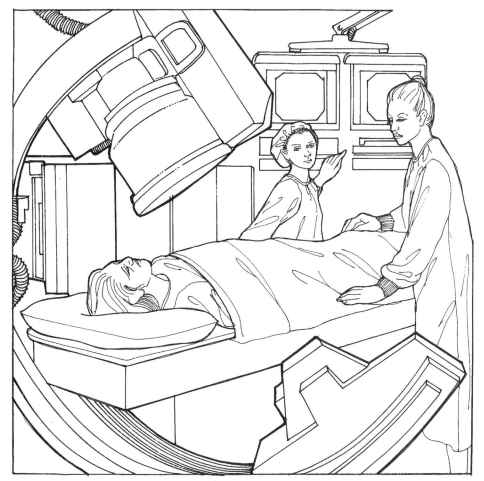

Figure A2 Angiography
Angiography provides important information about the blood vessels throughout the body. In this procedure, a catheter is inserted into a vein in either the arm (if only the vessels of the upper body are to be examined) or the groin area (for a whole-body angiogram) and passed through the vessel into the heart. A contrast medium is then injected through the catheter, and X-rays are used to see the movement of blood flow. The procedure allows the detection of abnormalities such as blockage or narrowing of the blood vessels.

from side to side. They are then examined for signs of lumps or masses. Small deposits of calcium may also be detected, which (depending on their pattern) may necessitate further evaluation.

Screening

When mammography is performed in women who do not have symptoms or risk factors, it is called screening mammography and is used to search for unsuspected cancers. It can also be used to evaluate specific problems related to the breast, such as a lump, to determine whether it is benign or malignant. This is a diagnostic mammogram.

Angiography

The arteries and veins throughout the body and head can be examined by inserting catheters into them and injecting contrast material. To image the contrast as it is rapidly moving in the vessels, movies or rapid sequence images are taken using X-rays. This visualization of the vessels is called angiography (See Fig. A.2).

The equipment to obtain these images has become very sophisticated, so that images can be obtained simultaneously at 90 degrees to each other (see equipment in figure). This is important as it allows accurate determination in two dimensions as to whether a vessel is diseased, narrowed or dilated.

Nuclear Medicine

Nuclear Scans

When radioisotopes are injected into a vein, they are taken up by the organs. Different organs take up different contrast agents. Specific compounds are used to view the liver, spleen, bones, brain, thyroid, kidneys, and heart. To create an image of the structure, scintillation scanners (gamma cameras) are used. This scanning gives a two-dimensional view of the gamma rays emitted by the radioisotope, revealing its concentration in a specific part of the body.

The time required for imaging depends on the compound being used and the part of the body being scanned. An image of the liver and spleen may be obtained within 30 minutes of injection, whereas images of radioisotope uptake in the bones are obtained at least 3 to 4 hours after injection.

PET Scans

Positron emission tomography (PET) is another form of nuclear medicine. It also involves injection of radioactive compounds into the blood. It utilizes specialized compounds, primarily for imaging the brain and heart. It is also extremely expensive and currently is used mainly for investigational procedures.

Ultrasonography

Ultrasound was derived from the sonar technique first used during World War II to detect submarines. It uses the physical characteristics of sound waves to send and receive signals as they pass through a medium. If there is no medium, no sound can be heard.

High-frequency sound waves are sent into the body by a device called a transducer. These sound waves bounce off parts of the body and are returned as echoes. The transducer also acts as a receiver of the echoes reflected from the tissues encountered by the sound waves. The return of the echoes is timed to map the area. The returning echoes are used to construct the image of the part of the body being studied.

Sound waves can also be used without creating an image. In Doppler ultrasound, sound waves create audible signals to evaluate motion. This technique analyzes the flow of blood in the veins and arteries and reveals if there is an obstruction or blood clot in the vessels. Doppler ultrasound is also used to monitor the heartbeat of a baby during labor.

Different transducers are used for different organs, because the frequency of the sound waves determines how deep they can penetrate and the degree of resolution of the image. For women, an ultrasound exam can be done with an abdominal transducer (passed over the abdomen) or with a vaginal transducer (inserted into the vagina) to study the pelvic organs. Ultrasound can be used to obtain good images of the liver, gallbladder, pancreas, spleen, kidneys, bladder, uterus, and ovaries. The air in the lungs limits the use of ultrasound for examinations of the chest. However, ultrasound is very useful in examining the heart (echocardiogram). It can show how well the heart muscle contracts and also how well the valves in the heart are working.

Ultrasound does not use ionizing radiation, so there is no known risk from the test. It has been used for more than 25 years and there is as yet no confirmed biologic effect at the levels used for most examinations. Because this test is considered to be safe, it is used to view a developing fetus. Although it can be of value in assessing some problems and in confirming the growth of the fetus, the test should not be used routinely.

Computed Tomography

For a CT scan, the patient is placed on a table that is then moved into the scanner (See Fig. A.3). The table advances during the procedure, while the stationary scanner acquires the images. The X-rays are generated by tubes within the scanner.

CT studies are used to examine the head, neck, chest, abdomen, pelvis, and extremities (arms and legs). The technique is very precise and can pick up anatomic details smaller than 1 millimeter. Because CT images show depth, soft tissues, muscles, nerves, blood vessels, bones, and different organs can be viewed without having one structure superimposed on another (as seen in radiographs). A CT scan allows one organ to be distinguished from another and is able to detect abnormalities within organs.

Depending on the condition being evaluated and the body area to be examined, intravenous, oral, or rectal contrast agents may be used during the procedure. Intravenous contrast agents are given to show problems in blood vessels. Abnormalities in surrounding soft tissues, such as lymph nodes next to blood

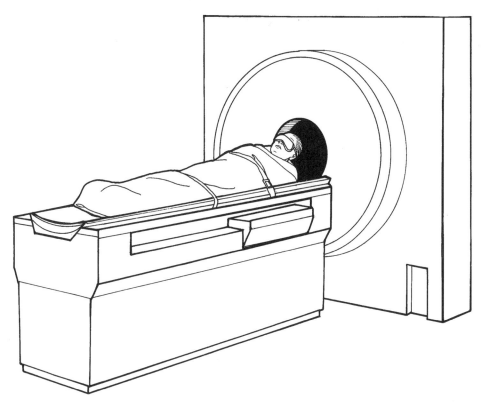

Figure A3 Computed Tomography
Computed tomography (CT) allows the visualization of soft tissue, including muscles, nerves, organs, and blood vessels. For a CT scan, the patient lies on a long, narrow platform that is then moved into a hollow, tunnellike machine. Depending on what part of the body is to be viewed, the platform may be moved part or all of the way into the scanner. Often a contrast medium, given orally, intravenously, or anally, is used to enhance the body part or area being examined. Inside the scanner, X-ray tubes can allow the detection of structures within the body of less than a millimeter in diameter. The resolution and detail provided by CT scanning makes it preferable to conventional X-rays in certain circumstances.

vessels, also can be studied in this manner. Oral contrast agents are used to highlight the gastrointestinal system, including the esophagus, stomach, and small and large bowels. Sometimes these agents are introduced into the rectum so the lower part of the large bowel can be better viewed.

CT scanning can be used to guide other procedures. A sample of tissue from inside the body can be obtained more safely when the doctor is being guided by the CT scan. The image shows the body's internal structure, so the doctor can direct the biopsy instruments to a specific site while avoiding other tissues.

The latest generation of CT scanners obtains images very quickly. An examination of the entire chest can be completed within a single breath held for 20 seconds. Total examination time, however, includes introduction of the contrast agents (if necessary) and setting up the equipment for the test, so the actual scan time is highly variable.

Magnetic Resonance Imaging

Radio waves within magnetic fields are used to create images of the head and body with magnetic resonance imaging. Although MRI scanners look similar to CT scanners on the outside, the MRI scanners contain a strong magnet, whereas CT scanners contain X-ray tubes. When placed in a magnetic field, certain molecules in the body will be affected and align themselves with the magnet. Radio waves (similar to those used in a standard radio) are then directed through the patient. This causes the molecules which are aligned with the magnet to change their direction. These molecules then emit radio waves of their own, which are picked up by a coil (antenna) within the scanner. This creates a signal which is then analyzed by a sophisticated computer to form an image. Information on the makeup of body tissues and blood flow can be obtained from the strength of the magnetic field and the sequence of the radio wave pulses, from which the computer creates an image.

The test is performed similarly to CT scanning. The patient lies on a table, which is then moved slowly into the MRI scanner. This surrounds the patient with a magnetic field, while radio waves are pulsed through the body and the computer analyzes the return signals, creating an image.

The images displayed via MRI are similar to those obtained from CT scanning, but they can show a greater variety of views. Unlike CT scans, blood flow can be studied without using a contrast agent. Specialized types of MRI equipment can give very detailed views of the joints, and are very useful for looking at cartilage, ligaments, and tendons. Depending on the problem, MRI may be used to supplement a CT study. For certain diseases of the nervous system, MRI can give information not obtained by CT scanning and is often the only examination necessary.

Associations and Organizations

1. A New National Focus on Women's Health

Office of Research on Women's Health, Building 1, Room 201, National Institutes of Health, 9000 Rockville Pike, Bethesda, Maryland 20892, 301-402-1770

Office on Women's Health, 200 Independence Avenue, SW, Washington, DC 20201, 202-690-7650

Women's Health & Fertility Branch, National Center for Chronic Disease Prevention and Health Promotion, 1600 Clifton Road, NE, Atlanta, Georgia 30333, 404-329-3286

2. How to Cope with the Health Care System

American Hospital Association, 840 North Lake Shore Drive, Chicago, Illinois 60611, 800-242-2626 or 312-280-6000

American Medical Association, 515 North State Street, Chicago, Illinois 60610, 800-262-3211 or 312-464-5000

Health Care Financing Association, 200 Independence Avenue, SW, Room 428-H, Washington, DC 20201, 202-245-6145

Health Resources and Services Administration, 5600 Fishers Lane, Parklawn Building, Room 14-05, Rockville, Maryland 20857, 301-443-2216

Joint Commission on the Accreditation of Healthcare Organizations, 1 Renaissance Boulevard, Oakbrook Terrace, Illinois 60181, 708-916-5600

3. Diet, Nutrition, and Healthy Weight

American Dietetic Association, 216 West Jackson Boulevard, Suite 800, Chicago, Illinois 60606, 312-899-0040

Institute of Medicine, 2101 Constitution Avenue, NW, Washington, DC 20418, 202-334-2169

The National Agricultural Library, Food and Nutrition Information Center, Room 304, Beltsville, Maryland 20705, 301-504-5472

Human Nutrition Information Service, US Department of Agriculture, Hyattsville, Maryland 20782, 301-436-7725

4. Exercise and Physical Fitness

American College of Sports Medicine, PO Box 1440, Indianapolis, Indiana 46206, 317-637-9200

Sports Gynecology Society, c/o Mona M. Shangold, MD, Department of Ob-Gyn, Hahneman University - MS 958, 1427 Vine Street, Suite 315, Philadelphia, Pennsylvania 19102, 212-762-6866

5. Living in a Healthy Environment

See Chapter 5, "Health Watch"

6. Working in a Healthy Environment

Association of Occupational and Environmental Clinics, 1010 Vermont Avenue, NW, Suite 513, Washington, D.C. 20005, 202-347-4976

CHEMTREC, 2501 M Street, NW, Washington, D.C. 20037, 800-262-8200

Equal Employment Opportunity Commission, 7 World Trade Center, 18th Floor, New York, NY 10048, 800-669-4000

National Institute for Occupational Safety and Health, 4676 Columbia Parkway, Cincinnati, OH 45226-1998, 800-356-4674

Occupational Safety and Health Administration, U.S. Department of Labor, 200 Constitution Avenue, NW, Washington, D.C. 20210, 202-219-8151

Office of Occupational Medicine, U.S. Department of Labor, 200 Constitution Avenue, NW, Washington, D.C. 20210, 202-219-5003

7. Chemical Dependencies

Alcoholics Anonymous (World Services), 475 Riverside Drive, New York, NY 10163, 212-870-3400

Al-Anon (Family Group Headquarters), PO Box 862, Midtown Station, New York, NY 10018, 212-302-7240

Al-Ateen, check your local listing for nearest branch

COCAINE Hotline, 800-262-2463

Narcotics Anonymous, PO Box 9999, Van Nuys, CA 91409, 818-780-3951

National Association for Children of Alcoholics, 11426 Rockville Pike, Suite 100, Rockville, MD 20852, 301-468-0985

National Institute on Drug Abuse, 800-662-HELP (English); 800-662-AYUDA (Spanish)

8. Mental Health

American Psychiatric Association, 1400 K Street, NW, Washington, DC 20005, 202-682-6000
American Psychological Association, 750 First Street, NW, Washington, DC 20002, 202-336-5500
National Institute of Mental Health, 5600 Fishers Lane, Room 15C-05, Rockville, Maryland 20857, 301-443-4513
National Mental Health Association, 1021 Prince Street, Alexandria, Virginia 22314-2971, 703-684-7722

9. Staying Healthy in Spite of Stress

American Institute of Stress, 124 Park Avenue, Yonkers, New York 10703, 914-963-1200 or 800-24-RELAX
International Society for Traumatic Stress Studies, 435 North Michigan Avenue, Suite 1717, Chicago, Illinois 60611, 312-644-0828
International Stress Management Association, 10455 Pomerado Road, San Diego, California 92131, 619-693-4698

10. Violence and Women

National Center on Women and Family Law, 799 Broadway, Room 402, New York, New York 10033, 212-674-8200
National Coalition Against Domestic Violence, PO Box 18749, Denver, Colorado 80218, 303-839-1852
National Coalition Against Sexual Assault, PO Box 21378, Washington, DC 20009, 202-483-7165
National Crime Prevention Council, 1700 K Street, NW, 2nd Floor, Washington, DC 20006, 202-466-6272

11. Aging

Alzheimer's Association, Inc., 919 North Michigan Avenue, Suite 1000, Chicago, Illinois 60611-1676, 800-272-3900 or 312-355-8700
American Association for Retired Persons, 601 E Street, NW, Washington, DC 20024, 202-434-2277
American Geriatrics Society, 770 Lexington Avenue, Suite 300, New York, New York 10021, 212-308-1414
American Society on Aging, 833 Market Street, Suite 512, San Francisco, California 94103, 415-882-2910
The Gerontological Society of America, 1275 K Street, NW, Suite 350, Washington, DC 20005, 202-842-1275
National Council on the Aging, Inc., 409 Third Street, SW, 2nd floor, Washington, DC 20024, 800-424-9046
National Institute on Aging, 9000 Rockville Pike, Bethesda, Maryland 20892

12. Sexuality

American Association of Sex Educators, Counselors and Therapists, 435 Michigan Avenue, Suite 1717, Chicago, Illinois 60611, 312-644-0828
Council for Sex Information and Education, 2272 Colorado Boulevard, No. 1228, Los Angeles, California 90041

13. Genetics

American Board of Medical Genetics, 9650 Rockville Pike, Bethesda, Maryland 20814, 301-571-1825

14. Genetic Counseling

Alliance of Genetic Support Groups, 35 Wisconson Circle, Suite 440, Chevy Chae, MD 20815, 800-336-GENE; 301-652-5553
March of Dimes Birth Defects Foundation, 1275 Mamaroneck Avenue, White Plains, NY 10605, 914-428-7100
Metabolic Information Network, P.O. Box 670847, Dallas, TX 75367-08547, 214-696-2188; 945-2188
National Center for Education in Maternal & Child Health, 2000 15th Street North, Suite 701, Arlington, VA 22201-2617, 703-524-7802
National Organization for Rare Disorders, P.O. Box 8923, New Fairfield, CT 06812-1783, 203-746-6518; 800-999-NORD
National Society of Genetic Counselors, 233 Canterbury Drive, Wallingford, PA 19086, 215-872-7608

15. The Reproductive System

American College of Obstetricians and Gynecologists, 409 12th Street, SW, Washington, DC 20024, 800-673-8444 or 202-638-5577
American Urological Association, 112 North Charles Street, Baltimore, Maryland 21201, 410-727-1100
Association of Reproductive Health Professionals, 2401 Pennsylvania Avenue, NW, Suite 350, Washington, DC 20037, 202-466-3825

16. Understanding Your Fertility

American College of Obsetricians and Gynecologists, 409 12th Street, NW, Washington, DC 20024, 800-673-8444 or 638-5577
American Fertility Society, 1209 Montgomery Highway, Birmingham, Alabama 35216, 205-978-5000
Society for the Prevention of Human Infertility, 877 Park Avenue, New York, New York 10021, 212-288-3737

17. Pregnancy and Childbirth

American College of Nurse Midwives, 1522 K Street, NW, Suite 1000, Washington, DC 20005, 202-289-0171
American College of Obstetricians and Gynecologists, 409 12th Street, NW, Washington, DC 20024, 800-673-8444 or 638-5577
International Childbirth Education Association, PO Box 20024, Minneapolis, Minnesota 55420, 800-624-4934

18. Breastfeeding

Human Lactation Center, 666 Sturges Highway, Westport, Connecticut 06880, 203-259-5995
La Leche League International, PO Box 1209, Franklin Park, Illinois 60131, 708-455-7730 or 800-LA LECHE

19. Sexually Transmitted Diseases

American College of Obstetrics and Gynecology, 409 12th Street, SW, Washington, DC 20024, 800-673-8444 or 202-638-5577

American Social Health Association, PO Box 13827, Research Triangle Park, North Carolina 27709, 919-361-8400

Centers for Disease Control and Prevention, 1600 Clifton Road, NE, Atlanta, Georgia 30333

20. AIDS and Women

National AIDS Hotine, 800-342-AIDS (English); 800-344-AIDS (Spanish); 800-AIDS-TTY (deaf access)

CDC National AIDS Clearinghouse, P.O. Box 6003, Rockville, MD 20849-6003

21. Accidents and Emergencies

American Red Cross, 431 18th Street, NW, Washington, DC 20006, 202-737-8300

American Trauma Society, 8903 Presidential Parkway, Suite 512, Upper Marlboro, Maryland 20772, 800-556-7890 or 301-420-4189

22. The Nervous System

American Association of Neurologic Surgeons, 22 South Washington Street, Park Ridge, Illinois 60068, 708-692-9500

American Brain Tumor Association, 3725 North Talman Avenue, Chicago, Illinois 60618, 800-866-2282 or 312-286-5571

American Parkinson's Disease Association, 60 Bay Street, Suite 401, Staten Island, New York 10301, 800-223-2732

Brain Tumor Society, 258 Harvard Street, Suite 308, Brookline, Massachusetts 02146, 617-243-4229

Epilepsy Foundation of America, 4351 Garden City Drive, Suite 406, Landover, Maryland 20785, 800-EFA-1000 or 301-459-3700

The National Head Injury Foundation, Inc. 1140 Connecticut Avenue, NW, Suite 812, Washington, DC 20036, 800-444-NHIF or 202-296-6443

National Headache Foundation, 4242 North Western Avenue, Chicago, Illinois 60625, 800-843-2256 or 312-878-7715

National Institute of Neurological Disorders and Stroke, Office of Scientific and Health Reports, PO Box 5801, Bethesda, Maryland 20824, 800-352-9424 or 301-496-5751

National Spinal Cord Injury Association, 600 West Cummings Park, Suite 2000, Qovuen, Massachusetts 01801, 800-962-9629 or 617-935-2722

23. The Eyes

American Academy of Ophthalmology, 655 Beach Street, San Francisco, California 94109, 415-561-8500

American Foundation for the Blind, 15 West 16th Street, New York, New York 10011, 800-232-4563 or 212-620-2000

American Optometric Association, 243 North Lindbergh Boulevard, St. Louis, Missouri 63141, 314-991-4100

Glaucoma Support Network, Foundation for Glaucoma Research, 490 Post Street, Suite 830, San Francisco, California 94102

National Eye Institute, 9000 Rockville Pike, Bethesda, Maryland 20892, 301-496-2234

24. Ears, Nose, and Throat

American Academy of Otolaryngology-Head and Neck Surgery, One Prince Street, Alexandria, Virginia 22314, 703-936-4444

American Speech-Language-Hearing Association, 10801 Rockville Pike, Rockville, Maryland 20852, 800-638-5700 or 301-571-0457

American Tinnitus Association, PO Box 5, Portland, Oregon 97207, 503-248-9985

Better Hearing Institute, PO Box 1840, Washington, DC 20013, 800-327-9355

The Deafness Research Foundation, 9 East 38th Street, New York, New York 10016, 800-535-3323

National Association for the Deaf, 814 Thayer Avenue, Silver Spring, Maryland 20910, 301-587-1788 or 301-587-1789 (TDD)

National Information Center on Deafness, Gallaudet University, 800 Florida Avenue, NE, Washington DC 20002, 202-651-5051 or 202-651-5052 (TDD)

National Institute on Deafness and Other Communication Disorders, 9000 Rockville Pike, Building 31, Room 3C-35, Bethesda, Maryland 20892 301-496-7243 or 301-402-0252 (TDD)

25. The Breast

National Alliance of Breast Cancer Organizations, 1180 Avenue of the Americas, 2nd Floor, New York, New York 10036, 212-719-0154

Society for the Study of Breast Disease, 3409 Worth, Suite 300, Sammons Tower, Dallas, Texas 75246, 214-821-2962

26. The Respiratory System

American Lung Association, 1740 Broadway, New York, New York 20019, 800-LUNG-USA

National Heart, Lung, and Blood Institute, PO Box 30105, Bethesda, Maryland 20824, 301-251-1222

National Institute of Allergy and Infectious Diseases, Building 31, Room 7A-32, Bethesda, Maryland 20892, 301-496-5717

27. The Cardiovascular System

American College of Cardiology, 9111 Old Georgetown Road, Bethesda, Maryland 2081-1699, 800-253-4636 or 302-897-9745

American Heart Association, 7320 Greenville Avenue, Dallas, Texas 75231, 800-AHA-8721

National Heart, Lung, and Blood Institute, PO Box 30105, Bethesda, Maryland 20824, 800-352-9424 or 301-496-5751

National Rehabilitation Information Center, 8455 Colesville Road, Suite 935, Silver Spring, Maryland 800-34-NARIC (voice/TDD) or 301-588-9284

28. Hypertension

American College of Cardiology, 9111 Old Georgetown Road, Bethesda, Maryland 2081-1699, 800-253-4636 or 302-897-9745

American Society of Hypertension, 515 Madison Avenue, Suite 1515, New York, New York 10022, 212-644-0650

American Heart Association, 7320 Greenville Avenue, Dallas, Texas 75231-4599, 214-373-6300

National Heart, Lung, and Blood Institute, Information Center, PO Box 30105, Bethesda, Maryland 20824, 301-951-3260

National Hypertension Association, 324 East 30th Street, New York, New York 10016, 212-889-3557

29. The Blood and Lymphatic System

International Center for Control of Nutritional Anemia, 3901 Rainbow Boulevard, Kansas City, Kansas 66160, 913-588-7037

National Association for Sickle Cell Disease, 3345 Wilshire Boulevard, Suite 1106, Los Angeles, California 90010, 800-421-8453 or 203-736-5455 (in California)

National Heart, Lung, and Blood Institute, Information Center, PO Box 30105, Bethesda, Maryland 20824, 301-951-3260

30. The Endocrine System

American Diabetes Association, 1660 Duke Street, Alexandria, Virginia 22314, 800-ADA-DISC or 703-232-3472

The Thyroid Foundation of American, Inc., Massachusetts General Hospital, Ruth Sleeper Hall, Room 350, Boston, Massachusetts 02114, 617-726-8500

Endocrine Society, 9650 Rockville Pike, Bethesda, Maryland 20814, 301-571-1800

National Institute of Diabetes and Digestive and Kidney Diseases, National Institutes of Health, 900 Rockville Pike, Bethesda, Maryland 20892, 301-496-5877

North American Menopause Society, 4074 Abington Road, Cleveland, Ohio 44106, 216-844-3334

31. The Immune System and Allergies

American Academy of Allergy and Immunology, 611 East Wells Street, Milwaukee, Wisconsin 53202, 800-822-2762 or 414-272-6071

American Allergy Association, PO Box 7273, Menlo Park, California 94026, 415-328-2295

Asthma and Allergy Foundation of America, 1125 15th Street, NW, Suite 502, Washington, DC 20005, 800-7ASTHMA or 202-466-7643

National Institute of Allergy and Infectious Diseases, Building 31, Room 7A-32, Bethesda, Maryland 20892, 301-496-5717

32. The Kidneys and the Urinary System

American Urological Association, 1120 North Charles Street, Baltimore, Maryland 21201, 410-727-1100

The National Kidney and Urologic Diseases Information Clearinghouse, PO Box NKUDIC, 9000 Rockville Pike, Bethesda, Maryland 20892 (contact by mail)

National Kidney Foundation, 30 East 33rd Street, New York, anew York 10016, 800-622-9010 or 212-889-2210

33. The Digestive System

American Liver Foundation, 1425 Pompton Avenue, Cedar Grove, New Jersey 07009, 800-223-2550 or 201-256-3214

Center for Digestive Disorders, 550 East Washington Street, West Chicago, Illinois 60185, 708-260-2685

Crohn's and Colitis Foundation of American, Inc., 444 Park Avenue South, New York, New York 10016, 800-343-3637 or 212-685-3440

National Digestive Diseases Information Clearinghouse, PO Box NDDIC, 9000 Rockville Pike, Bethesda, Maryland 20892 (contact by mail)

National Institute of Diabetes and Digestive and Kidney Diseases, National Institutes of Health, 900 Rockville Pike, Bethesda, Maryland 20892, 301-496-5877

34. The Musculoskeletal System

American Academy of Orthopaedic Surgeons, 222 South Prospect Avenue, Park Ridge, Illinois 60068, 800-346-AAOS, 708-823-7186

American Lupus Society, 3914 Del Amo Boulevard, #922, Torrance, California 90503, 310-542-8891

Arthritis Foundation, PO Box 19000, Atlanta, Georgia 30326, 800-283-7800 ot 404-872-7100

National Arthritis and Musculoskeletal and Skin Diseases Information Clearinghouse, PO Box AMS, 9000 Rockville Pike, Bethesda, Maryland 20892, 301-495-4484

35. Skin, Hair, Nails

American Academy of Dermatology, PO Box 4014, Schaumberg, Illinois 60168-4014, 708-330-0230

National Arthritis and Musculoskeletal and Skin Diseases Information Clearinghouse, PO Box AMS, 9000 Rockville Pike, Bethesda, Maryland 20892, 301-495-4484

National Psoriasis Foundation, 6443 SW Beaverton Highway, Suite 210, Portland, Oregon 97221, 503-297-1545

36. Reconstructive and Plastic Surgery

American Academy of Facial Plastic and Reconstructive Surgery, 1101 Vermont Ave., NW, Suite 220, Washington, D.C. 20005, 202-842-4500

American Board of Plastic Surgery, 7 Penn Center, Suite 400, 1635 Market Street, Philadelphia, PA 19103, 215-587-9322

American Society for Aesthetic Plastic Surgery, 3922 Atlantic Avenue, Long Beach, CA 90807, 310-595-4275

American Society of Plastic and Reconstructive Surgeons, 444 East Algonquin Road, Suite 110, Arlington Heights, IL 60005, 708-228-9900

37. Cancer in Women

American Cancer Society, Inc., 1599 Clifton Road, NE, Atlanta, Georgia 30329,800-ACS-2345 or 404-320-3333

Cancer Research Institute, Inc., 133 East 58th Street, New York, New York 10022, 212-688-7515

National Cancer Institute, Public Inquiries Office, 9000 Rockville Pike, Building 31, Room 10A24, Bethesda, Maryland 20892, 800-4-CANCER

Society of Gynecologic Oncologists, 401 North Michigan Avenue, Chicago, Illinois 60611, 312-644-6610

38. Pain Evaluation and Management

American Academy of Pain Medicine, 5700 Old Orchard Road, 1st Floor, Skokie, Illinois 60077, 708-966-9510

American Chronic Pain Association, PO Box 850, Rocklin, California 95677, 916-632-0922

American Society of Anesthesiologists, 520 North Northwest Highway, Park Ridge, Illinois 60068, 708-825-5586

39. Managing Medication

American Pharmaceutical Association, 2215 Constitution Avenue, NW, Washington, DC 20037, 202-628-4410 or 800-237-APHA

Food and Drug Administration, Center for Biologics Evaluation and Research, 8800 Rockville Pike, Building 29-NIH Campus, Bethesda, Maryland 20852, 301-295-8228

Pharmaceutical Manufacturers Association, 1100 15th Street, NW, Washington, DC 20005, 202-835-3400

Appendix: Diagnostic Tests

American College of Radiology, 1891 Preston White Drive, Reston, Virginia 22092, 703-648-8900

Editors and Contributors

MEDICAL CO-EDITORS

Roselyn Payne Epps, M.D., M.P.H., M.A., F.A.A.P., is an expert at the National Institutes of Health, Bethesda, Maryland, and a Professor at Howard University College of Medicine, Washington, D.C. She is recognized nationally and internationally in areas of health policy and research, health promotion and disease prevention, and medical education and health service delivery. As a pioneer and leader in numerous professional and community organizations, she served, in 1991, as the first African-American president of AMWA and the founding president of the AMWA Foundation.

Susan Cobb Stewart, M.D., F.A.C.P., is an internist and gastroenterologist, and is presently Associate Medical Director at J.P. Morgan in New York, where she delivers general medical care, specialty consultations, and preventive services. She is Clinical Assistant Professor of Medicine at SUNY, Brooklyn. Since serving as President of AMWA in 1990, Dr. Stewart has continued to help AMWA shape and focus its mission in the area of women's health.

CONTRIBUTORS

Elizabeth A. Abel, M.D., F.A.A.D., is in private practice in Mountain View, California, and is a Clinical Associate Professor of Dermatology at Stanford University School of Medicine. Dr. Abel is Assistant Editor of the *Journal of the American Academy of Dermatology* and a member of the Medical Advisory Board of the National Psoriasis Foundation.

Diane L. Adams, M.D., M.P.H., is the medical officer in the Office of Science and Date Technology, U.S. Agency for Health Care Policy and Research. She is also an Associate Professor at the University of Maryland, Eastern Shore. Her research activities have focused on occupational and environmental health, rural health, and minority and women's health.

Judith C. Ahronheim, M.D., F.A.C.P., a nationally recognized specialist in geriatrics, is Attending Physician at Mount Sinai Medical Center in New York. She is also Associate Professor of Medicine and Associate Professor of Geriatrics at Mount Sinai School of Medicine. Dr. Ahronheim serves on the Ethics Committee of the American Geriatrics Society.

Jeanne F. Arnold, M.D., F.A.A.F.P., is Director of the Malden Hospital Family Practice Residency Program in Boston, Massachusetts. She is a Clinical Assistant Professor at the Boston University School of Medicine. She has served on the Board of Directors of the American Academy of Family Physicians and has chaired the Research Committee and the Committee on Women in Medicine.

Penny A. Asbell, M.D., F.A.C.S., is an Associate Professor of Ophthalmology at Mount Sinai School of Medicine and Director of the Cornea Service at Mount Sinai Medical Center in New York. Dr. Asbell is a certified investigator in the Herpetic Eye Disease Study. Currently, Dr. Asbell is the president-elect of the Contact Lens Association for Ophthalmologists and the past president and founder of Women in Ophthalmology, Inc.

Susan Aucott Ballagh, M.D., has advanced training in reproductive endocrinology and is Director of the Stanford Women's Group, Stanford Health Services. She is an Assistant Professor of Obstetrics and Gynecology at Stanford University School of Medicine, Palo Alto, California.

Claudia R. Baquet, M.D., M.P.H., serves as Visiting Scholar in Health Policy and Assistant Dean for Health Affairs at the University of Maryland School of Medicine in Baltimore, Maryland. She developed and implemented the first national cancer prevention and control intervention research program that focuses solely on African-American and Native American populations.

Barbara Bartlik, M.D., is a psychiatrist in private practice in New York City and is on staff at the Human Sexuality Teaching Program at New York Hospital-Cornell Medical Center. She has expertise in the psychiatric aspects of disorders related to the female reproductive system.

Ana Bartolomei Aguilera, M.D., is in private practice in ophthalmology in San Juan, Puerto Rico. She has advanced training in cornea and external diseases of the eye at Mount Sinai Medical Center in New York.

Doris Gorka Bartuska, M.D., F.A.C.P., F.A.C.E., is Director, Division of Endocrinology, Diabetes, and Metabolism at the Medical College of Pennsylvania and Hahnemann University, where she is Professor of Medicine. She is on the Board of Directors of the American Association of Clinical Endocrinologists. She is a past president of AMWA (1988).

Tamara G. Bavendam, M.D., F.A.C.S., is Director of Female Urology at the University of Washington School of Med-

Seattle, where she is an Assistant Professor of Urology. She has developed a multispecialty, multidisciplinary approach to urological problems in women.

Susan J. Blumenthal, M.D., M.P.A., F.A.P.A., serves as Assistant Surgeon General and Rear Admiral in the United States Public Health Service and as a Clinical Professor of Psychiatry at Georgetown School of Medicine. She was recently appointed the country's first Deputy Assistant Secretary for Women's Health. Dr. Blumenthal is cofounder and served as Scientific Director of the Society for the Advancement of Women's Health Research.

Marjorie Braude, M.D., is a psychiatrist in private practice in Los Angeles, California. She has chaired the Domestic Violence Subcommittee of AMWA, and she chairs the City of Los Angeles Domestic Violence Task Force.

Carolyn Barley Britton, M.D., M.S., is an Associate Professor of Clinical Neurology and an Associate Attending at Columbia Presbyterian Medical Center. She is Director of Ambulatory Care for the Department of Neurology. She has served on the New York State Advisory Council to the AIDS Institute.

Linda M. Brzustowicz, M.D., is currently an Assistant Professor at the Center for Molecular and Behavioral Neuroscience of Rutgers University. She is also an Assistant Professor in the Department of Psychiatry of the University of Medicine and Dentistry of New Jersey. Her research focuses on genetic factors in psychiatric conditions and treatment.

Karen Laurie David, M.D., M.S., F.A.A.P., Diplomate of the American Board of Pediatrics, Diplomate of the American Board of Medical Genetics, has served since 1978 as Chief of the Section of Genetics in the Department of Obstetrics and Gynecology at the Brooklyn Hospital Center. She is also an Attending Physician in the Departments of Pediatrics, Obstetrics and Gynecology, and Pathology. Dr. David is a Clinical Associate Professor of Pediatrics at New York University Medical Center and School of Medicine.

Leah J. Dickstein, M.D., F.A.P.A., is a Professor in the Department of Psychiatry and Behavioral Sciences and Associate Dean for Faculty and Student Advocacy at the University of Louisville School of Medicine. She is a past president of AMWA (1992) and has served as vice-president of the American Psychiatric Association.

Zoe Diana Draelos, M.D., F.A.A.D., is in private practice at the Central Carolina Dermatology Clinic, Inc., in High Point, North Carolina. She is a Clinical Assistant Professor at Bowman Gray School of Medicine, Wake Forest University. She specializes in cosmetic dermatology.

Patricia G. Engasser, M.D., F.A.A.D., practices dermatology in northern California. Dr. Engasser is a Clinical Professor of Dermatology at Stanford University and an Associate Clinical Professor of Dermatology at University of California at San Francisco. Presently, she serves on the Executive Committee of the Board of Directors of the American Academy of Dermatology.

Elaine Bossak Feldman, M.D., F.A.C.P., is Professor Emerita of Medicine and Physiology and Endocrinology and Chief

Emerita of the Section of Nutrition at the Medical College of Georgia in Augusta. In addition, she is Director Emerita at the Georgia Institute of Human Nutrition and a former member of the Bureau of Scientific Counselors of the National Cancer Institute.

Kathleen M. Foley, M.D., is Attending Neurologist at both Memorial Sloan-Kettering Cancer Center and New York Hospital. She is a Professor of Neurology and Neuroscience and of Clinical Pharmacology at Cornell University Medical College. Further, she serves as a Consultant at Rockefeller University Hospital and Calvary Hospital.

Jean L. Fourcroy, M.D., PH.D., is a urologist with a primary interest in male reproductive endocrinology and toxicology. She is medical officer in the Division of Endocrinology and Metabolic Drug Products of the Food and Drug Administration. She is also an Assistant Professor of Surgery at the University of Health Sciences—F. Edward Hebert School of Medicine and the founder of Women in Urology. Dr. Fourcroy will serve as AMWA President in 1996.

Janet Emily Freedman, M.D., is the Acting Medical Director of Rehabilitation Medicine at Bellevue Hospital in New York. She is Assistant Professor of Rehabilitation Medicine at New York University Medical Center.

Anne Geller, M.D., a neurologist, is Chief of the Smithers Addiction, Treatment, and Training Center in New York. She is Senior Attending Physician in Medicine at St. Luke's/Roosevelt Hospital Center and Associate Professor of Clinical Medicine at Columbia College of Physicians and Surgeons. She is the 1993-1995 president of the American Society of Addiction Medicine.

Leslie Carroll Grammer, M.D., F.A.C.P., a specialist in allergy and immunology, is a Professor of Medicine at Northwestern University Medical School and Attending Physician at Northwestern Memorial Hospital in Chicago. She also serves on the FDA Advisory Committee for Pulmonary and Allergy Drugs. She served as Chairman of the American Academy of Allergy and Immunology in 1991.

Jean A. Hamilton, M.D., is a Professor of Psychology, Social and Health Sciences, and Women's Studies at Duke University and an Associate Professor in Psychiatry and Consultant to the general internal medicine section's "Women's Health Program" at Duke University Medical Center, Durham, North Carolina. She cofounded and served as Director of the Institute for Research on Women's Health.

Claudia I. Henschke, M.D., PH.D., is a Professor of Radiology at Cornell University Medical College in New York. She is also Attending Radiologist and Chief of the Division of Chest and Abdominal Imaging at the New York Hospital—Cornell Medical Center.

Debra R. Judelson, M.D., F.A.C.P., F.A.C.C., is a cardiologist and internist in private practice and a senior partner with the Cardiovascular Medical Group of Southern California. She is Chair of the Subcommittee on Cardiovascular Disease in Women for AMWA.

Lynn C. Kase, M.A., C.C.C.-A., owns the Dunshaw Hearing Aid Centers in New York. She is a member of the American

Speech and Hearing Association and a Fellow of the Academy of Dispensing Audiologists.

Lois Anne Katz, M.D., F.A.C.P., is Associate Chief of Staff for Ambulatory Care and Associate Chief of Nephrology at the New York Veterans Affairs Medical Center. She is an Associate Professor of Clinical Medicine at New York University School of Medicine.

Satty Gill Keswani, M.D., F.A.C.O.G., is a practicing reproductive endocrinologist in Livingston, New Jersey, specializing in infertility, and a Clinical Assistant Professor of Obstetrics and Gynecology at the University of Medicine and Dentistry of New Jersey, Newark. She is the AMWA representative to the United Nations.

Gwen S. Korovin, M.D., is an otolaryngologist who is in private practice in New York. She is an Attending Physician at Lenox Hill Hospital and is a consultant at the Ames Vocal Dynamics Laboratory, specializing in the care of the voice.

Ruth A. Lawrence, M.D., F.A.A.P., is a Professor of Pediatrics and Professor of Obstetrics and Gynecology at the University of Rochester. A national and international authority on lactation, she is a Consultant to the Breastfeeding Advisory Group of the State of New York Department of Health and to the International Childbirth Education Association.

Sandra P. Levison, M.D., F.A.C.P., is a Professor and Associate Chair of the Department of Medicine, Chief of the Division of Nephrology of the Medical College of Pennsylvania and Hahnemann University, and serves as Program Director of the Nephrology Fellowship Program and Co-Director of the Dialysis Unit. She is a founding member and past president of Women in Nephrology.

Joan A. Lit, M.D., practices endocrinology and internal medicine at the Henry Avenue Clinic in Philadelphia. She is an Assistant Professor of Medicine at the Medical College of Pennsylvania and Hahnemann University.

Katherine A. O'Hanlan, M.D., F.A.C.O.G., F.A.C.S., is an Assistant Professor of Gynecology and Obstetrics at Stanford University School of Medicine in California and Associate Director of the Gynecological Cancer Service at Stanford Medical Center.

Janet Rose Osuch, M.D., F.A.C.S., is an Associate Professor of Surgery and Medical Director of the Comprehensive Breast Health Clinic at Michigan State University. She is Chair of the Breast Cancer Subcommittee of AMWA and is American Cancer Society Breast Cancer Subcommittee Chair and National Spokesperson on breast cancer.

Melissa Susan Pashcow, M.D., F.A.C.S., an otolaryngologist and facial plastic surgeon, is an Associate Attending in the Department of Otolaryngology at the New York Eye and Ear Infirmary and a Clinical Instructor in the Department of Otolaryngology at New York Medical College.

Jane A. Petro, M.D., F.A.C.S., is an Associate Professor of Surgery at New York Medical College, where she serves also as the Chief of Microsurgery. She is Associate Director of the Burn Center at the Westchester County Medical Center and Chief of Pediatric Plastic Surgery at St. Agnes Children's Hospital in White Plains.

Judith J. Petry, M.D., F.A.C.S., is a former Assistant Professor of Plastic and Reconstructive Surgery at the University of Massachusetts Medical School. She has recently retired from the private practice of plastic surgery in Massachusetts and now resides in Vermont.

Linda G. Phillips, M.D., F.A.C.S., is Chief of the Division of Plastic Surgery and Director of the Plastic and Reconstructive Surgery Residency Program at the University of Texas Medical Branch, Galveston, where she is also an Associate Professor of Surgery. She is a past president of the Association of Women Surgeons.

Claudia S. Plottel, M.D., F.C.C.P., is a pulmonary specialist at Tisch Hospital of New York University Medical Center and in the Department of Medicine, Division of Pulmonary and Critical Care of the Bellevue Hospital Medical Center. She is a Clinical Assistant Professor of Medicine at New York University School of Medicine.

Christina Gertrud Rehm, M.D., F.A.C.S., is an Assistant Professor of Surgery at the University of Medicine and Dentistry of New Jersey/Robert Wood Johnson Medical School at Camden. She is an Assistant on the Traumatology Staff and Medical Co-Director of the Trauma Intensive Care Unit at the Southern New Jersey Regional Trauma Center.

June K. Robinson, M.D., F.A.A.D., is currently a Professor of Dermatology and Surgery at Northwestern University Medical School. She is immediate past president of the Women's Dermatological Society, serves on the Board of Directors of the American Academy of Dermatology, and is currently President of the American Society for Dermatologic Surgery.

Maj-Britt Rosenbaum, M.D., F.A.P.A., is Director of the Human Sexuality Center of Long Island Jewish Medical Center. She is also an Associate Clinical Professor of Psychiatry at Albert Einstein College of Medicine of Yeshiva University in New York. Dr. Rosenbaum is a Charter Member and Executive Board Member of the Society for Sexual Therapy and Research.

Marjorie S. Sirridge, M.D., M.A.C.P., A hematologist, is Director of the Office of Medical Humanities at Truman Medical Center and a Professor of Medicine at the University of Missouri in Kansas City. She has special expertise in the field of hemostasis and thrombosis.

Diane Sixsmith, M.D., M.P.H., F.A.C.E.P., is Chairperson of the Department of Emergency Medicine at the New York Hospital Medical Center of Queens and Clinical Associate Professor and Director of the Division of Emergency Medicine at the Cornell University Medical College, New York.

Rosemary K. Sokas, M.D., M.O.H., F.A.C.P., is an Associate Professor of Medicine and of Health Care Sciences at George Washington University in Washington D.C., where she directs the Environmental/Occupational Health Program and the Occupational Medicine Residency Program.

Jeanne Spurlock, M.D., F.A.P.A., is a Clinical Professor of Psychiatry at George Washington and Howard Universities. She has been in private practice in Washington, D.C., since 1974. She is a former Deputy Medical Director and Director of the Office of Minority/National Affairs of the American Psychiatric Association.

Penny Steiner-Grossman, Ed.D., M.P.H., is a specialist in health education, primarily in the area of chronic disease. She is currently Assistant Professor of the Department of Family Medicine at Albert Einstein College of Medicine of Yeshiva University in New York.

Frances J. Storrs, M.D., F.A.A.D., is a Professor of Dermatology in the Department of Dermatology at the Oregon Health Sciences University. She will serve as the president of the American Contact Dermatitis Society in 1995.

Francesca Morosani Thompson, M.D., F.A.A.O.S., is Associate Attending Surgeon at St. Luke's/Roosevelt Hospital Center and Chief of the Adult Orthopaedic Foot Clinic at Roosevelt Hospital in New York. She is also an Assistant Clinical Professor of Orthopaedic Surgery at the College of Physicians and Surgeons of Columbia University. Dr. Thompson is on the Board of Directors of the American Orthopaedic Foot and Ankle Society.

Laura L. Tosi, M.D., F.A.A.O.S., is an Assistant Professor of Pediatrics and Orthopaedic Surgery at the George Washington School of Medicine and the Children's National Medical Center in Washington, D.C. She was the second woman to be elected to the Board of Directors of the American Academy of Orthopaedic Surgeons. She is also a past president of the Ruth Jackson Orthopaedic Society.

Patience White, M.D., F.A.A.P., is Director of the Adult and Pediatric Rheumatology Division at George Washington University Hospital and Children's National Medical Center, Washington, D.C. She is a Professor of Medicine and Pediatrics at George Washington University Medical School.

Carol Widrow, M.D., is currently an Assistant Professor of Medicine in the Division of Infectious Diseases at the Albert Einstein College of Medicine of Yeshiva University in New York. The major focus of her work is the care of those infected with HIV.

Kimberly A. Yonkers, M.D., trained in psychiatry and psychopharmacology, currently works in the Departments of Psychiatry and Obstetrics and Gynecology at the University of Texas Southwestern Medical Center, Dallas. Her work is focused on elucidating hormonal influences on affective disorders in women.

DESIGNER

Leon Bolognese

ILLUSTRATOR

Wendy Frost

EDITORS

Rebecca Rinehart
Mary Mitchell
Lisa Healy
Julie Henderson
Eileen McGrath, J.D., C.A.E.
Leslie Schnur
Patricia Barnes-Svarney
Maryanne Bucknum Brinkley
Eleanor Dienstag
Gay Norton Edelman
Tanya Nadas
Carolyn Pugh, Ph.D.
Constance Schrader
Deborah Schuman
Linda Lee Small

COPY EDITORS

Candace Levy
Jack Roberts
Beth Wilson
Clare Wulker

PRODUCTION STAFF

Diane Bartoli
Sharon Deokule
Stephanie Knox
Kristin Kiser
Nina Neimark
Joyce Nolan
Anne Pierce
Claudia HCQ Sorsby
Naomi Starr
Molleen Theodore
Alda Trabucchi
Mitchell Waters

ABBREVIATIONS OF DEGREES

C.A.E.	Certified Association Executive
C.C.C.-A.	Certificate of Clinical Competence-Audiology
D.Ed.	Doctor of Education
J.D.	Doctor of Jurisprudence
M.A.	Master of Arts
M.D.	Doctor of Medicine
M.O.H.	Master of Occupational Health
M.P.A.	Master of Public Administration
M.P.H.	Master of Public Health
M.S.	Master of Science
Ph.D.	Doctor of Philosophy

ABBREVIATIONS OF HONORARY TITLES IN ORGANIZATIONS

F.A.A.P.	Fellow, American Academy of Pediatrics
F.A.A.O.S.	Fellow, American Academy of Orthopaedic Surgeons
F.A.A.D.	Fellow, American Academy of Dermatology
F.A.A.F.P.	Fellow, American Academy of Family Physicians
F.A.C.C.	Fellow, American College of Cardiology
F.A.C.E.	Fellow, American College of Endocrinology
F.A.C.E.P.	Fellow, American College of Emergency Physicians
F.A.C.O.G.	Fellow, American College of Obstetricians and Gynecologists
F.A.C.P.	Fellow, American College of Physicians
F.A.C.S.	Fellow, American College of Surgeons
F.C.C.P.	Fellow, American College of Chest Physicians
M.A.C.P.	Master, American College of Physicians

Index

Note: Italicized page numbers indicate main discussion.